Handbook of Research on Data Science for Effective Healthcare Practice and Administration

Elham Akhond Zadeh Noughabi
University of Calgary, Canada

Bijan Raahemi
University of Ottawa, Canada

Amir Albadvi
Tarbiat Modares University, Iran

Behrouz H. Far
University of Calgary, Canada

A volume in the Advances in Healthcare
Information Systems and Administration (AHISA)
Book Series

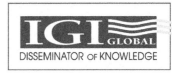

www.igi-global.com

Published in the United States of America by
  IGI Global
  Medical Information Science Reference (an imprint of IGI Global)
  701 E. Chocolate Avenue
  Hershey PA, USA 17033
  Tel: 717-533-8845
  Fax: 717-533-8661
  E-mail: cust@igi-global.com
  Web site: http://www.igi-global.com

Library of Congress Cataloging-in-Publication Data

Names: Noughabi, Elham Akhond Zadeh. | Raahemi, Bijan, 1964- editor. |
  Albadvi, Amir, 1961- editor. | Far, Behrouz H., 1959- editor.
Title: Handbook of research on data science for effective healthcare practice
  and administration / Elham Akhond Zadeh Noughabi, Bijan Raahemi, Amir
  Albadvi, Behrouz H. Far, editors.
Description: Hershey, PA : Medical Information Science Reference, [2017]
Identifiers: LCCN 2017004940| ISBN 9781522525158 (hardcover) | ISBN
  9781522525165 (ebook)
Subjects: | MESH: Medical Informatics Applications | Research Design | Data
  Collection
Classification: LCC R852 | NLM W 20.5 | DDC 610.72--dc23 LC record available at https://lccn.loc.gov/2017004940

This book is published in the IGI Global book series Advances in Healthcare Information Systems and Administration (AHISA) (ISSN: 2328-1243; eISSN: 2328-126X)

British Cataloguing in Publication Data
A Cataloguing in Publication record for this book is available from the British Library.

All work contributed to this book is new, previously-unpublished material. The views expressed in this book are those of the authors, but not necessarily of the publisher.

For electronic access to this publication, please contact: eresources@igi-global.com.

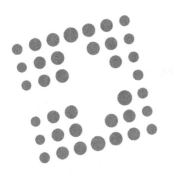

Advances in Healthcare Information Systems and Administration (AHISA) Book Series

Anastasius Moumtzoglou

Hellenic Society for Quality & Safety in Healthcare and P. & A.
Kyriakou Children's Hospital, Greece

ISSN:2328-1243
EISSN:2328-126X

MISSION

The **Advances in Healthcare Information Systems and Administration (AHISA) Book Series** aims to provide a channel for international researchers to progress the field of study on technology and its implications on healthcare and health information systems. With the growing focus on healthcare and the importance of enhancing this industry to tend to the expanding population, the book series seeks to accelerate the awareness of technological advancements of health information systems and expand awareness and implementation.

Driven by advancing technologies and their clinical applications, the emerging field of health information systems and informatics is still searching for coherent directing frameworks to advance health care and clinical practices and research. Conducting research in these areas is both promising and challenging due to a host of factors, including rapidly evolving technologies and their application complexity. At the same time, organizational issues, including technology adoption, diffusion and acceptance as well as cost benefits and cost effectiveness of advancing health information systems and informatics applications as innovative forms of investment in healthcare are gaining attention as well. **AHISA** addresses these concepts and critical issues.

COVERAGE

- Decision support systems
- Virtual health technologies
- IS in Healthcare
- Management of Emerging Health Care Technologies
- Measurements and Impact of HISA on Public and Social Policy
- Rehabilitative Technologies
- Medical informatics
- Nursing Expert Systems
- IT security and privacy issues
- Pharmaceutical and Home Healthcare Informatics

IGI Global is currently accepting manuscripts for publication within this series. To submit a proposal for a volume in this series, please contact our Acquisition Editors at Acquisitions@igi-global.com or visit: http://www.igi-global.com/publish/.

Titles in this Series

For a list of additional titles in this series, please visit: www.igi-global.com/book-series

Design, Development, and Integration of Reliable Electronic Healthcare Platforms
Anastasius Moumtzoglou (P&A Kyriakou Children's Hospital, Greece)
Medical Information Science Reference • copyright 2017 • 357pp • H/C (ISBN: 9781522517245) • US $205.00 (our price)

Cloud Computing Systems and Applications in Healthcare
Chintan M. Bhatt (Charotar University of Science & Technology, India) and S. K. Peddoju (Indian Institute of Technology Roorkee, India)
Medical Information Science Reference • copyright 2017 • 282pp • H/C (ISBN: 9781522510024) • US $205.00 (our price)

Handbook of Research on Healthcare Administration and Management
Nilmini Wickramasinghe (Epworth HealthCare, Australia & Deakin University, Australia)
Medical Information Science Reference • copyright 2017 • 825pp • H/C (ISBN: 9781522509202) • US $345.00 (our price)

Reshaping Medical Practice and Care with Health Information Systems
Ashish Dwivedi (University of Hull, UK)
Medical Information Science Reference • copyright 2016 • 399pp • H/C (ISBN: 9781466698703) • US $150.00 (our price)

M-Health Innovations for Patient-Centered Care
Anastasius Moumtzoglou (P&A Kyriakou Children's Hospital, Greece)
Medical Information Science Reference • copyright 2016 • 438pp • H/C (ISBN: 9781466698611) • US $235.00 (our price)

Improving Health Management through Clinical Decision Support Systems
Jane D. Moon (The University of Melbourne, Australia) and Mary P. Galea (The University of Melbourne, Australia)
Medical Information Science Reference • copyright 2016 • 425pp • H/C (ISBN: 9781466694323) • US $225.00 (our price)

Maximizing Healthcare Delivery and Management through Technology Integration
Tiko Iyamu (Cape Peninsula University of Technology, South Africa) and Arthur Tatnall (Victoria University, Australia)
Medical Information Science Reference • copyright 2016 • 378pp • H/C (ISBN: 9781466694460) • US $235.00 (our price)

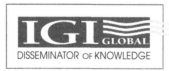

www.igi-global.com

701 East Chocolate Avenue, Hershey, PA 17033, USA
Tel: 717-533-8845 x100 • Fax: 717-533-8661
E-Mail: cust@igi-global.com • www.igi-global.com

List of Contributors

Table of Contents

Section 1
Mathematical Techniques and Operation Research

Section 4
Big Data

Section 5
Other Topics in Data Science

Detailed Table of Contents

Section 1
Mathematical Techniques and Operation Research

The support services of health care organizations, such as maintenance, have not traditionally been considered important from the perspective of care quality. Nevertheless, the degree of excellence in maintenance significantly influences availability, maintenance costs and safety of facilities, medical equipment, patients and care staff. Thus, it would be of great importance for health care organizations to apply benchmarking to their maintenance processes, as do other processing companies, in order to determine the quality of maintenance provided, and compare it to other, similar, organizations. This would also allow all the continuous improvement processes to be controlled, and actions for radical improvement to be carried out by comparing performance with that of companies in other sectors. This chapter describes a multicriteria model integrating a fuzzy Analytic Hierarchy Process with utility theory to obtain a valuation for the Maintenance Service of a Health Care Organization over time.

Chapter 2

Maintenance decisions by medical staff play an essential role in achieving availability, quality and safety in care services provided. This has, in turn, an effect on the quality of care perceived by patients. Nonetheless, despite its importance, there is a serious deficiency in models facilitating optimization of maintenance decisions in critical care equipment. This chapter shows a decision support system (DSS) for choosing the best combination of maintenance policies, together with other actions for improvement, such as the increase in the number of back-up devices used in the assisted breathing unit in the Neonatology Service of a hospital. This DSS is combined with an innovative form of continuous time Markov chains, and the multicriteria Measuring Attractiveness by a Categorical Based Evaluation Technique (MACBETH). The result is a ranking of the various maintenance alternatives to be applied. Finally, the real implications for availability and quality of care of applying the best solution are described.

Chapter 3

Mahsa Yousefi Sarmad, Iran University of Science and Technology, Iran
Mir Saman Pishvaee, Iran University of Science and Technology, Iran

Pharmaceutical industry is considered as a global industry because of its effects on the human life. Many researchers used optimization tools to manage the pharmaceutical supply chain (PSC) efficiently. A supply chain may be defined as an integrated process where several business entities work together to produce goods and/or services and deliver them to the end customer. The issue of PSC which includes strategic, tactical and operational decisions, is still a quite hot issue. The intended mission of this chapter is to introduce and discuss the recent developments of procurement, production and distribution management of pharmaceutical products in order to pave the way for the readers who are interested in this area of research. Notably, the focus of the chapter is on quantitative OR-based models which enable the decision makers to appropriately coordinate and manage the whole pharmaceutical industry.

Chapter 4

Arzu Eren Şenaras, Uludag University, Turkey
Hayrettin Kemal Sezen, Uludag University, Turkey

This study aims to analyze resource effectiveness through developed model. Changing different number of resources and testing their response, appropriate number of resources can be identified as a basis of resource balancing through what-if analysis. The simulation model for emergency department is developed by Arena package program. The patient waiting times are reduced by the tested scenarios. Health care system is very expensive sector and related costs are very high. To raise service quality, number of doctor and nurse are increased but system target is provided by increased number of register clerk. Testing different scenarios, effective policy can be designed using developed simulation model. This chapter provides the readers to evaluate healthcare system using discrete event simulation. The developed model could be evaluated as a base for new implementations in other hospitals and clinics.

Chapter 5

Soraia Oueida, American University of the Middle East, Kuwait
Seifedine Kadry, Beirut Arab University, Lebanon
Pierre Abichar, American University of the Middle East, Kuwait
Sorin Ionescu, Politehnica of Bucharest, Romania

A recent study carried out an empirical investigation of the quality of healthcare delivered to adults and found out that only $54.9\pm0.6\%$ adult received recommended care. Huge variation in the quality of care depends on patient's condition. In fact, the literature on healthcare is laden with articles like these that emphasize on the importance of the systems view of healthcare problems. Healthcare is a very vast and complex system where different departments interact with each other in order to deliver a certain service to arriving patients. Emergency departments (EDs) are the busiest units of healthcare. Existing problems and their cascading effect will be highlighted by a literature review of a bunch of researches. The purpose of this work is to study, in specific, the emergency department of a hospital with the existing problems and how simulation modeling can interfere in order to solve these problems, increase patient satisfaction and reduce cost. Simulation has emerged as a popular decision support in the domains of manufacturing and services industries.

Chapter 6

Zohreh Dadi, University of Bojnord, Iran

Human T-cell lymphotropic virus type I (HTLV-I) infects a type of white blood cell called a T lymphocyte. HTLV-I infection is seen in diverse region of the world such as the Caribbean Islands, southwestern Japan, southeastern United States, and Mashhad (Iran). This virus is the etiological agent of two main types of disease: HTLV-I-associated myelopathy/tropical spastic paraparesis and adult T cell leukemia. Also, the role of HTLV-I in the pathogenesis of autoimmune diseases such as HTLV-I associated arthropathy and systemic lupus erythematosus is under investigation. In this chapter, the author considers an ODE model of T-cell dynamics in HTLV-I infection which was proposed by Stilianakis and Seydel in 1999. Mathematical analysis of the model with fixed parameters has been done by many researchers. The author studies dynamical behavior (local stability) of this model with interval uncertainties, called interval system. Also, effective parameters in the local dynamics of model are found. For this study, interval analysis and particularly of Kharitonov's stability theorem are used.

Chapter 7

Zohreh Dadi, University of Bojnord, Iran

By clinical data, drug treatment sometimes is ineffective to eradicate the infection completely from the host in some human pathogens such as human immunodeficiency virus (HIV), hepatitis B virus (HBV), hepatitis C virus (HCV), and human T cell lymphotropic virus type I. Therefore, mathematical modeling can play a significant role to understand the interactions between viral replication and immune response. In this chapter, the author investigates the global dynamics of antiviral immune response in an immunosuppressive infection model. In this model, the global asymptotic stability of an immune control equilibrium point is proved by using the Poincare–Bendixson property, Volterra–Lyapunov stable matrices, properties of monotone dynamical systems and geometric approach. The analysis and results which are presented in this chapter make building blocks towards a comprehensive study and deeper understanding of the dynamics of immunosuppressive infection model.

Section 2
Statistical Analysis Techniques

Chapter 8

This chapter discusses applications of analytics at the strategic level of health system planning in the province of Ontario, Canada. To supplement the strategic priorities of the Ontario Renal Plan I, a roadmap developed by the Ontario Renal Network to guide its directions in coordinating renal care province-wide, an interactive user-friendly analytical capacity planning model was developed to forecast the growth of the prevalent chronic dialysis patient population and estimate consequent future need for hemodialysis stations at Ontario's dialysis facilities. The model also projects operational funding to care for dialysis patients, vascular surgeries to achieve arteriovenous fistula targets, peritoneal dialysis catheter insertions to achieve peritoneal dialysis prevalence targets, and incident dialysis patients to be sent home to achieve prevalent home dialysis targets. The model uses a variety of analytical methods, including time series analysis, mathematical optimization, geo-spatial analysis and Monte Carlo simulation.

Chapter 9

The assumption of Gaussian distribution of population does not always hold strongly in health studies. The sample size may not be large enough due to the limited nature of observations such as biopsies taken during kidney transplantation, the distribution of sample may not be Gaussian, or the observation may not even be possible for the far ends of a Gaussian distribution. In such cases, an alternative approach, called nonparametric tests can be applied. In this study, a non-parametric single center retrospective analysis of adult kidney transplant is performed to compare histological outcomes among three different groups of deceased kidney donors, based on the biopsies taken before and after kidney transplant at months 1, 3, and 12. A total of 107 transplants were observed in this study with 310 surveillance biopsy taken then classified based on the Banff 97 adequacy assessment. It is concluded that the recipient's internal condition after kidney transplant is as important as the donor's risk factors.

Chapter 10

Monitoring medical processes gained importance and researchers attempted to reduce death rates by quick detection mortality rate of surgical outcomes in recent years. The patient time until death (survival time) depends on risk factor of each patient, which reflects the patients' health condition prior to surgery. Ignoring differences in risk factors among specific patients, risk adjusted control charts could be considered as a corrective tool to minimize false alarms related to inhomogeneity in patients' health condition. A number of risk adjusted charting procedures have been developed on both phase I & II monitoring of aforementioned outcomes. This chapter will review both models and focus on phase-I risk-adjustment models in medical setting with a particular emphasis on monitoring for surgical context and describe each method's unique properties.

Section 3
Machine Learning and Data Mining

Precision medicine is an emerging medical model based on the customization of medical decisions and treatments to individuals. In personalized cancer therapy, tailored optimal therapies are selected depending on patient response to treatment rather than just using a one-size-fits-all approach. To this end, the field has witnessed significant advances in cancer response monitoring early after the start of therapy administration by using functional medical imaging modalities, particularly quantitative ultrasound (QUS) methods to monitor cell death at microscopic levels. This motivates the design of computer-assisted technologies for cancer therapy assessment, or computer-aided-theragnosis (CAT) systems. This chapter elaborates recent advances in the design and development of CAT systems based on QUS technologies in conjunction with advanced texture analysis and machine learning techniques with the aim of providing a framework for the early assessment of cancer responses that can potentially facilitate switching to more efficacious treatments in refractory patients.

Data mining techniques are increasingly used in clinical decision making and help the physicians to make more accurate and effective decisions. In this chapter, a classification of data mining applications in clinical decision making is presented through a systematic review. The applications of data mining techniques in clinical decision making are divided into two main categories: diagnosis and treatment. Early prediction of medical conditions, detecting multi-morbidity and complications of diseases, identifying and predicting the chronic diseases and medical imaging are the subcategories which are defined in the diagnosis part. The Treatment category is composed of treatment effectiveness and predicting the average length of stay in hospital. The majority of the reviewed articles are related to diagnosis and there is only one article which discusses the determination of drug dosage in successful treatment. The classification model is the most commonly practical model in the clinical decision making.

Chapter 13

Toktam Khatibi, Tarbiat Modares University (TMU), Iran
Mohammad Mehdi Sepehri, Tarbiat Modares University (TMU), Iran
Mohammad Javad Soleimani, Iran University of Medical Sciences (IUMS), Iran
Pejman Shadpour, Iran University of Medical Sciences (IUMS), Iran

Shock wave lithotripsy (SWL) is a noninvasive and safe treatment for small renal stones. In unsuccessful cases, retreatment procedures are needed after SWL. According to the previous studies, patient and stone descriptors are good predictors of SWL success. Some stone and kidney descriptors are measured from renal Non-Contrast Computed Tomography (NCCT) images. It is a tedious, time-consuming and error-prone process with large inter-user variability when performed manually. In this study, novel features are proposed automatically extracted from NCCT images to describe morphology and location of renal stones and kidneys to predict retreatments after SWL. The proposed features can distinguish between different kidney and stone morphologies and locations while being less sensitive to image segmentation errors. These features are added to other stone and patient features to predict retreatment within 3 months after SWL. The experimental results show that using the proposed stone features extracted from NCCT images can improve the accuracy of predicting retreatment.

Chapter 14

Toktam Khatibi, Tarbiat Modares University (TMU), Iran
Mohammad Mehdi Sepehri, Tarbiat Modares University (TMU), Iran
Pejman Shadpour, Iran University of Medical Sciences (IUMS), Iran
Seyed Hessameddin Zegordi, Tarbiat Modares University (TMU), Iran

Laparoscopy is a minimally-invasive surgery using a few small incisions on the patient's body to insert the tools and telescope and conduct the surgical operation. Laparoscopic video processing can be used to extract valuable knowledge and help the surgeons. We discuss the present and possible future role of processing laparoscopic videos. The various applications are categorized for image processing algorithms in laparoscopic surgeries including preprocessing video frames by laparoscopic image enhancement, telescope related applications (telescope position estimation, telescope motion estimation and compensation), surgical instrument related applications (surgical instrument detection and tracking), soft tissue related applications (soft tissue segmentation and deformation tracking) and high level applications such as safe actions in laparoscopic videos, summarization of laparoscopic videos, surgical task recognition and extracting knowledge using fusion techniques. Some different methods have been proposed previously for each of the mentioned applications using image processing.

Section 4
Big Data

Chapter 15

Leveraging Applications of Data Mining in Healthcare Using Big Data Analytics: An Overview ... 345

Mohammad Hossein Tekieh, University of Ottawa, Canada
Bijan Raahemi, University of Ottawa, Canada
Eric I. Benchimol, University of Ottawa, Canada

Big data analytics has been introduced as a set of scalable, distributed algorithms optimized for analysis of massive data in parallel. There are many prospective applications of data mining in healthcare. In this chapter, the authors investigate whether health data exhibits characteristics of big data, and accordingly, whether big data analytics can leverage the data mining applications in healthcare. To answer this interesting question, potential applications are divided into four categories, and each category into sub-categories in a tree structure. The available types of health data are specified, with a discussion of the applicable dimensions of big data for each sub-category. The authors conclude that big data analytics can provide more advantages for the quality of analysis in particular categories of applications of data mining in healthcare, while having less efficacy for other categories.

Chapter 16

Overview of Big Data in Healthcare 360

Mohammad Hossein Fazel Zarandi, Amirkabir University of Technology (Tehran Polytechnic), Iran
Reyhaneh Gamasaee, Amirkabir University of Technology (Tehran Polytechnic), Iran

Big data is a new ubiquitous term for massive data sets having large, more varied and complex structure with the complexities and difficulties of storing, analyzing and visualizing for further processes or results. The use of Big Data in health is a new and exciting field. A wide range of use cases for Big Data and analytics in healthcare will benefit best practice development, outcomes analysis, prediction, and surveillance. Consequently, the aim of this chapter is to provide an overview of Big Data in Healthcare systems including two applications of Big Data analysis in healthcare. The first one is understanding disease outcomes through analyzing Big Data, and the second one is the application of Big Data in genetics, biological, and molecular fields. Moreover, characteristics and challenges of healthcare Big Data analysis as well as technologies and software used for Big Data analysis are reviewed.

Section 5
Other Topics in Data Science

Chapter 17

Notifiable Disease Databases for Client Management and Surveillance 386

Ann M. Jolly, University of Ottawa, Canada
James J. Logan, University of Ottawa, Canada

The spread of certain infectious diseases, many of which are preventable, is widely acknowledged to have a detrimental effect on society. Reporting cases of these infections has been embodied in public health laws since the 1800s. Documenting client management and monitoring numbers of cases are the primary goals in collecting these data. A sample notifiable disease database is presented, including database structure, elements and rationales for collection, sources of data, and tabulated output. This chapter is a comprehensive guide to public health professionals on the content, structure, and processing of notifiable disease data for regional, provincial, and federal use.

The brain-machine interface (BMI) is a very recent development in the area of the human machine interaction (HCI) and emerged as the sister technology of BCI. A physiological signal related to these electrical potentials in response of the mental thoughts is known as Electroencephalogram (EEG) signals. The BMI is most commonly known as the BCI because there is a direct communication between the brain and the external machine via a computer, which analyses and interprets the incoming physiological signals, which contain the shadow of the mental activity and the different types of artefacts. A multi-channel recording of the electromagnetic waves emerging from the neural currents in the brain generate a large amounts of the EEG data. The neural activity of the human brain recorded non-invasively is sufficient to control the external machine, if advanced methods of signal analysis and feature extraction are used in combination with the machine learning techniques either supervised or unsupervised.

Asthma is a chronic disease of the airways in the lungs. The differentiation between asthma, COPD and bronchiectasis in the early stage of disease is very important for the adoption of appropriate therapeutic measures. In this research, a case-based-reasoning (CBR) model is proposed to assist a physician to therapy. First of all, features and symptoms are determined and patients' data is gathered with a questionnaire, then CBR algorithm is run on the data which leads to the asthma diagnosis. The system was tested on 325 asthmatic and non-asthmatic adult cases and the accuracy was eighty percent. The consequences were promising. This study was performed in order to determine risk factors for asthma in a specific society and the results of research showed that the most important variables of asthma disease are symptoms hyper-responsive, frequency of cough and cough.

Preface

The quantity of available healthcare data is increasing at a phenomenal rate, in structured and semi-structured formats. With this growth, there is an obvious need to develop efficient tools, skills and techniques for analyzing this data for useful and actionable knowledge. Since healthcare data is characterized by its complexity, high volume and high dimensionality, extensive use of data science is needed for managing and analyzing this data.

"Data science" is an interdisciplinary field of science and technology, used to extract novel and useful information from large volumes of data. Techniques and theories are drawn from many fields within mathematics, statistics, information science, and computer science, including signal processing, probability models, machine learning, statistical learning, data mining, database systems, data engineering, pattern recognition and learning, visualization, predictive analytics, uncertainty modeling, data warehousing, data compression, computer programming, artificial intelligence, and high performance computing. Data science applications span a wide range in engineering (examples include intrusion detection and network security, flow classification, web mining), business (fraud detection, decision support systems, risk analysis, market trend forecasting), medicine (population health, study of drug implications, epidemiology), bioinformatics (protein interactions, gene sequence analysis), and environmental science (flood prediction).

Methods for understanding, analyzing, and managing healthcare systems include data preparation, statistics, predictive modeling and machine learning. The healthcare industry can reap significant benefits from such efforts. Examples: healthcare insurers detecting fraud; healthcare organizations making decisions for better patient relationship management; physicians evaluating the effectiveness of treatment for specific diseases; early prediction of medical conditions; detecting multi-morbidity and complications of diseases, and identifying and controlling chronic diseases. Data science can also be helpful in managing problems associated with delivering hospital services, such as patient recovery, resource planning, facility utilization, logistics, vaccination, and emergency response, including dealing with bioterrorism. The cumulative result is people receiving better and more affordable healthcare services.

Despite the important current and potential value of data science in healthcare and medical decision-making, thus far there is a lack of an organized textbook in this area. Accordingly, this handbook provides healthcare professionals and practitioners a systematic framework with practical examples and solutions on how to use data science methods and tools. Readers can use this knowledge and experience to gain useful insights and novel actionable information from their own vast amounts of data.

In this handbook, the contributing authors survey various techniques and tools of data science, and explain application in the domains of healthcare and medical decision-making. The methods are illustrated with case studies, and the implementation of common relevant tools and software programing frameworks are discussed in some chapters.

The Handbook will help healthcare professionals and practitioners to understand the benefits of data science in healthcare, and understand where a particular method or tool would be useful.

The main value and contribution of this handbook lies first in its comprehensive presentation of a framework of the field. Second, it is suitable for training and supporting healthcare professionals to become intelligent users and consumers of various data science methods, and thus bridge the gap between technical specialists and healthcare managers. Our hope is that the Handbook can be a source of encouragement and guidance for healthcare students, professionals and practitioners, providing them with a better understanding of the applications of data science in healthcare.

TARGET AUDIENCE

This handbook is designed for those who are interested in applying data science to improve healthcare and medical decision-making. In particular, the Handbook focuses on developing skills and techniques for improvement in the domain of healthcare. The Handbook is suitable as a reference for a course on data science in healthcare and medical decision-making at the graduate level (master's or doctoral), particularly for medical or health systems students. In addition, the Handbook is a valuable source for self-study in data science, and as a learning tool for healthcare and medical practitioners, academics and managers in public health, research, governmental agencies, and the pharmaceutical industry. Students of data science, computer science, information technology, mathematics and statistics who would like to conduct research in healthcare are also a target audience of this handbook.

STRUCTURE OF THE HANDBOOK

In this handbook, various topics of data science are categorized into five main sections: "Mathematical Techniques and Operation Research", "Statistical Analysis Techniques", "Machine Learning and Data Mining", "Big Data" and "Other Topics in Data Science". Each section includes overview chapters that present a comprehensive literature review on the application of related techniques in healthcare and medicine. There are also supplementary chapters in each section with original research or case studies discussing the application of a specific technique or group of methods in a specific area of healthcare. The associated tools and software are briefly explained in each chapter, toward helping medical students and practitioners understand the potential benefits, and know when a particular approach would be useful for their specific cases. An overview of the five sections is presented below:

Section 1: Mathematical Techniques and Operation Research

Among the different quantitative methods which have been used in healthcare, mathematical methods and operation research have received considerable attention during the last few decades. Various optimization problems in the field have been addressed. Resource planning, facility utilization, vaccination, bioterrorism, emergency department management, production and distribution management are some examples. The section covers these techniques with seven chapters describing the application of different methods of optimization, multi-criteria decision-making, simulation and the use of nonlinear dynamic models in healthcare (e.g. maintenance in healthcare systems, production and distribution management of pharmaceutical products, and management of an emergency department) including:

Benchmarking of Maintenance Service in Health Care Organizations

It is of a great interest to healthcare organizations to apply benchmarking to their maintenance processes in order to determine the quality of the provided services, and improve it further. In this chapter, Carnero uses a collection of fuzzy Analytic Hierarchy Process (AHP), utility theory and Monte Carlo simulation together with a benchmarking approach to evaluate the maintenance service of a healthcare organization.

Optimization of Maintenance in Critical Equipment in Neonatology

Maintenance decisions by medical staff play an essential role in achieving availability, quality and safety and affect the quality of services. Nonetheless, despite its importance, there is a serious deficiency in models facilitating optimization of maintenance decisions. In this regard, the chapter proposes a decision support system (DSS) for choosing the best combination of maintenance policies and improvement actions in the neonatology services of a hospital. The DSS combines Markov Chains and Categorical Based Evaluation Technique (MACBETH) methods. The result is a ranking of various maintenance alternatives and real implications of applying the best solution.

Applications of Operations Research in Production and Distribution Management of Pharmaceutical Products

Pharmaceutical industry is considered as a global industry because of its effects on the human life. Many researchers have used optimization tools to manage the pharmaceutical supply chain (PSC) efficiently. The issue of PSC, which includes strategic, tactical and operational decisions, is an active research area. In this chapter, Sarmad and Pishvaee introduce and discuss the recent developments of procurement, production and distribution management of pharmaceutical products. The main focus is on quantitative Operation Research (OR)-based models which enable the decision makers to appropriately coordinate and manage the whole pharmaceutical industry.

A Simulation Model for Resource Balancing in Healthcare Systems

In this chapter, Şenaras and Sezen aim to analyze resource effectiveness and identify efficient hospitalization admission policies for an emergency department in Turkey. They test different scenarios by using the discrete event simulation modeling to design the effective policy. The developed model could be used as a base for new implementations in other hospitals and clinics.

The Applications of Simulation Modeling in Emergency Departments: A Review

Emergency Departments (EDs) are the busiest units of healthcare system. This review chapter presents a comprehensive overview of the applications of simulation modeling in the management of EDs. The authors study the potential problems of emergency departments and discuss how simulation modeling can interfere in order to solve these problems, improve patient satisfaction and reduce cost.

Analyzing Interval Systems of Human T-Cell Lymphotropic Virus Type I Infection of CD4+ T-Cells

Human T-cell lymphotropic virus type I (HTLV-I) infects a type of white blood cell called T lymphocyte. In this chapter, T-cell dynamics in HTLV-I infection are studied which were proposed by Stilianakis and Seydel (1999). This model is defined by a system of ordinary differential equations. Then, dynamical behaviors of this system with interval uncertainties are studied. To achieve this objective, interval analysis and Kharitonov's stability theorem are used.

Global Dynamics of an Immunosuppressive Infection Model Based on a Geometric Approach

In this chapter, an immunosuppressive infection model is considered which was studied by Dadi and Alizade (2016) from the view point of bifurcation theory. The authors investigate the global dynamics of antiviral immune response in this model. To this end, Poincare-Bendixon property, the properties of monotone dynamical systems and a geometric approach are used.

Section 2: Statistical Analysis Techniques

Statistical analysis has been extensively applied in many areas of health studies. Three chapters are included in this section discussing the statistical analysis techniques. The first two chapters of this section present the application of time-series analysis and other analytic methods, as well as non-parametric statistical analysis in the cases of provincial capacity-planning for dialysis and histologic outcomes of kidney transplantation, respectively. The section concludes with an overview chapter on the applications of regression-based methods in monitoring surgical performance.

Strategic Analytics to Drive Provincial Dialysis Capacity Planning: The Case of Ontario Renal Network

This chapter discusses applications of analytics at the strategic level of health system planning in the province of Ontario, Canada. To supplement the strategic priorities of the Ontario Renal Plan I, a roadmap and an interactive user-friendly analytical capacity planning model were developed to forecast the growth of the prevalent chronic dialysis patient population and estimate consequent future need for hemodialysis stations at Ontario's dialysis facilities. The model uses a variety of analytical methods including time series analysis, mathematical optimization, geo-spatial analysis and Monte Carlo simulation.

Non-Parametric Statistical Analysis of Rare Events in Healthcare: Case of Histological Outcome of Kidney Transplantation

This chapter recommends using non-parametric tests in the statistical analysis of health studies as the assumption of the Gaussian distribution of population may not hold strongly in such cases. The authors present a non-parametric single-center retrospective analysis of kidney transplants to compare histological outcomes among different deceased donors, based on consecutive biopsies. A total of 310 surveillance biopsies were taken, and classified based on the Banff 97 adequacy assessment. It is concluded that the recipient's physiological condition after kidney transplant is as important as the donor's risk factors.

Regression-Based Methods of Phase-I Monitoring Surgical Performance Using Risk-Adjusted Charts: An Overview

This chapter focuses on monitoring phase-I risk-adjustment models in surgical context which have been presented in medical setting and discuss the unique properties of each method. Results show that the overall probability of Type-I error has affected from the number of hypothesis tests for each patient. Furthermore, ignoring the important categorical operational covariates may lead to poorer performance in detecting possible changes in the reviewed models.

Section 3: Machine Learning and Data Mining

Artificial intelligence techniques have been implemented in recent years. Among these tools, machine learning and data mining are becoming increasingly popular, if not increasingly essential. These techniques are becoming of interest and importance for healthcare practice and research. Various descriptive and predictive methods are effetely employed in the areas of clinical decision making, public health, and administration and policies. This section includes two survey and two supplementary chapters:

Machine Learning Applications in Cancer Therapy Assessment and Implications on Clinical Practice

In personalized cancer therapy, tailored optimal therapies are selected depending on patient response to treatment. In this regard, significant advances in cancer response monitoring early after the start of therapy administration have been emerged. This chapter elaborates recent advances in the design and development of computer-aided-theragnosis (CAT) systems based on quantitative ultrasound (QUS) technologies in conjunction with advanced texture analysis and machine learning techniques. The purpose is providing a framework for the early assessment of cancer responses that can potentially facilitate switching to more efficacious treatments in refractory patients.

Application of Data Mining Techniques in Clinical Decision Making: A Literature Review and Classification

With regards to the benefits of data mining techniques in clinical decision making, Ameri, Alizadeh and Akhond Zadeh Noughabi present a systematic literature review in the field. The applications of data mining techniques in clinical decision making are classified into two main categories including diagnosis and treatment and discussed in the detected sub-categories. The results of review indicate that the majority of the articles are related to diagnosis; the classification model is also the most commonly practical model in clinical decision making.

New Features Extracted From Renal Stone NCCT Images to Predict Retreatment After Shock Wave Lithotripsy (SWL)

In this chapter, novel features are proposed which are automatically extracted from Non-Contrast Computed Tomography (NCCT) images to describe morphology and location of renal stones and kidneys to predict retreatments after Shock wave lithotripsy (SWL). Novel image segmentation and feature selection methods are implemented to obtain this objective.

Applications of Image Processing in Laparoscopic Surgeries: An Overview

Khatibi, Sepehri, Shadpour and Zegordi discuss the applications of image processing in laparoscopic surgeries through a review study. The various applications include preprocessing video frames by laparoscopic image enhancement, telescope related applications (telescope position estimation, telescope motion estimation and compensation), surgical instrument related applications (surgical instrument detection and tracking), soft tissue related applications (soft tissue segmentation and deformation tracking) and high level applications such as safe actions in laparoscopic videos, summarization of laparoscopic videos, surgical task recognition and extracting knowledge using fusion techniques. The corresponding techniques are also discussed in various applications.

Section 4: Big Data

Using big data analytics in healthcare is a nascent field. The emergence of massive datasets in the healthcare sector and advances in information technology offer great opportunities for the use of big data analytics in healthcare. This section presents two overview chapters on the advantages and applications of big data analytics in healthcare:

Leveraging Applications of Data Mining in Healthcare Using Big Data Analytics: An Overview

There are many prospective applications of data mining in healthcare. In this chapter, the authors investigate whether health data exhibits characteristics of big data, and accordingly whether big data analytics can leverage data mining applications in healthcare. To answer this interesting question, potential applications of data mining in healthcare and the available types of health data are specified, with a discussion of the applicable dimensions of big data for each category of applications. The results indicate that big data analytics can provide more advantages for the quality of analysis in particular categories of data mining applications in healthcare, while having less efficacy for other categories.

Overview of Big Data in Healthcare

Zarandi and Gamasaee review big data applications in healthcare in this chapter. The focus is on two major applications including "understanding disease outcomes" and "genetics, biological, and molecular fields". Moreover, characteristics and challenges of big data analysis in healthcare, as well as its technologies and soft wares are discussed.

Section 5: Other Topics in Data Science

Finally, this section discusses additional related topics of data science in healthcare in three chapters:

Notifiable Disease Databases for Client Management and Surveillance

The requirement to report cases of infectious diseases has been embedded in public health laws since the 1800s. Documenting client management and monitoring numbers of cases are the primary goals in collecting these data. In this chapter, a sample notifiable disease database is presented, including database structure, elements and rationales for collection, sources of data, and tabulated output. This study is a comprehensive guide to public health professionals on the content, structure, and processing of notifiable disease data for regional, provincial, and federal use.

Brain-Machine Interface: Human-Computer Interaction

Many patients who become afflicted with neurological conditions or neurodegenerative diseases may lose all their abilities to control their muscles. One option to address this problem is to provide the brain with a new and non-muscular output channel, a brain–computer interface (BCI) for conveying the user's intent to the external world. This chapter discusses the advantages of using data analytics methods in this area. The results indicate that the neural activity of the human brain recorded non-invasively is sufficient to control the external machine, if advanced methods of signal processing and feature extraction are used in combination with the machine learning techniques.

A Case-Based-Reasoning System for Feature Selection and Diagnosing Asthma

The differentiation between asthma as a chronic disease, COPD and bronchiectasis in the early stage of disease is very important for the adoption of appropriate therapeutic measures. In this research, a case-based-reasoning (CBR) model is proposed to diagnose the disease and assist a physician to therapy. The most important risk factors for asthma were detected as symptoms hyper responsive, frequency of cough and cough.

Elham Akhond Zadeh Noughabi
University of Calgary, Canada

Bijan Raahemi
University of Ottawa, Canada

Amir Albadvi
Tarbiat Modares University, Iran

Behrouz H. Far
University of Calgary, Canada

Acknowledgment

We express our sincere thanks to all contributors, reviewers, and authors for their significant contribution for the preparation of this handbook. We would also like to thank the editorial advisory board for their detailed review of the manuscripts, and providing constructive comments to the authors. Without their dedication, we would not be able to prepare this handbook. We wish to thank Bernard Marrocco, Noah Raahemi, and Fadwa Al-Azab for proof reading the manuscripts. Their contributions greatly enhanced presentation of the chapters. A big thanks goes to Mohammad Saeedi for the formatting and consistency job on the chapters. We also express special thanks to the publishing board of the IGI Global for their continuous support along this exciting journey. Without their support, we would not be able to publish the Handbook. And finally, we would also like to thank the sponsors and funding agencies. This work is partially supported by Alberta Innovates Technology Futures (AITF), Natural Sciences and Engineering Research Council of Canada (NSERC), and University of Calgary's EyesHigh program.

We hope that this handbook stimulates the development of new ideas and efficient solutions in the area of data science for effective healthcare practice and administration.

Section 1
Mathematical Techniques and Operation Research

Chapter 1
Benchmarking of the Maintenance Service in Health Care Organizations

María Carmen Carnero
University of Castilla-La Mancha, Spain & University of Lisbon, Portugal

ABSTRACT

The support services of health care organizations, such as maintenance, have not traditionally been considered important from the perspective of care quality. Nevertheless, the degree of excellence in maintenance significantly influences availability, maintenance costs and safety of facilities, medical equipment, patients and care staff. Thus, it would be of great importance for health care organizations to apply benchmarking to their maintenance processes, as do other processing companies, in order to determine the quality of maintenance provided, and compare it to other, similar, organizations. This would also allow all the continuous improvement processes to be controlled, and actions for radical improvement to be carried out by comparing performance with that of companies in other sectors. This chapter describes a multicriteria model integrating a fuzzy Analytic Hierarchy Process with utility theory to obtain a valuation for the Maintenance Service of a Health Care Organization over time.

INTRODUCTION

The support services of health care organizations, such as maintenance, have not traditionally been considered important from the perspective of care quality. Nevertheless, the degree of excellence in maintenance significantly influences availability, maintenance costs and safety of facilities, medical equipment, patients and care staff (Carnero & Gómez, 2016). Therefore, it would be very important to devise continuous improvement procedures for the level of maintenance applied in Health Care Organizations. A very useful tool for developing these continuous improvement processes is benchmarking (Wireman, 2004).

DOI: 10.4018/978-1-5225-2515-8.ch001

Benchmarking may be defined as the process of continuously comparing and measuring the activity of an organization with respect to others, to obtain information about the practices, processes and methodologies, which will help the organization to improve its performance (APQC, 2013).

Thus, it would be of great importance for health care organizations to apply benchmarking to their maintenance processes, as other companies do, in order to determine the quality of maintenance provided, and compare it to other similar organizations. This would also allow all the continuous improvement processes to be controlled, and actions for radical improvement to be carried out by comparing performance with that of companies in other sectors. This chapter describes a multi-criteria model integrating a Fuzzy Analytic Hierarchy Process (FAHP) with utility theory to obtain a valuation for the maintenance service of a health care organization over time.

The paper is structured as follows. First, there is a review of the literature on benchmarking in maintenance. Then the model for maintenance benchmarking is described, including the structure of the model, the weighting process and the valuation of alternatives. Next, the results obtained from applying the model to a health care organization in the years 2000, 2005 and 2010 are given, followed by future research directions, conclusions and references.

BACKGROUND

There are four types of benchmarking (Kelessidis, 2000):

1. **Competitive Benchmarking:** Benchmarking is carried out against competing companies and the data analysis is intended to determine the reasons behind the superior performance of the competition. This has the advantage that there is a series of exogenous variables, which affect the organization and its competitors equally if they all belong to the same economic sector. Nonetheless, it is unlikely that competing businesses will cooperate unless, for example, they compete in different markets.
2. **Internal Benchmarking:** This is applied between units of departments belonging to multinational companies with branches, manufacturing operations or sales offices spread over different countries or geographical areas.
3. **Process Benchmarking:** This compares processes with some degree of similarity but in companies from different sectors.
4. **Generic Benchmarking:** This analyses technological aspects, comparing companies from the same or from different sectors.

The benchmarking application process has the following stages (Dunn, 1999):

- Establish the scope.
- Develop the project plan.
- Select the key performance variables to benchmark.
- Identify potential participant companies.
- Measure performance of reference company.
- Measure performance of benchmarking participants.
- Communicate your results.

- Compare current data.
- Identify best practices and enablers.
- Formulate the strategy.
- Implement a plan.
- Monitor results.
- Plan for problem solving.

There is a great deal of literature about benchmarking in different fields; however, in the field of maintenance application has been very limited (Carnero, 2014a). Among the contributions to apply benchmarking to maintenance the following are noteworthy; Luxhej et al. (1997) compared the level of maintenance in companies in Denmark, Norway, Sweden, and Finland with US companies analysed by Wireman (1990). Dunn (1999) set out ranks and best practice values in maintenance for a variety of indicators typically reported by organizations. Dunn (2001) gives 15 maintenance indicators used in processing and manufacturing industries and the values obtained for the organizations with superior maintenance performance. Wireman (2004) surveyed more than 100 US companies about aspects of maintenance such as: preventive maintenance, predictive maintenance, maintenance inventory and purchasing, maintenance outsourcing, document management, etc. A similar study was carried out by Pinjala et al. (2006) among Belgian and Dutch companies and, by Alsyouf (2009), in Swedish companies. Svantesson (2006) analysed the performance of 15 Key Performance Indicators (KPI) for maintenance used as a benchmark and applied to organizations in the pharmaceutical and food industries, and diverse industries in a number of European countries. Conde (2007) described a number of maintenance benchmarks specific to petrochemical plants, such as total maintenance costs, ratio of labour costs for maintenance to overall maintenance costs, percentage of cost of materials and parts against overall maintenance costs, percentage of overtime costs against labour costs, level of availability present at the petrochemical plant, percentage of corrective, preventive and predictive maintenance applied, etc. Wheelhouse (2009) performed benchmarking in petrochemical plants with regard to maintenance costs by class of assets: fixed plant and equipment account for 40-50% of the total maintenance costs, the rotating equipment 15-20%, instruments and control 15% and electrical systems 10%. Muchiri et al. (2010) carried out a survey and subsequent analysis on the use of KPI's in maintenance management in Belgium industries; it can be observed that in few cases the results of the KPI are used to take decisions. Anvari and Edwards (2011) set out a model for measuring overall equipment effectiveness in capital intensive industries, which could be used as a benchmark to achieve world-class standard. Fumagalli and Macchi (2009) analysed the state of the art of condition based maintenance in 59 Italian companies from different sectors and of different sizes; 69% of those surveyed had a predictive maintenance system in place, and this was especially true of the chemical, mechanical and steel sectors. A similar study was carried out in Carnero (2012) among Spanish small and medium enterprises, showing excessively high levels of corrective maintenance, poor control of the costs and time involved in the different types of maintenance, low standards of university education among those in charge of maintenance, and underuse of Computerised Maintenance Management Systems (CMMS).

Most studies of maintenance benchmarking in the literature were applied to processing plants and manufacturing companies; the only studies carried out in service companies are Lai and Yik (2008), which described maintenance cost benchmarks for luxury hotels. Wang et al. (2010) proposed a three-step aeroengine health assessment evaluation model problem. This model combines FAHP and fuzzy preference programming (FPP) to calculate the weights of multiple evaluation criteria and synthesize the ratings of candidate aeroengines. The technique for order performance by similarity to ideal solution (TOPSIS) is used to find the overall performance value for each alternative. Carnero (2014a), which looks at the large building sector, including Health Care Organizations. Shafii et al. (2015) carried out a performance analysis on hospital managers. They used FAHP to obtain the weightings of the criteria: functional, professional, organizational, individual and human. Fuzzy TOPSIS was used to obtain the performance of a total of 407 senior and middle managers from 10 hospitals in Iran. Azam et al. (2015) built a model with AHP to evaluate quality of care, assessing three Health Care Organizations from Northern India.

A key concern in benchmarking studies is to find normalized indicators; European Federation of National Maintenance Societies (EFNMS), through its standard Maintenance Key Performance Indicators (EN15341, 2007), therefore defines 71 indicators, classified as economic, technical or organizational. The Society for Maintenance & Reliability Professionals (SMRP), on the other hand, has defined 70 best maintenance practice indicators. Although there is a process of harmonization of indicators, which involves both organizations, there are still difficulties with the thresholds recommended for these indicators (Kahn et al., 2009).

Generally, maintenance benchmarking compares average values for a given industrial sector with those an organization; it is therefore necessary to have values for all the indicators in all sectors. However, there are too many exogenous variables which can influence the final result, such as the amount of production equipment, the downtime costs to production, the usage rate of production equipment, or technological factors (Komonen, 2002).

An analysis of maintenance benchmarking should simultaneously consider strategic, tactical, technical, economic, safety, organizational and environmental factors; in many cases, some will clash with others. It is also necessary to use a technique that considers the points of view of the different stakeholders and which can provide objective results acceptable to the management of Health Care Organizations. These requirements are satisfied by the use of Multi-Criteria Decision Analysis (MCDA) techniques (Huang, Keisler & Linkov, 2011). Thus, for example, Parameshwaran et al. (2009) applied a FAHP joint Data Envelopment Analysis model to measure the efficiency of automobile repair shops. Joshi et al. (2011) used Delphi to identify, synthesize and prioritize key performance factors, an Analytic Hierarchy Process (AHP) for a cold-chain performance evaluation of an organization with respect to its competitors and a Technique for Order Preference by Similarity to Ideal Solution (TOPSIS) based assessment of possible alternatives for the continuous improvement of the company's cold-chain performance. Carnero (2014b) developed a model using FAHP, utility functions and discrete probability distributions for the application of competitive and generic benchmarking in small and medium enterprises. It is, nonetheless, necessary to develop specific models for Health Care Organizations, as the sector they are in is a key area for building a maintenance benchmarking model.

MODEL FOR MAINTENANCE BENCHMARKING IN HEALTH CARE ORGANIZATIONS

Using the surveys carried out by the Spanish Maintenance Association (SMA) a process was designed to structure the choice of criteria, sub-criteria and alternatives pertinent to the problem. Then FAHP was applied, to acquire weightings for the criteria and sub-criteria. FAHP was chosen over other fuzzy multi-criteria methods because it is the only one which uses a hierarchy structure involving goals, criteria, sub-criteria and alternatives. This is especially important in a study analysing up to 50 different aspects of an organization. In addition, the use of pairwise comparisons allows more accurate information to be obtained about the preferences of the decision makers (Bozbura, Beskese, & Kahraman, 2007).

A descriptor was defined for each sub-criterion. AHP was used to obtain the weightings for the scale levels of each descriptor. These weightings were converted into utilities to homogenize the scales of the various descriptors.

The alternatives were defined by calculating the probabilities for each scale level of each descriptor in the service and buildings sector for companies with over 500 employees in 2000, 2005 and 2010. A discrete probability distribution function was derived from these probabilities, for each sub-criterion.

The final valuation of each alternative is calculated via a multi-measure utility function. Uncertainty in the results is calculated by means of a Monte Carlo simulation.

We now describe each stage of the model in more detail.

Structuring

The model is based on data collected by the SMA in surveys carried out in 2000, 2005 and 2010 (SMA, 2000; 2005; 2010) in large companies (more than 500 employees) and in the buildings sector, which includes Health Care Organizations. The 2000 survey includes, rather than the buildings sector, data from the service sector, which includes state and commercial organizations, financial service companies, department stores, large food companies, hotel chains, tourism and public services, and so it is here that health care organizations are to be found. The number of surveys competed by large companies in these sectors was 22 in 2000, 11 in 2005 and 10 in 2010.

Firstly, a full analysis of the questions included in the survey was carried out, and those that did not satisfy the requirements stipulated by Keeney (2006) for the definition of decision criteria and sub-criteria were detached, modified or discarded. These requirements are that criteria and sub-criteria should be: exhaustive, non-redundant, concise, made operational with descriptors of performance, and independent. Within each criterion, a set of relevant sub-criteria were defined. We now list the criteria and sub-criteria, together with (in brackets) the codes used in the maintenance benchmarking model:

1. Maintenance Manager (MMA):
    a. Time in post of the maintenance manager (TMM).
    b. Academic Degree (ADE).
    c. Experience in maintenance positions (EMP).
    d. Frequency of presence outside working hours (FPO).
    e. Payment for overtime work or work outside normal hours (POW).
    f. Attendance at congresses, conferences, group sessions, etc. about maintenance (ACM).
    g. Regular reading of Spanish technical journals of maintenance (RSJ).
    h. Regular reading of international technical journals of maintenance (RIJ).
    i. Use of the Internet to find out about and keep up to date with maintenance (UIM).
2. Training (TRA):
    a. Training courses (TCU).
    b. Trends in training (TTR).
    c. Versatility of maintenance workers (VMW).
    d. Specialities with most requirements for future training (SRF).

3. Maintenance Computerization (COM):
    a. Subjects to which computerization is applied (SCA).
    b. Type of computerized maintenance management system used (TCM).
    c. Hardware operating the maintenance software (HMS).
    d. Assessment of satisfaction with the use of computerization (ASC).
    e. Forecast for applying integrated economical-technical maintenance management (FMM).

4. Control (CON):
    a. Organization of work into work orders (OWO).
    b. Distribution of in-house work (DIW).
    c. Percentage of urgent work received (PUW).
    d. Workload pending (WPE).
    e. Regularity of information gathered on maintenance costs (RMC).
    f. Delay in the gathering of cost data (DCD).
    g. Areas into which maintenance costs are arranged (AMC).
    h. Systematic control indices for maintenance management (SCI).

5. Outsourcing Maintenance (OMA):
    a. Type of higher cost outsourced work (TCO).
    b. Percentage of preventive maintenance outsourced (PPM).
    c. Percentage of corrective maintenance outsourced (PCM).
    d. Percentage of programmed stoppage work outsourced (PPS).
    e. Quality of outsourced work (QOW).
    f. Trend in outsourcing (TOU).
    g. Percentage of outsourced personnel (POP).

6. Maintenance Costs (MCO):
    a. Annual budget of maintenance department (ABM).
    b. Percentage of annual cost of spares and consumables (PAS).
    c. Percentage of annual cost of outsourced work (PAO).
    d. Percentage of annual cost of in-house staff (PAI).
    e. Trend in maintenance costs (TMC).

7. Maintenance Organization (MOR):
    a. Existence of a maintenance department (EMD).
    b. To whom the maintenance manager reports (MMR).
    c. Responsibilities of the maintenance manager (RMM).
    d. Existence of organized, specialized work groups (EWG).
    e. Number of workers in maintenance department (NWM).
    f. Trend in staff hiring (TSH).
    g. Incidents outside working hours (IOW).
    h. Use of Total Productive Maintenance (TPM).
    i. Trend in cooperation of production staff with maintenance (TCP).

8. Quality, Environment and Safety Standards (QES):
    a. Certification to ISO 9000 (CI9).
    b. Certification to ISO 14000 (CI1).
    c. Compliance with Health and Safety legislation (CHS).

The hierarchy of the maintenance benchmarking model is shown in Figure 1.

A descriptor has been defined for each sub-criterion. A descriptor is an ordered set of impact levels that can measure, quantitatively or qualitatively, the level of satisfaction of a fundamental viewpoint (Bana e Costa, Correa, De Corte, & Vansnick, 2002). The descriptors defined for this model are constructed, and are generally qualitative although in some cases they are quantitative

Once the criteria, sub-criteria and descriptors have been defined, they were used to produce a questionnaire that could be completed by the head of maintenance of the health care organization.

Weighting Process

The use of fuzzy set theory introduced by Zadeh (1965) allows uncertainty (doubt, hesitancy, vagueness and ambiguous situations) associated with the mapping of a judgement to a number, to be included in the decision process. Otherwise, the results obtained can be misleading. Furthermore, decision makers sometimes feel more confident providing interval judgements rather than crisp judgements (Isaai, Kanani, Tootoonchi, & Afzali, 2011). A fuzzy set is characterized by a membership function, which assigns to each object a grade of membership (Cebeci, 2009). A special type of trapezoidal fuzzy number is the triangular fuzzy number (TFN), widely used in the literature. The TFNs $\tilde{a} = (l, m, u)$ are defined mathematically via the membership function $\mu_{\tilde{a}}(x) : \Re \longrightarrow [0,1]$ in Equation (1) (Chang, 1996).

$$\mu_{\tilde{a}}(x) = \begin{cases} \dfrac{x-l}{m-l}, & \text{if } l \leq x \leq m \\ \dfrac{u-x}{u-m}, & \text{if } m \leq x \leq u \\ 0 & \text{otherwise} \end{cases} \tag{1}$$

Where l and u are the lower and upper bounds of the fuzzy number and m is the median value, where $l \leq m \leq u$.

Although various fuzzy scales have been proposed, this study uses the triangular fuzzy conversion scale given in Table 1.

Table 1. Fuzzy scale

Linguistic Scale	Triangular Fuzzy Numbers	Reciprocal Triangular Fuzzy Numbers
Just equal	(1, 1, 1)	(1, 1, 1)
Very weakly important	(1/2, 1, 3/2)	(2/3, 1, 2)
Weakly important	(1, 3/2, 2)	(1/2, 2/3, 1)
Moderately more important	(3/2, 2, 5/2)	(2/5, 1/2, 2/3)
Strongly more important	(2, 5/2, 3)	(1/3, 2/5, 1/2)
Absolutely more important	(5/2, 3, 7/2)	(2/7, 1/3, 2/5)

(Bozbura et al., 2007)

Figure 1. Hierarchy
(Created by the author)

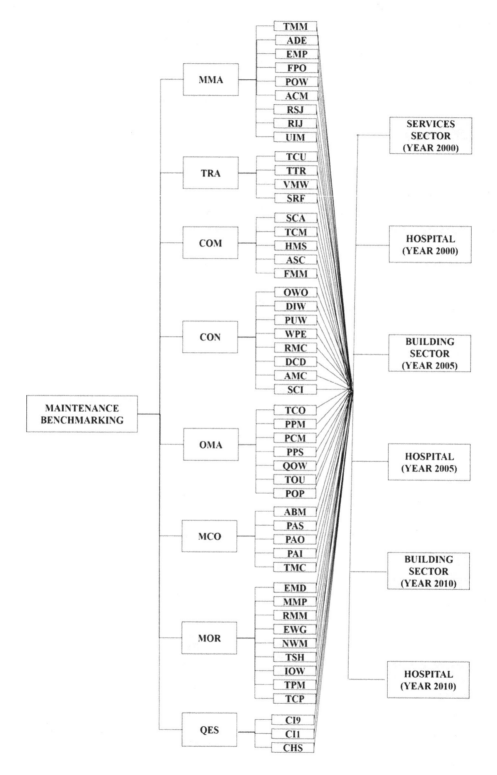

Different techniques may be used for weighting the criteria. In addition to the methodology to be explained here, using FAHP, the best-worst and entropy methods are worthy of mention.

In the best-worst method, for a series of criteria C_1, C_2, ..., C_n associated with a decision problem, the decision maker must identify the best and the worst criterion. Next, the preference of the best criterion over the rest is calculated using a scale from 1 to 9. This gives a vector $A_B = (a_{B1}, a_{B2}, ..., a_{Bn})$. A value a_{Bj} shows the preference of the best criterion B over a criterion j. Then a preference is identified for all the criteria over the worst criterion, using a scale from 1 to 9. This gives the vector $A_W = (a_{1W}, a_{2W} ..., a_{nW})^T$. Each element, a_{jW} of this vector shows the preference of the criterion j over the worst criterion W. The optimal weightings $(w_1{}^*, w_2{}^*, ..., w_n{}^*)$ are found by calculating, for each pair of w_B/w_j and w_j/w_W, a solution for which the maximum absolute differences $|(w_B/w_j)\text{-}a_{Bj}|$ and $|(w_j/w_W)\text{-}a_{jW}|$ for all j are minimized (Reza, 2015).

Weighting by entropy uses a matrix $X=(x_{ij})_{nxm}$ which evaluates n objects with respect to m criteria. Normalizing this matrix gives the matrix $R=(r_{ij})_{nxm}$ where r_{ij} is the data from the jth object evaluated in the criterion. If the criterion is of the "the bigger the better" type, then (Zou, Yun, & Sun, 2006):

$$r_{ij} = \frac{x_{ij} - \min\{x_{ij}\}}{\max\{x_{ij}\} - \min\{x_{ij}\}}$$

While if it is of the "the smaller the better" type, then:

$$r_{ij} = \frac{\max\{x_{ij}\} - x_{ij}}{\max\{x_{ij}\} - \min\{x_{ij}\}}$$

The entropy of the ith criterion is defined as:

$$H_i = -k\sum_{j=1}^{n} f_{ij} Ln f_{ij}, \; i=1, 2, ..., n$$

and $f_{ij} = r_{ij} \Big/ \sum_{j=1}^{n} r_{ij}$, $k = Ln \, n$ and supposing $f_{ij}=0$ then $Ln f_{ij} =0$.

The weighting of the ith criterion may be defined as:

$$w_i = \frac{1 - H_i}{m - \sum_{i=1}^{m} H_i}$$

So that the weighting has values between 0 and 1 and the sum of the weightings of all the criteria is equal to 1.

Different FAHP methodologies have been described in the literature. Van Laarhoven and Pedrycz (1983) broadened the AHP method, using triangular fuzzy numbers and the logarithmic least squares method proposed by Lootsma to obtain fuzzy weights and fuzzy performance scores. Nonetheless, there is a problem with this method: the priorities obtained can change and even lead to rank reversal (Zhu, 2012). Buckley (1985) used trapezoidal fuzzy numbers and the geometric mean to derive fuzzy weights and performance scores. Boender et al. (1989) modified the method proposed by Van Laarhoven and Pedrycz (1983) and obtain a more robust methodology for the normalization of local priorities. Chang (1996) follows the methodology used by crisp AHP, using triangular fuzzy numbers to perform the pairwise comparison. It also uses the extent analysis method to obtain the synthetic degree values of the weightings. Cheng (1996) represents the performance scores via membership functions and uses the concept of entropy to obtain aggregate weights. Entropy is used when the probability distributions are known, using both probability and possibility values (Büyüközkan et al. 2004).

These methods are distinguished by their computational cost, which is very high for the methods developed by Van Laarhoven and Pedrycz (1983), Buckley (1985) and Boender et al. (1989). With the methods designed by Laarhoven and Pedrycz (1983) and Chang (1996), only triangular fuzzy numbers can be used (Bozbura, Beskese, & Kahraman, 2007).

Chang's extent analysis method has been successfully used in a significant number of cases in the literature, and is therefore the one used in this study. The description of Chang's extent analysis method may be found in Chang (1996), Meixner, (2009), Isaai et al. (2011), SeongKon et al. (2011), Durán, (2011) and Lima et al. (2014).

Once the hierarchy is constructed, incorporating the decision problem, the criteria, sub-criteria and alternatives, the fuzzy judgement matrix $\tilde{A}$ shown in Equation (2), is obtained. The elements of this matrix $\tilde{a}_{ij}$ are the fuzzy comparison values which express the decision maker's opinion about the relative importance of a criterion or sub-criterion i over another j at the same level of the hierarchy.

$$\tilde{A} = \begin{bmatrix} (1,1,1) & (l_{12},m_{12},u_{12}) & \cdots & (l_{1n},m_{1n},u_{1n}) \\ (l_{21},m_{21},u_{21}) & (1,1,1) & \cdots & (l_{2n},m_{2n},u_{2n}) \\ \cdot & \cdot & \cdot & \cdot \\ \cdot & \cdot & \cdots & \cdot \\ \cdot & \cdot & & \cdot \\ (l_{n1},m_{n1},u_{n1}) & (l_{n2},m_{n2},u_{n2}) & \cdots & (1,1,1) \end{bmatrix} \quad (2)$$

Where $\tilde{a}_{ij} = (l_{ij},m_{ij},u_{ij})$ and $\tilde{a}_{ij}^{-1} = (\frac{1}{u_{ij}},\frac{1}{m_{ij}},\frac{1}{l_{ij}})$ for $i,j=1,2,...,n$ and $i\neq j$.

To obtain pairwise comparison matrices, the study uses two decision makers, widely experienced experts in maintenance and in particular in health care organizations. The decision makers used the fuzzy scale from Table 1 to create the pairwise comparisons between the criteria and sub-criteria. The judgements of the two experts were aggregated using the geometric mean, giving triangular fuzzy numbers as a result. As an example, Table 2 shows the pairwise comparison matrix for the aggregated judgements of the experts in the sub-criteria included in the criterion Maintenance organization.

Next, the value of the fuzzy synthetic extent with respect to the i-object $\tilde{S}_i$ is obtained by applying equation (3) (Chang, 1996).

Table 2a. The pairwise comparison matrix of the sub-criteria of the criterion maintenance organization

Sub-Criteria	EMD			MMP			RMM			EWG			NWM		
	l_{ij}	m_{ij}	u_{ij}	l_{ij}	m_{ij}	u_{ij}	l_{ij}	m_{ij}	u_{ij}	l_{ij}	m_{ij}	u_{ij}	l_{ij}	m_{ij}	u_{ij}
EMD	1.000	1.000	1.000	0.500	1.000	1.500	0.707	1.225	1.732	1.000	1.500	2.000	1.000	1.500	2.000
MMP	0.667	1.000	2.000	1.000	1.000	1.000	0.707	1.000	1.225	0.500	1.000	1.500	0.500	1.000	1.500
RMM	0.577	0.816	1.414	0.816	1.000	1.414	1.000	1.000	1.000	0.707	1.000	1.225	0.707	1.000	1.225
EWG	0.500	0.667	1.000	0.667	1.000	2.000	0.816	1.000	1.414	1.000	1.000	1.000	1.000	1.000	1.000
NWM	0.500	0.667	1.000	0.667	1.000	2.000	0.816	1.000	1.414	1.000	1.000	1.000	1.000	1.000	1.000
TSH	0.309	0.365	0.447	0.365	0.447	0.577	0.408	0.516	0.707	0.500	0.667	1.000	0.500	0.667	1.000
IOW	0.400	0.500	0.667	0.408	0.516	0.707	0.447	0.577	0.816	0.516	0.707	1.155	0.516	0.707	1.155
TPM	0.400	0.500	0.667	0.408	0.516	0.707	0.447	0.577	0.816	0.516	0.707	1.155	0.516	0.707	1.155
TCP	0.286	0.333	0.400	0.365	0.400	0.500	0.365	0.447	0.577	0.447	0.577	0.816	0.447	0.577	0.816

Table 2b. (continuation). The pairwise comparison matrix of the sub-criteria of the criterion maintenance organization

Sub-Criteria	TSH			IOW			TPM			TCP		
	l_{ij}	m_{ij}	u_{ij}	l_{ij}	m_{ij}	u_{ij}	l_{ij}	m_{ij}	u_{ij}	l_{ij}	m_{ij}	u_{ij}
EMD	2.236	2.739	3.240	1.500	2.000	2.500	1.500	2.000	2.500	2.500	3.000	3.500
MMP	1.732	2.236	2.739	1.414	1.936	2.449	1.414	1.936	2.449	2.000	2.500	3.000
RMM	1.414	1.936	2.449	1.225	1.732	2.236	1.225	1.732	2.236	1.732	2.236	2.739
EWG	1.000	1.500	2.000	0.866	1.414	1.936	0.866	1.414	1.936	1.225	1.732	2.236
NWM	1.000	1.500	2.000	0.866	1.414	1.936	0.866	1.414	1.936	1.225	1.732	2.236
TSH	1.000	1.000	1.000	0.577	0.816	1.414	0.577	0.816	1.414	0.707	1.000	1.225
IOW	0.707	1.225	1.732	1.000	1.000	1.000	1.000	1.000	1.000	0.707	1.000	1.414
TPM	0.707	1.225	1.732	0.500	1.000	1.500	1.000	1.000	1.000	0.707	1.000	1.414
TCP	0.816	1.000	1.414	0.707	1.000	1.414	0.707	1.000	1.414	1.000	1.000	1.000

$$\tilde{S}_i = \sum_{j=1}^{m} \tilde{a}_{g_i}^j \otimes \left[\sum_{i=1}^{n} \sum_{j=1}^{m} \tilde{a}_{g_i}^j \right]^{-1} \tag{3}$$

where g_i are the goals of the hierarchy and $\tilde{a}_{g_i}^j$ is a triangular fuzzy number of the fuzzy comparison matrix $\tilde{A}$ with n objects and m goals.

The values of the fuzzy synthetic extents obtained for the sub-criteria of the criterion Maintenance organization are:

$$\tilde{S}_{EMD} = \left(\frac{11.943}{119.749}, \frac{15.963}{78.262}, \frac{19.972}{68.151} \right) = (0.100, 0.204, 0.293)$$

$$\tilde{S}_{MMP} = \left(\frac{9.934}{119.749}, \frac{13.609}{78.262}, \frac{17.862}{68.151} \right) = (0.083, 0.174, 0.262)$$

$$\tilde{S}_{RMM} = \left(\frac{9.940}{119.749}, \frac{12.453}{78.262}, \frac{15.938}{68.151} \right) = (0.079, 0.159, 0.234)$$

$$\tilde{S}_{EWG} = \left(\frac{9.940}{119.749}, \frac{10.727}{78.262}, \frac{14.523}{68.151} \right) = (0.066, 0.137, 0.213)$$

$$\tilde{S}_{NWM} = \left(\frac{9.940}{119.749}, \frac{10.727}{78.262}, \frac{14.523}{68.151} \right) = (0.066, 0.137, 0.213)$$

$$\tilde{S}_{TSH} = \left(\frac{4.944}{119.749}, \frac{6.295}{78.262}, \frac{8.785}{68.151} \right) = (0.041, 0.080, 0.129)$$

$$\tilde{S}_{IOW} = \left(\frac{5.702}{119.749}, \frac{7.233}{78.262}, \frac{9.646}{68.151} \right) = (0.048, 0.092, 0.142)$$

$$\tilde{S}_{TPM} = \left(\frac{5.202}{119.749}, \frac{7.233}{78.262}, \frac{10.146}{68.151} \right) = (0.043, 0.092, 0.149)$$

$$\tilde{S}_{TCP} = \left(\frac{5.141}{119.749}, \frac{6.335}{78.262}, \frac{8.353}{68.151} \right) = (0.043, 0.081, 0.123)$$

Then the degree of possibility of $\tilde{S}_j = (l_j, m_j, u_j) \geq \tilde{S}_i = (l_i, m_i, u_i)$ is calculated from Equation (4) (Durán, 2011).

$$V(\tilde{S}_j \geq \tilde{S}_i) = hgt(\tilde{S}_i \cap \tilde{S}_j) = \mu_{\tilde{s}_j}(d) = \begin{cases} 1 & \text{If } m_j \geq m_i \\ 0 & \text{If } l_i \geq u_j \\ \dfrac{l_i - u_j}{(m_j - u_j) - (m_i - l_i)} & \text{otherwise} \end{cases} \tag{4}$$

Where d is the abscissa of the cut point of $\tilde{S}_i$ and $\tilde{S}_j$. In order to compare $\tilde{S}_i$ and $\tilde{S}_j$ it is necessary to calculate $V(\tilde{S}_j \geq \tilde{S}_i)$ and $V(\tilde{S}_i \geq \tilde{S}_j)$.

The degrees of possibility of $V(\tilde{S}_j \geq \tilde{S}_i)$ corresponding to the sub-criteria of Maintenance organization are shown in Table 3.

The minimum degree of possibility of $V(\tilde{S}_j \geq \tilde{S}_i)$ for $i,j=1,2, ..., k$ is calculated from the previous results by means of Equation (5).

$$V(\tilde{S}_j \geq \tilde{S}_1, \tilde{S}_2, ..., \tilde{S}_k) = V(\tilde{S}_j \geq \tilde{S}_1) \text{ and } V(\tilde{S}_j \geq \tilde{S}_2) \text{ and } ... V(\tilde{S}_j \geq \tilde{S}_k) = \min V(\tilde{S}_j \geq \tilde{S}_i) \qquad (5)$$

for $i=1,2, ..., k$.

Table 3. Degrees of possibility $V(\tilde{S}_j \geq \tilde{S}_i)$ of maintenance organization sub-criteria

Degrees of Possibility	Degrees of Possibility	Degrees of Possibility
$V(\tilde{S}_{EMD} \geq \tilde{S}_{MMP}) = 1.000$	$V(\tilde{S}_{EWG} \geq \tilde{S}_{EMD}) = 0.629$	$V(\tilde{S}_{IOW} \geq \tilde{S}_{EMD}) = 0.273$
$V(\tilde{S}_{EMD} \geq \tilde{S}_{RMM}) = 1.000$	$V(\tilde{S}_{EWG} \geq \tilde{S}_{MMPD}) = 0.779$	$V(\tilde{S}_{IOW} \geq \tilde{S}_{MMP}) = 0.418$
$V(\tilde{S}_{EMD} \geq \tilde{S}_{EWG}) = 1.000$	$V(\tilde{S}_{EWG} \geq \tilde{S}_{RMM}) = 0.859$	$V(\tilde{S}_{IOW} \geq \tilde{S}_{RMM}) = 0.486$
$V(\tilde{S}_{EMD} \geq \tilde{S}_{NWM}) = 1.000$	$V(\tilde{S}_{EWG} \geq \tilde{S}_{NWM}) = 1.000$	$V(\tilde{S}_{IOW} \geq \tilde{S}_{EWG}) = 0.628$
$V(\tilde{S}_{EMD} \geq \tilde{S}_{TSH}) = 1.000$	$V(\tilde{S}_{EWG} \geq \tilde{S}_{TSH}) = 1.000$	$V(\tilde{S}_{IOW} \geq \tilde{S}_{NWM}) = 0.628$
$V(\tilde{S}_{EMD} \geq \tilde{S}_{IOW}) = 1.000$	$V(\tilde{S}_{EWG} \geq \tilde{S}_{IOM}) = 1.000$	$V(\tilde{S}_{IOW} \geq \tilde{S}_{TSH}) = 1.000$
$V(\tilde{S}_{EMD} \geq \tilde{S}_{TPM}) = 1.000$	$V(\tilde{S}_{EWG} \geq \tilde{S}_{TPM}) = 1.000$	$V(\tilde{S}_{IOW} \geq \tilde{S}_{TPM}) = 1.000$
$V(\tilde{S}_{EMD} \geq \tilde{S}_{TCP}) = 1.000$	$V(\tilde{S}_{EWG} \geq \tilde{S}_{TCP}) = 1.000$	$V(\tilde{S}_{IOW} \geq \tilde{S}_{TCP}) = 1.000$
$V(\tilde{S}_{MMP} \geq \tilde{S}_{EMD}) = 0.844$	$V(\tilde{S}_{NWM} \geq \tilde{S}_{EMD}) = 0.629$	$V(\tilde{S}_{TPM} \geq \tilde{S}_{EMD}) = 0.306$
$V(\tilde{S}_{MMP} \geq \tilde{S}_{RMM}) = 1.000$	$V(\tilde{S}_{NWM} \geq \tilde{S}_{MMP}) = 0.779$	$V(\tilde{S}_{TPM} \geq \tilde{S}_{MMP}) = 0.447$
$V(\tilde{S}_{MMP} \geq \tilde{S}_{EWG}) = 1.000$	$V(\tilde{S}_{NWM} \geq \tilde{S}_{RMM}) = 0.859$	$V(\tilde{S}_{TPM} \geq \tilde{S}_{RMM}) = 0.513$
$V(\tilde{S}_{MMP} \geq \tilde{S}_{NWM}) = 1.000$	$V(\tilde{S}_{NWM} \geq \tilde{S}_{EWG}) = 1.000$	$V(\tilde{S}_{TPM} \geq \tilde{S}_{EWG}) = 0.649$
$V(\tilde{S}_{MMP} \geq \tilde{S}_{TSH}) = 1.000$	$V(\tilde{S}_{NWM} \geq \tilde{S}_{TSH}) = 1.000$	$V(\tilde{S}_{TPM} \geq \tilde{S}_{NWM}) = 0.649$
$V(\tilde{S}_{MMP} \geq \tilde{S}_{IOW}) = 1.000$	$V(\tilde{S}_{NWM} \geq \tilde{S}_{IOW}) = 1.000$	$V(\tilde{S}_{TPM} \geq \tilde{S}_{TSH}) = 1.000$
$V(\tilde{S}_{MMP} \geq \tilde{S}_{TPM}) = 1.000$	$V(\tilde{S}_{NWM} \geq \tilde{S}_{TPM}) = 1.000$	$V(\tilde{S}_{TPM} \geq \tilde{S}_{IOW}) = 1.000$

continued on following page

Table 3. Continued

Degrees of Possibility	Degrees of Possibility	Degrees of Possibility
$V(\tilde{S}_{MMP} \geq \tilde{S}_{TCP}) = 1.000$	$V(\tilde{S}_{NWM} \geq \tilde{S}_{TCP}) = 1.000$	$V(\tilde{S}_{TPM} \geq \tilde{S}_{TCP}) = 1.000$
$V(\tilde{S}_{RMM} \geq \tilde{S}_{EMD}) = 0.749$	$V(\tilde{S}_{TSH} \geq \tilde{S}_{EMD}) = 0.191$	$V(\tilde{S}_{TCP} \geq \tilde{S}_{EMD}) = 0.157$
$V(\tilde{S}_{RMM} \geq \tilde{S}_{MMP}) = 0.911$	$V(\tilde{S}_{TSH} \geq \tilde{S}_{MMP}) = 0.330$	$V(\tilde{S}_{TCP} \geq \tilde{S}_{MMP}) = 0.299$
$V(\tilde{S}_{RMM} \geq \tilde{S}_{EWG}) = 1.000$	$V(\tilde{S}_{TSH} \geq \tilde{S}_{RMM}) = 0.390$	$V(\tilde{S}_{TCP} \geq \tilde{S}_{RMM}) = 0.360$
$V(\tilde{S}_{RMM} \geq \tilde{S}_{NWM}) = 1.000$	$V(\tilde{S}_{TSH} \geq \tilde{S}_{EWG}) = 0.525$	$V(\tilde{S}_{TCP} \geq \tilde{S}_{EWG}) = 0.501$
$V(\tilde{S}_{RMM} \geq \tilde{S}_{TSH}) = 1.000$	$V(\tilde{S}_{TSH} \geq \tilde{S}_{NWM}) = 0.525$	$V(\tilde{S}_{TCP} \geq \tilde{S}_{NWM}) = 0.501$
$V(\tilde{S}_{RMM} \geq \tilde{S}_{IOW}) = 1.000$	$V(\tilde{S}_{TSH} \geq \tilde{S}_{IOW}) = 0.872$	$V(\tilde{S}_{TCP} \geq \tilde{S}_{TSH}) = 1.000$
$V(\tilde{S}_{RMM} \geq \tilde{S}_{TPM}) = 1.000$	$V(\tilde{S}_{TSH} \geq \tilde{S}_{TPM}) = 0.877$	$V(\tilde{S}_{TCP} \geq \tilde{S}_{IOW}) = 0.876$
$V(\tilde{S}_{RMM} \geq \tilde{S}_{TPC}) = 1.000$	$V(\tilde{S}_{TSH} \geq \tilde{S}_{TCP}) = 0.994$	$V(\tilde{S}_{TCP} \geq \tilde{S}_{TPM}) = 0.873$

Supposing $d'(A_j) = \min V(\tilde{S}_j \geq \tilde{S}_i)$ $i=1,2, ..., n$ and $i \neq j$, the weighting vector W' is calculated by applying Equation (6).

$$W' = (d'(A_1), d'(A_2), ..., d'(A_n))^T \tag{6}$$

Finally, this vector must be normalized to obtain the crisp weighting vector W.

The weighting vector obtained for the sub-criteria of the criterion Maintenance organization is W' = (1.000, 0.844, 0.749, 0.629, 0.629, 0.191, 0.273, 0.306, 0.157).

And the normalized vector W' = (0.209, 0.177, 0.157, 0.132, 0.132, 0.040, 0.057, 0.064, 0.033).

A similar process is applied to the sub-criteria associated with each criterion and for the group of criteria. The remaining non-fuzzy weight vectors obtained are shown in Table 4.

A pairwise comparison matrix has been produced between the scale levels of each descriptor. In this case crisp numbers and AHP were used to calculate the utilities of each scale level. This is due to the high degree of complexity that is already in the model with 50 sub-criteria and the 50 discrete probability distribution functions to be calculated. Each sub-criterion could also have four, five, six or more scale levels, thus the degree of computational complexity that it would add to the model is very high. Table 5 shows an example of the scale levels for the sub-criterion Application of Total Productive Maintenance and the resulting utilities after applying AHP.

Table 4. Non-fuzzy weight vectors

Weight Vector of Criteria/Sub-Criteria	Non-Fuzzy Weight Vectors
W = (MMA, TRA, COM, CON, OMA, MCO, MOR, QES)	W = (0.124, 0.053, 0.096, 0.134, 0.022, 0.262, 0.135, 0.174)
W = (TMM, ADE, EMP, FPO, POW, ACM, RSJ, RIJ, UIM)	W = (0.260, 0.228, 0.179, 0.144, 0.084, 0.032, 0.024, 0.019, 0.030)
W = (TCU, TTR, VMW, SRF)	W = (0.268, 0.201, 0.291, 0.240)
W = (SCA, TCM, HMS, ASC, FMM)	W = (0.204, 0.197, 0.197, 0.204, 0.197)
W = (OWO, DIW, PUW, WPE, RMC, DCD, AMC, SCI)	W = (0.128, 0.122, 0.125, 0.124, 0.127, 0.127, 0.123, 0.125)
W = (TCO, PPM, PCM, PPS, QOW, TOU, POP)	W = (0.271, 0.124, 0.145, 0.129, 0.207, 0.012, 0.113)
W = (ABM, PAS, PAO, PAI, TMC)	W = (0.252, 0.209, 0.209, 0.307, 0.022)
W = (CI9, CI1, CHS)	W = (0.213, 0.045, 0.742)

Table 5. Scale levels and associated utilities for the sub-criterion Application of Total Productive Maintenance (TPM)

Scale Levels	Utilities
A TPM programme exists	1.0000
Care staff are assigned routine maintenance tasks	0.5800
Care staff help maintenance staff during stoppages for preventive maintenance	0.3138
Care staff carry out minor repairs in the absence of maintenance staff	0.1470
Care staff help occasionally with no fixed rules	0.0536
Care staff do not cooperate in any way with maintenance staff	0.0000

Finally, the consistency of the judgements made by the decision makers must be evaluated. This is done by calculating the Consistency Ratio (*CR*) defined by Saaty (1980). Saaty showed that for a consistent reciprocal matrix, the largest eigenvalue λ_{max} is equal to the size of the judgement matrix *n*, i.e. $\lambda_{max} = n$. The *CR* is calculated as the coefficient of the Consistency Index (*CI*) and the Random Consistency Index *(RCI)* for a matrix of similar size (Forman and Selly, 2001). The *CI* is calculated from (7) (Saaty, 1980).

$$CI = \frac{\lambda_{max} - n}{n - 1} \tag{7}$$

The *RCI* was obtained by Saaty from a simple of 500 randomly generated reciprocal matrices (Saaty, 1980). The average *RCI's* for different matrix sizes are shown in Table 6.

Table 6. Random Consistency Index

n	1	2	3	4	5	6	7	8	9	10
RCI	0	0	0.58	0.9	1.12	1.24	1.32	1.41	1.45	1.49

If CR is less than 0.05 for a 3x3 matrix, 0.08 for a 4x4 matrix and 0.1 for matrices of higher order, then the judgement matrix is consistent (Saaty, 2001). As these are fuzzy pairwise comparison matrices, the mean value of the fuzzy elements of the matrix has been considered (Duran, 2011). For example, the judgment matrix for the sub-criteria included in the criterion Maintenance organization gives the following CI and CR.

$$CI = \frac{9.040 - 9}{9 - 1} = 0.005$$

$$CR = \frac{0.005}{1.45} = 0.00345 < 0.1$$

All the fuzzy pairwise comparison matrices used in the maintenance benchmarking model show consistency ratios below the limits set by Saaty according to the rank of each matrix. Table 7 shows the CR obtained from the different judgement matrices when the criteria and sub-criteria in the first column of the Table are compared.

Definition of Alternatives

The alternatives considered are the service sector for the evaluation of 2000, and the buildings sector for 2005 and 2010. In all these cases, organizations with more than 500 workers are considered, since Health Care Organizations generally have a higher number of human resources than this, between the care and non-care staff.

Furthermore, as many alternatives should be included as Health Care Organizations the model is intended to evaluate.

The data from the surveys carried out by the SMA (SMA, 2000; 2005, 2010) have been converted into probabilities that are then associated with each scale level of each descriptor. The probabilities associated with the different scale levels of a descriptor constitute a discrete probability distribution function. In all, 50 discrete probability distribution functions were calculated.

Table 7. Consistency ratio obtained for judgement matrices of criteria and sub-criteria

Criteria/Sub-Criteria in the Judgement Matrix	CR
MMA, TRA, COM, CON, OMA, MCO, MOR, QES	0.00288
TMM, ADE, EMP, FPO, POW, ACM, RSJ, RIJ, UIM	0.00476
TCU, TTR, VMW, SRF	0.00813
SCA, TCM, HMS, ASC, FMM	0.00075
OWO, DIW, PUW, WPE, RMC, DCD, AMC, SCI	0.01470
TCO, PPM, PCM, PPS, QOW, TOU, POP	0.00350
ABM, PAS, PAO, PAI, TMC	0.00457
EMD, MMP, RMM, EWG, NWM, TSH, IOW, TPM, TCP	0.00345
CI9, CI1, CHS	0.00288

An example of the discrete probability distribution used in the model is shown in Figure 2. The Monte Carlo simulation is a method for estimating uncertainty in a variable which is a complex function of one or more probability distributions. In order to apply the Monte Carlo simulation, 5,000 trials were considered, and a random number seed of 10,000.

SOLUTIONS AND RECOMMENDATIONS

The following procedure was used to calculate the valuation or final utility of each alternative. If $p(x)$ is the probability associated with each scale level of a descriptor in an alternative y, and $U(x)$ the utility associated with that level, then the equivalent uncertainty level for each alternative is calculated by adding the expected utility $p(x) * U(x)$ for all the levels x with non-zero probability in the probability distribution function. The final utility of a criterion in an alternative is calculated via a multi-measure utility function. This function is obtained by multiplying the weightings of each sub-criterion by the $U(y)$ previously obtained for each sub-criterion.

For example, if w_1, w_2, w_3, w_4, w_5, w_6, w_7, w_8 and w_9 are the weightings of the sub-criteria included in the criterion maintenance organization, the final utility of the criterion is calculated by applying Equation (8).

$$Utility\ (MOR) = w_1 {}^*U_{EMD}(y) + w_2 {}^*U_{MMR}(y) + w_3 {}^*U_{RMM}(y) + w_4 {}^*U_{EWG}(y) + w_5 {}^*U_{NWM}(y) + w_6 {}^*U_{TSH}(y) + w_7 {}^*U_{IOW}(y) + w_8 {}^*U_{TPM}(y) + w_9 {}^*U_{TCP}(y) \tag{8}$$

Figure 2. Discrete probability distribution function of the sub-criterion application of Total Productive Maintenance (TPM) in the year 2010
(Created by the author)

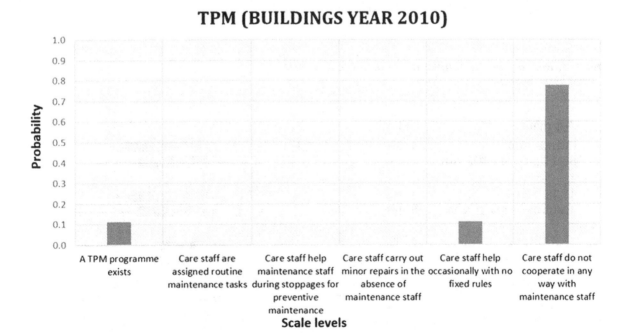

With $U_{EMD}(y)$ = *utility (best scale level)*probability+...+ utility (worst scale level)*probability.*

The benchmarking model was evaluated by applying it to the maintenance department of the University General Hospital of Ciudad Real (UGHCR). This is a Spanish public-general Health Care Organization built in 2005. The UGHCR serves a population of 590,000 inhabitants, although the nuclear medicine, eating disorders and infant and child short stays units make it a regional centre of reference.

The maintenance manager of the UGHCR filled out the questionnaire at set intervals, in order to assess the scale level of each descriptor relevant to the hospital.

The benchmarking model included alternatives corresponding to the state of maintenance at UGHCR in 2000, 2005 and 2010.

Figure 3 shows the results obtained with maintenance benchmarking model for the sector (services and buildings) and for UGHCR in the years 2000, 2005 and 2010. In the sections which represent the contribution of each criterion to the evaluation of alternatives, the criteria are arranged in each of the years under assessment, firstly, in white, Maintenance costs, followed by Quality, environment and safety standards, Maintenance organization, Control, Maintenance manager, Maintenance computerization, Training and Outsourcing. Note that for the year 2000 there were no available data for the criterion Quality, environment and safety standards, and so this criterion is not included in the Figure 3 for that year.

When the results of 2000 for the service sector and the hospital are compared, the hospital can be seen to have a utility over 3.11%. Nonetheless, among the areas where the hospital performed more poorly than its sector are the absence of maintenance budgets, and factors relating to the computerization of maintenance, since the type of CMMS used, and the satisfaction arising, give lower utilities than the sector overall. For example, in the case of satisfaction with the CMMS applied, the sector returns 100% of those surveyed as satisfied or very satisfied, whereas the experience at the hospital was unsatisfactory. The frequency with which the maintenance manager is summoned outside working hours is 2 or 3 times a month, while the most likely result for the sector is 1 to 3 times a year. The versatility of maintenance staff also needs to be improved, as while 61.91% of those surveyed has a mostly versatile staff, the hospital only has this in a few specialities. Poor behaviour can also be seen with respect to

Figure 3. Ranking of alternatives in 2000, 2005, and 2010
(Created by the author)

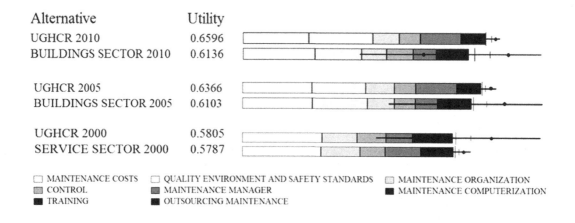

the delay with which information about maintenance costs is received, from 2 weeks to a month in the hospital, whereas the most likely result in the sector is between 1 and 2 weeks.

Comparison between the buildings sector and the hospital for 2005 shows an increase in utility of 4.31% for the HCO. It can also be seen that the utilities, both in the sector and in the hospital have improved since 2000. However, the deficiencies found in the hospital in 2000 are mostly still present, essentially in the areas of budgeting, versatility of maintenance staff and satisfaction with the CMMS. On the other hand, it is notable how in 2005 the hospital carried out a training programme for most of the staff, which only occurs in 30% of those surveyed in the sector. Incidents outside working hours also shows improvement with respect to the sector and the year 2000, as these are resolved by maintenance staff working in shifts, while 64.29% of those surveyed in the sector use other, less efficient systems. Questions such as the experience in the post, the training, and the experience in performing maintenance work of the maintenance manager, continue to have, over time, higher utilities in the HCO than in the sector in general.

Comparing the results for the buildings sector with those for the hospital in 2010, it can be seen that the HCO has utility above 7.50%. This is largely due to improved behaviour in compliance with Health and Safety Law and the gaining of the ISO 9000 certificate. Also, the level of excellence of the management of the maintenance department is well above the sector, as while in the hospital experience is over 25 years, 60% of those surveyed in the sector had less than 15 years, and the mode was between 11 and 15 years. The training of the maintenance manager also gives higher utility; while the manger in the hospital has a higher degree in Industrial Engineering, in 60% of cases in the sector the manager has only a first degree. The time in post of the maintenance manager at the hospital is over 20 years, while in the sector, 70% of those surveyed had not been in post as long. Other areas in which the HCO has a better showing than its sector is in the number of incidents outside normal working hours, and percentage of costs associated with in-house staff, spares and consumables. On the other hand, the hospital needs to work on the matters of costs, such as budgeting and the costs associated with outsourcing. It is true, however, that Health Care Organizations increasingly outsource maintenance of high-tech equipment to the manufacturer, meaning in this case that the result may be justified. There is also a need to improve the frequency with which the maintenance manager is required on-site outside normal working hours, which is monthly in this case, while 70% of those surveyed in the sector were only required 4 to 10 times a year, or even less. Questions about control of maintenance also need to be improved at UGHCR; in particular, the number of urgent jobs received is very high, as is the regularity at which information about costs is transmitted, and the delay in receiving it, as well as the number of maintenance indices used to take decisions.

In any case, the trend over time in improvements at UGHCR is faster than the rhythm achieved by the sector in general. This is very positive, and it also leads one to think that the results for UGHCR should be compared with other sectors, more competitive than buildings, such as the automobile and related industries, or the transport sector.

FUTURE RESEARCH DIRECTIONS

Future research includes the expectation of obtaining a number of surveys on maintenance completed by different Health Care Organizations. This would allow a comparison to be made between an HCO and another with similar characteristics, making the results of the benchmarking model more accurate. This is because at the moment valuations of the survey include HCO's, but also other types of organization such as shopping centres, government buildings, etc., which tend to have less demanding maintenance requirements.

The intention is to use fuzzy numbers and fuzzy AHP to obtain the utilities associated with the scale levels of each descriptor. The model proposed in this research will be validated by means of other methods, for example Fuzzy Measuring Attractiveness by a Categorical Based Evaluation Technique (MACBETH) approach.

CONCLUSION

Contributions analysing the level of maintenance applied in Health Care Organizations are virtually non-existent. However, this type of organization has requirements for availability, quality of performance of medical equipment, and safety, far higher than other organizations. It should be borne in mind that the consequences of a breakdown may be very serious for patients or for care staff. To solve this problem, therefore, this chapter sets out a benchmarking model which allows the level of excellence of maintenance applied by a Health Care Organization to be assessed in comparison with the rest of the sector it belongs to. This means that anomalous behaviours and possibilities for improvement may be found more readily. It also allows a comparison over time of the level of maintenance carried out by a hospital, making it easier to control the consequences of improvement actions or decisions taken.

The benchmarking model described in this chapter combines the use of FAHP with utility theory to obtain a ranking of the service and buildings sectors, and of the Health Care Organizations to be evaluated. The probabilities of each scale level of each descriptor associated with each sub-criterion were calculated from Spanish surveys on the state of maintenance in the service and buildings sectors. A Monte Carlo simulation was used to estimate the resulting uncertainty when a number of probability distribution functions are combined.

ACKNOWLEDGMENT

This research was supported by the Junta de Comunidades de Castilla-La Mancha and the European Regional Development Fund under Grant number PPII-2014-013-P.

REFERENCES

Alsyouf, I. (2009). Maintenance practices in Swedish industries: Survey results. *International Journal of Production Economics*, *121*(1), 212–223. doi:10.1016/j.ijpe.2009.05.005

Anvari, F., & Edwards, R. (2011). Maintenance engineering in capital-intensive manufacturing systems. *Journal of Quality in Maintenance Engineering*, *17*(4), 351–370. doi:10.1108/13552511111180177

APQC (American Productivity & Quality Center). (2013). *Benchmarking*. Retrieved May 22, 2013, from http://www.apqc.org/benchmarking

Azam, M., Qureshi, M. N., & Talib, F. (2015). AHP Model for Identifying Best Health Care Establishment. *International Journal of Productivity Management and Assessment Technologies*, *3*(2), 34–66. doi:10.4018/IJPMAT.2015070104

Bana e Costa, C. A., Correa, E., De Corte, J. M., & Vansnick, J. C. (2002). Facilitating bid evaluation in public call for tenders: A socio-technical approach. *Omega*, *30*(3), 227–242. doi:10.1016/S0305-0483(02)00029-4

Boender, C. G. E., de Grann, J. G., & Lootsma, F. A. (1989). Multicriteria decision analysis with fuzzy pairwise comparison. *Fuzzy Sets and Systems*, *29*(2), 133–143. doi:10.1016/0165-0114(89)90187-5

Bozbura, F. T., Beskese, A., & Kahraman, C. (2007). Prioritization of human capital measurement indicators using fuzzy AHP. *Expert Systems with Applications*, *32*(4), 1100–1112. doi:10.1016/j.eswa.2006.02.006

Buckley, J. J. (1985). Fuzzy hierarchical analysis. *Fuzzy Sets and Systems*, *17*(3), 233–247. doi:10.1016/0165-0114(85)90090-9

Büyüközkan, G., Kahraman, C., & Ruan, D. (2004). A fuzzy multicriteria decision approach for software development strategy selection. *International Journal of General Systems*, *33*(2-3), 259–280. doi:10.1080/03081070310001633581

Carnero, M. C. (2012). Condition Based Maintenance in small industries. In *Proceeding of the 2nd International Workshop on Advanced Maintenance Engineering*, 21-23.

Carnero, M. C. (2014a). A Decision Support system for Maintenance Benchmarking in big buildings. *European Journal of Industrial Engineering*, *8*(3), 388–420. doi:10.1504/EJIE.2014.061064

Carnero, M. C. (2014b). Multicriteria model for Maintenance Benchmarking. *Journal of Manufacturing Systems*, *33*(2), 303–321. doi:10.1016/j.jmsy.2013.12.006

Carnero, M. C., & Gómez, A. (2016). A multicriteria decision making approach applied to improving maintenance policies in healthcare organizations. *BMC Medical Informatics and Decision Making*, *16*(1), 47. doi:10.1186/s12911-016-0282-7 PMID:27108234

Cebeci, U. (2009). Fuzzy AHP-based decision support system for selecting ERP systems in textile industry by using balanced scorecard. *Expert Systems with Applications*, *36*(5), 8900–8909. doi:10.1016/j.eswa.2008.11.046

Chang, D. Y. (1996). Applications of the extent analysis method on fuzzy AHP. *European Journal of Operational Research*, *95*(3), 649–655. doi:10.1016/0377-2217(95)00300-2

Cheng, C. H. (1996). Evaluating naval tactical missile systems by fuzzy AHP based on the grade value of membership function. *European Journal of Operational Research*, *96*(2), 343–350. doi:10.1016/S0377-2217(96)00026-4

Conde, R. (2007). El benchmarking en la industria química. In *Proceedings of the Jornada sobre Benchmarking en Mantenimiento Industrial*. Madrid: Spanish Maintenance Association.

Dunn, R. L. (1999). *Basic guide to maintenance benchmarking*. Retrieved June 3, 2016, from http://www.plantengineering.com

Dunn, R. L. (2001). Benchmarking maintenance. *Plant Engineering, 55,* 68–70.

Durán, O. (2011). Computer-aided maintenance management systems selection based on a fuzzy AHP approach. *Advances in Engineering Software, 42*(10), 821–829. doi:10.1016/j.advengsoft.2011.05.023

EN15341. (2007). *Maintenance. Maintenance key performance indicators.* CEN.

Fumagalli, L., & Macchi, M. (2009). A state of the art of CBM in the Italian industry. *Proceedings of the 22nd International Congress on Condition Monitoring and Diagnostic Engineering Management - COMADEM,* 173-180.

Huang, I. B., Keisler, J., & Linkov, I. (2011). Multi-criteria decision analysis in environmental sciences: Ten years of applications and trends. *The Science of the Total Environment, 409*(19), 3578–3594. doi:10.1016/j.scitotenv.2011.06.022 PMID:21764422

Isaai, M. T., Kanani, A., Tootoonchi, M., & Afzali, H. R. (2011). Intelligent timetable evaluation using fuzzy AHP. *Expert Systems with Applications, 38*(4), 3718–3723. doi:10.1016/j.eswa.2010.09.030

Joshi, R., Banwet, D. K., & Shankar, R. A. (2011). Delphi-AHP-TOPSIS based benchmarking framework for performance improvement of a cold chain. *Expert Systems with Applications, 38*(8), 10170–10182. doi:10.1016/j.eswa.2011.02.072

Kahn, J., Svantesson, T., Olver, D., & Poling, A. (2009). Global Maintenance and Reliability Indicators: Fitting the Pieces Together (2nd ed.). European Federation of National Maintenance Societies and the Society of Maintenance & Reliability Professionals.

Kahraman, C., Cebeci, U., & Ruan, D. (2004). Multi-attribute comparison of catering service companies using fuzzy AHP: The case of Turkey. *International Journal of Production Economics, 87*(2), 171–184. doi:10.1016/S0925-5273(03)00099-9

Keeney, R. L. (1996). *Value-focused Thinking: A Path to Creative Decision making.* Cambridge, MA: Harvard.

Kelessidis, V. (2000). *Benchmarking.* Report produced for the EC funded project INNOREGIO: dissemination of innovation management and knowledge techniques.

Komonen, K. (2002). A cost model of industrial maintenance for profitability analysis and benchmarking. *International Journal of Production Economics, 79*(1), 15–31. doi:10.1016/S0925-5273(00)00187-0

Lai, J. H. K., & Yik, F. W. H. (2008). Benchmarking operation and maintenance costs of luxury hotels. *Journal of Facilities Management, 6*(4), 279–289. doi:10.1108/14725960810908145

Lee, S. K., Mogi, G., Lee, S. K., & Kim, J. W. (2011). Prioritizing the weights of hydrogen energy Technologies in the sector of the hydrogen economy by using a fuzzy AHP approach. *International Journal of Hydrogen Energy, 36*(2), 1897–1902. doi:10.1016/j.ijhydene.2010.01.035

Lima, F. R., Osiro, L., & Carpinetti, L. C. R. (2014). A comparison between Fuzzy AHP and Fuzzy TOPSIS method to suplier selection. *Applied Soft Computing, 21,* 194–209. doi:10.1016/j.asoc.2014.03.014

Luxhej, J., Riis, J. O., & Thorsteinsson, U. (1997). Trends and Perspectives in Industrial Maintenance Management. *Journal of Manufacturing Systems, 16*(6), 437–453. doi:10.1016/S0278-6125(97)81701-3

Meixner, O. (2009). Fuzzy AHP Group Decision Analysis and its Application for the Evaluation of Energy Sources. In *Proceedings of the 10th International Symposium on the Analytic Hierarchy/Network Process*. Pittsburgh, PA: University of Pittsburgh.

Muchiri, P., & Pintelon, L. (2008). Performance measurement using overall equipment effectiveness (OEE): Literature review and practical application discussion. *International Journal of Production Research*, *46*(13), 3517–3535. doi:10.1080/00207540601142645

Parameshwaran, R., Srinivasan, P. S. S., Punniyamoorthy, M., Charunyanath, S. T., & Ashwin, C. (2009). Integrating fuzzy analytical hierarchy process and data envelopment analysis for performance management in automobile repair shops. *European Journal of Industrial Engineering*, *3*(4), 450–467. doi:10.1504/EJIE.2009.027037

Pinjala, S. K., Pintelon, L., & Vereecke, A. (2006). An empirical investigation on the relationship between business and maintenance strategies. *International Journal of Production Economics*, *104*(1), 214–229. doi:10.1016/j.ijpe.2004.12.024

Rezaei, J. (2015). Best-worst multi-criteria decision-making method. *Omega*, *53*, 49–57. doi:10.1016/j.omega.2014.11.009

Saaty, T. L. (1980). *The Analytic Hierarchy Process*. New York, NY: McGraw Hill.

Saaty, T. L. (2001). *Decision Making with Dependence and Feedback: The Analytic Network Process*. Pittsburgh, PA: RWS Publications.

Shafii, M., Hosseini, S. M., Arab, M., Asgharizadeh, E., & Farzianpour, F. (2015). Performance Analysis of Hospital Managers Using Fuzzy AHP and Fuzzy TOPSIS: Iranian Experience. *Global Journal of Health Science*, *8*(2), 137–155. doi:10.5539/gjhs.v8n2p137 PMID:26383216

SMA (Spanish Maintenance Association). (2000). *El Mantenimiento en España*. Barcelona: Spanish Maintenance Association.

SMA (Spanish Maintenance Association). (2005). *El Mantenimiento en España*. Barcelona: Spanish Maintenance Association.

SMA (Spanish Maintenance Association). (2010). *El Mantenimiento en España*. Barcelona: Spanish Maintenance Association.

Svantesson, T. (2006). Benchmarking in Europe. Proceedings of EuroMaintenance.

van Laarhoven, P. J. M., & Pedrycz, W. (1983). A fuzzy extension of Saatys priority theory. *Fuzzy Sets and Systems*, *11*(1-3), 229–241. doi:10.1016/S0165-0114(83)80082-7

Wang, J., Fan, K., & Wang, W. (2010). Integration of fuzzy AHP and FPP with TOPSIS methodology for aeroengine health assessment. *Expert Systems with Applications*, *37*(12), 8516–8526. doi:10.1016/j.eswa.2010.05.024

Wheelhouse, P. J. (2009). Benchmarking Maintenance & Asset Management for Performance Improvement. *Proceedings of the 22nd International Congress on Condition Monitoring and Diagnostic Engineering Management - COMADEM 2009*, 81-87.

Wireman, T. (1990). *World Class Maintenance Management*. New York, NY: Industrial Press Inc.

Wireman, T. (2004). *Benchmarking best practices in maintenance management*. New York, NY: Industrial Press Inc.

Zadeh, L. A. (1965). L. A. Fuzzy sets. *Information and Control, 8*(3), 338–353. doi:10.1016/S0019-9958(65)90241-X

Zhu, K. (2012). *The Invalidity of Triangular Fuzzy AHP: A Mathematical Justification. Electronic Journal*. doi:10.2139/ssrn.2011922

Zou, Z. H., Yun, Y., & Sun, J. N. (2006). Entropy method for determination of weight of evaluating indicators in fuzzy synthetic evaluation for water quality assessment. *Journal of Environmental Sciences (China), 18*(5), 1020–1023. doi:10.1016/S1001-0742(06)60032-6 PMID:17278765

ADDITIONAL READING

Alsyouf, I. (2007). The role of maintenance in improving companies productivity and profitability. *International Journal of Production Economics, 105*(1), 70–78. doi:10.1016/j.ijpe.2004.06.057

Chan, K. T., Lee, R. H. K., & Burnett, J. (2001). Maintenance performance: A case study of hospitality engineering systems. *Facilities, 19*(13/14), 494–503. doi:10.1108/02632770110409477

Chang, D. Y. (1992). *Extent analysis and Synthetic Decision, Optimization Techniques and Applications* (Vol. 1, p. 352). Singapore: World Scientific.

Eti, M. C., Ogaji, S. O. T., & Probert, S. D. (2006). Strategic maintenance-management in Nigerian industries. *Applied Energy, 83*(3), 211–227. doi:10.1016/j.apenergy.2005.02.004

Holgeid, K. K., Krogstie, J., & Sjøberg, D. I. K. (2000). A study of development and maintenance in Norway: Assessing the efficiency of information systems support using functional maintenance. *Information and Software Technology, 42*(10), 687–700. doi:10.1016/S0950-5849(00)00111-7

Ikhwan, M. A. H., & Burney, F. A. (1994). Maintenance in Saudi Industry. *International Journal of Operations & Production Management, 14*(7), 70–80. doi:10.1108/01443579410062194

Jamasb, T., & Pollitt, M. (2003). International benchmarking and regulation: An application to European electricity distribution utilities. *Energy Policy, 31*(15), 1609–1622. doi:10.1016/S0301-4215(02)00226-4

Kaufmann, A., & Gupta, M. M. (1988). *Fuzzy Mathematical Models in Engineering and Management Science*. Amsterdam: North Holland.

Kaufmann, A., & Gupta, M. M. (1991). *Introduction to Fuzzy Arithmetic*. New York, NY: Van Nostrand.

Krogstie, J. (1995). On the distinction between functional development and functional maintenance. *Journal of Software Maintenance: Research and Practice, 7*(6), 383–403. doi:10.1002/smr.4360070603

Muthu, S., Devadasan, S. R., Ahmed, S., Suresh, P., & Baladhandayutham, R. (2000). Benchmarking for strategic maintenance quality improvement. *Benchmarking: An International Journal*, 7(4), 292–303. doi:10.1108/14635770010378927

Wireman, T. (2005). *Developing Performance indicator for managing maintenance*. New York, NY: Industrial Press Inc.

Yam, R. C. M., Tse, P., Ling, L., & Fung, F. (2000). Enhancement of maintenance management through benchmarking. *Journal of Quality in Maintenance Engineering*, 6(4), 224–240. doi:10.1108/13552510010373419

KEY TERMS AND DEFINITIONS

Activity Sector: Classification of economic activity into groups which have common characteristics in the production processes carried out in each of them, and which distinguish them from other groupings.

Analytic Hierarchy Process: A multi-criteria technique developed by Thomas Saaty in 1980 by which a ranking of alternatives is calculated based on the principles of comparison by pairs, decomposition and synthesis. A hierarchy must be constructed to establish the relationship between the goal, criteria, sub-criteria and alternatives; to determine the relative importance of the alternatives with regard to each of the criteria or between criteria, linguistic terms are used that include the judgements of the decision maker.

Benchmarking: A continuous improvement process consisting of seeking, comparing and adapting best practice in other organizations to one's own, by using indicators or benchmarks to achieve the highest level of performance.

Fuzzy Analytic Hierarchy Process: The inability of AHP to deal with imprecision and subjectivity in the judgements given by the decision maker is solved using fuzzy AHP. It is, therefore, a multi-criteria technique, based on AHP, but using range of values to incorporate the uncertainty of the decision maker. A number of different methodologies have been developed for applying it, e.g.; the algorithm designed by Van Laarhoven and Pedrycz, which is a direct extension of the original AHP method; the Buckley method for incorporating fuzzy comparison ratios into the methodology; other methodologies used are Chang's Extent Analysis Method and Cheng's entropy-based Fuzzy AHP.

Fuzzy Logic: A technique of computational intelligence introduced by Lotfy A. Zadeh in 1965 which allows the imprecision, uncertainty, vagueness, etc., which characterize human judgements and thought to be included. It represents knowledge, which is primarily linguistic and qualitative, in mathematical language, by the use of fuzzy sets and associated characteristic functions.

Maintenance: A set of technical and management actions carried out to operate, preserve, improve and adapt machines and/or facilities in an organization over their lifetime, so as to support the aims established by the company at minimum cost.

Monte Carlo Simulation: A method for estimating uncertainty in a variable which is a complex function of one or more probability distributions; it uses random numbers to provide an estimate of the distribution and a random number generator to produce random samples from the probabilistic levels.

Chapter 2
Optimization of Maintenance in Critical Equipment in Neonatology

María Carmen Carnero
University of Castilla-La Mancha, Spain & University of Lisbon, Portugal

Andrés Gómez
University of Castilla-La Mancha, Spain

ABSTRACT

Maintenance decisions by medical staff play an essential role in achieving availability, quality and safety in care services provided. This has, in turn, an effect on the quality of care perceived by patients. Nonetheless, despite its importance, there is a serious deficiency in models facilitating optimization of maintenance decisions in critical care equipment. This chapter shows a decision support system (DSS) for choosing the best combination of maintenance policies, together with other actions for improvement, such as the increase in the number of back-up devices used in the assisted breathing unit in the Neonatology Service of a hospital. This DSS is combined with an innovative form of continuous time Markov chains, and the multicriteria Measuring Attractiveness by a Categorical Based Evaluation Technique (MACBETH). The result is a ranking of the various maintenance alternatives to be applied. Finally, the real implications for availability and quality of care of applying the best solution are described.

INTRODUCTION

Maintenance decisions by medical staff play an essential role in achieving availability, quality and safety in care services. This has, in turn, an effect on the quality of care perceived by patients. Nonetheless, despite its importance, there is a serious deficiency in models facilitating optimization of maintenance decisions in health care organizations. There is, however, literature analysing the choice of maintenance policies in manufacturing, transport, processing, energy companies, etc., which shows how little importance has been attached to these logistical processes in hospitals.

DOI: 10.4018/978-1-5225-2515-8.ch002

Also, most of the literature dealing with the choice of the most suitable maintenance policy to be used in industrial settings does not consider the fact that in common practice organizations apply a combination of maintenance policies rather than just one.

This chapter shows a Decision Support System (DSS) for choosing the best combination of maintenance policies, together with other actions for improvement, such as an increase in the number of back-up devices used, in the assisted breathing unit in the Neonatology Service of a hospital. This DSS uses an innovative combination of continuous time Markov chains and the multi-criteria Measuring Attractiveness by a Categorical Based Evaluation Technique (MACBETH) approach. This involved using judgements given by a decision group made up of those in charge of different areas of the hospital.

The result is a ranking of the various maintenance alternatives to be applied. Finally, the real implications for availability and quality of care of applying the best solution are described. This is the first study aimed at optimizing decisions about the maintenance policies to be used in such critical systems as the assisted breathing unit in a Neonatology Service.

This chapter is structured as follows: Firstly, there is a review of the literature on maintenance policy selection. Then the DSS developed for the optimization of maintenance in the assisted breathing unit in a Neonatology Service is described; this includes the application of Markov chains to this system, as well as the construction of the multi-criteria model using the MACBETH approach. It also shows the full classification of the alternatives obtained as a result, and the sensitivity analysis of the model. Finally future lines of research, acknowledgements and conclusions are presented.

BACKGROUND

Although there are many mathematical models and optimization techniques applied to maintenance in the literature, they mostly optimize a single maintenance policy, and are mathematically so complex that to put them into practice in organizations is extremely difficult.

Choosing a maintenance policy in an organization is a complex decision, as it is necessary to analyse technical aspects, related to machinery and facilities, at the same time as organizational and strategic matters. This decision affects availability of machinery and facilities, plant and staff safety, quality of the product or service, and maintenance costs.

It is therefore necessary to take into account a variety of criteria, both quantitative and qualitative, when taking this decision, which is why the use of Multi-Criteria Decision Analysis (MCDA) techniques is justified (Carnero, 2014). In fact, Almeida and Bohoris (1995) and Martorell et al. (2005) underlined the benefits of using multi-criteria techniques in the field of maintenance, especially when reliability, maintainability, availability and safety are involved in the decision.

Despite its importance to organizations, there are few studies analysing maintenance policies (Wang, Chu, & Wu, 2007). Among the literature analysing choice of maintenance policies with multi-criteria techniques, Bevilacqua and Braglia (2000) used Analytic Hierarchy Process (AHP) to choose the best maintenance policy in an Integrated Gasification and Combined Cycle plant, is particularly worth of note. Azaiez (2002) uses multi-attribute utility theory to choose an optimal replacement policy. Al-Najjar and Alsyouf (2003) applied a fuzzy multi-criteria decision-making methodology to find that Total Quality Maintenance using vibration analysis is the best maintenance policy to use in a paper mill. Emblemsvåg and Tonning (2003) used AHP to identify the best maintenance policy for weapons system of the Norwegian Army. Bertolini and Bevilacqua (2006) applied AHP and goal programming to identify the best maintenance policy for a set of the 10 most critical centrifugal pumps operating in an Italian oil refinery. Carnero (2005) presented a model which integrates AHP and factor analysis for the choice of diagnostic techniques and instrumentation in predictive maintenance policy. Gómez de León and Ruiz (2006) suggested the use of a multi-criteria method for the classification of critical equipment, in order to calculate a criticality index which allows the most suitable maintenance policy to be assigned to each machine. Wang et al. (2007) applied a modified fuzzy AHP to boilers in a thermal power plant. Carnero (2007) used AHP to choose the most suitable predictive technique, from vibration analysis, lubricant analysis and the integration of both techniques, in the petrochemical, food, pharmaceutical and machinery manufacturing industries. Shyjith et al. (2008) and Ilangkumaran and Kumanan (2009) combined AHP and Technique for Order Preference by Similarity to Ideal Solution (TOPSIS) to choose the best maintenance policy in a textile industry. Ahmadi et al. (2010) used AHP, TOPSIS, the Compromise Ranking method (VIKOR) and benefit-cost ratio, in an aircraft system, and identify the pros and cons of each maintenance policy. Arunraj and Maiti (2010) combined AHP and goal programming, considering the risk in the machines and the costs of the maintenance policy. Vahdani et al. (2010) applied fuzzy VIKOR to the choice of maintenance policies. Ghosh and Roy (2010) used fuzzy AHP and a goal programming model to optimize the objectives risk reduction and cost minimization. Shahin et al. (2012) applied the Analytic Network Process (ANP) to the choice of the most suitable maintenance policy in a mining company, while Zaim et al. (2012) applied AHP and ANP for the same purpose in a local newspaper printing facility. Fouladgar et al. (2012) used fuzzy AHP to calculate the weightings of the criteria, while the ranking of alternatives is calculated by fuzzy set theory and the COmplex PRoportional ASsessment (COPRAS) technique. Cavalcante and Lopes (2015) used a multi-attribute value function to analyse the application of opportunistic maintenance for a cogeneration system in a power plant. Goossens and Basten (2015) used AHP to choose a maintenance policy for naval ships. Kirubakaran and Ilangkumaran (2016) applied fuzzy AHP, grey relational analysis and TOPSIS technique to choose, from among corrective maintenance, predictive maintenance, time-based preventive maintenance, and condition-based maintenance, the policy to apply to the pumps of a paper manufacturing plant. In Tajadod et al. (2016) a comparison among different Multiple Criteria Decision Making techniques, such as AHP, FAHP, ANP or fuzzy ANP was carried out in a dairy factory to rank the maintenance policies. Predictive maintenance was selected as the most suitable maintenance policy. In addition, there are literature reviews on the application of MCDA to the choice of maintenance policies in Carnero (2014) and Shafiee (2015). Zhang et al. (2017) suggested a methodology to evaluate, compare and improve the sustainability of the maintenance strategies applied in port infrastructures using Markov chains.

Most of these contributions choose a single maintenance policy from among the possible options. However, organization in actual practice combines a variety of maintenance policies, and so the models developed lose a certain amount of applicability to real situations.

In all the previous contributions, the decision is applied to manufacturing, processing, transport industries, etc.; however, the number of studies which seek to choose maintenance policies in service organizations, and in particular, Health Care Organizations, is very limited. This is a serious problem, as the influence of maintenance of medical facilities and apparatus on time and quality of health care, in diagnosis and treatment, and therefore on the lives of patients, is very significant.

The criteria most frequently applied in the existing literature are spare part cost or minimizing inventories, followed by investment cost, reliability or Mean Time Between Failures (MTBF), maintenance cost, training cost, safety of personnel, maintainability or Mean Time To Repair (MTTR), product quality, and safety of equipment and facilities (Carnero, 2014). Although many criteria are used in the literature, they clearly lean towards the use of technical maintenance criteria related to availability of the systems analysed, such as MTBF and MTTR, and cost factors. The research in this chapter, however, uses quality of care as the most important criterion, since, if the improvements obtained by the hospital from a change in maintenance strategy to that suggested by the DSS are evident, the Health Care Organization will seek ways to prioritize resources and introduce new policies.

It should be noted that in Spain, most Health Care Organizations are state-owned and run, and do not pursue profit, but rather to achieve acceptable levels of health and of quality of life of patients. The criteria used in manufacturing enterprises cannot, therefore, be generally applied to the criteria used in Health Care Organizations. Thus, the criteria recommended in this research are unique and specific to this type of organization. The decision was also taken to include a decision group comprising those in charge of different care and non-care sectors, due to the implications for both areas and the way they are interrelated.

Only in Taghipour et al. (2011) and Carnero and Gómez (2016) this question is analysed for Health Care Organizations. Taghipour et al. (2011) prioritized medical devices according to their criticality using a multi-criteria model built with AHP. Depending on the criticality value obtained for each medical device, a priority is established for maintenance actions carried out on them. Thus, devices in the high criticality class are assigned proactive, predictive or time-based maintenance. Those of medium criticality have the options proactive or time-based maintenance. Devices with low criticality are assigned corrective maintenance.

Carnero and Gómez (2016) combined continuous time Markov chains with the MACBETH approach, to obtain the best combination of maintenance policies to be applied to the dialysis systems for chronic and acute patients infected with hepatitis C and hepatitis B. In all cases, the maintenance policy obtained consists of applying corrective and preventive maintenance plus two reserve machines. Carnero and Gómez (2017) selected the most suitable maintenance policies for use in the different subsystems of an operating theatre. So, for power supply, air conditioning subsystems and operating theatre lighting, corrective, preventive and predictive maintenance policies are suggested. In the sterile water subsystem, corrective and preventive maintenance is proposed. In medicinal gases subsystem corrective and predictive maintenance is recommended.

It is therefore necessary to do more research into the choice of maintenance policies in clinical apparatus and facilities, due to the peculiarities which make their needs more critical, as well as the characteristics of medical equipment itself, which is very different from the situation in other organizations.

DECISION SUPPORT SYSTEM FOR OPTIMIZATION OF MAINTENANCE IN THE ASSISTED BREATHING UNIT IN THE NEONATOLOGY SERVICE

Figure 1 shows a flow chart with the methodology applied in this study. The following sections describe firstly the application of Markov Chain to the assisted breathing system in neonatology. This gives suitable alternatives and the mean availability of the system to include in the multi-criteria MACBETH approach.

Figure 1. Flow chart of the methodology applied in this research
(Created by the authors)

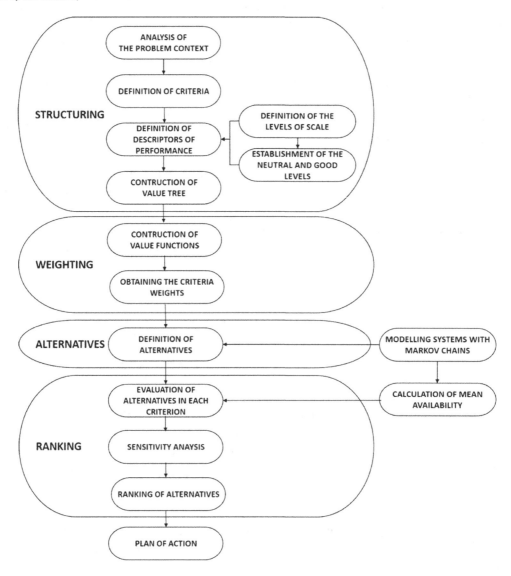

Markov Chain for the Assisted Breathing Unit

A neonatal ventilator is the device responsible for mixing air and oxygen and providing the resulting gas to the new-born baby in the right conditions of heat and humidity. In turn, this generates positive pressure in the breathing tubes which replaces the active stage of the breathing cycle.

The Neonatal Service of the University General Hospital of Ciudad Real (UGHCR) has eight ventilators. Under normal conditions six are in use, with two in reserve, available for use. The system is considered to have failed when two ventilators are not working.

The methodology for applying Markov chains is widely known and may be reviewed in Taha (2011), Hillier and Lieberman (2002) and in standard CEI IEC 61165:2006.

Two failure scenarios are considered: failure of accessory elements, and breakdown of the module controlling the breathing function. λ_1 and μ_1, are, respectively, the failure and repair rates. Three alternatives are considered for improving availability, consisting of adding one, two or three machines to the set. The availability of the original system is defined as D_{0m} and D_{1m}, D_{2m} and D_{3m} are the availabilities for eight, nine and ten ventilators, respectively. Replacement time is held to be virtually zero.

Figure 2 shows the Markov graph of the original system.

The transition matrix D_{0m} corresponding to the Markov graph is shown in Equation (1).

$$D_{0m} = \begin{pmatrix} -8\lambda_1 & 8\lambda_1 & 0 & 0 & 0 & 0 & 0 & 0 & 1 \\ \mu_1 & -7\lambda_1 - \mu_1 & 7\lambda_1 & 0 & 0 & 0 & 0 & 0 & 1 \\ 0 & \mu_1 & -6\lambda_1 - \mu_1 & 6\lambda_1 & 0 & 0 & 0 & 0 & 1 \\ 0 & 0 & \mu_1 & -5\lambda_1 - \mu_1 & 5\lambda_1 & 0 & 0 & 0 & 1 \\ 0 & 0 & 0 & \mu_1 & -4\lambda_1 - \mu_1 & 4\lambda_1 & 0 & 0 & 1 \\ 0 & 0 & 0 & 0 & \mu_1 & -3\lambda_1 - \mu_1 & 3\lambda_1 & 0 & 1 \\ 0 & 0 & 0 & 0 & 0 & \mu_1 & -2\lambda_1 - \mu_1 & 2\lambda_1 & 1 \\ 0 & 0 & 0 & 0 & 0 & 0 & \mu_1 & -\lambda_1 - \mu_1 & 1 \\ 0 & 0 & 0 & 0 & 0 & 0 & 0 & \mu_1 & 1 \end{pmatrix}$$

$$(1)$$

Solving the system of equations in Equation (2) by considering the matrix of Equation (1) and defining $(p_0, p_1, \ldots p_{m-1}, p_m)$ as the vector p of probabilities in the stationary state,

Figure 2. Markov graph for the assisted breathing system in Neonatology
(Created by the authors)

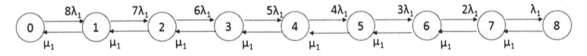

State 0: normal operation.
State 1: failure of first ventilator.
State 2: failure of second ventilator. Failure of the subsystem.
State 3: failure of third ventilator. Failure of the subsystem.
State 4: failure of fourth ventilator. Failure of the subsystem.
State 5: failure of fifth ventilator. Failure of the subsystem.
State 6: failure of sixth ventilator. Failure of the subsystem.
State 7: failure of seventh ventilator. Failure of the subsystem.
State 8: failure of eighth ventilator. Failure of the subsystem.

$$(p_0, p_1, ..., p_{m-1}, p_m) * \begin{pmatrix} d_{00} & d_{01} & \cdots & d_{0m-1} & 1 \\ d_{10} & d_{11} & \cdots & d_{1m-1} & 1 \\ \cdot & \cdot & & \cdot & \cdot \\ \cdot & \cdot & & \cdot & \cdot \\ \cdot & \cdot & & \cdot & \cdot \\ d_{m-10} & d_{m-11} & \cdots & d_{m-1m-1} & 1 \\ d_{m0} & d_{m1} & \cdots & d_{mm-1} & 1 \end{pmatrix} = (0, 0, ..., 0, 1) \tag{2}$$

gives the mean availability for the original subsystem $D_{0m}=p_0+p_1$, and for each improvement alternative with one two and three spares: $D_{1m}=p_0+p_1+p_2$, $D_{2m}=p_0+p_1+p_2+p_3$, $D_{3m}=p_0+p_1$, where p_i are the coefficients obtained by solving Equation (2) for each alternative. The system of equations in Equation (2) was solved using a recursive approach with Matlab software for each alternative. The resulting mean availabilities are shown in Table 1.

Structuring

MACBETH (Bana e Costa & Vansnick, 1997) is a decision-aid approach to multi-criteria value measurement. MACBETH uses only qualitative judgements of difference in attractiveness to obtain value scores for alternatives and weightings for criteria via mathematical programming. Additionally, it appears especially suitable for the aggregation of evaluation criteria when absolute and relative is required; this allows the alternatives to be assessed by considering specific targets (Montignac, Noirot, & Chaudourne, 2009).

M-MACBETH software (www.m.macbeth.com) has been used in this research to create the additive value model, to simulate challenges due to hesitation in choosing between two or more categories of difference in attractiveness and to perform the sensitivity analysis on the results obtained.

To construct the DSS described in this chapter, a multi-disciplinary decision group was interviewed to obtain the scales of attractiveness v_i and the weightings of the criteria w_i. The decision group is made up of those in charge of these areas of UGHCR: Programming and Admissions, Central Clinical Services and Supervisors of Medical Areas, Maintenance of Facilities, Maintenance of Electro-medical Equipment, Environment, and Health and Safety. The facilitator of the decision group was the Sub-director of Technical Services at UGHCR, as he has deep knowledge of decision making and different multi-criteria techniques, including MACBETH.

To choose the criteria, the decision group analysed the currently-existing literature; however, due to its deficiency, criteria specifically adapted to the needs of UGHCR were chosen.

A descriptor was associated with each criterion or sub-criterion to make an operational description. A descriptor is an ordered set of plausible performance levels (quantitative or qualitative) to describe the impacts of alternatives objectively with respect to one criterion (Bana e Costa, & Carvalho, 2002).

A performance scale was designed for each descriptor in order of decreasing attractiveness; firstly, two reference levels were defined: neutral (N), considered by the decision group to be neither a satisfactory nor unsatisfactory level, and good (G), considered by the decision group to be a fully satisfactory level (Bana e Costa, & Carvalho, 2002); then additional levels were included to cover the plausible range of performances. Each level of performance was defined to avoid subsequent ambiguous or erroneous interpretation.

The value tree with the hierarchy structure is shown in Figure 3. For each criterion a descriptor was defined with an associated scale, in which the reference levels neutral (N) and (good (G) were identified, which is necessary to apply the MACBETH approach. The criteria and scales of the descriptors are as follows:

1. **Economic Criteria:** These include the costs both direct and indirect, generated by each alternative. These criteria include the sub-criteria:
   a. **Investment Costs (IC):** This includes annual costs dedicated to introducing each alternative. The scale levels of the descriptor are:
      i. Level 1. €0 (G).
      ii. Level 2. €2,500.
      iii. Level 3. €5,000.
      iv. Level 4. €7,500 (N).
      v. Level 5. €10,000.
   b. **Maintenance Costs (MC):** These are the annual labour and material costs associated with a given alternative for each subsystem analysed. The scale levels of the descriptor associated with this criterion are:
      i. Level 1. €10,000 (G).
      ii. Level 2. €15,000.
      iii. Level 3. €20,000 (N).
      iv. Level 4. €25,000.
      v. Level 5. €30,000.
2. **Acceptance by Staff (AP):** This measures the level of technical satisfaction of the operation of the subsystem. That is, it considers safety when giving fault diagnoses, and the level of programming of corrective action. The descriptor associated with the criterion is the capacity for fault diagnosis and to programme corrective action. The scale levels of the descriptor are:
   a. **Level 1:** The staff member is certain of the diagnoses of the faults analysed. Corrective action can be programmed jointly with other subsystems involved (G).
   b. **Level 2:** The staff member is certain of the diagnoses of the faults analysed, and corrective action must be programmed in the subsystem.
   c. **Level 3:** The staff member is certain of the diagnoses of the faults analysed, and corrective action must be undertaken in the subsystem immediately (N).
   d. **Level 4:** The staff member is not certain on some occasions of the diagnoses of the faults analysed, informing his superiors of the need to decide whether to take immediate corrective action in the subsystem.
   e. **Level 5:** The staff member is not certain of the diagnoses of the faults analysed, and immediate corrective action must be taken in the subsystem.
3. **Quality of Care (QC):** This measures the impact on care, by mean availability and the consequences on attention to patients, caused by interruptions, stoppages or cancelling of care activity. The descriptor associated with this criterion takes into account mean availability and the time the system is off-line. The scale levels of the descriptor associated with this criterion are:
   a. **Level 1:** Mean availability of the system is greater than 0.9990. There is no pause or decrease in health care services (G).

Figure 3. Value tree
(Created by the authors)

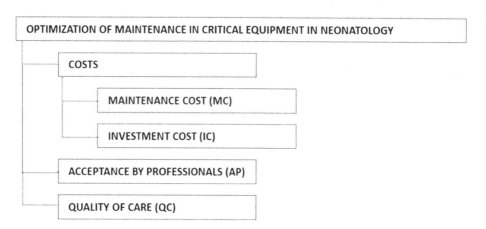

b. **Level 2:** Mean availability of the system is between 0.9981 and 0.9990. There is a small pause, which does not require the process to be stopped.

c. **Level 3:** Mean availability of the system is between 0.9971 and 0.9980. There is a pause, requiring intervention of maintenance staff, although the process is not interrupted, the basic functions are maintained and the process is supervised by care staff until restarted automatically (N).

d. **Level 4:** Mean availability of the system is between 0.9961 and 0.9970. There is a pause, and the level of service of the system must be reduced below normal operation.

e. **Level 5:** Mean availability of the system is below 0.9960. There is a stoppage in the subsystem, and the service provided by the system must be reduced to a level considered critical.

Weighting

A value function is required to assign value scores to the performance levels of a descriptor relative to the fixed scores of 0 and 100 assigned to the neutral and good reference levels. Value functions can either be discrete or continuous. These value functions are constructed by comparing the relative attractiveness of defined impact descriptor levels. Once a criterion's value function is defined it can be used to convert the level of impact any alternative into a value score.

MACBETH only needs qualitative judgements to provide value functions, overcoming the scepticism created by the use of numerical judgements (Gurmankin, Baron, & Armstrong, 2004). To provide comparison judgements between scale levels or criteria, the following categories of attractiveness were used: no difference, very weak difference, weak, moderate, strong, very strong and extreme. In addition, in the case of disagreement or hesitation between two or more consecutive categories, other than indifference, they may all be chosen.

To construct a value function for the investment cost criterion, the facilitator asked the decision group to judge the differences in attractiveness between the performance levels of the maintenance cost descriptor (see Table 1). The decision group considered that the difference between level 1 (most preferred level) and level 5 (least preferred level) was strong. Next, the decision group was asked about the difference in attractiveness between level 2 and level 5, giving, unanimously, a value of very strong. The decision group was asked repeatedly until the last column of the judgement matrix in Figure 4 was completed; then, the first row of the matrix, the diagonal above the main diagonal and the remaining judgments were also completed. For each judgment included in the matrix, M-MACBETH software tested the consistency of all the judgments already formulated and pointed out any situations of inconsistency. Figure 4 shows the final judgment matrix of the qualitative judgments of the decision group. In this case the matrix obtained is consistent. This matrix was processed in M-MACBETH by means of linear programming to build a value function for each criterion or sub-criterion, as appropriate. The linear programming problem solved by M-MACBETH to obtain the value functions is shown in Equation (3) (Bana e Costa, De Corte, & Vansnick, 2011):

$$Min \ [v(x^+)-v(x^-)] \tag{3}$$

Subject to:

$v(x^-)=0$ by means of arbitrary assignment.

$v(x)-v(y)=0 \ \forall x, y \in C_0$

$v(x)-v(y) \geq i, \ \forall x, y \in C_i \cup ... \cup C_s$

with $i, s \in \{1,2,3,4,5,6\}$, $i \leq s$ and with the six categories of difference of attractiveness C_0 (no difference), C_1 (very weak), C_2 (weak), C_3 (moderate), C_4 (strong), C_5 (very strong) and C_6 (extreme).

$v(x)-v(y) \geq v(w)-v(z)+i-s', \ \forall x, y \in C_i \cup ... \cup C_s$ and $\forall w, z \in C_{i'} \cup ... \cup C_{s'}$ with $i, s, i', s' \in \{1,2,3,4,5,6\}$ and $i \leq s$, $i' \leq s'$ and $i > s'$.

For X a finite set of elements corresponding to the different performance levels under evaluation and $v(x)$ the score assigned to element x of X, x^+ is at least as attractive as any other element of X and x^- is at most as attractive as any other element of X.

M-MACBETH software performs all the calculations related to the application of linear programming and provides the value functions that can be seen in Figures 4 to 7.

Once the value functions had been obtained, the decision group assessed their cardinality; this was done by analysing the proportions of the resulting scale intervals to ensure that their relative size correctly captured the value judgements of the decision group. Figure 4 shows how the value function has two sections with different slopes; this implies a discontinuity in the scale levels: 0 to 7,500 and 7,500 to 10,000. However, no changes in the original value function were proposed by the group.

The same process was applied to the remaining criteria. Figure 5 shows the judgement matrix and normalized value function for the criterion Maintenance cost. In this case, when the decision group compared the preferred level (€10,000) with level 4 (€25,000), half the decision group considered the value to be strong and the other half very strong; thus, the value strong-very strong is associated with this comparison in the judgement matrix. The matrix obtained is consistent, and gives a linear value function over the range of Maintenance costs.

Figure 4. MACBETH Judgement matrix and value function for the criterion investment costs
(Created by the authors)

IC	0	2,500	5,000	7,500	10,000
0	no	moderate	strong	strong	very strong
2,500		no	moderate	strong	very strong
5,000			no	moderate	strong
7,500				no	moderate
10,000					no

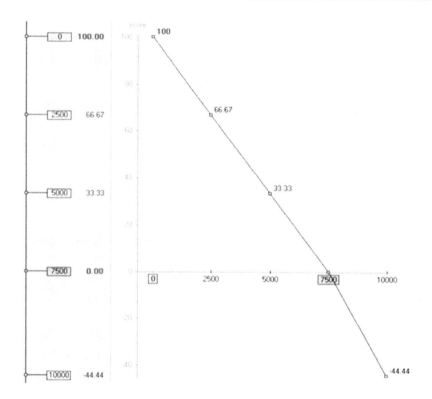

The judgement matrix and value function for Acceptance by staff and Quality of care are shown in Figure 6 and Figure 7 respectively. In both cases the judgement matrices are consistent. Validation of all the value functions was carried out by the decision group, and all the original judgements were maintained.

The weightings of the criteria were obtained by assessing the possibility of an alternative being at the neutral level in all criteria. The decision group was asked to give a qualitative judgement, using the MACBETH semantic categories, of the increase in overall attractiveness provided by a swing from the neutral level to the most attractive impact level, in each of the criteria under consideration. Next, a comparison is made of the extent to which the change from the neutral to the good level in the first criterion is preferable to the change from the neutral to the good level in the second criterion. This judgement was repeated comparing the first and third criteria, and so on. The remaining elements of the matrix were obtained by comparing the swings pairwise, using the MACBETH semantic categories. The resulting judgement matrix and the relative weightings are shown in the bar chart in Figure 8.

Figure 5. MACBETH Judgement matrix and value function for the criterion maintenance costs (*Created by the authors*)

MC	10,000	15,000	20,000	25,000	30,000
10,000	no	moderate	strong	strong-very strong	very strong
15,000		no	moderate	strong	very strong
20,000			no	moderate	strong
25,000				no	moderate
30,000					no

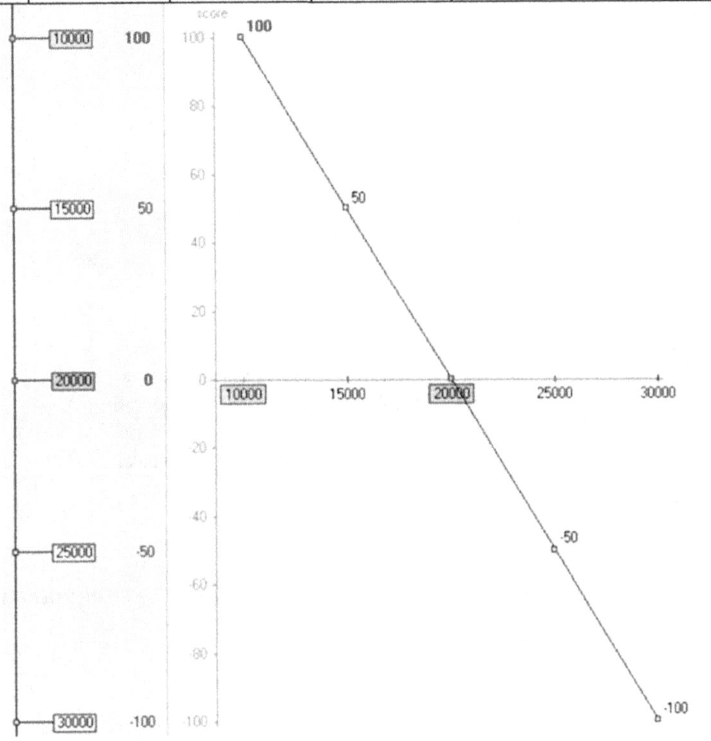

Alternatives

Having obtained a Markov graph, the possible alternatives are considered. These represent a combination of the various maintenance policies to be used in the assisted breathing unit in the Neonatology Service of the UGHCR.

The following alternatives are considered:

- Corrective and preventive maintenance (CM+PM). Corrective maintenance is carried out at two levels: a first level performed by the care staff before each treatment, and a second level, outsourced to and carried out by the official technicians. An annual, contracted preventive check-up, also performed by the official technicians, should be added to this. This is the alternative which is currently being used at UGHCR.

Figure 6. MACBETH Judgement matrix and value function for the criterion acceptance by staff
(Created by the authors)

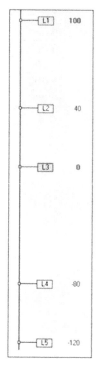

	Level 1	Level 2	Level 3	Level 4	Level 5
Level 1	no	weak	moderate	strong	strong
Level 2		no	weak	moderate	moderate
Level 3			no	moderate	moderate
Level 4				no	weak
Level 5					no

Figure 7. MACBETH Judgement matrix and value function for the criterion quality of care
(Created by the authors)

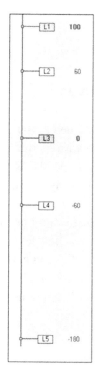

	L1	L2	L3	L4	L5
L1	no	weak	moderate	strong	very strong
L2		no	moderate	strong	strong
L3			no	moderate	strong
L4				no	strong
L5					no

Figure 8. Weighted judgement matrix and bar chart
(Created by the authors)

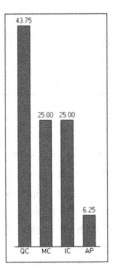

	QC	MC	IC	AP
QC	no	weak-moderate	moderate	moderate-strong
MC		no	no	moderate
IC				weak-moderate
AP				no

- Corrective and preventive maintenance plus a reserve ventilator (CM+PM+1RR). This achieves the same results as the previous alternative, plus the possibility of having a reserve ventilator in perfect working order, included in the plan for corrective and preventive maintenance.
- Corrective and preventive maintenance with two reserve ventilators (CM+PM+2RR). This alternative is the same as before, but includes two reserve ventilators.
- Corrective and preventive maintenance with three reserve ventilators (CM+PM+3RR). This alternative is the same as before, but includes three reserve ventilators.

SOLUTIONS AND RECOMMENDATIONS

The evaluation of an alternative is carried out by simple additive aggregation from bottom to top in the value tree. If n decision criteria are being considered, the performance $V(x)$ of an alternative x is calculated using Equation (4) (Bana e Costa, De Corte, & Vansnick, 2012).

$$V(x) = \sum_{i=1}^{n} w_i v_i(x) \tag{4}$$

With $\sum_{i=1}^{n} w_i = 1$, $w_i > 0$ and $\begin{cases} v_i(good) = 100 \\ v_i(neutral) = 0 \end{cases}$ and w_i are the relative weights of the criteria and v_i(impact of x on criterion i) is the value score of x in criterion i.

To evaluate the alternatives for the criterion Quality of care, it is necessary to know the mean availability of the assisted breathing system in Neonatology for each alternative. Table 1 shows the mean

Table 1. Mean availability for each alternative

Alternative	Mean availability
CM+PM	0.9969
CM+ PM+RR1	0.9997
CM+PM+ RR2	1
CM+PM+RR3	1

(Created by the authors)

availability obtained for each alternative, where the failure rate λ_1=0.000217 failures/hour, and the repair rate μ_1= 0.010 repairs/hour.

Table 2 shows the impacts of the alternatives on the various decision criteria.

Applying Equation (4) which multiplies the per unum weighting of each criterion shown in Figure 8 by the value each alternative has in this criterion, summing over the criteria, gives the following global scores for each alternative.

$$V(CM+PM) = 0.4375*-60.00+0.25*80.00+0.25*100.00+0.0625*-80.00=13.75$$

$$V(CM+PM+RR1) = 0.4375*100.00+0.25*65.00+0.25*66.67+0.0625*0.00=76.67$$

$$V(CM+PM+RR2) = 0.4375*100.00+0.25*50.00+0.25*33.33+0.0625*40.00=67.08$$

Table 2. Impact of the alternatives on the criteria

Criterion	Alternative	Level of impact
Investment cost (IC)	CM+PM	€0
	CM+ PM+RR1	€2,500
	CM+PM+ RR2	€5,000
	CM+PM+RR3	€7,500
Maintenance costs (MC)	CM+PM	12,000
	CM+ PM+RR1	13,500
	CM+PM+ RR2	15,000
	CM+PM+RR3	16,00
Degree of acceptance by staff (AC)	CM+PM	L4
	CM+ PM+RR1	L3
	CM+PM+ RR2	L2
	CM+PM+RR3	L1
Quality of care (QC)	CM+PM	L4
	CM+ PM+RR1	L1
	CM+PM+ RR2	L1
	CM+PM+RR3	L1

(Created by the authors)

$V(CM+PM+RR3) = 0.4375*100.00+0.25*35.00+0.25*0.00+0.0625*100.00=58.75$

For example, in the case of the alternative CM+PM, the impact of this alternative on the criterion Quality of care is L4, as shown in Table 2. Figure 7, which shows the value functions for this criterion, also shows that to scale level L4 of the descriptor there is assigned a value of -60 in the value function. This value -60 is multiplied by the weighting 0.4375 obtained for the criterion Quality of care. It is necessary to turn the percentage weightings into per unum weightings, since the sum of the weightings of the criteria must be equal to 1. Likewise for the other criteria, and then the sum is taken of the contributions from each of them, giving the global score.

Figure 9 shows the classification of alternatives obtained for the assisted breathing system in Neonatology. The model recommends the application of Corrective and Preventive Maintenance plus a reserve ventilator (CM+PM+1RR)

Figure 9. Ranking of maintenance policies for the assisted breathing system in Neonatology
(*Created by the authors*)

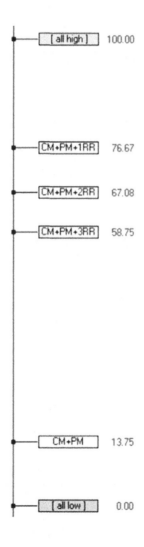

A sensitivity analysis was then carried to assess the implications that a logical modification of the weightings of the decision criteria would have on the classification. Figure 10 shows the trends in the alternatives when the weightings assigned to each criterion are modified. The current weighting of each criterion is shown by a vertical line. It can be seen that it would require changes in the weightings of more than 100% to alter the ranking of the alternatives. This level of variation of the weightings for the criteria is not considered remotely feasible, and so the model is robust.

Currently, UGHCR applies corrective maintenance together with preventive maintenance (CM+PM). Mean availability with this alternative is 0.9969. On the other hand, by applying CM+PM+1RR, mean availability would be 1.

The current alternative has maintenance costs of €12,000/year; switching to CM+PM+1RR would lead to a slight increase in costs, as maintenance costs would be €13,000/year, plus €2,500 in invest-

Figure 10. Sensitivity analysis for the criteria: Maintenance cost, investment cost, acceptance by staff and quality of care (from left to right and top to bottom)
(Created by the authors)

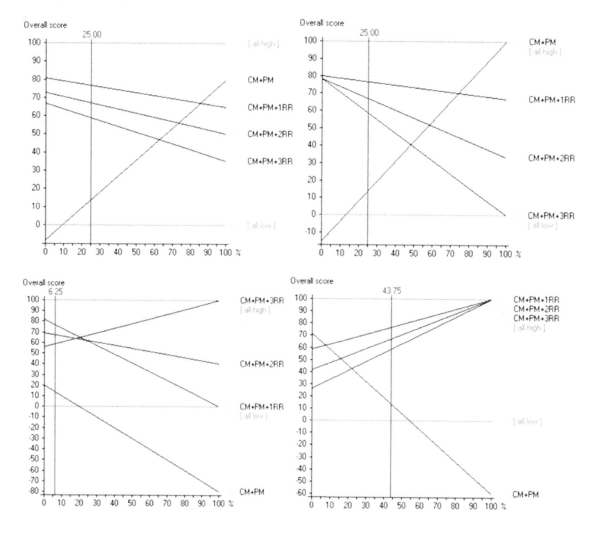

ment costs. However, this small increase in costs is compensated by the operational effects on quality of care produced by the change of alternative. CM+PM can have problems which may involve a potential risk to the babies who are on assisted breathing. With CM+PM+1RR, however, although there may be problems, they would not have consequences for the babies. UGHCR, therefore, determined a need to change the alternative applied to the subsystem, with criticality 1 (the highest possible), and gave 15 days as the time necessary for the introduction of the new alternative.

FUTURE RESEARCH DIRECTIONS

The DSS set out here is a dynamic model which should be reviewed after a certain amount of time, as it may be necessary to include other decision criteria in the model, or the possibility may arise of new improvement alternatives, other than the existing ones. Therefore, it would be necessary to review the model after a period of time to confirm its suitability to new economic conditions and care requirements.

It is also important to control how the change in the combination of maintenance policies in the Neonatology assisted breathing system affects care quality, not only in terms of availability, but through surveys of care staff, who can make a qualitative assessment of the level of service provided by the equipment with the proposed improvements.

The multi-criteria model will be updated to include the point of view of patients at the UGHCR. A decision group of patients will be formed to establish the descriptor associated with the criterion Quality of care and the various scale levels that form it. They will also be asked to give judgements which will be used to construct the value function for the criterion Quality of care. The results obtained will be compared with those obtained by the decision group made up of the heads of section of the Hospital, and the effect on the final ranking of the alternatives will be assessed.

CONCLUSION

Despite its importance for quality of health care, the number of studies analysing choice of maintenance policies in Health Care Organizations is very small. This chapter therefore describes an innovative DSS which combines continuous time Markov chains with the MACBETH approach to obtain the best combination of maintenance policies to apply in the assisted breathing unit of the Neonatology Service at UGHCR.

A multi-disciplinary decision group, made up of those in charge of different areas of the Technical and Care Services of the Hospital, participated in the construction of the DSS. This was intended to guarantee the applicability of the results obtained by the DSS.

It should be noted that the alternatives assessed, as well as combining different maintenance policies, incorporate improvements that are not considered by other decision models, involving other actions of broader scope and with specifically measurable results, such as the introduction of additional spare equipment. The alternatives proposed in this study thus provide real solutions to the problem posed.

ACKNOWLEDGMENT

This research was supported by the Junta de Comunidades de Castilla-La Mancha and the European Regional Development Fund under Grant number PPII-2014-013-P.

REFERENCES

Ahmadi, A., Gupta, S., Karim, R., & Kumar, U. (2010). Selection of maintenance strategy for aircraft systems using multi-criteria decision making methodologies. *International Journal of Reliability Quality and Safety Engineering, 17*(3), 223–243. doi:10.1142/S0218539310003779

Al-Najjar, B., & Alsyouf, I. (2003). Selecting the most efficient maintenance approach using fuzzy multiple criteria decision making. *International Journal of Production Economics, 84*(1), 85–100. doi:10.1016/S0925-5273(02)00380-8

Almeida, A. T., & Bohoris, A. T. (1995). Decision theory in maintenance decision making. *Journal of Quality in Maintenance Engineering, 1*(1), 39–45. doi:10.1108/13552519510083138

Arunraj, N. S., & Maiti, J. (2010). Risk-based maintenance policy selection using AHP and goal programming. *Safety Science, 48*(2), 238–247. doi:10.1016/j.ssci.2009.09.005

Azaiez, M. N. (2002). A multi-attribute preventive replacement model. *Journal of Quality in Maintenance Engineering, 8*(3), 213–225. doi:10.1108/13552510210439793

Bana e Costa, C. A., & Carvalho, R. (2002). Assigning priorities for maintenance, repair and refurbishment in managing a municipal housing stock. *European Journal of Operational Research, 138*(2), 380–391. doi:10.1016/S0377-2217(01)00253-3

Bana e Costa, C. A., De Corte, J. M., & Vansnick, J. C. (2011). MACBETH (Measuring Attractiveness by a Categorical Based Evaluation Technique). In J. J. Cochran, L. A. Cox Jr, P. Keskinocak, J. P. Kharoufeh, & J. C. Smith (Eds.), *Encyclopedia of Operations Research and Management Science*. New York, NY: John Wiley & Sons. doi:10.1002/9780470400531.eorms0970

Bana e Costa, C. A., De Corte, J. M., & Vansnick, J. C. (2012). MACBETH. *International Journal of Information Technology & Decision Making, 11*(2), 359–387. doi:10.1142/S0219622012400068

Bana e Costa, C. A., & Vansnick, J. C. (1997). Applications of the MACBETH approach in the framework of an additive aggregation model. *Journal of Multi-Criteria Decision Analysis, 6*(2), 107–114. doi:10.1002/(SICI)1099-1360(199703)6:2<107::AID-MCDA147>3.0.CO;2-1

Bertolini, M., & Bevilacqua, M. (2006). A combined goal programming-AHP approach to maintenance selection problem. *Reliability Engineering & System Safety, 91*(7), 839–848. doi:10.1016/j.ress.2005.08.006

Bevilacqua, M., & Braglia, M. (2000). The analytic hierarchy process applied to maintenance strategy selection. *Reliability Engineering & System Safety, 70*(1), 71–83. doi:10.1016/S0951-8320(00)00047-8

Carnero, M. C. (2005). Selection of diagnostic techniques and instrumentation in a predictive maintenance program. A case study. *Decision Support Systems*, *38*(4), 539–555. doi:10.1016/j.dss.2003.09.003

Carnero, M. C. (2007). Model for the selection of predictive maintenance techniques. *INFOR*, *45*(2), 83–94.

Carnero, M. C. (2014). MCDA Techniques in Maintenance Policy Selection. In J. Wang (Ed.), *Encyclopedia of Business Analytics and Optimization* (Vol. III, pp. 406–415). Hershey, PA: IGI Global.

Carnero, M. C., & Gómez, A. (2016). A multicriteria decision making approach applied to improving maintenance policies in healthcare organizations. *BMC Medical Informatics and Decision Making*, *16*(1), 47. doi:10.1186/s12911-016-0282-7 PMID:27108234

Carnero, M. C., & Gómez, A. (2017). Multicriteria model for the selection of maintenance policies in subsystems of an operating theatre. In Optimum decision making in asset management. IGI Global.

Cavalcante, C. A. V., & Lopes, R. S. (2015). Multi-criteria model to support the definition of opportunistic maintenance policy: A study in a cogeneration system. *Energy*, *80*, 32–40. doi:10.1016/j.energy.2014.11.039

CEI IEC 61165:2006. (n.d.). *Application of Markov techniques, International Electrotechnical Commission*. IEC.

Emblemsvag, J., & Tonning, L. (2003). Decision support in selecting maintenance organization. *Journal of Quality in Maintenance Engineering*, *9*(1), 11–24. doi:10.1108/13552510310466765

Fouladgar, M. M., Yazdani-Chamzini, A., Lashgari, A., Zavadskas, E. K., & Turskis, Z. (2012). maintenance strategy selection using AHP and COPRAS under fuzzy environment. *International Journal of Strategic Property Management*, *16*(1), 85–104. doi:10.3846/1648715X.2012.666657

Ghosh, D., & Roy, S. (2010). A decision-making framework for process plant maintenance. *European Journal of Industrial Engineering*, *4*(1), 78–98. doi:10.1504/EJIE.2010.029571

Gómez de León, F. C., & Ruiz, J. J. (2006). Maintenance strategy based on a multicriterion classification of equipments. *Reliability Engineering & System Safety*, *91*(4), 444–451. doi:10.1016/j.ress.2005.03.001

Goossens, A. J. M., & Basten, R. J. I. (2015). Exploring maintenance policy selection using the Analytic Hierarchy Process; An application for naval ships. *Reliability Engineering & System Safety*, *142*, 31–41. doi:10.1016/j.ress.2015.04.014

Gurmankin, A. D., Baron, J., & Armstrong, K. (2004). The effect of numerical statements of risk on trust and comfort with hypothetical physician risk communication. *Medical Decision Making*, *24*(3), 265–271. doi:10.1177/0272989X04265482 PMID:15155015

Hillier, F., & Lieberman, G. (2002). *Introduction to operations research*. New York, NY: McGraw-Hill Science.

Ilangkumaran, M., & Kumanan, S. (2009). Selection of maintenance policy for textile industry using hybrid multi-criteria decision making approach. *Journal of Manufacturing Technology Management*, *20*(7), 1009–1022. doi:10.1108/17410380910984258

Kirubakaran, B., & Ilangkumaran, M. (2016). Selection of optimum maintenance strategy based on FAHP integrated with GRA-TOPSIS. *Annals of Operations Research, 245*(1), 285–313. doi:10.1007/s10479-014-1775-3

Martorell, S., Villanueva, J. F., Carlos, S., Nebot, Y., Sanchez, A., Pitarch, J. L., & Serradell, V. (2005). RAMS+C informed decision-making with application to multiobjective optimization of technical specifications and maintenance using genetic algorithms. *Reliability Engineering & System Safety, 87*(1), 65–75. doi:10.1016/j.ress.2004.04.009

Montignac, F., Noirot, I., & Chaudourne, S. (2009). Multi-criteria evaluation of on-board hydrogen storage technologies using the MACBETH approach. *International Journal of Hydrogen Energy, 34*(10), 4561–4568. doi:10.1016/j.ijhydene.2008.09.098

Shafiee, M. (2015). Maintenance strategy selection problem: An MCDM overview. *Journal of Quality in Maintenance Engineering, 21*(4), 378–402. doi:10.1108/JQME-09-2013-0063

Shahin, A., Shirouyehzad, H., & Pourjavad, E. (2012). Optimum maintenance strategy: A case study in the mining industry. *International Journal of Services and Operations Management, 12*(3), 368–386. doi:10.1504/IJSOM.2012.047626

Shyjith, K., Ilangkumaran, M., & Kumanan, S. (2008). Multi-criteria decision-making approach to evaluate optimum maintenance strategy in textile industry. *Journal of Quality in Maintenance Engineering, 14*(4), 375–386. doi:10.1108/13552510810909975

Taghipour, S., Banjevic, D., & Jardine, A. K. S. (2011). Prioritization of medical equipment for maintenance decisions. *The Journal of the Operational Research Society, 62*(9), 1666–1687. doi:10.1057/jors.2010.106

Taha, H. A. (2011). *Operations research. An introduction.* New York, NY: Prentice Hall.

Tajadod, M., Abedini, M., Rategari, A., & Mobin, M. (2016). A Comparison of Multi-Criteria Decision Making Approaches for Maintenance Strategy Selection (A Case Study). *International Journal of Strategic Decision Sciences, 7*(3), 51–69. doi:10.4018/IJSDS.2016070103

Vahdani, B., Hadipour, H., Sadaghiani, J. S., & Amiri, M. (2010). Extension of VIKOR method based on interval-valued fuzzy sets. *International Journal of Advanced Manufacturing Technology, 47*(9-12), 1231–1239. doi:10.1007/s00170-009-2241-2

Wang, L., Chu, J., & Wu, J. (2007). Selection of optimum maintenance strategies based on a fuzzy analytic hierarchy process. *International Journal of Production Economics, 107*(1), 151–163. doi:10.1016/j.ijpe.2006.08.005

Zaim, S., Turkyílmaz, A., Acar, M. F., Al-Turki, U., & Demirel, O. F. (2012). Maintenance strategy selection using AHP and ANP algorithms: A case study. *Journal of Quality in Maintenance Engineering, 18*(1), 16–29. doi:10.1108/13552511211226166

Zhang, Y., Kim, C. W., Tee, K. F., & Lam, J. S. L. (2017). Optimal sustainable life cycle maintenance strategies for port infrastructures. *Journal of Cleaner Production, 142*(4), 1693–1709. doi:10.1016/j.jclepro.2016.11.120

ADDITIONAL READING

Bana e Costa, C. A., Carnero, M. C., & Duarte, M. (2012). A multi-criteria model for auditing a Predictive Maintenance Programme. *European Journal of Operational Research, 217*(2), 381–393. doi:10.1016/j.ejor.2011.09.019

Bana e Costa, C. A., De Corte, J. M., & Vansnick, J. C. (2011). MACBETH (Measuring Attractiveness by a Categorical Based Evaluation Technique). In J. J. Cochran, L. A. Cox Jr, P. Keskinocak, J. P. Kharoufeh, & J. C. Smith (Eds.), *Encyclopedia of Operations Research and Management Science*. New York, NY: John Wiley & Sons. doi:10.1002/9780470400531.eorms0970

Bashiri, M., Badri, H., & Hejazi, T. H. (2011). Selecting optimum maintenance strategy by fuzzy interactive linear assignment method. *Applied Mathematical Modelling, 35*(1), 152–164. doi:10.1016/j.apm.2010.05.014

Ciarapica, F. E., Giacchetta, G., & Paciarotti, C. (2008). Facility management in the healthcare sector: Analysis of the Italian situation. *Production Planning and Control, 19*(4), 327–341. doi:10.1080/09537280802034083

Iung, B., Véron, M., Suhner, M. C., & Muller A. (2005). Integration of maintenance strategies into prognosis process to decision-making aid on system operation. *CIRP Annals - Manufacturing Technology, 54*(1), 5-8.

Rani, N. A. A., Baharum, M. R., Akbar, A. R. N., & Nawawi, A. H. (2015). Perception of Maintenance Management Strategy on Healthcare Facilities. *Procedia: Social and Behavioral Sciences, 170*(27), 272–281. doi:10.1016/j.sbspro.2015.01.037

Regattieri, A. A., Gamberi, G. M., & Gamberini, R. (2015). An innovative method to optimize the maintenance policies in an aircraft: General framework and case study. *Journal of Air Transport Management, 44-45*, 8–20. doi:10.1016/j.jairtraman.2015.02.001

Wild, C., & Langer, T. (2008). Emerging health technologies: Informing and supporting health policy early. *Health Policy (Amsterdam), 87*(2), 160–171. doi:10.1016/j.healthpol.2008.01.002 PMID:18295925

Wolf, M. (2008). Strategic management of medical equipment. Starting and operating a TSC. *Proceedings of the 20th Congress of the International Federation of Hospital Engineering.*

KEY TERMS AND DEFINITIONS

Corrective Maintenance: A maintenance policy consisting of carrying out unplanned maintenance activity to return a machine or facility to the desired state, after a fault has occurred and the machine has ceased to perform its function.

MACBETH: Multicriteria decision-making approach created by Carlos Antonio Bana e Costa, Jean-Marie de Corte and Jean-Claude Vansnick in 1997. From a structuring of the problem in value trees, the construction of descriptors associated to each criterion, the weighting of criteria and the construction of value functions from the qualitative judgements of a group or individual decision maker, an additive model provides a complete ranking of alternatives. This method can be applied with the help of M-MACBETH software.

Markov Chains: A stochastic process in which, if the current state and the previous states are known, the probability of a future state depends only on the current state and not on the previous states.

Neonatal Ventilator: This is a medical device which mixes air and oxygen and provides the resulting warm, wet gas to the new born baby. In turn, this generates positive pressure in the breathing tubes which replaces the active stage of the breathing cycle.

Neonatology: Branch of paediatrics dealing with diagnosis and treatment of illness during the first 28 days of life of newborns who are ill or require special care because they are of low weight, are premature or suffer from severe complications.

Preventive Maintenance: Maintenance policy consisting of carrying out, in advance of the appearance of faults, periodic revisions and repairs of machinery and facilities with the aim of anticipating these faults and increasing the life cycle of assets.

Chapter 3
Applications of Operations Research in Production and Distribution Management of Pharmaceutical Products

Mahsa Yousefi Sarmad
Iran University of Science and Technology, Iran

Mir Saman Pishvaee
Iran University of Science and Technology, Iran

ABSTRACT

Pharmaceutical industry is considered as a global industry because of its effects on the human life. Many researchers used optimization tools to manage the pharmaceutical supply chain (PSC) efficiently. A supply chain may be defined as an integrated process where several business entities work together to produce goods and/or services and deliver them to the end customer. The issue of PSC which includes strategic, tactical and operational decisions, is still a quite hot issue. The intended mission of this chapter is to introduce and discuss the recent developments of procurement, production and distribution management of pharmaceutical products in order to pave the way for the readers who are interested in this area of research. Notably, the focus of the chapter is on quantitative OR-based models which enable the decision makers to appropriately coordinate and manage the whole pharmaceutical industry.

INTRODUCTION

Pharmaceutical industry is a system which consists of processes, operations and organizations involved in the discovery, development, production and distribution of drugs and medications (Shah, 2004). Economically, medicine is the second profitable industry after crude oil. Pharmaceutical supply chain aims to deliver safe and high quality pharmaceutical products at the right time and place to final consumers. Namely, (1) discovery, (2) development, (3) production and (4) distribution are the main stages needed for a drug to reach the market successfully. The efficient management of the product flow through these

DOI: 10.4018/978-1-5225-2515-8.ch003

four stages plays an important role in the competitiveness of pharmaceutical supply chains. Accordingly, integrated planning of procurement, production and distribution processes can lead to cost saving and more amount of profit. One significant issue which should be considered by decision makers and managers is the risk of failure within the mentioned four stages. Notably, the rate of success is less than 1 per 1000 and 1 per 5 in discovery and development stages, respectively (Tollman et al., 2011). Moreover, the production and distribution stages also include operational and environmental uncertainties which may disrupt the drug flow from pharmaceutical companies to market.

Pharmaceutical products have some special features which differentiate them from the other products. One of these features goes back to perishable nature of pharmaceutical products. Perishable products such as drugs have a maximum allowable usage time (Sazvar et al., 2013); therefore, they should stock carefully in wholesalers and retailers to prevent any waste product and/or possible damage to consumers.

The aim of this chapter is to introduce and discuss the recent developments of procurement, production and distribution management of pharmaceutical products in order to pave the way for the readers who are interested in this area of research. Accordingly, a systemic review on the relevant models is provided and a several mathematical models as well as a case study are described and analyzed in this chapter.

Importance and Drivers

The importance of modern pharmaceutical industry is declared because three of the eight main goals set by the United Nations for development in the millennium are related to pharmaceutical industry (Narayana et al., 2012). (1) Decreasing child's death, (2) improving mother's health and (3) fighting with AIDS, Malaria and other diseases are depending on the access to medications. Notably, one of the millennium development goals includes the cooperation with pharmaceutical companies in order to achieve affordable access to essential medicines in developing countries.

One of the key factors related to this goal is the effective and efficient management of pharmaceutical supply chain (Susarla & Karimi, 2012). In addition, irreversible globalization, increasing environmental rules and new scientific progress may lead to renewed operational organization in sketch of drugs and medicines, business, pharmaceutical industry, production, stock, distribution, products checking mechanism and medications delivery. To face these challenges and remaining competitive in the market, companies are looking for integrated tools for managing operations and control resources. The objectives are to minimize the operational and development costs and maximizing profits in accordance with environmental rules.

Nowadays, the importance of inventory control is one of the vital issues in all parts of supply chain management and pharmaceutical industry. Surveying business reports shows that, total investment in inventory in the United States is more than 1.3 trillion dollars (Nahmias, 2011). Therefore, it is obvious that the use of appropriate and efficient methods for inventory control can decrease costs and smooth the flow of materials, goods and services from suppliers to end-customers. Accordingly, many researchers made effort to develop decision-making tools to manage inventory through the pharmaceutical supply chain. However, most of these researches assumed that, products have unlimited life and their quality and application do not change during the time. In fact, pharmaceutical products are categorized in the class of perishable products. The perishability of pharmaceutical products is an important issue which should be taken into account while making different supply chain planning decisions such as inventory decisions (Goyal & Giri, 2001).

Definition and Scope

Managing pharmaceutical supply chain aims to create integrated relationships among the suppliers, producers, distributors and customers to convert raw material into drugs and medications and distribute them into hospitals, clinics and pharmacies (Shah, 2004). A pharmaceutical supply chain includes one or more nodes in kind of:

1. Primary manufacturing centers;
2. Secondary manufacturing centers;
3. Distribution centers (Main & Local DCs) and;
4. Clinics/hospitals/pharmacies.

The primary manufacturing centers (PMC) produce active ingredient or active pharmaceutical ingredient (AI or API). This is the first stage of pharmaceutical supply chain. In addition, the quality of material should be checked and controlled in PMCs. Thereafter, the produced active ingredients are sent to secondary manufacturing centers (SMC). In SMCs, the active ingredient is converted to end product (i.e., drugs & medications) by the aid of some production processes. It should be noted that in most of the cases the number of SMCs is more than primary ones.

Distribution centers including both main and local ones form the third layer of pharmaceutical supply chain. Products are sent to main DCs after production from secondary manufacturing centers and stocked in these facilities. Also, the amount of drugs needed to fulfill the local requirement and customer demands is stocked in local distribution centers. The last layer includes the customer zones which consists of clinics, hospitals and pharmacies. The final product is sent to them from local distribution centers.

Main Management Challenges

Pharmaceutical supply chain ensures the delivery of appropriate medications and drugs to those in need at the right place and time. Because of the direct link between pharmaceutical industry and the peoples' health and safety, managing of pharmaceutical supply chain is quite important and critical. Pharmaceutical supply chain confronts with some important challenges such as parallel trade of fake medications and drugs, visibility through the extensive supply chain (including foreign suppliers and distributors) and pricing which should be taken into account during the planning process. In the past, pharmaceutical companies were highly depended on introduction of new medications and drugs and they had a tendency toward storing high-level of medication inventory. However, in recent decades, companies try to decrease the costs and improve the effectiveness through managing the product flow and inventory level within the supply chain layers (Sursala & Karimi, 2012). Privett & Gonsalvez (2014) count ten important challenges of pharmaceutical supply chain as follows:

Lack of Coordination

Lack of coordination among pharmaceutical supply chain members is the most important challenge in todays' drug industry. Most of the times, pharmaceutical supply chain members have some conflicting goals and objectives with each other and their own decision may not be optimal for the entire supply chain. In this situation, using coordination tools such as buy-back contracts or delayed payments can eliminate the conflicts and improve the total performance of the pharmaceutical supply chain.

Inventory Management

Inventory management is the second challenge in the management of pharmaceutical supply chain. Large number and various types of medications and drugs besides the perishability of medications and imprecise information about them are the main issues which make this challenge more complex.

Demand Information

The complete information about demand is rarely available in pharmaceutical marketplace. Given that, the demand for medications are related to human's health and prevalence of diseases, it is hard to predict the amount of demand for future time-periods. Moreover, since upstream members such as manufacturers and distributors get orders from downstream members with a specific amount of delay, they will predict real demands in market by mistakes.

Human Resources Dependency

Human resources dependency is a significant issue in the planning of pharmaceutical supply (Dowling, 2011). Therefore, the production and distribution planning decisions should be made according to availability of relevant human resources (Sridhar et al., 2008).

Order Management

According to long delivery time and lack of knowledge about the exact demand information, the order management becomes more complex in the context of pharmaceutical supply chain.

Shortage Avoidance

Shortage is not allowed in almost all pharmaceutical supply chains since it may significantly affect the health of consumers. In other words, it can be said that preparing appropriate medications for patients has strong relationship with society's health and security. Therefore, medicine is categorized as a strategic good.

Expiration

Expiration of drugs beside the shortage avoidance makes the planning of pharmaceutical supply chain more complex. Poor warehouse management and lack of employee training are the significant causes of expiration. To deal with such issues, most of the practitioners use the FEFO (First-Expired-First-out) system in the management of drug inventory (Spicer et al., 2010).

Warehouse Management

Warehouse management is another important challenge which is related to some critical decisions such as warehouse design and drug storage management.

Temperature Control

Temperature failure is one the challenges in pharmaceutical supply chain that causes a lot of risks to patients and decreasing efficiency and effectiveness of medications (Grayling, 1999).

Shipment Visibility

Tracing and Tracking of drugs within the supply chain are difficult when a shipment leaves producers. Often, when orders arrive recipients have no information and this may cause some problems.

REVIEW AND CLASSIFICATION OF PLANNING PROBLEMS IN PROCUREMENT, PRODUCTION, AND DISTRIBUTION OF PHARMACEUTICAL PRODUCTS MANAGEMENT

In this section, the pharmaceutical procurement, production and distribution planning problems are reviewed and classified according to some important characteristics.

Classification of Planning Problems in Procurement, Production and Distribution of Pharmaceutical Products Management

The existing pharmaceutical supply chain planning problems can be categorized with respect to different planning horizons. They range from long-term decision problems to short-term ones. Decisions related to supply chain design and development with long-term effects (e.g. five up to ten years) can be considered as strategic level decisions. These decisions include network design, location-allocation, strategic sourcing and supplier selection decisions. Short-term decisions also concern about a number of operational decisions such as scheduling of production facilities and human resources. Last but not the least, mid-term or tactical level decisions can be considered as a mediocrity in terms of time that is one up to two years and include a variety of procurement, production and distribution planning decisions (Gupta & Maranas, 2000; Stadtler & Kilger, 2008; Chopra & Meindl, 2004). Figure 1 illustrates the pharmaceutical supply chain's hierarchical planning matrix.

Review of the Relevant Literature

As discussed before, strategic decisions of pharmaceutical supply chain deal with the long-term decisions. In this territory, Grunow et al. (2003) presented a plant coordination model within pharmaceutics supply networks. They considered total inventory startup and cleanout, production and transportation costs and solved the developed model by aggregation techniques. Oh & Karimi (2004) developed a strategic decision making model under uncertain condition, which considers both the manufacturing, and holding

Figure 1. Planning matrix for pharmaceutical supply chain
(adopted form Stadtler & Kilger, 2008)

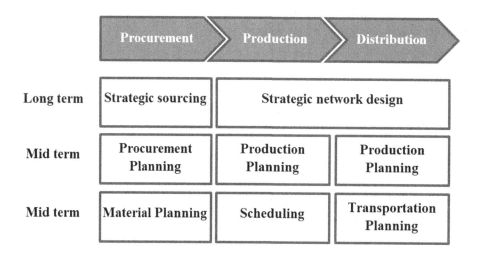

costs. Leachman et al. (2014) proposed an integrated production and distribution planning model for the pharmaceutical supply chain. The model tries to minimize manufacturing, holding and transportation costs. In addition, Mousazadeh et al. (2015) proposed a bi-objective mixed integer linear programming (BOMILP) model for the pharmaceutical supply chain network design (PSCND) problem. To handle the epistemic uncertainty of uncertain parameters, they used robust possibilistic programming approach.

As the literature shows, the majority of pharmaceutical supply chain researches focus on tactical level problems. Gupta and Maranas (2000) proposed a multi-period, multi-product production planning model for a drug producer. Meijboom and Obel (2005) presented a multi-objective optimization model to minimize transportation, holding and manufacturing costs in a tactical PSC planning problem. Lejeune (2005) proposed a multi-product and multi-period mathematical programming model to deal with a tactical level pharmaceutical supply chain (PSC) planning problem. They minimized the manufacturing and holding costs as an objective function and solved the model by a metaheuristic algorithm. Sundaramoorthy et al. (2006) developed a mixed integer multi-product, multi-period mathematical programming model in order to determine the inventory and transportation decisions within a PSC. Papageorgiou (2009) presented a mixed integer linear programming (MILP) model for long-term, multi-site capacity planning of a pharmaceutical firm under uncertainty while considering the trading structure of the company. Fengqi et al. (2010) proposed a multi-stage, multi-period and multi-product model for tactical planning of a PSC. They solved the proposed model by both exact and heuristic methods. In another paper, Terraz et al. (2010) presented a deterministic, multi-agent model to deal with a PSC planning problem. A metaheuristic algorithm is used to solve the proposed model. Sousa et al. (2011) proposed an integrated production and distribution planning model. Moreover, Susarla and Karimi (2012) studied the problem of the integrated procurement, production and distribution pharmaceutical products while accounting for tax differential, material shelf-lives, inventory holding costs and waste treatment.

A thin part of the relevant literature is dedicated to operational level problems in the area of PSC planning problems. Orcaun et al. (2001) proposed a continuous time model for optimal scheduling of pharmaceutical production activities. The model tries to minimize the raw material and manufacturing costs. Last but not the least, Blomer & Gunther (2000) presented a MILP model for scheduling of chemical batch processes. The proposed model is solved by a heuristic algorithm.

Systemic Classification of the Existing Works

To provide a systemic view on the PSC planning literature, we have classified and tabulated some of the important published papers in Table 1.

Table 1. Classification of some selected papers

Author	Costs	Planning	Horizon of decision	Solution approach	Certainty /Uncertainty	Type of uncertainty	Uncertain parameters/ Variables
Gupta & Maranas (2000)	Manufacturing, Holding, Transportation	Production	Tactical	Metaheuristic	Uncertain	Data/ Epistemic	Demand
Orcun et al. (2001)	Cost associated with operator, Raw material, Manufacturing	Production, Scheduling	Operational	Exact	Certain	-	-
Gatica et al. (2003)	Manufacturing, Holding	Capacity, Production	Tactical	Exact	Uncertain	Data/ Epistemic	Cost and Production capacity
Grunow et al. (2003)	Holding, Start-up and Clean-out, Production	Production, Distribution	Strategic	Metaheuristic/ Aggregation techniques	Certain	-	-
Oh & Karimi (2004)	Manufacturing, Holding	Capacity, Production	Strategic	Exact	Uncertain	Data/ Epistemic	Problem parameters
Lejeun (2006)	Manufacturing, Transportation, Holding	Production, Distribution	Tactical	Metaheuristic	Certain	-	-
Sundaramoorthy et al. (2006)	Manufacturing, Holding, Transportation	Production, Distribution	Tactical	Metaheuristic	Certain	-	-
Meijboom & Obel (2007)	Manufacturing, Transportation	Production, Distribution	Tactical	Heuristic	Uncertain	Data/ Epistemic	Demand, Production and Procurement capacity
Varma et al. (2008)	-	Scheduling and Resource allocation	Tactical	Metaheuristic	Certain	-	-
Colvin & Marvalias (2008)	Cost of trial, Total development cost	Research and Development	Tactical	Exact	Uncertain	Randomness (Stochastic)	Total development cost, Future (open) revenue, Revenue from drugs successfully passing PIII, etc.
Amaro & Barbosa-Po'voa (2008)	Manufacturing, Holding, Transportation	Production, Distribution	Tactical	Exact	Certain	-	-
Blomer & Gunther (2000)	-	Scheduling	Operational	Heuristic	Certain	-	-
Colvin & Marvalias (2010)	Cost to perform trial	Scheduling	Tactical	Metaheuristic	Uncertain	Randomness (Stochastic)	Expected future Revenue, Costs associated with Scenario, Revenue from successfully completed drug, etc.

continued on following page

Table 1. Continued

Author	Costs	Planning	Horizon of decision	Solution approach	Certainty /Uncertainty	Type of uncertainty	Uncertain parameters/ Variables
Peidro et al. (2009)	Manufacturing, Transportation, Marketing	Production, Distribution	Tactical	Exact/Heuristic	Certain	-	-
Alemany et al. (2009)	Manufacturing, Holding, Transportation	Production, Distribution	Tactical	Exact	Certain	-	-
Fengqi et al., (2011)	Manufacturing, Transportation	Production, Distribution	Tactical	Exact/ Metaheuristic	Certain	-	-
Terraz et al. (2010)	Manufacturing, Holding, Transportation	Production, Distribution	Tactical	Exact/ Metaheuristic	Certain	-	-
Sousa et al. (2011)	Manufacturing, Holding, Transportation	Production, Distribution	Tactical	Metaheuristic	Certain	-	-
Mirzapour et al. (2011)	Manufacturing, Holding, Transportation	Production	Tactical	Exact/ Metaheuristic	Uncertain	Data/ Epistemic	Cost and Demand
Fengqi & Grossman (2011)	Manufacturing, Holding	Production	Tactical	Exact/ Metaheuristic	Certain	-	-
Kelle et al. (2012)	Storage, Holding, Refill	Distribution	Tactical	Metaheuristic	Certain	-	-
Vila-Parrish et al. (2012)	Manufacturing, Holding and Shortage	Production, Distribution	Tactical	Exact	Uncertain	Randomness	Production
Susala & Karimi (2012)	Manufacturing, Holding, Transportation	Production, Distribution	Tactical	LP–MILP algorithm	Certain	-	-
Uthayakumar & Priyan (2013)	Manufacturing, Holding, Transportation	Capacity	Tactical	Metaheuristic	Certain	-	-
Leachman et al. (2014)	Manufacturing, Holding, Transportation	Production, Distribution	Strategic	Exact	Certain	-	-
Mousazadeh et al. (2015)	Manufacturing, Holding, Transportation	Production, Distribution	Strategic	Exact	Uncertain	Data/ Epistemic	Demand, Manufacturing cost, Transportation and Transshipment costs and Safety stock levels

According to existing papers in the context of pharmaceutical supply chain planning, it is obvious that this area becomes more attractive in recent years as more papers are dedicated to PSC planning problems. However, still the literature suffers from some deficiencies such as lack of efficient quantitative decision making tools which can integrate the procurement, production and distribution planning decisions. Moreover, with respect to importance of uncertainty in PSC management problems more powerful decision making methods are needed to cope with such issue.

SELECTED OR MODELS

In this section we discuss three selected pharmaceutical supply chain planning models in detail. The first model is a production planning model which is able to determine the amount of production as well as the capacity and technology of production site. The second model focuses on distribution planning decisions and the third one deal with an integrated procurement, production and distribution planning problem of pharmaceutical products. The notations used here are somehow similar to the paper of Mousazadeh et al. (2015) to keep integrity and facilitate the reference to this paper.

OR Models for Production Planning of Pharmaceutical Products

In this part, a multi-product, multi-period production planning model of pharmaceutical products is presented which the notations used in is described in below.

Indices:

i index of manufacturing sites, $i \in \{1, 2, ..., I\}$
j index of customer zones including hospitals/clinics and pharmacies
mp index of production technologies for product family p, $mp \in \{1, 2, ..., Mp\}$
p index of product families, $p \in \{1, 2, ..., P\}$
t index of periods, $t \in \{1, 2, ..., T\}$

Parameters:

f_{ip}^{mp}: Fixed cost of opening manufacturing center i for production of product family p with production technology mp

mc_{ip}^{mp}: Unit manufacturing cost of product family p at manufacturing center i with production technology mp

d_{ipt}: Demand of customer zone j for product family p at period t

tr_{ijp}: Unit transportation cost of product family p between manufacturing center i and customer zone j

C_{ip}^{mp}: Required capacity for producing a unit of drug from product family p using technology mp

Variables:

q_{ijpt}^{mp}: quantity of product family p produced in manufacturing center i and transported to customer zone j in period t using technology mp

x_{ip}^{mp}: 1 if manufacturing center i for producing product family p using production technology mp is opened; and 0, otherwise

Using the aforementioned notations, the proposed model is formulated as follows:

$$MinZ = \sum_{i,p,mp} f_{ip}^{mp} x_{ip}^{mp} + \sum_{i,mp,p,t} (mc_{ip}^{mp} + tr_{ijp}) q_{ijpt}^{mp} \tag{1}$$

$$\sum_{mp,i} q_{ijpt}^{mp} \geq d_{jpt} \quad \forall j,p,t \tag{2}$$

$$\sum_{j,mp} q_{ijpt}^{mp} \leq c_{ip}^{mp} x_{ip}^{mp} \quad \forall i,p,t \tag{3}$$

$$\sum_{mp} x_{ip}^{mp} \leq 1 \quad \forall i,p, \tag{4}$$

$$x_{ip}^{mp} \in \{0,1\} \quad \forall i,mp,p \tag{5}$$

$$q_{ijpt}^{mp} \geq 0 \quad \forall i,j,p,mp,t. \tag{6}$$

The objective function (1) includes the fixed opening cost of manufacturing centers, manufacturing and transportation costs. Constraints (2) demonstrate the satisfaction demand. Constraints (3) ensure that the quantity of products manufactured in each manufacturing sites at each period must be less than or equal to the production capacity. Constraints (4) guarantee that only one production technology for each product family must be used in each opened manufacturing sites. Finally, Constraints (5) and (6) declare the type of decision variables.

OR Models for Distribution Planning of Pharmaceutical Products

In this part, we discuss about a distribution planning problem of pharmaceutical products. According to Figure 2, the concerned supply chain is a multi-product, multi-period, two-echelon pharmaceutical supply chain which includes main and local distribution centers as well as customer zones including hospitals, clinics and pharmacies. The main decisions to be determined in this problem comprised of inventory levels at both main and local distribution centers as well as the amount of shipments between network facilities.

Figure 2. Distribution planning of pharmaceutical products

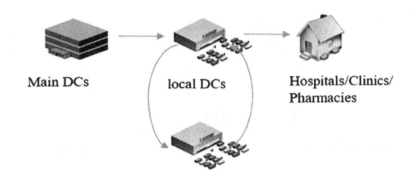

Indices:

h Index of transportation modes, $h \in \{1, 2, ..., H\}$
j Index of locations for main DCs, $j \in \{1, 2, ..., J\}$
k Index of locations for local DCs, $k \in \{1, 2, ..., K\}$
l Index of customer zones including hospitals/clinics and pharmacies, $l \in \{1, 2, ..., L\}$
n Index of possible capacity levels for main DCs, $n \in \{1, 2, ..., N\}$
p Index of product families, $p \in \{1, 2, ..., P\}$
t Index of periods $t \in \{1, 2, ..., T\}$

Parameters:

tr_{jkp}^{h} : unit transportation cost of product family p from main DC j to local DC k via Transportation mode h

$d_{l,p,t}$: demand of customer zone l for product family p at period t

tr'_{klp}^{h} : unit transportation cost of product family p from local DC k to customer zone l via transportation mode h

fj_{j}^{n} : fixed cost of opening main DC j with capacity level n

fk_{k} : fixed cost of opening local DC k

sj_{jp} : unit storage cost of product family p at the end of each period in main DC j

sk_{kp} : unit storage cost of product family p at the end of each period in local D k

$tr''_{k'kp}^{h}$: unit transshipment cost of product family p from local DC k to local DC k' via transportation mode h

cj_{j}^{n} : storage capacity of main DC j established by the capacity level n

ck_k : storage capacity available at local DC k

π_p : relative importance of product family p

Variables:

I_{jpt} : inventory level of product family p at main DC j at the end of period t

I'_{kpt} : inventory level of product family p at local DC k at the end of period t

q^h_{jkpt} : quantity of product family p shipped from main DC j to local DC k in period t using transportation mode h

q'^h_{klpt} : quantity of product family p shipped from local DC k to customer l in period t using transportation mode h

$q''^h_{k'kpt}$: quantity of product family p transshipped from local DC k' to k in period t using transportation mode h

x^n_j : 1 if potential main DC j with capacity level n is opened; and 0, otherwise

y_k : 1 if potential local DC k is opened; and 0, otherwise

Using the aforementioned notations, the proposed model is formulated as follows:

$$MinZ1 = \sum_{j,n} fj^n_j x^n_j + \sum_{k} fk_k y_k + \sum_{j,k,h,p,t} tr^h_{jkp} q^h_{jkpt} + \sum_{k,k'} tr''^h_{k'kp} q''^h_{k'kpt} + \sum_{k,l,h,p,t} tr'^h_{klp} q'^h_{klpt}$$
$$+ \sum_{j,p,t} sj_{jp} I_{jpt} + \sum_{k,p,t} sk_{kp} I'_{kpt} \qquad (7)$$

$$Minz2 = Max_{l,p,t}(\pi_p(d_{l,p,t} - \sum_{k,h} q'^h_{klpt})) \qquad (8)$$

$$I_{jpt} = I_{jpt-1} - \sum_{k,h} q^h_{jkpt} \quad \forall j, p, t \qquad (9)$$

$$I'_{kpt} = I'_{kpt-1} + \sum_{j,h} q^h_{jkpt} - \sum_{l,h} q'^h_{klpt} + \sum_{k',h} q''^h_{k'kpt} - \sum_{k',h} q''^h_{kk'pt} \quad \forall k, p, t \qquad (10)$$

$$\sum_{p} I_{jpt-1} \leq \sum_{n} x_{j}^{n} cj_{j}^{n} \; \forall j, t \tag{11}$$

$$\sum_{p} (I'_{kpt-1} + \sum_{j,h} q_{jkpt}^{h} + \sum_{k',k} q''_{k'kpt}^{h}) \leq y_{k} ck_{k} \; \forall k, t \tag{12}$$

$$\sum_{n} x_{j}^{n} \leq 1 \; \forall j \tag{13}$$

$$x_{j}^{n}, y_{k} \in \{0,1\} \; \forall j, k, n, p, \tag{14}$$

$$q_{jkpt}^{h}, q'_{klpt}^{h}, I_{jpt}, I'_{kpt}, q''_{k'kpt}^{h} \geq 0 \; \forall j, k, l, h, p, t. \tag{15}$$

The first objective function (7) includes the fixed opening cost of main distribution centers (Main DCs) and local distribution centers (Local DCs), transportation/transshipment costs and inventory holding cost in the main and local DCs. The second objective function (8) aims to minimize the maximum differences between demand and quantity of products shipped from local DC to customer zone of all product families in all periods. Constraints (9) and (10) ensure inventory and flow balance at both main and local DSc, respectively. Constraints (11) and (12) enforce the capacity limitations of the main and local DC in each time period, respectively. Constraints (13) guarantee that only one capacity level for each opened main DC is assigned. Finally, Constraints (14) and (15) declare the types of decision variables.

Linearization of the Proposed Model

As the second objective function is nonlinear due to its Min-Max structure, the following formulation can be used to convert this term into linear form.

$$Minz2 = \nu \tag{16}$$

s.t.

$$\nu \geq (\pi_{p}(d_{l,p,t} - \sum_{k,h} q'^{h}_{klpt})) \; \forall l, p, t \tag{17}$$

(7), (9) to (15)

OR Models for Integrated Procurement, Production and Distribution Planning of Pharmaceutical Products

The integrated procurement, production and distribution planning of pharmaceutical supply chain is recently studied by Mousazadeh et al. (2015). They also present a robust possibilistic approach to cope with the uncertainty of the input data in such problem. In this section we present a modified version of the model proposed by Mousazadeh et al. (2015). The model is developed by considering perishability of drugs. In comparison with the base paper, we restrict our attention to the tactical planning decisions rather than strategic ones as well as using credibility measure instead of necessity to convert fuzzy mathematical programming model into equivalent crisp one.

Figure 3 is an illustration of the studied pharmaceutical supply chain and the existing relations among its different facilities. According to this illustration, products are manufactured in secondary drug manufacturing centers with a special manufacturing technology. Thereafter products are shipped to main distribution centers. Then, medications are shipped to local distribution centers and there are lateral transshipment flows between the local DCs. Finally, products are shipped to hospitals, clinics and pharmacies.

The model aims to minimize the total cost and unfulfilled demands simultaneously. The following notations are used to address the mathematical formulation of the proposed model (Yousefi Sarmad & Pishavee, 2016):

Indices:

h- index of transportation modes, $h \in \{1, 2, ..., H\}$
i- index of candidate locations for manufacturing sites, $i \in \{1, 2, ..., I\}$
j- index of candidate locations for main DCs, $j \in \{1, 2, ..., J\}$
k- index of candidate locations for local DCs, $k \in \{1, 2, ..., K\}$
l- index of customer zones including hospitals/clinics and pharmacies, $l \in \{1, 2, ..., L\}$
mp- index of potential production technologies for product family p, $mp \in \{1, 2, ..., Mp\}$
n- index of possible capacity levels for main DCs, $n \in \{1, 2, ..., N\}$
p -index of product families, $p \in \{1, 2, ..., P\}$
t- index of periods, $t \in \{1, 2, ..., T\}$

Figure 3. Integrated procurement, production and distribution planning of pharmaceutical products

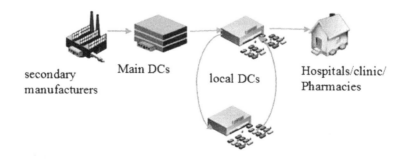

secondary
manufacturers

Main DCs

local DCs

Hospitals/clinic/
Pharmacies

Parameters:

a_{jkp}^{h} : Unit transportation cost of product family p from main DC j to local DC k via transportation mode h

c_{ijp}^{h} : Unit transportation cost of product family p from manufacturing site i to main DC j via transportation mode h

$d_{l,p,t}$: Demand of customer zone l for product family p at period t

e_{klp}^{h} : Unit transportation cost of product family p from local DC k to customer zone l via transportation mode h

sc_{jp} : Unit storage cost of product family p at the end of each period in main DC j

sc'_{kp} : Unit storage cost of product family p at the end of each period in local DC k

ss_{kpt} : Safety stock of product p in local DC k at the end of period t

$tr_{k'kp}^{h}$: Unit transshipment cost of product family p from local DC k to local DC k' via transportation mode h

δ_{j}^{n} : Storage capacity of main DC j established by the capacity level n

γ_{k} : Storage capacity available at local DC k

π_{p} : Relative importance of product family p

ρ_{ip}^{mp} : Unit manufacturing cost of product family p at manufacturing site i with production technology mp

τ_{i}^{mp} : Production capacity of manufacturing site i for product family p using technology mp

λ_{i} : Lost capacity of manufacturing center i

λ_{j} : Lost capacity of main DC j

λ_{k} : Lost capacity of main DC k

μ_{p} : Marketing costs for product p

v_{p} : Sales price of product p

T_{Maxp} : Maximum time period for product p that drug can be used and stocked

Variables:

I'_{jpt1t} : Stocked inventory level of product family p at time period $t1$ at main DC j at the end of period t

I_{jpt} : Inventory level of product family p at main DC j at the end of period t

II'_{kpt1t} : Stocked inventory level of product family p at time period $t1$ at main DC k at the end of period t

II_{kpt} : Inventory level of product family p at local DC k at the end of period t

o'^{h}_{klpt1t} : Quantity of product family p that is manufactured in time period $t1$ shipped from local DC k to customer l in period t using transportation mode h

o^{h}_{klpt} : Quantity of product family p shipped from local DC k to customer l in period t using transportation mode h

q'^{h}_{jkpt1t} : Quantity of product family p that is manufactured in time period $t1$ shipped from main DC j to local DC k in period t using transportation mode h

q^{h}_{jkpt} : Quantity of product family p shipped from main DC j to local DC k in period t using transportation mode h

u'^{mph}_{ijpt1t} : Quantity of product family p that is manufactured in time period $t1$ shipped from manufacturing center i to main DC j in period t using transportation mode h

u^{mph}_{ijpt} : Quantity of product family p shipped from manufacturing center i to main DC j in period t using transportation mode h and technology mp

$v'^{h}_{k'kpt1t}$: Quantity of product family p that is manufactured in time period $t1$ transshipped from local DC k' to k in period t using transportation mode h

$v^{h}_{k'kpt}$: Quantity of product family p transshipped from local DC k' to k in period t using transportation mode h

s_{ptl} : Amount of product p sold at time t at customer zone l

Using the aforementioned notations, the proposed model is formulated as follows:

$$Minz1 = \sum_{i,j,mp,h,p,t} (\rho^{mp}_{ip} + c^{h}_{ijp})u^{mph}_{ijpt} + \sum_{j,k,h,p,t} a^{h}_{jkp}q^{h}_{jkpt} + \sum_{k,k',h,p,t} tr^{h}_{k'kp}v^{h}_{k'kpt} + \sum_{k,l,h,p,t} e^{h}_{klp}o^{h}_{klpt}$$
$$+ \sum_{j,p,t} sc_{jp}I_{jpt} + \sum_{k,p,t} sc'_{kp}II_{kpt} + \sum_{p,t,l} \mu_{p}v_{p}s_{ptl} - \sum_{p,t,l} v_{p}s_{ptl} \tag{18}$$

$$Minz2 = Max_{l,p,t}(\pi_{p}(d_{l,p,t} - \sum_{k,h} o^{h}_{klpt})) \tag{19}$$

$$Minz2 = \nu \tag{19a}$$

$$\nu \geq \left(\pi_p \left(d_{l,p,t} - \sum_{k,h} o^h_{klpt} \right) \right) \tag{19b}$$

$$I'_{jpt1t} = I'_{jpt1t-1} + \sum_{i,mp,h,t1 \leq t2 \leq t} q'^h_{jkpt1t2} - \sum_{k,h,t1 \leq t2 \leq t} q'^h_{jkpt1t2} \quad \forall j,p, t - T_{Maxp} \leq t1 \leq t \tag{20}$$

$$I_{jpt} = \sum_{t1 \leq t} I'_{jpt1t} \quad \forall j,p,t \tag{21}$$

$$II'_{kpt1t} = II'_{kpt1t-1} + \sum_{j,h,t1 \leq t2 \leq t} q'^h_{jkpt1t2} - \sum_{l,h,t1 \leq t2 \leq t} o'^h_{klt1t2} \quad \forall k,p, t - T_{Maxp} \leq t1 \leq t$$
$$+ \sum_{k',h,t1 \leq t2 \leq t} v'^h_{k'kpt1t2} - \sum_{k',h,t1 \leq t2 \leq t} v'^h_{kk'pt1t2'} \tag{22}$$

$$II_{kpt} = \sum_{t1 \leq t} II'_{kpt1t} \quad \forall k,p,t \tag{23}$$

$$\sum_{t1 \leq t} u'^{mph}_{ijpt1t} \leq u^{mph}_{ijpt} \quad \forall i,j,p,t,h \tag{24}$$

$$\sum_{t1 \leq t} q'^h_{jkpt1t} \leq q^h_{jkpt} \quad \forall j,k,p,t,h \tag{25}$$

$$\sum_{t1 \leq t} v'^h_{k'kpt1t} \leq v^h_{k'kpt} \quad \forall k',k,p,t,h \tag{26}$$

$$\sum_{t1 \leq t} o'^h_{klt1t} \leq o^h_{klpt} \quad \forall k,l,p,t,h \tag{27}$$

$$\sum_{k,k',h} \left(v'^h_{k'kpt1t} + v'^h_{kk'pt1t} \right) + \sum_{k,l,h} o'^h_{klt1t} + \sum_{j,k,h} q'^h_{jkpt1t} + \sum_{i,j,h,mp} u'^{mph}_{ijpt1t} = 0 \quad \forall p,t,t1 \prec t - T_{Maxp} \tag{28}$$

$$\sum_k II'_{kpt1t} = 0 \ \forall p,t,t1 \prec t - T_{Maxp} \tag{29}$$

$$\sum_j I'_{jpt1t} = 0 \ \forall p,t,t1 \prec t - T_{Maxp} \tag{30}$$

$$\sum_{j,h,mp} u^{mph}_{ijpt} \leq \tau^{mp}_i (1-\lambda_i) \ \forall i,p,t \tag{31}$$

$$\sum_p (I_{jpt-1} + \sum_{i,mp,h} u^{mph}_{ijpt}) \leq \sum_n \delta^n_j (1-\lambda_j) \ \forall j,t \tag{32}$$

$$\sum_p (II_{kpt-1} + \sum_{j,h} q^h_{jkpt} + \sum_{k',k} v^h_{k'kpt}) \leq \gamma_k (1-\lambda_k) \ \forall k,t \tag{33}$$

$$II_{kpt} \geq ss_{kpt} \ \forall k,p,t \tag{34}$$

$$s_{ptl} = \sum_{k,h} o^h_{klpt} \ \forall p,t,l \tag{35}$$

$$u^{mph}_{ijpt}, u'^{mph}_{ijpt1t}, q^h_{jkpt}, q'^h_{jkpt1t}, o^h_{klpt}, o'^h_{klt1t}, I_{jpt}, I'_{jpt1t}, II_{kpt}, II'_{kpt1t}, v^h_{k'kpt}, v'^h_{k'kpt}, s_{ptl} \geq 0 \ \forall i,j,k,l,mp,h,p,t. \tag{36}$$

The first objective function (18) includes manufacturing costs, transportation/ transshipment costs, inventory holding cost in the main and local DCs as well as sales revenue and also marketing costs that are assumed to be proportional to the product amounts sold over time period t at customer zone l. The second objective function (19) aims to minimize the maximum differences between demand and quantity of products shipped from local DC to customer zone of all product families in all periods. As discussed before, this objective is nonlinear and the linearization of this model is the same as the second model (19a) and (19b). Constraints (20) and (22) are inventory and flow balance at both main and local DSc, respectively. Constraints (21) and (23) guarantee that the total stocked inventory for product family p in period t is equals with total inventories for those products. Constraints (24) to (27) determine the amount of flow from manufacturing center to main DC, main DC to local DC and local DC to local DC and local DC to hospitals, clinics and pharmacies, respectively. Eqs. (28) guarantee that if the difference between manufacturing period $t1$ and t is more than maximum time period for product p, the total flow of all centers should equal to zero in order to avoid the shipment of perishable products. Also, Constraints (29) and (30) show that if the difference between t and $t1$ is greater than maximum time period for product p, the inventory can't be stocked because products will be spoiled and discarded. Eqs. (31) guarantee that the level of total production for each product family does not exceed the production capacity. Constraints (32) and (33) ensure that the level of total inventory for each product from last period in addition inputting data to main and local DC in each time period mustn't exceed the admissible capacity.

Eqs. (34) ensure that the inventory of each product family is equal to or greater than safety stock in each time-period at each local DC. Constraint (35) indicate that amount of product p sold at time t at customer zone l equals with quantity of product family p shipped from local DC k to customer l in period t using transportation mode h. Constraints (36) declare the types of decision variables.

Coping With Uncertainty

The reason of uncertainty in procurement, production and distribution planning of pharmaceutical products goes back to dynamic and imprecise nature of data. Dubois et al. (2003) classified uncertainty into two categories. The first one is uncertainty in data and the second one is flexibility in goals and constraints. Uncertainty in data can be happened in two forms: (1) randomness and (2) epistemic uncertainty. Randomness is coming from the random nature of the input parameters and epistemic uncertainty is related to lack of knowledge about the model parameters. Epistemic uncertainty can be formulated by fuzzy numbers. To handle the epistemic uncertainty in model parameters possibilistic programming approaches can be used (Pishvaee et al. 2012a; Pishvaee et al., 2012b; Mousazadeh et al., 2014).

In the procurement, production and distribution planning of pharmaceutical products, demand, manufacturing costs, marketing costs, safety stock and transportation costs are the input parameters which may be tainted by epistemic uncertainty (Shah, 2004; Laínez et al., 2012). Here a credibility-based possibilistic programming model is used to cope with uncertainty in the concerned problem.

Proposed Credibility-Based Fuzzy Chance Constrained Programming Model (CBCCP)

In the studied problem the demands, manufacturing costs, transportation and transshipment costs, safety stock levels and marketing costs over the planning horizons are assumed as uncertain parameters. According to lack of historical data about these parameters, expert's opinions are used to estimate the value of the imprecise parameters. Accordingly, trapezoidal fuzzy numbers are used to model the uncertain parameters as follows:

$$\tilde{d}_{lpt} = \left(d_{lpt(1)}, d_{lpt(2)}, d_{lpt(3)}, d_{lpt(4)} \right)$$

$$\tilde{\rho}_{ip}^{mp} = \left(\rho_{ip(1)}^{mp}, \rho_{ip(2)}^{mp}, \rho_{ip(3)}^{mp}, \rho_{ip(4)}^{mp} \right)$$

$$\tilde{c}_{ijp}^{h} = \left(c_{ijp(1)}^{h}, c_{ijp(2)}^{h}, c_{ijp(3)}^{h}, c_{ijp(4)}^{h} \right)$$

$$\tilde{a}_{jkp}^{h} = \left(a_{jkp(1)}^{h}, a_{jkp(2)}^{h}, a_{jkp(3)}^{h}, a_{jkp(4)}^{h} \right)$$

$$t\tilde{r}_{k'kp}^{h} = \left(tr_{k'kp(1)}^{h}, tr_{k'kp(2)}^{h}, tr_{k'kp(3)}^{h}, tr_{k'kp(4)}^{h} \right)$$

$$\tilde{e}_{klp}^{h} = \left(e_{klp(1)}^{h}, e_{klp(2)}^{h}, e_{klp(3)}^{h}, e_{klp(4)}^{h} \right)$$

$$s\tilde{s}_{kpt}^{h} = \left(ss_{kpt(1)}, ss_{kpt(2)}, ss_{kpt(3)}, ss_{kpt(4)} \right)$$

$$\tilde{\mu}_{p} = \left(\mu_{p(1)}, \mu_{p(2)}, \mu_{p(3)}, \mu_{p(4)} \right)$$

Here, a credibility-based chance constrained programming approach is used to form the proposed model. Notably, Possibility and necessity measures aren't self-dual but the credibility measure has self-duality (Li & Liu, 2006). In the other words, when the credibility value is equal to 1, it shows that the fuzzy event will be happen definitely and when it is 0, it won't happen at all. Credibility-based chance constrained programming was firstly introduced by Liu and Liu (2002) and then extended by Liu (2004).

Now you can suppose that $\tilde{\xi}$ is a fuzzy variable with membership function $\mu(x)$ and r is a real number. According to Liu and Liu (2002) credibility measure is stated as follows:

$$\text{Cr}\{\tilde{\xi} \leq r\} = \frac{1}{2} \left(\sup_{x \leq r} \mu(x) + 1 - \sup_{x > r} \mu(x) \right). \tag{37}$$

It is notable that because $\text{Nec}\{\tilde{\xi} \leq r\} = 1 - \sup_{x > r} \mu(x)$ *and* $\text{Pos}\{\tilde{\xi} \leq r\} = \sup_{x \leq r} \mu(x)$ therefore, credibility measure is stated as follows:

$$\text{Cr}\{\tilde{\xi} \leq r\} = \frac{1}{2} \left(\text{Pos}\{\tilde{\xi} \leq r\} + \text{Nec}\{\tilde{\xi} \leq r\} \right). \tag{38}$$

$$\text{Pos}\{\tilde{\xi} \leq r\} = \begin{cases} 1, & r \in (\xi_{(2)}, +\infty], \\[2mm] \dfrac{r - \xi_{(1)}}{(\xi_{(2)} - \xi_{(1)})}, & r \in (\xi_{(1)}, \xi_{(2)}], \\[2mm] 0, & r \in (-\infty, \xi_{(1)}], \end{cases} \tag{39}$$

$$\text{Nec}\{\tilde{\xi} \leq r\} = \begin{cases} 1, & r \in (\xi_{(4)}, +\infty], \\ \dfrac{r - \xi_{(3)}}{(\xi_{(4)} - \xi_{(3)})}, & r \in (\xi_{(3)}, \xi_{(4)}], \\ 0, & r \in (-\infty, \xi_{(3)}], \end{cases} \tag{40}$$

Accordingly, credibility measure is considered as an average of possibility and necessity measures. Also, expected value ξ is formulated below:

$$\text{E}[\tilde{\xi}] = \int\limits_{0}^{\infty} \text{Cr}\{\tilde{\xi} \geq r\} \ \mathrm{d}r - \int\limits_{-\infty}^{0} \text{Cr}\{\tilde{\xi} \leq r\} \ \mathrm{d}r. \tag{41}$$

If ξ is a trapezoidal fuzzy number $\tilde{\xi} = (\xi_{(1)}, \xi_{(2)}, \xi_{(3)}, \xi_{(4)})$ according the last formulation expected value ξ is as follows:

$$(\xi_{(1)} + \xi_{(2)} + \xi_{(3)} + \xi_{(4)}) / 4$$

Thus, credibility measure is formulated below:

$$\text{Cr}\{\tilde{\xi} \leq r\} = \begin{cases} 0, & r \in (-\infty, \xi_{(1)}], \\ \dfrac{r - \xi_{(1)}}{2(\xi_{(2)} - \xi_{(1)})}, & r \in (\xi_{(1)}, \xi_{(2)}], \\ \dfrac{1}{2}, & r \in (\xi_{(2)}, \xi_{(3)}], \\ \dfrac{r - 2\xi_{(3)} + \xi_{(4)}}{2(\xi_{(4)} - \xi_{(3)})}, & r \in (\xi_{(3)}, \xi_{(4)}], \\ 1, & r \in (\xi_{(4)}, +\infty], \end{cases} \tag{42}$$

$$\text{Cr}\{\tilde{\xi} \geq r\} = \begin{cases} 1, & r \in (-\infty, \xi_{(1)}], \\ \dfrac{2\xi_{(2)} - \xi_{(1)} - r}{2(\xi_{(2)} - \xi_{(1)})}, & r \in (\xi_{(1)}, \xi_{(2)}], \\ \dfrac{1}{2}, & r \in (\xi_{(2)}, \xi_{(3)}], \\ \dfrac{\xi_{(4)} - r}{2(\xi_{(4)} - \xi_{(3)})}, & r \in (\xi_{(3)}, \xi_{(4)}], \\ 0, & r \in (\xi_{(4)}, +\infty], \end{cases} \tag{43}$$

It can be proven that if ε is a trapezoidal fuzzy number and $\alpha > 0.5$ so the formulation is as follows (see Pishvaee et al, 2012a):

$$Cr\{\tilde{\xi} \leq r\} \geq \alpha \Leftrightarrow r \geq (2 - 2\alpha)\xi_{(3)} + (2\alpha - 1)\xi_{(4)}, \tag{44}$$

$$Cr\{\tilde{\xi} \geq r\} \geq \alpha \Leftrightarrow r \leq (2\alpha - 1)\xi_{(1)} + (2 - 2\alpha)\xi_{(2)}. \tag{45}$$

Now consider the following fuzzy mathematical programming problem.

$$Min Z = \tilde{f}.y + \tilde{c}.x \tag{46}$$

$$s.t \, A.x \geq \tilde{d} \tag{47}$$

$$S.x \leq \tilde{N}.y \tag{48}$$

$$B.x = e \tag{49}$$

$$y \in \{0,1\}, x \geq 0 \tag{50}$$

Based on *Eqs.* (44) and (45) the crisp equivalent model can be formulated as follows:

$$Min E[Z] = (\frac{f^1 + f^2 + f^3 + f^4}{4}).y + (\frac{c^1 + c^2 + c^3 + c^4}{4}).x \tag{51}$$

$$s.t \, A.x \geq (2 - 2\beta)d^3 + (2\alpha - 1)d^4 \tag{52}$$

$$S.x \leq (2\beta - 1)N^1.y + (2 - 2\beta)N^2.y \tag{53}$$

$$B.x = e \tag{54}$$

$$y \in \{0,1\}, x \geq 0 \tag{55}$$

It should be noted that $0.5 \prec \alpha, \beta \leq 1$ control the minimum satisfaction degree of chance constraints and they can be determined by the decision maker according to desired conservatism level. Therefore, the crisp equivalent model of Constraints (18) to (36) can be formulated as follows.

$$Min \left\{ \sum_{i,j,mp,h,p,t} \begin{bmatrix} (\dfrac{\rho_{ip}^{1mp} + \rho_{ip}^{2mp} + \rho_{ip}^{3mp} + \rho_{ip}^{4mp}}{4} + \dfrac{c_{ijp}^{1h} + c_{ijp}^{2h} + c_{ijp}^{3h} + c_{ijp}^{4h}}{4}) u_{ijpt}^{mph} \\ + \sum_{j,k,h,p,t} \dfrac{a_{jkp}^{1h} + a_{jkp}^{2h} + a_{jkp}^{3h} + a_{jkp}^{4h}}{4} q_{jkpt}^{h} \\ + \sum_{k,k',h,p,t} \dfrac{tr_{k'kp}^{1h} + tr_{k'kp}^{2h} + tr_{k'kp}^{3h} + tr_{k'kp}^{4h}}{4} v_{k'kpt}^{h} \\ + \sum_{k,l,h,p,t} \dfrac{e_{klp}^{1h} + e_{klp}^{2h} + e_{klp}^{3h} + e_{klp}^{4h}}{4} o_{klpt}^{h} + \\ \sum_{j,p,t} sc_{jp} I_{jpt} + \sum_{k,p,t} sc'_{kp} II_{kpt} \\ + \sum_{p,t,l} \dfrac{\mu_{p}^{1} + \mu_{p}^{2} + \mu_{p}^{3} + \mu_{p}^{4}}{4} v_{p} s_{ptl} \end{bmatrix} \right\} \tag{56}$$

s.t.

$$II_{kpt} \geq (2 - 2\alpha) ss_{kpt}^{3} + (2\alpha - 1) ss_{kpt}^{4} \quad \forall k, p, t \tag{57}$$

$$\nu \geq \pi_p \{ (2 - 2\beta) d_{lpt}^{3} + (2\beta - 1) d_{lpt}^{4} - \sum_{k,h} o_{klpt}^{h} \} \quad \forall l, p, t \tag{58}$$

(20) to (33), (35) -(36)

CASE STUDY

To demonstrate the usefulness of the integrated procurement, production and distribution planning model of pharmaceutical products presented in this chapter, a real case study is provided here. The model presented in 3.3 is implemented by the use of the data of a real case study, i.e., Hakim Pharmaceutical Company. Hakim Pharmaceutical Company is one of the largest and most well-known companies in Iran. This company has continuously experienced growth and expansion during the last five decades. Currently, Hakim is capable of manufacturing various dosage forms such as coated and uncoated tablets, effervescent tablets, hard gelatin capsules, soft gelatin capsules, oral drops, syrups, oral suspensions, topical solutions, topical gels, topical creams and ointments. Hakim is continuously increasing its production capacities and is currently engaged in updating its sensitive laboratory equipment.

The production and distribution of a single drug is chosen as a case study due to limited access to data. This drug is called "MULTIKIM", which is used as a vitamin for children. This drug is manufactured in manufacturing centers and then transported to the main distribution centers. Thereafter, it is transported to local distribution centers and finally, is transshipped into hospitals, clinics and pharmacies. It is assumed that all the customer demands may not be fulfilled; but one of the considered objective functions aims to minimize the amount of unsatisfied demand.

It should be noted that there are two production centers, four customer zone, one main and five local distribution centers in the studied case. Moreover, two production technologies are available to produce MULTIKIM syrup in each center with production capacities of 16600 bottles. Furthermore, sales price of each syrup is 43150 Rials (Iranian currency), unit marketing cost is equal to 1000 and production cost of each manufacturing centers is between 6000 and 9000. In addition, storage cost is between 500 and 1000 in each distribution center. Table 2 represents the demands for three customer zones in three periods. The transportation costs between each two centers are between 2000 and 4000.

The results derived from implementing the model on the case study is illustrated in Table 3.

After representing initial results, sensitivity analysis is performed on some critical parameters to reveal effects on the model. Figure 4 shows the impact of marketing cost on objective functions. It's obvious that, objective function (1) (i.e., cost function) is growing up by increasing marketing cost and objective function (2) (i.e., unsatisfied demand) remains constant and marketing cost doesn't affect it.

CONCLUSION

This chapter studies the recent developments in procurement, production and distribution planning of pharmaceutical products in order to pave the way for the researchers and practitioners who are interested

Table 2. Demands of customer zone l at period t

l	d_{lt}		
	t		
	1	2	3
1	10000	8000	16000
2	9000	8500	14000
3	9500	8000	16000

Table 3. The summary of results

Objective Function Values		CPU Time
Z1(cost)	Z2 (max. unsatisfied demand)	
1.18372E+12	7004.658	662

Figure 4. The impact of marketing cost on objective functions

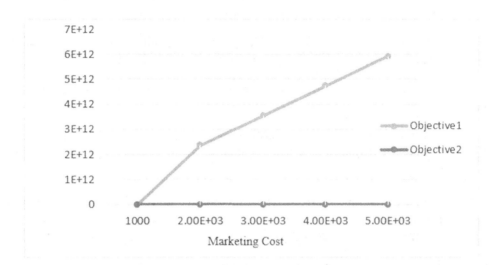

in the area of pharmaceutical supply chain management. The focus of the chapter is on quantitative mathematical programming models which enable the decision makers to appropriately adjust the planning decisions with in the pharmaceutical supply chain. A systemic literature review is provided through classification of relevant papers in the literature and then several mathematical programming models is discussed and analyzed. Finally, to show the practical value of quantitative decision making tools, a case study is provided and discussed.

Since mathematical programming models have a significant and explicit role in the efficient management of procurement, production and distribution processes of pharmaceutical products, there are various avenues for further research. Among them, we can refer to the following ones:

- Considering social aspects in the design and planning of is scarce in the current literature. Therefore, to move towards more sustainable procurement, production and distribution planning of pharmaceutical products, it is necessary to include the environmental and social aspects beside the economical dimensions.
- Since the size of most real life pharmaceutical supply chain planning problems are very large, the exact solution methods are unable to deal with such problems. Therefore, devising tailored solution approaches including heuristics, meta-heuristics or Mat-heuristics (the interoperation of meta-heuristics and mathematical programming techniques) would be of particular interest.
- According to importance of financial issues considering the cash follow in PSC beside physical flow would be attractive for future research efforts.

REFERENCES

Alemany, M. M. E., Boj, J. J., Mula, J., & Lario, F. (2009). Mathematical programming model for centralized master planning in ceramic tile supply chains. *International Journal of Production Research*, *48*(17), 5053–5074. doi:10.1080/00207540903055701

Amaro, A.C.S., & Barbosa-Po'voa, A.P.F.D. (2008). Planning and scheduling of industrial supply chains with reverse flows: A real pharmaceutical case study. *Computers and Chemical Engineering 32*, 2606-2625.

Blomer, F., & Gunther, H.-O. (2000). LP-based heuristics for scheduling chemical batch processes. *International Journal of Production Research, 38*(5), 1029–1051. doi:10.1080/002075400189004

Chopra, S., & Meindl, P. (2004). *Supply chain management: Strategy, planning, and operation*. Pearson, Prentice-Hall.

Colvin, M., & Maravelias, C. T. (2008). A stochastic programming approach for clinical trial planning in new drug development. *Computers & Chemical Engineering, 32*(11), 2626–2642. doi:10.1016/j.compchemeng.2007.11.010

Colvin, M., & Maravelias, C. T. (2010). Modeling methods and a branch and cut algorithm for pharmaceutical clinical trial planning using stochastic programming. *European Journal of Operational Research, 203*(1), 205–215. doi:10.1016/j.ejor.2009.07.022

Dowling, P. (2011). Health care supply chains in developing countries: Situational Analysis. Arlington, VA: Academic Press.

Fengqi, Y., Grossmann, I., & Wassick, J. (2003). Multi-Site Capacity, Production and Distribution Planning with Reactor Modifications: MILP Model, Bi-level Decomposition Algorithm vs. Lagrangean Decomposition Scheme. *Industrial & Engineering Chemistry Research, 50*(9), 4831–4849.

Gatica, G., Papageorigio, L. G., & Shah, N. (2011). Capacity Planning Under Uncertainty for the Pharmaceutical Industry. *Chemical Engineering Research & Design, 81*(6), 665–678.

Goyal, S. K., & Giri, B. C. (2001). Recent trends in modeling of deteriorating inventory. *European Journal of Operational Research, 134*(1), 1–16. doi:10.1016/S0377-2217(00)00248-4

Grayling, T. (1999). *Guidelines for safe disposal of unwanted pharmaceutical in and after emergencies*. Geneva: WHO.

Gorunow, M., Gunther, H.-O., & Yang, G. (2003). Plant co-ordination in pharmaceutics supply networks. *Operational Research Spectrum, 25*(1), 109–141. doi:10.1007/s00291-002-0117-z

Gupta, A., & Maranas, C. (2000). A Two-Stage Modeling and Solution Framework for Multisite Midterm Planning under Demand Uncertainty. *Industrial & Engineering Chemistry Research, 39*(10), 3799–3813. doi:10.1021/ie9909284

Kelle, P., Woosley, J., & Schneider, H. (2012). Pharmaceutical supply chain specifics and inventory solutions for a hospital case. *Operations Research for Health Care, 1*(2-3), 54–63. doi:10.1016/j.orhc.2012.07.001

Laínez, J. M., Schaefer, E., & Reklaitis, G. V. (2012). Challenges and opportunities in enterprise-wide optimization in the pharmaceutical industry. *Computers & Chemical Engineering, 47*, 19–28. doi:10.1016/j.compchemeng.2012.07.002

Leachman, R., Johnston, L., Li, S., & Shen, L. (2014). An automated planning engine for biopharmaceutical production. *European Journal of Operational Research, 238*(1), 327–338. doi:10.1016/j.ejor.2014.03.002

Lejeune, M. A. (2006). A variable neighborhood decomposition search method for supply chain management planning problems. *European Journal of Operational Research*, *175*(2), 959–976. doi:10.1016/j.ejor.2005.05.021

Liu, B., & Liu, Y. K. (2002). Expected value of fuzzy variable and fuzzy expected value models. *IEEE Transactions on Fuzzy Systems*, *10*(4), 445–450. doi:10.1109/TFUZZ.2002.800692

Liu, B. (2004). *Uncertainty theory: An introduction to its axiomatic foundations*. Berlin: Springer-Verlag. doi:10.1007/978-3-540-39987-2

Li, X., & Liu, B. (2006). A sufficient and necessary condition of credibility measure. *International Journal of Uncertainty & Knowledge-Based System*, *14*(5), 527–535. doi:10.1142/S0218488506004175

Meijboom, B., & Obel, B. (2007). Tactical coordination in a multi-location and multi-stage operations structure: A model and a pharmaceutical company case. *Omega*, *35*(3), 258–273. doi:10.1016/j.omega.2005.06.003

Mirzapour Al-e-hashem, S. M. J., Malekly, H., & Aryanezhad, M. B. (2011). A multi-objective robust optimization model for multi-product multi-site aggregate production planning in a supply chain under uncertainty. *International Journal of Production Economics*, *134*(1), 28–42. doi:10.1016/j.ijpe.2011.01.027

Mousazadeh, M., & Torabi, S. A. (2014). *Green and reverse logistics management under fuzziness.* In C. Kahraman & B. Öztaysi (Eds.), *Supply Chain Management Under Fuzziness, Studies in Fuzziness and Soft Computing* (Vol. 313, pp. 607–637). Springer-Verlag Berlin Heidelberg.

Mousazadeh, M., Torabi, S. A., & Zahiri, B. (2015). A robust possibilistic programming approach for pharmaceutical supply chain network design. *Journal of Computers and Chemical Engineering*, *82*, 115–128. doi:10.1016/j.compchemeng.2015.06.008

Nahmias, S. (2011). SEAC determines low bidders. *Technical News Bulletin*, *1954*, 38–179.

Narayana, S. A., Pati, R. K., & Vrat, P. (2012). Research on management issues in the pharmaceutical industry: A literature review. *International Journal of Pharmaceutical and Healthcare Marketing*, *6*(4), 351–375. doi:10.1108/17506121211283235

Oh, H. C., & Karimi, I. A. (2004). Regulatory factors and capacity-expansion planning in global chemical supply chains. *Industrial & Engineering Chemistry Research*, *43*(13), 3364–3380. doi:10.1021/ie034339g

Orcun, S., Altinel, I. K., & Hortacsua, Ö. (2001). General continuous time models for production planning and scheduling of batch processing plants: Mixed integer linear program formulations and computational issues'. *Computers & Chemical Engineering*, *25*(2-3), 371–389. doi:10.1016/S0098-1354(00)00663-3

Papageorgiou, L. G. (2009). Supply chain optimization for the process industries: Advances and opportunities. *Computers & Chemical Engineering*, *33*(12), 1931–1938. doi:10.1016/j.compchemeng.2009.06.014

Peidro, D., Mula, J., Poler, R., & Verdegay, J.-L. (2009). Fuzzy Optimization for Supply Chain Planning Under Supply, Demand and Process Uncertainties. *Fuzzy Sets and Systems*, *160*(18), 2640–2657. doi:10.1016/j.fss.2009.02.021

Pishvaee, M. S., Torabi, S. A., & Razmi, J. (2012a). Credibility-based fuzzy mathematical programming model for green logistics design under uncertainty. *Computers & Industrial Engineering, 62*(2), 624–632. doi:10.1016/j.cie.2011.11.028

Pishvaee, M. S., Razmi, J., & Torabi, S. A. (2012b). Robust possibilistic programming for socially responsible supply chain network design: A new approach. *Fuzzy Sets and Systems, 206*, 1–20. doi:10.1016/j.fss.2012.04.010

Privett, N., & Gonsalvez, D. (2015). The top ten global health supply chain issues. *Journal of Operations Research for Health Care.*

Sazvar, Z., Baboli, A., & Akbari Jokar, M. R. (2013). A replenishment policy for perishable products with non-linear holding cost under stochastic supply lead time. *International Journal of Advanced Manufacturing Technology, 64*(5-8), 1087–1098. doi:10.1007/s00170-012-4042-2

Shah, N. (2004). Pharmaceutical supply chains: Key issues and strategies for optimization. *Computers & Chemical Engineering, 28*(6-7), 929–941. doi:10.1016/j.compchemeng.2003.09.022

Sousa, T., Liu, S., Papageorgiou, L., & Shaha, N. (2011). Global supply chain planning for pharmaceuticals. *Chemical Engineering Research and Design, 8*(9), 2396–2409.

Spicer, N., Aleshkina, J., Biesma, R., Brugha, R., Caceres, C., Chilundo, B., & Ndubani, P. et al. (2010). National and subnational HIV/AIDS coordination: Are global health initiatives closing the gap between intent and practice?. *Globalization and Health, 6*(3). PMID:20196845

Srihar, D., & Batniji, R. (2008). Misfinancing global health: A case for transparency in disbursements and decision making. *Lancet, 372*(9644), 1185–119. doi:10.1016/S0140-6736(08)61485-3 PMID:18926279

Stadtler, H. (2005). Supply chain management and advanced planning—basics, overview and challenges. *European Journal of Operational Research, 163*(3), 575–588. doi:10.1016/j.ejor.2004.03.001

Stadtler, H., & Kilger, C. (2008). *Supply Chain Management and Advanced Planning* (4th ed.). Springer. doi:10.1007/978-3-540-74512-9

Sundaramoorthy, A., Xianming, X., Karimi, I. A., & Srinivasan, R. (2006). An integrated model for planning in global chemical supply chains. *16th European Symposium on Computer Aided Process Engineering and 9th International Symposium on Process Systems Engineering.* doi:10.1016/S1570-7946(06)80373-1

Susarla, N., & Karimi, I. A. (2012). Integrated supply chain planning for multinational pharmaceutical enterprises. *Computers & Chemical Engineering, 42*, 168–177. doi:10.1016/j.compchemeng.2012.03.002

Terrazas-Moreno, S., & Grossmann, I. (2011). A multiscale decomposition method for the optimal planning and scheduling of multisite continuous multiproduct plants. *Chemical Engineering Science, 66*(19), 4307–4318.

Tollman, P., Morieux, Y., Murphy, J., & Schulze, U. (2011). *Can R&D be fixed? Lessons from Biopharma outliers.* The Boston Consulting Group.

Uthayakumar, R., & Priyan, S. (2013). Pharmaceutical supply chain and inventory management strategies: Optimization for a pharmaceutical company and a hospital. *Operations Research for Health Care*, *2*(3), 52–64. doi:10.1016/j.orhc.2013.08.001

Varma, V. A., Pekny, J. F., Blau, G. E., & Reklaitis, G. V. (2008). A framework for addressing stochastic and combinatorial aspects of scheduling and resource allocation in pharmaceutical R&D pipelines. *Computers & Chemical Engineering*, *32*(4-5), 1000–1015. doi:10.1016/j.compchemeng.2007.05.006

Villa-Parish, A. R., Lvy, J., King, R. E., & Abel, S. R. (2012). Patient-based pharmaceutical inventory management: A two-stage inventory and production model for perishable products with Markovian demand. *Health Systems*, *1*(1), 69–83. doi:10.1057/hs.2012.2

Yousefi Sarmad, M., & Pishvaee, M. S. (n.d.). A robust possibilistic Tactical Planning Model for Pharmaceutical Supply Chain under Disruption considering Lateral Transshipment and Deterioration. *2nd International Conference on Industrial & Systems Engineering (ICIS)*, 394-401.

KEY TERMS AND DEFINITIONS

Active Ingredient: An active ingredient is the ingredient in pharmaceutical drug that is biologically active.

Epistemic Uncertainty: It is an uncertainty that is related to lack of knowledge about model parameters.

Healthcare Management: It describes the leadership and general management of hospitals and other healthcare centers in order to deliver healthcare services to people.

Perishable Products: A product with short shelf life or one that easily deteriorates. These items include fresh foods, dairy product and pharmaceutical.

Pharmaceutical Industry: The pharmaceutical industry discovers, develops, produces, and markets drugs or pharmaceutical drugs for use as medications.

Pharmaceutical Supply Chain: Integrated relationships among the suppliers, producers, distributors and customers to convert raw material into drugs and medications and distribute them into hospitals, clinics and pharmacies.

Chapter 4
A Simulation Model for Resource Balancing in Healthcare Systems

Arzu Eren Şenaras
Uludag University, Turkey

Hayrettin Kemal Sezen
Uludag University, Turkey

ABSTRACT

This study aims to analyze resource effectiveness through developed model. Changing different number of resources and testing their response, appropriate number of resources can be identified as a basis of resource balancing through what-if analysis. The simulation model for emergency department is developed by Arena package program. The patient waiting times are reduced by the tested scenarios. Health care system is very expensive sector and related costs are very high. To raise service quality, number of doctor and nurse are increased but system target is provided by increased number of register clerk. Testing different scenarios, effective policy can be designed using developed simulation model. This chapter provides the readers to evaluate healthcare system using discrete event simulation. The developed model could be evaluated as a base for new implementations in other hospitals and clinics.

INTRODUCTION

The growing costs of healthcare are a major concern for healthcare providers. As healthcare organizations move towards the goals of reducing costs, optimizing patient experience, and improving health of populations; operations research tools are becoming more important. These tools provide the ability to assess trade-offs between resource utilization, quality of service, and operating costs (Lal and Roh, 2013).

The Emergency Department (ED) is the service within hospitals responsible for providing care to life threatening and other emergency cases over 24 hours daily, 7 days a week. Therefore, such departments are highly frequented by patients and this frequency is continuously increasing (Weng et al. 2011, Saghafian et al. 2012, Ghanes et al. 2014).

DOI: 10.4018/978-1-5225-2515-8.ch004

Emergency Departments (ED) are one of the most complex parts of hospitals to manage, and yet a major entry point for patients. It deals with patients without an appointment and with a wide range of illnesses. Even if most patients arriving to an ED leave the hospital after having seen a physician at the ED, a significant part of them need to be hospitalized. In many hospitals, finding available beds for unscheduled patients is extremely complicated. Even if all patients arriving at the ED do not require the same level of care, many hospitals proceed with the following policy: accept any patient until no bed is available. However, more sophisticated policies, including bed booking strategies and dynamic decisions, can lead to significant improvement of overall hospital performance (Prodel et al., 2014).

Discrete event simulation (DES) is one of the most commonly used operations research tool in healthcare. Its unique ability to account for high levels of complexity and variability that exist in the real world, along with animation capability makes it easier to illustrate and gain buy-in from physicians and other clinical providers compared to other black-box mathematical models offered by operations research. However, DES also has some limitations. In scenarios where there is a large number of stochastic input decision variables and there is little information about the structure of output function using simulation modeling by itself can be tedious and complicated. In such cases, optimization via simulation can help to maximize or minimize measures of the performance by evaluating the system using discrete event simulation (Banks et al, 2004).

DES models for healthcare facilities commonly focus on improving wait time, patient flow and management of capacity (Hamrock et al. 2014; Jacobsen et al. 2006). Although DES is adept at modeling the complex queuing structure for patients in healthcare environments, transition process variation driven by organizational and human factors is more difficult to capture mathematically. For example, analyses of patient location data used to construct DES models may find that patients are consistently waiting for servers (e.g., beds, imaging suites, clinicians) at time-points despite their availability. In the DES, queued patients would efficiently shift to open servers. However in clinical practice, transition process factors such as inefficient communication, lack of awareness of server availability, complex administrative guidelines, interruptions, and cumbersome documentation create further delays (Shi et al. 2015; Armony et al. 2010). These delays are not inherent to queuing nor well understood from time-stamped patient flow data alone. To fully capture the dynamics of healthcare facilities or any flow-based sociotechnical system, transition process variability should be understood.

Not accounting for these processes can lead to results that severely under-estimate waiting. Moreover, DES wait time distributions may be difficult to validate against the observed healthcare system. To achieve sufficient validation, the model developer may be motivated to input additive time intervals to patients at transition points that are drawn from a distribution representing the difference between the current model and observed waits (Shi et al. 2015). A more in-depth approach, borrowed from lean methods, may motivate the model developer to map out the transition process and measure or elicit expert estimates of time distributions for each component; independent value of this investigation exists (Kang et al. 2014; Simon and Canacari 2012).

The aim of this paper is to develop methods to identify efficient hospitalization admission control policies for the emergency department patients.

LITERATURE REVIEW

It is impossible and impractical to have a whole hospital DES model that includes everything in a hospital: all models are simplifications (Pidd, 2003). An appropriate level of abstraction and scope must be chosen when attempting whole hospital simulation. The literature has very few examples of such studies. Surprisingly, though, Fetter and Thompson (1965) is a very early example of DES that reports a whole hospital simulation, with a special interest in maternity processes. The aim of this work was to give a decision support tool to hospital administrations to predict the consequences of design changes and alternative policies. They created three models of hospital subsystems: (1) maternity suite, (2) a surgical pavilion, and (3) an outpatient clinic. The maternity model was used to analyze patient load and bed occupancy (Gunal & Pidd, 2010: 46). Recent examples of application of this method in healthcare include study of Sundaramoorthi (2010), where this technique was used to plan nurse resource allocation to patients based on workload needs. Ahmed (2009) used simulation based optimization to design a decision support tool to determine the optimal number of doctors and other staff to maximize the number of patients seen. Ferrand et al. (2010) have compared two distinct resource-allocation policies to handle the flow of scheduled elective surgeries and unpredictable emergency surgeries. The flexible policy is the historical way of assigning patients to operating rooms. Under the flexible policy, emergency surgeries access any operating room and have priority over electives. The new policy provides the surgeon with more focus as the operating rooms are divided into two subsets and patients access the subset of rooms that corresponds to their type, either elective or emergency. Roberts (2011), recognizes that in healthcare it is often difficult to define a single performance characteristic. Especially in healthcare further investigation is often needed to understand how a change in the process leads to downstream impact. Hence simulation is considered an ideal technique to be used. Zhang (2012) applied this integrated approach to determine the staffing requirements of a long term care facility. Tan et al. (2013) presented an integrated framework for dynamic queue management from both demand and supply perspectives. Their experimental analysis showed that the demand-side strategies work seamlessly with both static and dynamic strategies of the supply-side. Likewise, supply-side strategies are performing well with each demand-side strategies. In addition, the dynamic staffing (supply of doctors) can adapt to demand surges or cut cost when demand is reduced. The integrated framework allows healthcare decision makers to play a role in achieving the desired service quality and select from a list of possible strategies that suit the operation needs of the ED. Ghanes et al (2014), proposed a Discrete Event Simulation (DES) model for an emergency department (ED). The model was developed in close collaboration with the French hospital Saint Camille, and is validated using real data. The objective of this model is to help ED managers better understand the behavior of the system and to improve the ED operations performance. Using DES in Arena software, they have built a realistic ED model taking into account all common structural and functional characteristics of at least French EDs. Their experiments focused on human staffing levels and provided useful insights to decision makers.

Espinoza et al. (2014) studied the impact of the model's ability to predict ER performance with a limited amount of input information, such that what-if questions may be asked to guide decision making. Towards this end, two input data scenarios are compared to a case of perfect information. One scenario considers only patient arrival times and the other assumes additional knowledge of patient care pathways. Although both generate similar performance measures, the case with least information yields a slightly worse estimate of patient care pathway composition. This project studies two different cases of real-time data obtained from an ER patient workflow, each representing less or more information useful to feed a discrete event simulation model of an emergency room. Moon et al. (2015) introduces EMSSim that is an agent-based simulation of emergency medical services during disasters. We developed EMSSim to encompass the disaster victims' pass-ways from their rescues to their definitive care. This modeling scope resulted that our model delivers the detailed geographical and medical modeling which are often modeled separately. This is an effort to fill the gap between the prehospital delivery and the in-hospital care over the disaster period. They specified the model with a variant of the dynamic DEVS formalism so that the complex models could be better understood and utilized by others. Also, we suggest a modeling approach to create a profile with mathematical modeling on the victims' survival rates, which would enable our models to simulate the effectiveness of the treatments by the responders. Finally, they provide a case study of virtual experiments that analyzes the sensitivity of rescue performances by varying the disaster response resources. Frank et al (2015) have compared two different configurations in two different geriatric hospitals. The integrated care scenario (Saint-Etienne hospital) means that Short Stay and Rehabilitative Care are both in the same department and separated scenario (Clermont-Ferrand hospital) means that both services are located in different departments. They used Discrete Event Simulation to evaluate both scenarios and a design of experiment to study the impact of the bed ratio in SS and RC. The model uses a data collection (one year of hospitalization) from the Saint-Etienne Hospital. Performance indicators are occupancy rates, admissions (admitted or refused), number of waiting patient, total LOS and total transfer time. Then a cost analysis considering the French hospital funding system was performed. The most interesting configuration is the one with integrated care. Lal et al (2015) discussed the methodology and applications of simulation based optimization, highlighting advantages, challenges and opportunities of using this method in healthcare. They summarized the needs of simulation based optimization in healthcare. They also introduce the key concepts and practical implications of using simulation based optimization to help the users identify the need and model the problems appropriately. Levin and Garifullin (2015) describe a novel method to integrate regression models for survival data in DES capable of quantifying the drivers of transition processes to estimate wait time. These methods are illustrated by example within a large hospital DES. Pepino et al. (2015) proposed a prototype simulation of a hospital ward which permits the study of the workload and task distribution among nursing and auxiliary personnel. In our study, we took both X a generic ward in a complex healthcare structure and a case study of a hospital immunology department as reference models. Both analyses were carried out together with a team of expert head nurses and following a specific simulation model developed in the Simul8 environment, which allowed the calculation of patient assistance timing as well as the efficiency of personnel use depending on the patient autonomy.

DISCRETE EVENT SIMULATION

We will define simulation as the process of designing a model of a real system and conducting experiments with this model for the purpose of understanding the behavior of the system and /or evaluating various strategies for the operation of the system. Thus it is critical that the model be designed in such a way that the model behavior mimics the response behavior of the real system to events that take place over time. The term's model and system are key components of our definition of simulation. By a model we mean a representation of a group of objects or ideas in some form other than that of the entity itself. By a system we mean a group or collection of interrelated elements that cooperate to accomplish some stated objective. One of the real strengths of simulation is the fact that we can simulate systems that already exist as well as those that are capable of being brought into existence, i.e. those in the preliminary or planning stage of development (Shannon, 1998: 7).

Simulation is one of the most powerful analysis tools available to those responsible for the design and operation of complex process or systems. In an increasingly competitive world, simulation has become a very powerful tool for the planning, design, and control of systems (Pegden, 1990).

We consider simulation to include both the construction of the model and the experimental use of the model for studying a problem. Thus, we can think of simulation modeling as an experimental and applied methodology, which seeks to (Shannon, 1998: 7):

- Describe the behavior of a system.
- Use the model to predict future behavior, i.e. the effects that will be produced by changes in the system or in its method of operation.

The majority of modern computer simulation tools implement a paradigm, called discrete-event simulation (DES). This paradigm is so general and powerful that it provides an implementation framework for most simulation languages, regardless of the user worldview supported by them (Altiok & Melamed, 2007: 11).

Discrete event systems simulation is the modeling of systems in which the state variable changes only at a discrete set of points in time (Banks et al, 2005: 13). In a discrete model, though, change can occur only at separated points in time, such as a manufacturing system with parts arriving and leaving at specific times, machines going down and coming back up at specific times, and breaks for workers (Kelton & Sadowski, 2004: 9).

The simulation event list is a means of keeping track of the different things that occur during a simulation run (Law & Kelton, 2000). Anything that occurs during the simulation run that can affect the state of the system is defined as an event. Typical events in a simple simulation include entity arrivals to the queue, the beginning of service times for entities, and the ending of service times for entities. These events change the state of the system because they can increase or decrease the number of entities in the system or queue or change the state of the resources between idle and busy. The event list is controlled by advances in the simulation clock. In our basic simulation model, the simulation clock advances in discrete jumps to each event on the event list. This type of model is called a discrete event simulation (Chung, 2004: 10).

A Discrete Event Simulation simulator executes the following algorithm (Altiok and Melamed, 2007: 12):

1. Set the simulation clock to an initial time (usually 0), and then generate one or more initial events and schedule them.
2. If the event list is empty, terminate the simulation run. Otherwise, find the most imminent event and unlink it from the event list.
3. Advance the simulation clock to the time of the most imminent event, and execute it (the event may stop the simulation).
4. Loop back to Step 2.

Although discrete event simulation could conceptually be done by hand calculations, the amount of data that must be stored and manipulated for most real-world systems dictates that discrete event simulations need to be done on a digital computer (Law & Kelton, 2000: 6).

Steps in Simulation Study

The essence or purpose of simulation modeling is to help the ultimate decision-maker solve a problem. Therefore, to learn to be a good simulation modeler, you must merge good problem solving techniques with good software engineering practice (Shannon, 1998: 9).

The steps in simulation study are as follows (Banks et al, 2005: 14-18; Shannon, 1998:9):

- **Problem Formulation:** Clearly defining the goals of the study so that we know the purpose, i.e. why are we studying this problem and what questions do we hope to answer? Every study should begin with a statement of the problem. If the statement is provided by the policymakers, or those that have the problem, the analyst must ensure that the problem being described is clearly understood. If a problem statement is being developed by the analyst, it is important that the policymakers understand and agree with the formulation.
- **Setting of Objectives and Overall Project Plan:** The objectives indicate the questions to be answered by simulation. At this point, a determination should be made concerning whether simulation is the appropriate methodology for the problem as formulated and objectives as stated.
- **Model Conceptualization:** The art of modeling is enhanced by an ability to abstract the essential features of a problem, to select and modify basic assumptions that characterize the system, and then to enrich and elaborate the model until a useful approximation results.
- **Data Collection:** There is a constant interplay between the construction of the model and the collection of the needed input data (Shannon, 1975). As the complexity of the model changes, the required data elements can also change. Also, since data collection takes such a large portion of the total time required to perform a simulation, it is necessary to begin it as possible, usually together with the early stages of model building.
- **Model Translation:** Most real-world systems result in models that require a great deal of information storage and cumputation, so the model be entered into a computer-recognizable format. We use the term "program" even though it is possible to accomplish the desired result in many instances with little or no actual coding.
- **Verified:** Verification pertains to the computer program prepared for the simulation model. Is the computer program performing properly? With complex models, it is difficult, if not impossible, to translate a model successfully in its entirety without a good deal of debugging; if the input parameters and logical structure of the model are correctly represented in the computer, verification has been completed.
- **Validated:** Validation usually is achieved through the calibration of the model, an iterative process of comparing the model against actual system behavior and using the discrepancies between the two, and the insight gained, to improve the model. This process is repeated until model accuracy is judged acceptable.
- **Experimental Design:** The alternatives that are to be simulated must be determined.
- **Production Runs and Analysis:** Production runs, and their subsequent analysis, are used to estimate measures of performance for the system designs that are being simulated.

- **More Runs:** Given the analysis of runs that have been completed, the analyst determines whether additional runs are needed and what design those additional experiments should follow.
- **Documentation and Reporting:** There are two types of documentation: program and progress. Program documentation is necessary for numerous reasons. If the program is going to be used again by the same or different analyst, it could be necessary to understand how the program operates. Musselman (1998) discuss progress reports that provide the important, written history of a simulation project. Project reports give a chronology of work done and decision made.
- **Implementation:** The success of the implementation phase depends on how well the previous 11 steps. It is also contingent upon how thoroughly the analyst has involved the ultimate model user during the entire simulation process.

Advantages and Disadvantages of Simulation

Simulation is a widely used and increasingly popular method for studying complex systems. Some possible advantages of simulation that may account for its widespread appeal are the following (Law and Kelton, 2000: 91-92):

- Most complex, real-world systems with stochastic elements cannot be accurately described by a mathematical model that can be evaluated analytically. Thus, a simulation is often the only type of investigation possible.
- Simulation allows us to estimate the performance of an existing system under some projected set of operating conditions.
- Alternative proposed system designs can be compared via simulation to see which best meets a specified requirement.
- In a simulation we can maintain much better control over experimental conditions than would generally be possible when experimenting with the system itself.
- Simulation allows us to study a system with a long time frame.

Simulation is not without its drawbacks. Some disadvantages are as follows:

- Each run of stochastic simulation model produces only estimates of a model's true characteristics for a particular set of input parameters. Thus, several independent runs of the model will probably be required for each set of input parameters to be studied. For this reason, simulation models are generally not as good at optimization as they are at comparing a fixed number of specified alternative system designs. On the other hand, an analytic model, if appropriate, can often easily produce the exact true characteristics of that model for a variety of sets of input parameters. Thus, if a "valid" analytic model is available or can easily be developed, it will generally be preferable to a simulation model.
- Simulation models are often expensive and time-consuming to develop.
- The large volume of numbers produced by a simulation study or the persuasive impact of a realistic animation often creates a tendency to place greater confidence in a study's results than is justified. If a model is not a "valid" representation of a system under study, the simulation results, no matter how impressive they appear, will provide little useful information about the actual system.

A Simulation Concept

Although there are several different types of simulation methodologies, we will limit our concerns to a stochastic, discrete, process oriented approach. In such an approach, we model a particular system by studying the flow of entities that move through that system. Entities can be customers, job orders, particular parts, information packets, etc. An entity can be any object that enters the system, moves through a series of processes, and then leaves the system. These entities can have individual characteristics which we will call attributes. An attribute is associated with the specific, individual entity. Attributes might be such things as name, priority, due date, required CPU time, ailment, account number etc. As the entity flows through the system, it will be processed by a series of resources. Resources are anything that the entity needs in order to be processed. For example, resources might be workers, material handling equipment, special tools, a hospital bed, access to the CPU, a machine, waiting or storage space, etc. Resources may be fixed in one location (e.g. a heavy machine, bank teller, hospital bed) or moving about the system (e.g. a forklift, repairman, doctor). A simulation model is therefore a computer program which represents the logic of the system as entities with attributes arrive, join queues to await the assignment of required resources, are processed by the resources, released and exit the system. In addition to the logic of how an entity flows through the system, the computer program keeps track of and advances time, as well as keeping track of resource utilization, time spent in queues, time in the system (processing time), and other desired statistics. Much of what happens in the system is probabilistic or stochastic in nature. For example the time between arrivals, the time for a resource to process the entity, the time to travel from one part of the system to another and whether a part passes inspection or not, are usually all random variables. It is these types of data for input to the model that are difficult to obtain (Shannon, 1998: 8).

Components and Organization of a Discrete Event Simulation

The following components will be found in most discrete event simulation models using the next event time advance approach programmed in a general purpose language (Law and Kelton, 2000):

- **System State:** The collection of state variables necessary to describe the system at a particular time.
- **Simulation Clock:** A variable giving the current value of simulated time.
- **Event List:** A list containing the next time when each type of event will occur.
- **Statistical Counters:** Variables used for storing statistical information about system performance.
- **Initialization Routine:** A subprogram to initialize the simulation model at time 0.
- **Timing Routine:** A subprogram that determines the next event from the event list and then advances the simulation clock to the time when that event is to occur.
- **Event Routine:** A subprogram that updates the system state when a particular type of event occurs (there is one event routine for each event type).
- **Library Routines:** A set of subprograms used to generate random observations from probability distributions that were determined as part of the simulation model.
- **Report Generator:** A subprogram that computes estimates (from the statistical counters) of the desired measures of performance and produces a report when the simulation ends.

- **Main Program:** A subprogram that invokes the timing routine to determine the next event and then transfers control to the corresponding event routine to update the system state appropriately. The main program may also check for termination and invoke the report generator when the simulation is over.

Areas of Application

The applications of simulation are vast. The Winter Simulation Conference (WSC) is an excellent way to learn more about the latest in simulation applications and theory. Some presentations, by area, from a recent WSC are listed next (Banks et al, 2005; Sezen and Günal, 2009):

- Manufacturing Applications
- Semiconductor Manufacturing
- Construction Engineering and Project Management
- Military Applications
- Logistics, Supply Chain, and Distribution Applications
- Transportation Modes and Traffic
- Business Process Simulation
- Health Care

CASE STUDY

In this study, an investigated emergency department is found in a second stage public hospital in Turkey. To begin our study, all patients who come to hospital are entity and our resources are doctors, nurses, and lab technicians, registration clerks and X ray technicians.

The hospital that is investigated in this study is located in a town. Its population is 157000. In this town there is only one state hospital. Apart from this state hospital, the town has two private hospitals.

Problem Description

To begin simulation study, conceptual understanding of the system must be done. When a patient arrives to emergency department, if there is a life-threatening condition, she/he is accepted to resuscitated zone without registration. If there isn't a life-threatening condition; registration of patient must be done. Pendant registration patient is classified as red or green and patient priority change according to this classification. When a patient is red, first nurse accepts patient and she realizes her first controls and medical examination is done by a doctor. After medical examination doctor asks patient to go to the lab or X-ray area, or ask nurse to apply a cure to patient. If patient's classification is green, than his priority is less then the patient whose classification is red; patient wait for a doctor and after doctor examination nurse can apply a cure according to the doctor decision or he can go to the lab or he can leave system.

If a patient goes to the lab or X-ray room, he/she waits in the queue. Patient waits also given her/his results. Then he/she returns to the examination room and doctor decides which cure nurse applies. After treatment patient passes observations room. In observation room, patient's keeping is done by nurses. When observation time is up, patient waits for doctor for last examination and then patient goes to the registration office and then leave system.

Simulation Model

Based on gathered data simulation model is built. System includes many stochastic variables such as arrivals time and service time. Some assumptions and simplification must be made. First in emergence department there is no appointment rule. Patient can arrive to emergency department through ambulance or by his own. Service time is in general triangular or normal. Based on gathered data arrivals time are fitted to exponential distribution with parameter 7.2 minutes. Patient with life threating condition is the %3,2 of patient. Service time for these patients is triangle with parameter 10, 20, 30. In fact after first intervention patient leaves system to enter intensive care department. Patients without life threating condition pass registration stage. Registration time is fitted to normal distribution with mean 3,2 and standard deviation 1,3. In registration, %23 of the patient are classified as red, the rest is green. For patient in red class, nurse service time is fitted to normal distribution with mean 3,2 and standard deviation is 0,5; doctor service time is fitted to triangular (4.2, 5.7, 9.1). %40 of this part of patient goes to lab and the rest wait for nurse to treat. Nurse service time is fitted to triangular (3.5, 7.5, 9.7) and patient passes to observation room. For patients in green class, their priority in queue is second. Their examination is realized by a doctor. Doctor service time is fitted to normal distribution with mean 7.3 mn and std is 2,5 mn. %40 of patients in green class leave system; %20 go to the lab and the rest wait for nurse to treat. Test and diagnosis part consists of Lab and X ray .X ray service time is fitted to normal (2.5, 0.8) and lab service time is fitted to normal distribution with parameter(10.1, 3.2) after lab operation ;we assume that patient must wait 15mn for test results. When patient takes results, patient returns to examination room to show his test results to doctor. Doctor's service time is fitted to triangular distribution (3.1, 7.2, 8.6). At the end of doctor examination, doctor decides either let patient to leave or send patient to observation room. In observation room, a nurse visits patient every 15 minutes and before patient leaves the observation rooms, a doctor gives approval. Doctor service time is fitted to triangular (1.8, 3.5, 5.6). To leave system, patient must visit registration office and registers clerk service time is fitted to normal distribution with parameter mean 5,2 minute and standard deviation is 2,1.

Simulation model was developed by Arena package program. The following commands are used in developed simulation model: Create, Assign, Branch, Seize, Release, Route, Delay, Station, Queue and Dispose.

Simulation Results

Simulation model runs for 1000 minutes and 100 minutes is assumed to warm up period. To initialize our system we begin with all resources with 1 capacity. Table 1 shows the number of resources for scenario 1.

Simulation model's results show that 118 patients came to the emergency service and 75 patients leave system during simulation. Table 2 shows the utilization rates of resources for scenario 1.

The Average number of patients waiting for doctor in green class for first examination is 8,5 . Then number of doctor is increased. Number of resources, utilization rate and number of patients that leave system are shown below. Table 3 shows the utilization rates of resources for scenario 2. 87 patient leave the system.

Table 1. Number of Resources for Scenario 1

Resource Name	Number of Resources
Doctor	1
Register Clerk	1
Nurse	1
X-ray technician	1
Lab.Tech	1

Table 2. Utilization rate for Scenario 1

Resource Name	Utilization
Doctor	% 94,96
Register Clerk	% 81,95
Nurse	% 89,70
X-ray technician	% 2,00
Lab. Tech	% 6,32

87 patients leave the system. Number of patients who wait for nurse in observation room is 5,23 in average and at the end of simulation 23 patients wait for nurse in this room. So number of nurses is increased. Table 4 shows the utilization rates of resources for scenario 3.

83 patients leave system. Number of nurse is increased one in scenario 3. Therefore utilization rate of nurse decreased to (1,15/2) 57,5. Number of doctor is increased to 3 in Scenario 4. Table 5 shows the utilization rates of resources for scenario 4.

89 patients leave system. Number of doctors is increased one in scenario 4. Therefore utilization rate of doctor is decreased to (1,15/3) 35. Table 6 shows the utilization rates of resources for scenario 5.

85 patients leave system. Number of nurse is increased one in scenario 5. Therefore utilization rate of doctor is decreased to (0,99/3) 33. Table 7 shows the utilization rates of resources for scenario 6. Number of nurses is increased one in scenario 6.

88 patients leave system. Table 8 shows the utilization rates of resources for scenario 7. Number of doctors is increased one in scenario 7.

Table 3. Utilization rate for Scenario 2

Resource Name	Number of Resources	Utilization
Doctor	2	1,10
Register Clerk	1	0,89
Nurse	1	0,94
X-ray technician	1	0,01
Lab.Tech	1	0,07

Table 4. Utilization rate for Scenario 3

Resource Name	Number of Resources	Utilization
Doctor	2	1,21
Register Clerk	1	0,86
Nurse	2	1,15
X-ray technician	1	0,01
Lab.Tech	1	0,04

Table 5. Utilization rate for Scenario 4

Resource Name	Number of Resources	Utilization
Doctor	3	1,15
Register Clerk	1	0,88
Nurse	2	1,02
X-ray technician	1	0,03
Lab.Tech	1	0,05

Table 6. Utilization rate for Scenario 5

Resource Name	Number of Resources	Utilization
Doctor	3	1,23
Register Clerk	1	0,90
Nurse	3	0,99
X-ray techniciantechnician	1	0,01
Lab.Tech	1	0,05

Table 7. Utilization rate for Scenario 6

Resource Name	Number of Resources	Utilization
Doctor	3	1,19
Register Clerk	1	0,89
Nurse	4	1,13
X-ray techniciantechnician	1	0,02
Lab.Tech	1	0,03

Table 8. Utilization rate for Scenario 7

Resource Name	Number of Resources	Utilization
Doctor	4	1,19
Register Clerk	1	0,88
Nurse	4	1,10
X-ray technician	1	0,01
Lab.Tech	1	0,04

86 patients leave system. Number of nurse is increased one in scenario 8. Table 9 shows the utilization rates of resources for scenario 8.

86 patients leave system. Number of nurse is increased one in scenario 9. Table 10 shows the utilization rates of resources for scenario 9.

86 patients leave system. Number of doctor is increased one in scenario 10. Table 11 shows the utilization rates of resources for scenario 10.

111 patients leave system. Number of register clerks is increased one in scenario 11. Table 12 shows the utilization rates of resources for scenario 11.

113 patients leave system. Number of doctors is decreased to three in scenario 12. Table 13 shows the utilization rates of resources for scenario 12.

114 patients leave system. Number of nurse is decreased to four in scenario 13. Table 14 shows the utilization rates of resources for scenario 13.

Table 9. Utilization rate for Scenario 8

Resource Name	Number of Resources	Utilization
Doctor	5	1,14
Register Clerk	1	0,88
Nurse	4	1,01
X-ray technician	1	0,01
Lab.Tech	1	0,04

Table 10. Utilization rate for Scenario 9

Resource Name	Number of Resources	Utilization
Doctor	5	1,14
Register Clerk	1	0,88
Nurse	5	1,01
X-ray technician	1	0,01
Lab.Tech	1	0,04

Table 11. Utilization rate for Scenario 10

Resource Name	Number of Resources	Utilization
Doctor	6	1,18
Register Clerk	1	0,88
Nurse	5	1,05
X-ray technician	1	0,02
Lab.Tech	1	0,03

Table 12. Utilization rate for Scenario 11

Resource Name	Number of Resources	Utilization
Doctor	6	1,22
Register Clerk	2	1,01
Nurse	5	1,06
X-ray technician	1	0,01
Lab.Tech	1	0,07

Table 13. Utilization rate for Scenario 12

Resource Name	Number of Resources	Utilization
Doctor	3	1,28
Register Clerk	2	1,03
Nurse	5	1,09
X-ray technician	1	0,03
Lab.Tech	1	0,07

Table 14. Utilization rate for Scenario 13

Resource Name	Number of Resources	Utilization
Doctor	3	1,30
Register Clerk	2	1,05
Nurse	4	1,15
X-ray technician	1	0,02
Lab.Tech	1	0,09

As a result of scenario 13; utilization rate of doctor is (1,3/3) %43, utilization rate of register clerk is %52,5, utilization rate of nurse is (1,15/4) %28,7, utilization rate of x-ray technician is %2, utilization rate of lab.tech is % 9.

CONCLUSION

The simulation model for emergency department is developed by Arena package program. The patient waiting times are reduced by the tested scenarios. This chapter provides the readers to evaluate healthcare systems using discrete event simulation. The developed model could be evaluated as a base for new implementations in other hospitals and clinics.

From scenario 1 to scenario 10, number of doctors and nurses are increased but service quality and number of patients does not increase. At scenario 11, number of register clerks is increased to 2 and service quality and number of patient who leave system rise. On the other hand utilization of X-ray technician and lab tech is very low. If it is possible, for 2 responsibilities using same staff will increase effectiveness of the system.

Health care system is very expensive sector and related costs are very high. To raise service quality, number of doctors and nurses are increased but system target is provided by increased number of register clerk. Testing different scenarios, effective policy can be designed using developed simulation model.

REFERENCES

Alessandro, P., Adriano, T., Annunziata, M., & Oscar, T. (2015). A Simulation Model For Analyzing The Nurse Workload In A University Hospital Ward. *Proceedings of the 2015 Winter Simulation Conference.*

Altiok, T., & Melamed, B. (2007). Simulation Modeling and Analysis with Arena. Academic Press.

Armony, M., Shlomo, I., Mandelbaum, A., Marmor, Y., Tseytlin, Y., & Yom-Tov, G. (2010). *On Patient Flow in Hospitals: A Data-Based Queuing-Science Perspective.* Working paper. New York University.

Banks, J., Carson, J. S., Nelson, B. L., & Nicol, D. M. (2004). *Discrete-Event System Simulation* (4th ed.). Upper Saddle River, NJ: Prentice-Hall, Inc.

Camila, E., Francisco, R., Jimena, P., & Daniel, B. (2014). Real-Time Simulation As A Way To Improve Daily Operations In An Emergency Room. *Proceedings of the 2014 Winter Simulation Conference.*

Chung, C. A. (2004). *Simulation Modeling Handbook A Practical Approach*. CRC Press.

Fetter, R. B., & Thompson, J. D. (1965). The Simulation Of Hospital Systems. *Opns Res*, *13*(5), 689–711. doi:10.1287/opre.13.5.689

Garifullin. (2015). *Simulating Wait Time In Healthcare: Accounting For Transition Process Variability Using Survival Analyses*. Academic Press.

Günal, M., & Pidd, M. (2010). Discrete event simulation for Performance Modelling in Health care: A review of the Literature. *Journal of Simulation*, *4*(1), 42–51. doi:10.1057/jos.2009.25

Hamrock, E., Paige, K., Parks, J., Scheulen, J., & Levin, S. (2012). Discrete Event Simulation for Healthcare Organizations: A Tool for Decision Making. *Journal of Healthcare Management*, *58*(2), 110–124. PMID:23650696

Il-Chul, M., Won, B. J., Junseok, L., Doyun, K., Hyunrok, L., Taesik, L., & Woon, K. G. et al. (2015). EMSSIM: Emergency Medical Service Simulator With Geographic And Medical Details. *Proceedings of the 2015 Winter Simulation Conference*.

Jacobsen, S., Hall, S., & Swisher, J. (2006). Discrete-Event Simulation of Health Care Systems. In R. Hall (Ed.), *Patient Flow: Reducing Delay in Healthcare Delivery* (pp. 211–252). Springer. doi:10.1007/978-0-387-33636-7_8

Kang, H., Nembhard, H., Rafferty, C., & DeFlitch, C. (2014). Patient Flow In The Emergency Department: A Classification And Analysis Of Admission Process Policies. *Annals of Emergency Medicine*, *64*(4), 335–342. doi:10.1016/j.annemergmed.2014.04.011 PMID:24875896

Karim, G., Oualid, J., Zied, J., Mathias, W., Romain, H., Valérie, T., & Ger, K. (2014). A Comprehensive Simulation Modeling Of An Emergency Department: A Case Study For Simulation Optimization Of Staffing Levels. *Proceedings of the 2014 Winter Simulation Conference*.

Kelton, W. D., Sadowski, R. P., & Sadowski, D. A. (2004). *Simulation with Arena*. McGraw Hill.

Lal Mohan, T., & Roh, T. (2013). Simulation in Healthcare. In J. A. Larson (Ed.), *A Book Management Engineering: A Guide to Best Practices for Industrial Engineering in Health Care* (1st ed.). Taylor and Francis Group.

Law, A. M. (2007). *Simulation Modeling and Analysis* (4th ed.). McGraw Hill.

Law, A. M., & Kelton, W. D. (2000). *Simulation Modeling and Analysis* (3rd ed.). New York: McGraw-Hill, Inc.

Martin, P., Vincent, A., & Xiaolan, X. (2014). Hospitalization Admission Control Of Emergency Patients Using Markovian Decision Processes And Discrete Event Simulation. *Proceedings of the 2014 Winter Simulation Conference*.

Mohan, L. T., Thomas, R., & Todd, H. (2015). Simulation Based Optimization: Applications In Healthcare. *Proceedings of the 2015 Winter Simulation Conference*.

Pegden, C. D. (1990). *Introduction to Simulation Using SIMAN*. McGraw-Hill, Inc.

Pidd, M. (2003). *Tools for Thinking: Modelling in Management Science* (2nd ed.). Chichester, UK: Wiley.

Roberts, S. D. (2011). Tutorial on the Simulation of Healthcare Systems. In *Proceedings of the 2011 Winter Simulation Conference*. Piscataway, NJ: Institute of Electrical and Electronics Engineers, Inc. doi:10.1109/WSC.2011.6147860

Saghafian, S., Hopp, W. J., Van Oyen, M. P., Desmond, J. S., & Kronick, S. L. (2012). Patient Streaming as a Mechanism for Improving Responsiveness in Emergency Departments. *Operations Research*, *60*(5), 1080–1097. doi:10.1287/opre.1120.1096

Sezen, H. K., & Günal, M. M. (2009). *Yöneylem Araştırmasında Benzetim*. Bursa: Ekin Yayınevi.

Shannon, R. E. (1975). *Systems Simulation: The Art and Science*. Prentice-Hall.

Shannon, R. E. (1998). Introduction To The Art And Science Of Simulation. *Proceedings of the 1998 Winter Simulation Conference*. doi:10.1109/WSC.1998.744892

Shi, P., Chou, M., Dai, J., Ding, D., & Sim, J. (2015). Models and Insights for Hospital Inpatient Operations: Time Dependent ED Boarding Time. *Management Science*, *24*, 13–14.

Simon, R., & Canacari, E. (2012). A Practical Guide to Applying Lean Tools and Management Principles to Health Care Improvement Projects. *Association of Perioperative Registered Nurses Journal*, *95*(1), 85–100. doi:10.1016/j.aorn.2011.05.021 PMID:22201573

Thomas, F., Regis, G., Vincent, A., Xiaolan, X., & Emilie, A. (2015). Performance Evaluation Of An Integrated Care For Geriatric Departments Using Discrete-Event Simulation. *Proceedings of the 2015 Winter Simulation Conference*.

Way, T. K., Lau, H. C., & Lee, F. C. Y. (2013). Improving Patient Length-Of-Stay In Emergency Department Through Dynamic Queue Management. *Proceedings of the 2013 Winter Simulation Conference*.

Weng, S.-J., Cheng, B.-C., Kwong, S. T., Wang, L.-M., & Chang, C.-Y. (2011). Simulation Optimization for Emergency Department Resources Allocation. In *Proceedings of the 2011 Winter Simulation Conference*. Piscataway, NJ: Institute of Electrical and Electronics Engineers. doi:10.1109/WSC.2011.6147845

Yann, F., Michael, M., & Uday, R. (2010). Comparing Two Operating Room Allocation Policies For Elective And Emergency Surgeries. *Proceedings of the 2010 Winter Simulation Conference*.

KEY TERMS AND DEFINITIONS

Computer Simulation: Reproducing the behavior of a system using a mathematical model.

Discrete Event Simulation: DES is the modeling of systems in which the state variable changes only at a discrete set of points in time.

Discrete Model: Change can occur only at separated points in time.

Event List: A list containing the next time when each type of event will occur.

Simulation Clock: A variable giving the current value of simulated time.

Validation: Validation usually is achieved through the calibration of the model, an iterative process of comparing the model against actual system behavior and using the discrepancies between the two, and the insight gained, to improve the model. This process is repeated until model accuracy is judged acceptable.

Verification: Verification pertains to the computer program prepared for the simulation model. Is the computer program performing properly? With complex models, it is difficult, if not impossible; to translate a model successfully in its entirety without a good deal of debugging; if the input parameters and logical structure of the model are correctly represented in the computer, verification has been completed.

Chapter 5
The Applications of Simulation Modeling in Emergency Departments:
A Review

Soraia Oueida
American University of the Middle East, Kuwait

Seifedine Kadry
Beirut Arab University, Lebanon

Pierre Abichar
American University of the Middle East, Kuwait

Sorin Ionescu
Politehnica of Bucharest, Romania

ABSTRACT

A recent study carried out an empirical investigation of the quality of healthcare delivered to adults and found out that only 54.9±0.6% adult received recommended care. Huge variation in the quality of care depends on patient's condition. In fact, the literature on healthcare is laden with articles like these that emphasize on the importance of the systems view of healthcare problems. Healthcare is a very vast and complex system where different departments interact with each other in order to deliver a certain service to arriving patients. Emergency departments (EDs) are the busiest units of healthcare. Existing problems and their cascading effect will be highlighted by a literature review of a bunch of researches. The purpose of this work is to study, in specific, the emergency department of a hospital with the existing problems and how simulation modeling can interfere in order to solve these problems, increase patient satisfaction and reduce cost. Simulation has emerged as a popular decision support in the domains of manufacturing and services industries.

DOI: 10.4018/978-1-5225-2515-8.ch005

INTRODUCTION

The medical sector has been growing largely over the last decade and healthcare services became more complex and costly, amplified by a poor healthcare delivery system. Healthcare is a highly interconnected dynamic environment where individuals and teams contribute in order to serve patients' demand. The main focus of this study is to discuss this revolution and take care of the whole medical community not only illness, but also improving patient safety, quality, and effectiveness of the healthcare system. This can be achieved by developing new methodologies to improve the health care systems available nowadays.

Many methodologies were presented over the literature in order to study healthcare problems. Some of them are listed as follows (Ceglowski, 2006):

- Patients are grouped by clinicians under several cases; where similar cases should be treated alike and should share the same type of resources every time the same case arises (see Palmer, 1996). This approach can be valuable only in case of few available cases such as in clinics not in large complex systems like ED.
- Time and motion studies were used by industrial engineering analysts in order to introduce enhancement to healthcare (see Hoffenberg et al., 2001).
- Prevention of high patient waiting times and ambulance diversions were discussed over the years and simulation was introduced in order to alleviate this risk (see Jun et al., 1999; Preater, 2002).
- The flow of data in the ED was studied by information science analysts in order to design a computer system that supports the doctors and nurses in their roles (see Nelson et al., 2004).
- ED data inspection for better knowledge of information retrieved.

As a result of the above, the first area to focus on in order to develop an efficient and effective healthcare system is developing systems perspective, where simulation modeling can be generated and a review can be achieved. Simulation modeling can be a solution to tackle this complexity and valuable in providing predictions to forecast the outcome of a change in strategies or policies. The computer simulation is a decision making technique that allows management to conduct experiments with models representing the real system of interest. Busy and complex healthcare systems provide big challenges to managers and decision makers who should be able to serve the high demands constrained by limited budget and high costs of healthcare services. The highest number of patients should be cared of within a limited period of time in order to insure patient satisfaction (reduce waiting time) and increase hospital's revenue (reduce cost).

The delivery of healthcare quality can vary depending on patient's conditions, affecting the recommended care and leading sometimes to urgent and critical health conditions. This huge variation opens the eye on the importance of reviewing the healthcare systems' problems and improving them.

Emergency department (ED) is the most complex, critical and busy unit of a hospital, where medical facility treatment is provided to patients without prior appointment. Other reasons for ED to be a complex system and chosen, specifically, for this study are the high increase in patients' number, the 24/7 operation of the ED, and the open facility to all type of illness and all level of patients. EDs interact with the majority of other departments of the healthcare system. Table 1 shows this interaction. A patient arriving to the ED may be transferred to any other unit of the hospital depending on the diagnosis (such as requiring extra facilities: laboratory, imaging, etc., admission to hospital, referring to surgery unit if a surgery is scheduled, referring to pediatric unit in case the patient arriving is a kid/baby, etc.).

Table 1. ED and interacting departments

	ED	Anesthetics	ICU	Surgery	Cardiology	Radiology	ENT	Genecology/Maternity	Pediatric	Laboratory	Hematology	Microbiology	Neonatal	Nephrology	Neurology	Oncology	Ophthalmology	Orthopedics	Physiotherapy	Dentistry	Dermatology	Gastroenterology	Nutrition	Pharmacy	Admission & Discharge
ED		x	x	x	x	x	x	x	x	x	x	x	x	x	x	x	x	x	x	X	x	x	x	x	x
Anesthetics	x		x	x																					
ICU	x	x		x						x														x	x
Surgery	x		x			x				x									x						x
Cardiology	x			x		x				x														x	x
Radiology	x																							x	
ENT	x			x		x				x														x	x
Genecology/Maternity	x									x									x					x	x
Pediatric	x									x														x	
Laboratory	x																								
Hematology	x									x														x	
Microbiology	x			x						x															
Neonatal	x							X		x														x	x
Nephrology	x			x						x														x	x
Neurology	x		x	x		x				x														x	x
Oncology	x			x		x				x														x	x
Ophthalmology	x			x																				x	x
Orthopedics	x			x		x													x					x	x
Physiotherapy	x					x																		x	
Dentistry	x																							x	
Dermatology	x																							x	
Gastro-enterology	x					x				x															
Nutrition	x																							x	
Pharmacy	x																								x
Admission& Discharge	x			x																					

Moreover, the flow of patient in the ED varies from patient to patient depending on the case and the type of patient. Once arrived to the ED, the patient follows certain assessments before taking the appropriate decision (such as triage, waiting for consultation or directly assigned to a doctor, etc.). However, some essential steps the patient must follow during his journey at the ED are: arrival, consultation, diagnosis, interpretation and decision and finally the process outcome (whether discharged or admitted to the hospital). The patient journey in the ED can be represented in Figure 1.

Due to this complexity and unplanned nature of patient surge, simulation modeling is proven by many researchers to be very effective in order to study the necessary changes needed for better performance. Therefore, predictive modeling, using simulation, is very useful and effective for achieving better results

Figure 1. Patient journey in the ED

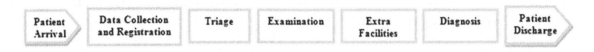

like controlling system costs, responding to new regulations and enhancing patient experience. Figure 2 presents a literature survey from 1997-2010 on the breakdown of the use of simulation. Most of the earlier simulation projects highlighted facility specific issues. Based on the papers reviewed and researches done before, only five percent dealt with multi-facility modeling (Gunal & Pidd, 2010).

Huge data amount will be resulting from the ED simulated system. New techniques should be developed in order to understand this data, and thus leading to the right and efficient information needed for improving the system. Data mining techniques are key factors used by many researchers and proved to be successful in healthcare (see Cullen, 2001; Chae, et al., 2003; Begg et al., 2006). These techniques also help researchers in identifying key measure variables and investigate the data available in hospital databases in order to understand the information that can be useful for the simulation. Since the data collected can be huge and classified under "data rich but information poor" (Han et al., 2001), data mining can be applied to improve the knowledge of important patterns and discover meaningful measures within the data that may lead to a better understanding of the information resulted from the simulation, and thus efficient enhancement can be proposed for the system.

The following section provides a literature review on the different problems facing the ED and how many researchers approached them in order to enhance the quality of care, and thus improve patients'

Figure 2. Simulation survey breakdown

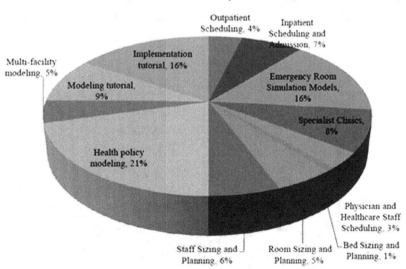

satisfaction. Section III presents a discussion over this literature in order to highlight the main solutions that can alleviate a certain problem in ED and how science management can interfere. Finally, Section IV presents a conclusion and future vision.

LITERATURE REVIEW

The healthcare is a very vast and complex system, where all departments interact with each other to offer care and service for patients. In this literature review, ED is the focus of our research, where complexity arises and prediction is highly needed. Improving EDs may lead to improving various services of the healthcare system and increasing revenue. The different problems studied by different researchers are presented along with some proposed solutions based on simulation modeling. At the end of this section a clear overview based on existing problems versus existing solutions can be achieved and discussed in section 3; leading to a chosen direction in order to improve the healthcare system as a future work.

An ED is the most complex unit of a hospital, where patients appear without any prior appointment, either by their own means or by ambulance. A patient suffering from an accident or a sudden injury, for example, will be directly addressed to the ED. Some of these appearing patients can be with critical cases and need immediate care and others may need a simple treatment. Once arrived to the ED, a patient should be observed before being admitted to the hospital or referred to another unit, like imaging, laboratory, etc. This scenario leads to overcrowding at some peak times and causing a large waiting time thus leading to dissatisfaction. Figure 3 shows an example of an ED.

There are several types of resources in an ED: Staff (doctors, nurses, physicians, and technicians), static resources (triage rooms, examination rooms, x-ray room) and equipment. The process includes in general: arrival to ED, registration, triage, examination, discharge/admission/tests; tests include blood tests or imaging. EDs usually lack sufficient resources in order to serve the unpredictable patient flow.

Most studies and surveys for the past years showed that EDs have a great impact on the healthcare system performance and quality of care. As EDs are linked to many other departments of the hospital, more attention should be addressed here. Thus, improving healthcare needs a recommended improvement in EDs, where patient flow should be monitored, waiting times and length of stay (LoS) should be

Figure 3. Emergency Department (ED)

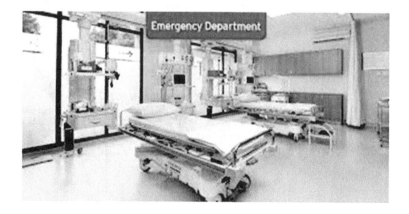

reduced (to satisfy patient) and revenue should be increased (to satisfy management). The most efficient way in order to approach these problems and find the optimal solution is to use simulation modeling.

Garcia et al. (1995) focused in their simulation modeling on the reduction of waiting time in ED for a hospital in Miami. Baesler F. et al. (2003) built a simulation model using Arena 4.0 in order to estimate the maximum increment rate of ED demands, a specific hospital in Chile could absorb it. The behavior of the variable patient's time in the system was predicted and the minimum number of human resources to serve this demand was defined. Nevertheless, the system should not exceed an acceptable waiting time level. The main focus of the hospital here was to understand the maximum extra demand their ED could absorb without facing problems, considering the patients waiting time, human resources limitations and maintaining the quality of service.

Samaha et al. (2003) studied the operation of a healthcare institution using the Arena simulation modeling. The main purpose of the model was to study the current operation and compare it to some suggested alternative scenarios that can reduce the length of stay patient spends in the ED. Each activity in the ED during a seven-day period, 24 hours a day was evaluated and used as input data to the constructed model. As a result, considerable time was saved without any additional costs. Alternative scenarios are suggestions proposed by the department staff in order to solve the issue of waiting time. Each scenario was implemented into the model in order to validate the output and study its efficiency. The main goal of the model was evaluating patient time, measuring patient throughput, evaluating resource utilization and determining queue sizes; these performance measures are essential in order to assess the effectiveness of the proposed scenarios. They are collected from the output of the model where it should be analyzed; leading to a clear decision on the optimal solution for the problem. Using this simulation model, the hospital improved its service without any unnecessary expenses by testing the proposed solutions via the model before implementing them in the actual running system (ED) (Centeno et al., 2003; Kelton et al., 2002).

Some physicians refer risky and urgent patients to EDs instead of providing care in their clinics (Berenson et al., 2003). As the 24/7 operation and the unneeded appointment make the ED the best option for medical care. Boarding or holding admitted patients until a bed is available, increases the percentage of crowding as well as the waiting time to see a physician; which restrict the system to respond to a patient surge in case of a disaster event. Boarding patients require monitoring, care and critical care procedures. A study about boarding patients considers them as a negative impact on other patient safety. Overcrowding can also cause ambulance diversion. Hospitals spending some time on diversion procedures urge patients to wait for a longer time for evaluation and treatment (Lewin Group, 2005).

Jacobson et al. (2006) presented an overview of DES (Discrete Event Simulation) modeling applications for healthcare clinics. Kolb et al.(2008) proved that the major cause of overcrowding of an ED is the waiting time patients spend in the emergency room waiting for in-patient assistance; which can block important ED resources. They improved patient and staff satisfaction through their design in this study. The design consisted of a discrete event simulation model for testing buffer alternatives in the patient flow. Park et al. (2008) proposed a forecasting model to predict patients' arrival to ED. Papers on treatment delays for high acuity patients (Schull et al., 2004; McCArthy et al., 2002), patient and staff dissatisfaction (Rowe et al., 2006; Abu-Laban (2006), patients left without being seen were reported over the years (Bullard et al., 2009).

Moreover, studies showed that to prevent this overcrowding and access block, many strategies and solutions can be followed; it requires a system level change by changing health policies. Access block, shown in Figure 4, is the delay waiting time that the patient suffers from once being admitted to the ED

Figure 4. Access block in ED

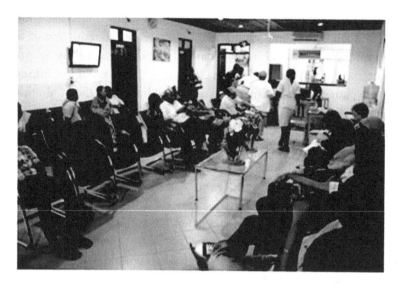

until he/she gains access to a dedicated bed. Jayaprakash (2009) studied the crowding of EDs in Europe. Access block is one of the main reasons of ED overcrowding and poor quality of care outcomes. Many studies from the UK, US, Canada and Australia have proven this (Forero et al., 2010; Sun et al., 2013).

Gunal and Pidd (2010) presented a literature review for DES models in healthcare where a number of important conclusions were drawn about simulation modelings such as issues faced during modeling from unit specific and facility-specific considerations. Paul et al. (2010) presented also a systematic review of ED simulation literature from 1970 to 2006. As a conclusion of their study, patient's perspective, environmental features and the role of information technology should be also incorporated in future simulation efforts in order to develop solutions to ED overcrowding.

Many solutions were suggested over the years in order to alleviate the overcrowding and access block in EDs and some are presented in the sections below. Solutions were classified under three general categories: modifying a process behavior in the ED, changing staffing levels and schedules and assessing the effect of external variables on the ED. These three categories are supported by simulation modeling techniques and optimization tools in order to find the optimal solution and guarantee the best performance of the ED.

Resource and Operational Rules Management

Reengineering and resource management of the ED consists of changing its aspect by adding specialized units responsible for specific tasks, relocating some equipment, beds, units and changing some hospital operation rules such as introducing the early discharge of patients, etc.

ED Re-Engineering

43% of hospital admissions originate in the ED, therefore the correlation between EDs and the several units of a hospital. A research linked America's ED overcrowding to hospitals restructuring, as a cause of financial pressures (Schull et al., 2001). Redesign or re-engineering of EDs including unit layout changes were presented by Miller et al. (2004), Mould et al. (2013), and Rado et al. (2014); other solutions were also studied by some researchers such as opening new units (Hannan et al., 1974) or expanding the ED capacity (Wiinamaki & Dronzek, 2003).

Kuo et al., 2016, proposed and analyzed the effect of relocating the ED in order to improve operation. They used simulation with Arena to build the system and apply the suggested changes.

Increasing Bed Capacity

Richmond et al. (1990) focused on the effect of bed capacity reduction into waiting times and explore the causes for these observed delays. The complex system was simulated using a dynamic model constructed on iThink software. The model studied the effect of policies changes on the performance of the system (such as controlling the roistering of ED doctors). The shortage in bed numbers may affect the elective admissions by increasing the number of cancellations. A research, proved that only 15-20% of patients arriving to ED require admission and the use of hospital beds (Audit Commission, 1996).

Bagust et al. (1998) used discrete-event stochastic simulation model in order to identify the dynamics of bed usage in emergency admissions. This study examined the relation between the available bed capacity and the unpredictable demand during an ED admission. The insufficient capacity for patients diagnosed for immediate admission may lead to a crisis. Statistics and analysis show that this trend will continue in the future, which indicates a significant increase in demands for beds. This fluctuation in emergency demand will affect the quality and efficiency of care in the hospital. Therefore, a deep understanding of these effects is required in order to apply the needed operational interventions and planning services for avoiding sudden problems leading to crisis. Lane et al. studied the impact of emergency demand on hourly basis emphasizing on the problem of waiting time for admissions (Lane et al., 2000). In this paper, an additional effect was taken into consideration; the random nature of the emergency demand admission affects the use of bed stock, that's why a discrete-event stochastic simulation modeling was used in order to investigate the complex system subject to this random effect. A relation was created between the fluctuating demands for emergency admission and the available in-patient bed capacity. The key output measures of system performance were:

1. Percentage rate of new arrivals to ED that cannot be admitted because of a lack of available beds;
2. Percentage rate of number of days in a year where a critical admission could not be accommodated (crisis day arises here);
3. Bed occupancy rates.

A possible intervention to alleviate the impact of rising emergency admission rates is a better management of existing resources and introducing early discharges which help in raising the bed availability rate. Other interventions can be by avoiding admission if it is not necessary or finding alternatives to admission (treating a patient in ED dedicated room, for example, without the need for hospital admission). As the emergency admissions are difficult to predict, this stochastic modeling proved that spare beds are essential for emergency admissions; where efficiency and a low level of patient risk are the goals.

Lane et al. study focused on the main factors behind the long waiting times for admission in an ED (Lane et al., 2000). Two significant insights, based on policy changes, were found: addition of resources reduce delays to patient demands and reduction in bed numbers do not increase the waiting times for emergency admissions. Bed shortage delays admission to the hospital and also causes cancellations of non-emergency admissions leading to additional future emergency cases.

One of the most significant factors affecting overcrowding is the bed shortage, where patients to be admitted should wait for hospital's bed availability (Derlet & Richards, 2000; Miro et al., 2003). In the UK, this bed shortage can affect even patients who are discharged from the hospital leading to patient dissatisfaction and bad economic events (Schneider et al., 2003). Derlet et al. (2001) met ED directors to define the crowding and evaluate the factors associated with this problem. This study highlights the link between overcrowding problems and nurse shortages. In their perspective, crowding is related to increase patient acuity, shortage in hospital's beds, insufficient space, laboratory/radiology delays, and examination delays, nursing/staff shortage and increasing ED volume. If waiting time spent by the patient in the ED exceeds the time taken to make a decision to admit a patient, then the clinical outcomes will be badly affected (Richardson, 2006; Cameron, 2006). McCarthy et al. (2008) presented a valid performance measure for crowding; which is the ED occupancy rate. This rate refers to the total number of patients divided by the total number of licensed beds.

More studies on this subject proved that modeling methods can improve the flow of patients in an ED by defining the peak times and key factors causing the access block and overcrowding. These models should take into consideration input data based on daily or weekly peak times in order to be able to distribute the admissions evenly across the week and to avoid any expected congestion (Moskop, 2009). Some techniques to be considered are the patient flow systems and bed capacity management. Martin et al. (2011) found that the waiting interval time of a patient from the time of admission request until the exit from ED to be admitted is the main cause of delay in patient flow. The best logical solution to avoid access block and emergency overcrowding is to increase the bed capacity in the hospital and dedicate the corresponding staff needed. When all solutions fail, the management should look upon this solution of increasing the capacity of the healthcare system. In order to alleviate the access block, government can also target some performance measures for the hospitals by introducing a strategy rule that must be followed by all healthcare organizations. Here, the bottleneck of the ED will be the whole organization's problem that must be solved and not just an ED issue. In this way, the emergency care is prioritized; which lead to a more efficient whole healthcare system since the ED interact with many other departments of the healthcare system as discussed earlier.

Hospital Specialization

The problem of ED overcrowding and patient boarding can be also alleviated by a proper assessment of the demographic needs including population age/density, historical trauma, emergency medicine trends and disaster preparedness. Care, is another valuable factor to ED problems, ad it should be provided based on specialization and not to depend on attracting the most number of patients. Therefore, hospitals should compete based on what they can do best. Medical outcomes were proved to be increased and cost to be reduced especially in the case of critical situations (Hillner et al., 2000).

Fast Track System

Yoon et al. (2003) suggested an efficient solution to the congestion problem by introducing the fast-track service in the EDs which is also cost-effective, safe and satisfactory for patients. In the UK, since 2002, this system was deployed under the principle of "see and treat" (Cooke et al., 2004). Chan et al. (2015) classified this problem into two categories: strategies addressing the ED overcrowding and strategies addressing access blocks. As per this study, solutions to these two main problems were, by introducing new concepts or strategies to the healthcare system. The fast-track service discussed here can be introduced in a dedicated area of the ED with a dedicated and efficient number of staff. It was proven to play a great role in alleviating the overcrowding problem. This concept can decrease the overall waiting time, eliminate the wastes and improve the patient flow. By decreasing the waiting time and shortening the length of stay in EDs, congestion issue can be reduced or even solved. Some studies in this area showed that also the rate of unseen patients was reduced. The key principal for this service to succeed is to have the competent and designated staff.

Triage System

Another initiative for reducing patient's complaints and increase satisfaction was conducted by Cooke et al. (2004), where an arriving patient follows the process of assessment at the triage stage, and then he/she will be directed to the appropriate service and staff based on the necessary needs. Therefore, triage system is also a significant way to reduce overcrowding. The triage system refers to a clinical assessment of the patient's medical status upon arrival to the ED; assessed by a primary triage nurse/ physician (Robertson-Steel, 2006).

O'Shea (2007) adopted the ED crisis of America's hospitals where factors are attributed to many reasons. In Maryland for example, non-urgent patients occupy over 40% of ED visits. A study showed that visits to EDs increased around 18%. One proposed solution can be by moving out non-emergency patients from emergency rooms leaving the space to urgent patients to be treated, thus decreasing overcrowding and misuse of ED facilities (Maryland Healthcare Commission, 2007).

Duguay and Chetouane (2007) also adopted a simulation model using Arena in order to improve the current operation of an ED by reducing patient waiting times and improving overall service delivery and system throughput. Resource availability is directly linked to patients waiting time. Key resources such as physicians, nurses, examination rooms are considered as control variables. Some features were taken into consideration while building the model such as the random flow of patients (seasonal illness or incident, fluctuates depending on days of the week and patient arrivals may increase during a specific peak time of a given day). Triage codes are a highly considered feature for the modeling system; where an arriving patient receives a triage code based on the severity of his case after being assessed by the triage nurse. The input data collected for model design and validation are based on time durations collected at different stages of the process in the ED. Time durations can be classified under the time spent by a patient during two consecutive activities (waiting duration) and the necessary time to complete an activity (activity duration). The time from registration to available exam room, was observed to be the largest waiting time in this system and therefore considered the main focus of this study. Based on the collected data observation, several alternative resource scenarios were proposed and studied in order to choose the best option to improve this time and apply it for this unit. These scenarios were designed in a way to increase staff/room capacity and decrease the waiting time within budgetary constraints and considering what-if analysis.

The 4-Hours and 3-Hours Rule

The UK NHS in 2004 introduced the 4-hour rule to be applied among all hospitals. The Department of Health launched a health service plan that states a clear policy which imposes an ED not to have a patient total waiting time more than four hours. The application of this policy was not easy, and many struggles were faced to achieve this target. The output of this policy was positive and major changes were resulted as per Cronin and Wright (2006). Munro et al. (2006) achieved a reduced waiting time in his study by applying this policy. Banerjee et al. (2008) stated "long waits in the ED are a thing of the past on the UK". Many factors were attributed to the overcrowding of ED, all leading to the same result of adverse clinical outcomes, patient dissatisfaction. Therefore, to figure out the best scenario and best solution, first the root of the problem should be determined not to affect the entire hospital operation based on the needs of individual regions.

All patients should be observed, admitted, discharged or transferred to another unit within the 4 hours only as presented by Letham and Gray (2012). A study was performed in this area in order to look at some performance measures on emergency overcrowding, access block and mortality rates by using as inputs: hospital data and patient data. This study showed results for pre and post introducing the 4-hours strategy. The results proved that sometimes patient care can be compromised in order to meet the time targets (Geelhoed & de Klerk, 2012).

Another 3-hours rule was suggested by some researchers in improve the total length of stay of the patient since he arrives until his departure from the ED. Discrete event simulation modeling was approached and many what-if scenarios were followed in order to reach this goal. As a result, 30% improvement of patient LoS was proven following this approach (Oh et al., 2016).

Due to the complexity of healthcare systems and the variation of systems from one country to another, the discussed solutions for reducing the overcrowding and access block cannot be applicable in some hospitals or can be less practicable. Nevertheless, the strategies and management approaches discussed above were developed and applied by many hospitals for many years with a proven evidence of efficiency and successful results. Therefore, more investigations and improvements should be taken into consideration on these solutions depending on the place and the type of system.

Early Discharge of In-Patients

Avoiding ED overcrowding and access block, can be achieved by early discharging in-patients; leading to an available bed capacity for new admitted patients. Usually, access block can increase the clinical risk of patients waiting for their turn to be admitted, that is why clinicians and managers should predict, categorize the levels of risks to discharge in-patients earlier and study the consequences behind this step when a sudden large bed capacity is demanded.

Kelen et al. (2006) described the process of discharging in-patients earlier by the "reverse triage", where patients should be safely selected with the lowest risk of consequences. Discharge lounges should be then dedicated for patients to wait for their discharge arrangements and some administrative paper work leading to a saving in bed hours and reducing the length of stay (Cowdell et al., 2002). This reverse triage system was fully described by an anecdotal report in 2012, putting in evidence the effective use of this system during an unexpected demand for beds (Satterthwaite & Atkinson, 2012).

Holding Units

The access block can be addressed to insufficient bed capacity, inefficient inpatient discharge and inefficient patient flow. In the US, reviews have proven that introducing holding units can reduce the access block and overcrowding by reducing the need for boarding or ambulance diversion (Institute of Medicine Committee, 2006). A study in Spain showed that providing a 16-bed observation unit in the ED of a 900-bed hospital improved the access block (Gómez-Vaquero et al., 2009). Holding units can also be referred as observation units or clinical decision units where the patient arriving to the ED can be examined and treated without the need for admission.

Moreover, a special observation unit should be dedicated for patients showing with low acuity symptoms such as chest pain, stomach ache etc. who may not need any hospital admission. A dedicated person should be assigned for the task of admission/discharge and responding to real-time demands for inpatients.

Other studies showed that the benefits of these holding units were not very efficient comparing to other hospital without any holding units (Schull et al., 2012); therefore, a carefully clinical management plan and adequate support staff should be incorporated in order to achieve a successful approach. Chan et al. (2015) also suggested these holding unit allowing early discharge and increasing capacity using political actions.

Human Resource Management

Resource management consists of adjusting the level of resources needed and capable of serving the maximum number of patients, assigning the appropriate resource to a certain task and editing resource schedules; thus leading to an increase in care demand and a reduction in the patient waiting time.

Optimizing the GP Role

Rieffe et al. (1999) proved that bypassing the general practitioner (GP) can lead to overusing the ED for minor complaints. This will decrease the service quality and increase the ED cost. Lee at al. (1999) conducted a study on ED attendees and found out that 57% were only primary cases. These primary cases can consult a GP instead of using the ED and thus causing additional patient flow. A study conducted by Van Uden et al. (2003) showed that a good way to optimize the GP role is to add after-hours services so they can be always available for primary care patients; thus reducing the inappropriate referrals to the ED.

Staffing Schedules

As discussed in many papers, researchers reached a conclusion where staff resources schedules can highly affect the operations of the ED and have great impact on many factors causing an ED crisis. Preparing these schedules are a complex task since large number of rules should be taken into consideration; such as number of consecutive shifts and weekly hours, conflicting timings, weekends, holidays, individual preferences (sick leaves, special occasions).

Rosetti et al. (1999) proposed a simulation model using Arena in order to determine an optimal attending physician staffing schedules. Since efficient allocation of staff resources is a common problem facing EDs in any hospital. A computer simulation was suggested in order to test alternative ED attending physician staffing schedules and then analyzing the results on the patient throughput and resource utilization. The suggested simulation can help even detecting any inefficiency in the actual system where patient flow, resources, layout and staffing changes can add a noticeable effect. It is agreed that the utilization of ED nurse and physician resources has a significant impact on patient throughput and system performance; therefore, an analysis was performed to reduce the staff idle time and operating expenses, and increase the resource utilization taking into consideration a constant patient quality of care. This can be done by looking at the patient showing up at ED as a function of hours/day, where peak times can be determined. Four different approaches were suggested and analyzed leading to the selection of the best approach where the overall waiting time of patient was significantly decreased as a daily/weekly basis. The approach focused on changing an existing double coverage shift of a current schedule by considering the patient arrival rates for the ED and assigning peak times during a day. Due to the complexity of the ED system and the understaffing, this procedure may increase the level of errors caused by overworked nurses and doctors. As a future work, a quality control analysis could be conducted before and after the implementation of this strategy to determine the problems and any potential solution. This improvement could be achieved by evaluating patient flow and layout designs in parallel with the suggested staff scheduling changes.

Hung (1995) presented a literature review on nurses scheduling using simulation modeling. Other researchers proved the success of these models in nurse scheduling problems using optimization techniques (Berrada, 1993; Weil et al., 1995; Jaumard et al., 1998; Komashi & Mousavi, 2005). Beaulieu et al. (2000) approached a mathematical programming to ensure a feasible performance of this task. The model constructs schedules for all staffing resources within a short period of time and less effort and proposes the best schedules since it takes into account all possible rules. Two major objectives should be considered while modeling: maximizing personnel satisfaction and minimizing salary cost.

Carter and Lapierre (2001) and Sinreich and Jabali (2007) adopted a simulation model to improve the ED operations by studying scheduling policies for physicians. Azadeh et al. (2013) applied fuzzy logic techniques in order to propose the optimal nursing scheduling. Centeno et al. (2003) also used simulation to help ED decision makers in their staff scheduling. The author of this paper presented a procedure that helps in efficiently estimating required parameters for model input data in case assumptions are needed (could not obtain sufficient data for simulation). This is for the reason that, while developing the simulation model for studying and improving the operations of the ED, two challenges were faced: the highly time-varying rate of the arrivals and data paucity (shortage of data). One of the model outputs implicated that by adding an extra doctor and adjusting shifts hours, the average waiting time of patients' consultations can be reduced by 10%. Using different what-if scenarios, that can be simulated using this model, to help hospital managers in taking their decisions for improving the quality of service (such as reducing waiting times) and to assure best allocation of resources. Wang et al. (2009) also focused in their study on the concept of resource allocation. Jerbi and Kamoun (2009) proposed a doctor's shift rescheduling.

Laroque et al. developed a simulation approach that analyzes how resource allocation can impact patient's journey in an ED. Based on some financial restrictions, hospital management cannot assure that resources are always available to fulfill service quality. Therefore, valuable resources (such as doctors and nurses) should be fully utilized. Another factor that should be highlighted is the non-urgent patients who may visit the ED. Increase of patient flow for routine consultation may increase the waiting times, and thus decreasing the quality of service and patient's satisfaction. Authors of this paper developed a simulation model in order to evaluate the impact of staffing and resource scheduling on patient demands, and to achieve insights about ED staffing policies.

Medical Resource Is the Driver

In most researches, the focus to improve the ED operation was the patient itself. Hay et al. (2006) proved that, in the contrary, the patient should not be the driver, but the medical resource should be considered as the main entity of study. It demonstrates the importance of assigning the appropriate doctor to a certain task (patient) along with the corresponding waiting time. Simulation modeling was used in this new approach highlighting three elements: the care paths (models including process and decision), operating priority (which is the clinical priority of the showing case and the waiting time of patient until the process is executed) and the skill sets (where the senior doctor can perform all tasks that a junior doctor can perform, but should not be called for simple tasks). Whenever a patient joins a queue, the operating priority gradually increases relatively to the waiting time. Choosing the right resource for a certain task depends on the severity of the patient's condition, waiting time of the patient and how busy is the hospital. Arena simulation was used with an integrated excel interface for easy configuration.

Subash et al., (2004) and Gunal and Pidd, (2006) classified patients in their study under three categories: "life-threatening", "Major" and "Minor". They studied the effect of junior/senior doctors in consulting patient. Senior doctors are experienced consultants who can spend less time with a patient to reach a clinical decision thus shortening the examination time, laboratory time, assessment time, radiology, discharge time; also, the total waiting time spent in the ED.

Part-Time Jobs and ENPs

The overcrowding can be related to the inappropriate usage of ED utilities by the primary care attendees. In the past several years, part time jobs were offered by some hospitals to general practitioners to serve ED low acuity type of cases leading to a congestion reduction. Theses general practitioners can also refer to senior doctors in the ED for an advice or discussion on the treatment which assure a high quality of care. Low acuity patients are those having minor injuries or minor illness and they constitute the majority of the ED crowding. Other studies showed that using emergency nurse practitioners (ENPs) may increase efficiency since patients will be more satisfied with the quality of care delivered. Carter and Chochnov (2007) performed a systematic review of ENPs working in the ED, concentrating on the outcome measures of this approach; which is the waiting time reduction, higher patient satisfaction, cost-effectiveness and high quality of care which can be equivalent to the same care provided by a junior doctor.

Alternative Staff Distribution

Ahmed and Alkhamis (2009) designed a decision support system simulation combined with optimization in order to determine the optimal number of resources needed to serve an ED in Kuwait taking into consideration management budget restrictions, maximum patient throughput and minimum patient waiting time in the system. The study was made for a public hospital in Kuwait, where decision makers should maximize resources (doctors, nurses, lab technicians) utilization and minimize the waiting time while maintaining the same level of care and a standard patient satisfaction rate. The current staff distribution was studied, and resources limitation was highlighted to figure out an alternative staffing distribution that can improve the ED and reach the target. Patients were classified into different categories based on the severity of their case and transferred to the required service accordingly. This simulation/optimization model focuses on the problem of how to choose the right distribution of resources based on the type of service and taking into consideration the constraints imposed by the system limitations. Many other researchers before Ahmad et al. highlighted the same problem using the simulation/optimization techniques over the past decades, like Swisher et al. (2001), Blasak et al. (2003) and Sinreich and Marmor (2005). These researchers reproduced the behavior of a healthcare system to evaluate its performance and analyze the outcome of different scenarios. Beaulieu et al. (2000) followed a mathematical programming approach in order to schedule doctors for an emergency room. Baesler et al. (2003) adopted a simulation model based on experiments to estimate the maximum capacity for an emergency room. Ahmed and Alkhamis (2009) method differs from all other models since it is not dealing with the mathematical model of the actual system, but by combining simulation with optimization. A complex stochastic objective function represents the optimization model which is subject to some stochastic constraints set by the management; these values can never be analytically evaluated and need simulation intervention. As a future author intention, an interface linkage between excel worksheet and SIMISCRIPT simulation software is intended. Input data for the simulation program will be taken from the excel sheets and accordingly necessary simulation analysis can be achieved. The number of receptionists, doctors, nurses, and lab technicians (etc.) are some of the input data required for evaluation purposes. The output of the simulation program are used for performance measures which includes staff cost, system throughput and average waiting time in the system along with detailed information about the queues formed for each type of service.

Marmor (2010) discussed the complexity of the ED of a hospital and pointed at the operational managerial challenges faced. For this reason, a simulation framework is necessary for realistic tracking of the EDs.

Considering External Factors

External factors such as requesting extra facilities from other units of the hospital, considering different insurance coverage types, predicting strain situations and forecasting disaster conditions affect the operation of the ED and may cause overcrowding or large waiting times. Patients arriving to the ED may be classified into different types of insurance coverage (private insurance, public health insurance, etc.). Also, some patients are uninsured and showed up to the ED for free diagnosis; even if they have a low severity case.

Most of the times, patients arriving to the ED are referred to other units in order to go through extra tests such as imaging or laboratory. These extra facilities help the doctor to come up with an accurate diagnosis and a final decision (whether a patient needs admission or no or whether to be referred to another unit in the hospital such as surgery, etc.). These referrals should be considered in the model for adequate results since patients may be accessing the corresponding units at the same time, thus leading to overcrowding and high waiting times in the ED. Moreover, predicting strain situations and forecasting disaster conditions are essential metrics for a successful ED operation. Thus, care demand can be predicted and the corresponding resource needs (material or human) can be forecasted for optimal operation of the ED during those peak times.

Considering the Lab Tests/Imaging Effect

During the last decade, most studies found in literature, impose an increase in the actual care process (Saunders et al., 1989; Komashie & Mousavi, 2005) or the size and operation of the ED (Samaha et al.,

2003; Ruohonen et al., 2006) in order to reach the desired service level (throughput) and reduce waiting times. Saunders et al. (1989) considered in his model, built with Siman/Cinema, several features such as lab tests, triage priorities, teaching aspects, communication delays and physicians' collaboration. Blood tests/results and patients were considered flowing entities in the modeling system; that means the turnaround time of these tests has direct effect on the patient throughput.

Komashie and Mousavi (2005) main objective was to determine the effect of key resources (beds, nurses, doctors) on key performance measures (waiting times, waiting queues and throughput). The Arena model designed was depending on variable service times that can vary depending on the case of the patient. In this study, several essential elements that may affect the process were not taken into consideration (lab tests, triage codes, imaging, etc.). Ruohonen et al. (2006) used Medmodel simulation software in order to evaluate, plan and redesign the healthcare systems. In his study, he introduced a new idea of adding a doctor with the nurse at the triage stage. Therefore, the lab tests can be ordered and medical diagnosis can be performed during the early stage of the process leading to an improvement in waiting times and system throughput. This method allows fast priority recognition and accurate treatment referral. The model adopted lab tests and resource shifts as flowing entities.

Emergency radiology has great impact on waiting time especially in case of trauma patients. Radiology results are needed for patient assessment and discharge. Delays in radiology can lead to unnecessary use of ED beds, increase in length of stay and an increase in patient dissatisfaction (Miele, 2006). Eskandari et al. (2011) proposed considering ED patients using other facilities in the hospital (such as MRI, CT scan etc.) as priority over non-ED patients along with adding financial personnel and five mobile inpatient beds. Paul and Lin (2012) related the long waiting times in EDs to the long waits in triage, delays in tests and receiving results, waiting for a physician or a shortage in nursing staff.

Considering Uninsured Patients

Another factor causing overcrowding can be the increase in the rate of uninsured patients since federal laws implicit any ED to adopt an urgent uninsured patient who lack access to regular primary care even if he is not able to pay the fees. Strunk and Cunningham (2002) highlighted additional factors contributing in the ED rising demand such as capacity constraints for private physicians and scheduling appointments, managed-care restrictions and some low insurance reimbursement rates.

Financial constraints and hospital profit also raise a good factor for ED crowding where some hospitals prefer to reserve a bed for an elective inpatient that is surely paying the necessary fees rather than referring it to an ED patient whose payment is uncertain. One solution presented was to urge a tax deduction for health insurance allowing families and individuals to purchase personal health insurance (Butler & Owcharenko, 2007). Private health plans limits patient showing up to the ED to those having emergency situations only; thus, improving outcomes and reducing costs.

Forecasting Disaster Conditions

More factors should be taken into consideration like managing unexpected catastrophic events discussed by other researchers as well (such as terrorist attacks, natural disasters, pandemic diseases). The Institute of Medicine, a branch of the National Academy of Sciences, recently announced America's emergency medical system to stretch beyond capacity, and thus lack preparedness to accommodate disaster events (Institute of Medicine, 2006).

The disaster events are linked to abnormal conditions that may disturb the normal life in society such as floods, volcanic eruptions, earthquakes, etc. Patvivatsiri (2006) presented a computer simulation model that analyzes patient throughput, assesses resources utilization, evaluates the effect of a terrorist attack and determines necessary staffing level for a corresponding scenario. Paul and Hariharan (2007) studied disaster event impact on ED capacity plan during a terrorist attack. Al Kattan (2009) developed two models to represent ED operations in both normal and disaster conditions. ED operations in earthquake disaster event were studied in Yi et al. (2010). In Joshi and Rys (2011), disaster events patient's arrival patterns and time durations were evaluated using Arena simulation and related to the ability of ED to treat these patients. Xiao et al. (2012) also focused on the optimization of work flow in EDs during extreme events using a DES framework.

Gul and Guneri (2015) carried out a literature review study on simulation modeling used for EDs in both normal and disaster conditions. The literature in this area is vast and expanding with time, but most published studies were based on daily normal conditions only and targeting ED KPIs (Key Performance Indicators) such as length of stay, resource utilization and patient throughput. The best DES model used by many researches in this area was Arena. As a future vision, many suggestions were presented such as considering the financial effects when developing simulation scenarios for improving the ED service or considering disaster times not only the normal period. Few studies only highlighted the costs control of an ED. Immediately after a disaster, the complexity of the ED grows dramatically therefore the need of simulation modeling to forecast the physical and human resources that will be needed. Using the simulation modeling, many scenarios can be proposed, evaluated, comparison and what-if analysis and optimization can be performed.

Considering Big Data Research

The complexity of the ED imposes sharing big data between different departments of the healthcare system in order to assess overcrowding. Halevy and al. showed that the more data provided as input to a simulation system the more scenarios can be conducted and predictions can be accurate; leading to decision making for an optimal solution, improving health service quality, efficiency and cost (Halevy et al., 2009). Big data research approach is proposed to manage the complexity and big volume of the healthcare existing data (Diebold et al., 2012). The increasing data storage capacity and diversity of data types are the main components of this research where healthcare services can be improved depending on the multiplicity of this data. The adoption of insights gained from big data analytics has the potential of saving lives, improve the care delivery process, align payment with performance and expand access to healthcare details (Belle et al., 2015).

In majority of emergency departments' simulations, the model is built upon incomplete data (such as missing arrival time, service times, etc.). Collecting reliable data for the system is a hard task which may often lead to invalid simulations. This problem can be solved by simulation optimization where the unavailable service time durations can be predicted through proposing new algorithms (Guo et al., 2016).

Predicting Strain Situations

As emergency departments have become the immediate and essential medical care unit in a hospital, efficient management of patient flow and predicting resources demand are urgent issues to focus on.

Kadri et al. (2014) studied in their research patient flow in the pediatric ED of a hospital in France using Arena simulation modeling taking into consideration strain situations and ED states (normal, degraded, critical) which was not defined in literature before 2012. Strain situations are defined as disequilibrium in the ED where care load flow and care production capacity exceed certain thresholds. To handle this patient influx, EDs require enough human and material resources which are at peak times limited; leading to ED overcrowding and strain situations. The purpose of this study is to build a simulation-based decision support system that takes as input data from the hospital database and based on interviews with healthcare staff in order to predict the strain situations. Inputs are information such as number of patient arrivals, means of arrival, arrival time, types and duration of each treatment, additional examinations, and destination after leaving the ED as well as information regarding the strain situations. Simulation output will help hospital management specifying strain situations, examine the relationship between them, propose correction actions and improve the service at ED. The main strain situations observed from the data collected were the influx of patients, long waits before receiving care, shortage in nursing staff, waiting for doctors, delays in additional examinations and the inability to transfer admitted patients. The simulation model was designed for every day of the week and Sundays were observed to be the most critical day where different scenarios were proposed as solutions, such adding a human resource (nurse/doctor) and material resources (adding an examination room with a doctor or/and a nurse). Results were examined and best scenario was chosen after deep analysis of waiting time reduction and decreasing in length of stay.

Adopting Simulation Techniques

Due to the complexity of the ED, simulation modeling was proven over the years to be a key solution to improve operations. Optimization techniques can be also integrated with simulation, and thus leading to an optimal solution for the arising and studied problem.

Using Queuing System Modeling

Siddharthan et al. (1996) presented a queuing policy in order to reduce the waiting times. Komashie and Mousavi (2005) investigated policy and decision making of an ED, where capacity was adopted by Baesler et al. (2003). Lim, Nye et al. (2012) and Lim, Worster et al. (2012) used mathematical modeling techniques-queuing models, DES, SD (System Dynamics) and ABS (Agent Based Simulation) in order to develop twenty nine scenarios for evaluating waiting time reduction. Abbas B. K. (2014) suggested a simulation model using different scenarios. This model studies the complexity of the ED in a hospital and assesses the patient's time interval process since his arrival to the ED until he receives the needed care. The minimum waiting time can be reached by considering a queuing system modeling. An arriving patient enters the system through the waiting room, shown in Figure 5, where he should pick a number and waits until nurse calls his name and transfers him into the screening room to assess his case (blood pressure, fever, etc.). Based on the patient case, he will be transferred to the examination room to receive the necessary care. Priority discipline should be taken into consideration; patients arriving by ambulance have to receive a priority and urgent care based on the severity of their case.

Figure 5. ED waiting room

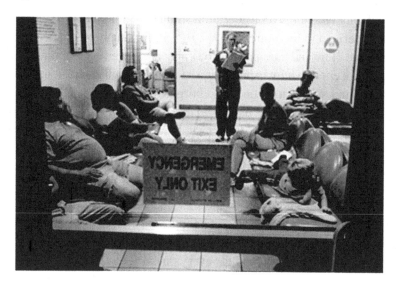

Integrating Optimization Tools With Simulation Modeling

Recently some studies proved that integration of other simulation method along with the simulation modeling is optimal to find the best solution (like using Opt Quest tool for optimization). Rico et al. (2007), Ahmed and Alkhamis (2009), and Weng et al. (2011) integrated the simulation modeling with optimization (Opt Quest tool) in order to reach the optimal solution. Balanced Scorecard (BSC) was integrated by Ismail, Abo-Hamad and Arisha (2013) with their simulation model to study the ED performance.

Medeiros et al. (2008), Jerbi and Kamoun(2009), Brenner et al. (2010), Taboada et al. (2011), Kuo et al. (2012), and Izady and Worthington (2012) studied staff scheduling in order to optimize the workload and cover patient demand. Morgareidge et al. (2014) demonstrated the advantage of using SSA with DES modeling for facilitating decision making regarding design, reducing costs and improving the ED performance.

INTERPRETATION

As ED is the most complex entity of the healthcare system, the most overcrowding unit and the main focus of our study. Table 2 presents a list of some problems that may affect the ED and some proposed solutions; which researchers should approach in order to alleviate the risk. This table is the result of the literature survey competed in section 2. Note that, due to the high interaction of the ED with several other departments in the hospital, the majority of the problems can lead to the same patient dissatisfaction factor, i.e.: long waiting times and high LoS in the ED. Therefore, the choice of the appropriate solution depends on the type of the problem, type of patients arriving to the ED (age, severity level, etc.), resource utilization levels and scheduling, budget constraints and management constraints.

For example, bed shortage in a hospital can directly affect a patient waiting in the ED for bed availability. Also, a patient referred to another unit for extra tests will have to wait in the ED until the results

Table 2. Some ED overcrowding problems/solutions

Problems	Bed shortage	Admission issues	Resource shortage (Doctors, Nurses, etc.)	Long Waiting times in queues	Admission & Discharge Process	Laboratory & Radiology	Different Insurance Coverage
Solutions	Add extra beds	Predict strain situations	Add resources	Introduce the Triage Category System	Add discharge lounges	Add resources in these units	Improve payment services
	Apply the rule of patient early discharge	Forecast disaster conditions and peak times	Change Staffing Schedules/ Shifts	Introduce the process of Fast-Track System	Add extra administrative staff	Add extra equipment for x-ray, CT-scan, MRI, etc.	Introduce tax deduction by law to push families to purchase private health insurance
	ED re-engineering (such as adding additional units, etc.)	Increase bed capacity	Increase resource utilization	Add Physicians	Hospital Physical Structure Change	Add rooms for extra capacity for these facilities	Limitation of insurance plan to emergency situations
	Introducing new operational rules	Consider Hospital Specialization	Assign part time jobs resources for low acuity patients	Assign the appropriate resource to the right patient			
		Add observation units	Add after-hours GPs/ ENPs for low severity cases	Apply the 4-hours rule			

are ready and, then only, the doctor can finalize his diagnosis and decide whether to treat the patient in the ED, admit him to the hospital or discharge him. Predicting and forecasting peak times can alleviate the risk of overcrowding. Introducing new operation rules and adding new units can improve also the process. New systems, like triage, fast track and assigning the right resource to the right arriving patient can accelerate the process of examination.

All these solutions, proposed earlier, should be integrated into a simulation modeling software in order to build a system close to the real ED and propose enhancement without the need of freezing the operation of the real system. Data mining algorithms can be applied to understand the huge amount of data resulted from the simulation. Moreover, optimization tools such as Opt Quest in Arena simulation software can be very efficient to reach the optimal solution for the best performance of the ED.

CONCLUSION

Healthcare is a large, dynamic and complex system where different units, teams, resources and patients interconnect to serve an activity. This inter-connection of facilities requires a multi-paradigm, flexible simulation modeling methodologies to capture this complexity and present a clear view on how to predict critical events and then reach an optimal decision making.

An ED is a medical treatment facility specializing in emergency medicine, the acute care of patients who present without prior appointment; either by their own means or by that of an ambulance. Most problems affecting the healthcare system are derived from the ED since patient flow is based on prediction without any prior appointment. This department is the biggest interacting unit within the hospital which makes it the most complex system as per the literature review. Studying the cascading effects and their direct link to the ED should be performed using a simulation platform.

As a result from this study, a future vision is deducted such as building a multi-facility platform, using simulation modeling, where the complex system is divided into simpler problems by creating a module for each queue or stage in the process and then combining all together to form the ED system.

Experimentation is the process of improving the system by applying some new changes or suggesting new rules. Three different aspects, discussed earlier in this study, will be the core of this experimentation (see Paul et al., 2010). One scenario can be achieved by changing staffing schedules and assessing the performance of the ED due to this change. Another scenario is modifying a process behavior in the ED (such as adding a new unit or proposing a new operation rule) or assessing the effect of external variables on the ED.

Using a simulation model, the whole complex system representing the real system of the ED will be built and then different scenarios will be created in order to validate this model. The proposed changes can be imposed on the modeled system without affecting the real system in process, and thus predictive analysis can be performed in order to evaluate the performance measures and find the optimal solution for any arising problem. Note that problems affecting ED may be different depending on the region, season, patient age, patient mentality, etc. From these several scenario runs, the optimal solution can be chosen, taking into consideration patient satisfaction (by decreasing waiting times) and increasing management revenue (by decreasing costs, increasing staff utilization, reducing hospital resources use). Therefore, the minimum number of resources required to serve the maximum demand should be predicted.

The computer simulation of the complex ED system will result in massive amount of data generation; where the information needs to be interpreted and analyzed in order to gain better knowledge of the system before experimentation can be suggested and applied. Therefore, efficient system knowledge can be achieved using data mining techniques. Approaching a certain data mining algorithm, useful information in the data collected can be potentially extracted for different processes in the system (Bruballa et al., 2014). Thus, prediction can be easily applied especially in peak times and disaster conditions.

To sum up, for a successful implementation of ED systems, simulation modeling should encourage multi-facilities investigations in order to cover up the complexity of these systems. A very common way to do so is to develop each facility separately (such as arrival, triage, radiology, examination, etc.) and then combine them together using a simulation model and therefore covering up the whole ED system model. This concept proposed earlier in Gunal and Pidd (2007), will be the focus of our research and it will be discussed in details in future work along with developing the required simulation and platform algorithms. Moreover, Majority of the studies reviewed in literature did not focus on the financial effects of the scenarios tested and approached only the normal periods without considering epidemic and disaster times (availability of sufficient medical staff). Therefore, our platform will aim to improve EDs considering as well both cost and epidemic periods during performance measuring.

After reviewing this large number of papers in the literature related to ED operations, Arena was found to be the most powerful simulation modeling tool which is used by majority of researchers, especially during disaster conditions. Most of these papers aim on reducing the waiting times and length of stay in all stages of the ED process, improving resource utilization, maintaining the quality of care either by suggesting different staffing schedules, hiring new staff, proposing new unit re-design; but the majority did not take into consideration the financial impact of these proposed scenarios which can be a highlighted point for our future study. Moreover, for studies of ED at the time of disasters, more focus should be related to the triage state where a new fast track strategy should be developed for patients with high acuity (victims). Studies showed that the impact of other departments of the hospital is worth to be taken into consideration while designing an ED simulation model (such as Mould et al., 2013, Ashour and Kremer, 2013, and Kang et al., 2014).

REFERENCES

Abbas, A. L. B. K. (2014). Simulation Models Of Emergency Department In Hospital. *Journal of Engineering and Development*, *18*(2).

Abo-Hamad, W., & Arisha, A. (2013). Simulation-based framework to improve patient experience in an emergency department. *European Journal of Operational Research*, *224*(1), 154–166. doi:10.1016/j.ejor.2012.07.028

Abu-Laban, R. B. (2006). The junkyard dogs find their teeth: Addressing the crisis of admitted patients in Canadian emergency departments. *Canadian Journal of Emergency Medical Care*, *8*(06), 388–391. doi:10.1017/S1481803500014160 PMID:17209487

Ahmed, M. A., & Alkhamis, T. M. (2009). Simulation optimization for an emergency department healthcare unit in Kuwait. *European Journal of Operational Research*, *198*(3), 936–942. doi:10.1016/j.ejor.2008.10.025

Al-Kattan, I. (2009). Disaster recovery plan development for the emergency department-Case study. *Public Administration and Management*, *14*(1), 75.

Ashour, O. M., & Kremer, G. E. O. (2013). A simulation analysis of the impact of FAHP–MAUT triage algorithm on the Emergency Department performance measures. *Expert Systems with Applications*, *40*(1), 177–187. doi:10.1016/j.eswa.2012.07.024

Audit Commission. (1996). By accident or design Improving A& E services in England and Wales. London: HMSO.

Azadeh, A., Rouhollah, F., Davoudpour, F., & Mohammadfam, I. (2013). Fuzzy modelling and simulation of an emergency department for improvement of nursing schedules with noisy and uncertain inputs. *International Journal of Services and Operations Management*, *15*(1), 58–77. doi:10.1504/IJSOM.2013.053255

Baesler, F. F., Jahnsen, H. E., & DaCosta, M. (2003, December). Emergency departments I: the use of simulation and design of experiments for estimating maximum capacity in an emergency room. *Proceedings of the 35th conference on Winter simulation: driving innovation*, 1903-1906.

Bagust, A., Place, M., & Posnett, J. W. (1999). Dynamics of bed use in accommodating emergency admissions: Stochastic simulation model. *BMJ (Clinical Research Ed.), 319*(7203), 155–158. doi:10.1136/bmj.319.7203.155 PMID:10406748

Banerjee, A., Mbamalu, D., &Hinchley, G. (2008). The impact of process re-engineering on patient throughput in emergency departments in the UK. *International Journal of Emergency Medicine, 1*(3), 189-192.

Beaulieu, H., Ferland, J. A., Gendron, B., & Michelon, P. (2000). A mathematical programming approach for scheduling physicians in the emergency room. *Health Care Management Science, 3*(3), 193–200. doi:10.1023/A:1019009928005 PMID:10907322

Begg, R., Kamruzzaman, J., & Sarkar, R. (2006). Neural Networks in Healthcare: Potential and Challenges. Idea Group Publishing.

Belle, A., Thiagarajan, R., Soroushmehr, S. M., Navidi, F., Beard, D. A., &Najarian, K. (2015). *Big Data Analytics in Healthcare.* BioMed Research International.

Berrada, I. (1993). *Planificationd'horaires du personnel infirmierdansunétablissementhospitalier* (Doctoral dissertation). Departement d''Inforrnatique et de RechercheOpe'rationnelle, Université de Montreal.

Blasak, R. E., Starks, D. W., Armel, W. S., & Hayduk, M. C. (2003, December). Healthcare process analysis: The use of simulation to evaluate hospital operations between the emergency department and a medical telemetry unit. *Proceedings of the 35th conference on Winter simulation: driving innovation,* 1887-1893.

Brenner, S., Zeng, Z., Liu, Y., Wang, J., Li, J., & Howard, P. K. (2010). Modeling and analysis of the emergency department at University of Kentucky Chandler Hospital using simulations. *Journal of Emergency Nursing: JEN, 36*(4), 303–310. doi:10.1016/j.jen.2009.07.018 PMID:20624562

Bruballa, E., Taboada, M., Cabrera, E., Rexachs, D., & Luque, E. (2014, August). Simulation and Big Data: A Way to Discover Unusual Knowledge in Emergency Departments: Work-in-Progress Paper. In *Future Internet of Things and Cloud (FiCloud), 2014 International Conference on* (pp. 367-372). IEEE. doi:10.1109/FiCloud.2014.65

Bullard, M. J., Villa-Roel, C., Bond, K., Vester, M., Holroyd, B. R., & Rowe, B. H. (2009). Tracking emergency department overcrowding in a tertiary care academic institution. *Healthcare Quarterly, 12*(3), 99–106. doi:10.12927/hcq.2013.20884 PMID:19553772

Butler, S. M., &Owcharenko, N. (2007). *Making Health Care Affordable: Bush's Bold Health Tax Reform Plan.* Heritage Foundation.

Cameron, P. (2006). Hospital overcrowding: A threat to patient safety?. *The Medical Journal of Australia, 184*(5), 203–204. PMID:16515426

Carter, A. J., & Chochinov, A. H. (2007). A systematic review of the impact of nurse practitioners on cost, quality of care, satisfaction and wait times in the emergency department. *Canadian Journal of Emergency Medical Care, 9*(04), 286–295. doi:10.1017/S1481803500015189 PMID:17626694

Carter, M. W., & Lapierre, S. D. (2001). Scheduling emergency room physicians. *Health Care Management Science*, *4*(4), 347–360. doi:10.1023/A:1011802630656 PMID:11718465

Ceglowski, A. (2006). *An investigation of emergency department overcrowding using data mining and simulation* (Doctoral dissertation). Monash University.

Centeno, A. P., Martin, R., & Sweeney, R. (2013, December). REDSim: A spatial agent-based simulation for studying emergency departments. In *Simulation Conference (WSC)* (pp. 1431-1442). IEEE. doi:10.1109/WSC.2013.6721528

Centeno, M. A., Giachetti, R., Linn, R., & Ismail, A. M. (2003, December). Emergency departments II: a simulation-ilp based tool for scheduling ER staff. *Proceedings of the 35th conference on Winter simulation: driving innovation*, 1930-1938.

Chae, Y. M., Kim, H. S., Tark, K. C., Park, H. J., & Ho, S. H. (2003). Analysis of Healthcare Quality Indicators Using Data Mining and Decision Support System. *Expert Systems with Applications*, *24*(2), 167–172. doi:10.1016/S0957-4174(02)00139-2

Chan, S. S., Cheung, N. K., Graham, C. A., & Rainer, T. H. (2015). Strategies and solutions to alleviate access block and overcrowding in emergency departments. *Hong Kong Medical Journal*, *21*(4), 345–352. PMID:26087756

Cooke, M., Fisher, J., Dale, J., McLeod, E., Szczepura, A., Walley, P., & Wilson, S. (2004). *Reducing attendances and waits in emergency departments: A systematic review of present innovations*. Academic Press.

Cowdell, F., Lees, B., & Wade, M. (2002). Discharge planning. *Armchair fan. The Health Service Journal*, *112*(5807), 28–29. PMID:12073514

Cronin, J. G., & Wright, J. (2006). Breach avoidance facilitator–managing the A&E 4-hour target. *Accident and Emergency Nursing*, *14*(1), 43–48. doi:10.1016/j.aaen.2005.11.005 PMID:16377191

Cullen, P. (2001). *Feature Selection Methods for Intelligent Systems Classifiers in Healthcare (PhD Dissertation)*. Chicago: Loyola University of Chicago.

Derlet, R. W., & Richards, J. R. (2000). Overcrowding in the nations emergency departments: Complex causes and disturbing effects. *Annals of Emergency Medicine*, *35*(1), 63–68. doi:10.1016/S0196-0644(00)70105-3 PMID:10613941

Derlet, R. W., Richards, J. R., & Kravitz, R. L. (2001). Frequent overcrowding in US emergency departments. *Academic Emergency Medicine*, *8*(2), 151–155. doi:10.1111/j.1553-2712.2001.tb01280.x PMID:11157291

Diebold, F. X., Cheng, X., Diebold, S., Foster, D., Halperin, M., Lohr, S., & Schorfheide, F. (2012). *A Personal Perspective on the Origin (s) and Development of "Big Data"*. The Phenomenon, the Term, and the Discipline.

Eskandari, H., Riyahifard, M., Khosravi, S., & Geiger, C. D. (2011, December). Improving the emergency department performance using simulation and MCDM methods. *Simulation Conference (WSC) Proceedings*, 1211–1222.

Forero, R., Hillman, K. M., McCarthy, S., Fatovich, D. M., Joseph, A. P., & Richardson, D. B. (2010). Access block and ED overcrowding. *Emergency Medicine Australasia*, 22(2), 119–135. doi:10.1111/j.1742-6723.2010.01270.x PMID:20534047

García, M. L., Centeno, M. A., Rivera, C., & DeCario, N. (1995, December). Reducing time in an emergency room via a fast-track. *In Simulation Conference Proceedings, 1995. Winter* (pp. 1048-1053). IEEE. doi:10.1109/WSC.1995.478898

Geelhoed, G. C., & de Klerk, N. H. (2012). Emergency department overcrowding, mortality and the 4-hour rule in Western Australia. *The Medical Journal of Australia*, 196(2), 122–126. doi:10.5694/mja11.11159 PMID:22304606

Gómez-Vaquero, C., Soler, A. S., Pastor, A. J., Mas, J. P., Rodriguez, J. J., & Virós, X. C. (2009). Efficacy of a holding unit to reduce access block and attendance pressure in the emergency department. *Emergency Medicine Journal*, 26(8), 571–572. doi:10.1136/emj.2008.066076 PMID:19625552

Gul, M., & Guneri, A. F. (2015). A comprehensive review of emergency department simulation applications for normal and disaster conditions. *Computers & Industrial Engineering*, 83, 327–344. doi:10.1016/j.cie.2015.02.018

Gunal, M. M., & Pidd, M. (2006, December). Understanding accident and emergency department performance using simulation. *In Simulation Conference, 2006. WSC 06. Proceedings of the Winter* (pp. 446-452). IEEE. doi:10.1109/WSC.2006.323114

Gunal, M. M., & Pidd, M. (2010). Discrete event simulation for performance modelling in healthcare: A review of the literature. *Journal of Simulation*, 4(1), 42–51. doi:10.1057/jos.2009.25

Guo, H., Goldsman, D., Tsui, K. L., Zhou, Y., & Wong, S. Y. (2016). Using simulation and optimisation to characterise durations of emergency department service times with incomplete data. *International Journal of Production Research*, 54(21), 6494–6511. doi:10.1080/00207543.2016.1205760

Halevy, A., Norvig, P., & Pereira, F. (2009). The unreasonable effectiveness of data. *IEEE Intelligent Systems*, 24(2), 8–12. doi:10.1109/MIS.2009.36

Han, J., & Kamber, M. (2001). *Data Mining: Concepts and Techniques Morgan Kaufmann*. San Francisco: International Thomson.

Hannan, E. L., Giglio, R. J., & Sadowski, R. S. (1974, January). A simulation analysis of a hospital emergency department. In *Proceedings of the 7th conference on winter simulation* (vol. 1, pp. 379-388). ACM. doi:10.1145/800287.811199

Hay, A. M., Valentin, E. C., & Bijlsma, R. A. (2006, December). Modeling emergency care in hospitals: a paradox-the patient should not drive the process. In *Simulation Conference, 2006. WSC 06. Proceedings* (pp. 439-445). IEEE.

Hillner, B. E., Smith, T. J., & Desch, C. E. (2000). Hospital and physician volume or specialization and outcomes in cancer treatment: Importance in quality of cancer care. *Journal of Clinical Oncology*, 18(11), 2327–2340. doi:10.1200/JCO.2000.18.11.2327 PMID:10829054

Hoffenberg, S., Hill, M. B., & Houry, D. (2001). Does Sharing Process Differences Reduce Patient Length of Stay in the Emergency Department? *Annals of Emergency Medicine*, *38*(5), 533–540. doi:10.1067/mem.2001.119426 PMID:11679865

Hung, R. (1995). Hospital nurse scheduling. *The Journal of Nursing Administration*, *25*(7-8), 21–23. doi:10.1097/00005110-199507000-00010 PMID:7636569

Institute of Medicine. (2006). *Emergency Medical Services: At the Crossroads*. Washington, DC: National Academies Press.

Institute of Medicine Committee on the Future of Emergency Care in the United States Health System. (2007). *Hospital-based emergency care: At the Breaking Point*. Washington, DC: National Academies Press. Available from: http://www.nap.edu/catalog/11621.html

Izady, N., & Worthington, D. (2012). Setting staffing requirements for time dependent queueing networks: The case of accident and emergency departments. *European Journal of Operational Research*, *219*(3), 531–540. doi:10.1016/j.ejor.2011.10.040

Jacobson, S. H., Hall, S. N., & Swisher, J. R. (2006). Discrete-event simulation of health care systems. In Patient flow: Reducing delay in healthcare delivery (pp. 211-252). Springer US. doi:10.1007/978-0-387-33636-7_8

Jaumard, B., Semet, F., & Vovor, T. (1998). A generalized linear programming model for nurse scheduling. *European Journal of Operational Research*, *107*(1), 1–18. doi:10.1016/S0377-2217(97)00330-5

Jayaprakash, N., O'Sullivan, R., Bey, T., Ahmed, S. S., &Lotfipour, S. (2009). Crowding and delivery of healthcare in emergency departments: the European perspective. *Western Journal of Emergency Medicine*, *10*(4).

Jerbi, B., & Kamoun, H. (2009). Using simulation and goal programming to reschedule emergency department doctors shifts: Case of a Tunisian hospital. *Journal of Simulation*, *3*(4), 211–219. doi:10.1057/jos.2009.6

Joshi, A. J., & Rys, M. J. (2011). Study on the effect of different arrival patterns on an emergency department capacity using discrete event simulation. *International journal of industrial engineering. Theory Applications and Practice*, *18*(1), 40–50.

Jun, J. B., Jacobson, S. H., & Swisher, J. R. (1999). Application of Discrete-Event Simulation in Health Care Clinics: A Survey. *The Journal of the Operational Research Society*, *50*(2), 109–123. doi:10.1057/palgrave.jors.2600669

Kadri, F., Harrou, F., Chaabane, S., & Tahon, C. (2014). Time series modelling and forecasting of emergency department overcrowding. *Journal of Medical Systems*, *38*(9), 1–20. doi:10.1007/s10916-014-0107-0 PMID:25053208

Kang, H., Nembhard, H. B., Rafferty, C., & DeFlitch, C. J. (2014). Patient flow in the emergency department: A classification and analysis of admission process policies. *Annals of Emergency Medicine*, *64*(4), 335–342. doi:10.1016/j.annemergmed.2014.04.011 PMID:24875896

Kelen, G. D., Kraus, C. K., McCarthy, M. L., Bass, E., Hsu, E. B., Li, G., & Green, G. B. et al. (2006). Inpatient disposition classification for the creation of hospital surge capacity: A multiphase study. *Lancet, 368*(9551), 1984–1990. doi:10.1016/S0140-6736(06)69808-5 PMID:17141705

Kelton, W. D., Sadowski, R. P., &Sadowski, D. A. (2002). *Simulation with ARENA*. McGraw-Hill, School Education Group.

Kolb, E. M., Schoening, S., Peck, J., & Lee, T. (2008, December). Reducing emergency department overcrowding: five patient buffer concepts in comparison. *Proceedings of the 40th conference on winter simulation*, 1516-1525. doi:10.1109/WSC.2008.4736232

Komashie, A., & Mousavi, A. (2005, December). Modeling emergency departments using discrete event simulation techniques. *Proceedings of the 37th conference on Winter simulation*, 2681-2685. doi:10.1109/WSC.2005.1574570

Kuo, Y. H., Leung, J. M., & Graham, C. A. (2012, December). Simulation with data scarcity: Developing a simulation model of a hospital emergency department. *Simulation Conference (WSC) Proceedings*, 1–12.

Kuo, Y. H., Rado, O., Lupia, B., Leung, J. M., & Graham, C. A. (2016). Improving the efficiency of a hospital emergency department: A simulation study with indirectly imputed service-time distributions. *Flexible Services and Manufacturing Journal, 28*(1-2), 120–147. doi:10.1007/s10696-014-9198-7

Lane, D. C., Monefeldt, C., & Rosenhead, J. V. (2000). Looking in the wrong place for healthcare improvements: A system dynamics study of an accident and emergency department. *The Journal of the Operational Research Society, 51*(5), 518–531. doi:10.1057/palgrave.jors.2600892

Laroque, C., Himmelspach, J., Pasupathy, R., Rose, O., & Uhrmacher, A. M. (2012). Simulation with data scarcity: developing a simulation model of a hospital emergency department. *WSC '12 Proceedings of the Winter Simulation Conference*.

Lee, A., Lau, F. L., Hazlett, C. B., Kam, C. W., Wong, P., Wong, T. W., & Chow, S. (1999). Measuring the inappropriate utilization of accident and emergency services? *International Journal of Health Care Quality Assurance, 12*(7), 287–292. doi:10.1108/09526869910287558 PMID:10724572

Letham, K., & Gray, A. (2012). The four-hour target in the NHS emergency departments: A critical comment. *Emergencias, 24*(1), 69–72.

Lewin Group. (2005). *TrendWatchChartbook 2005: Trends Affecting Hospitals and Health Systems*. American Hospital Association.

Lim, M. E., Nye, T., Bowen, J. M., Hurley, J., Goeree, R., & Tarride, J. E. (2012). Mathematical modeling: The case of emergency department waiting times. *International Journal of Technology Assessment in Health Care, 28*(02), 93–109. doi:10.1017/S0266462312000013 PMID:22559751

Lim, M. E., Worster, A., Goeree, R., & Tarride, J. E. (2012). PRM28 physicians as pseudo-agents in a hospital emergency department discrete event simulation. *Value in Health, 15*(4), A163. doi:10.1016/j.jval.2012.03.884

Marmor, Y. (2010). *Emergency-departments simulation in support of service-engineering: Staffing, design, and real-time tracking* (Doctoral dissertation).

Martin, M., Champion, R., Kinsman, L., & Masman, K. (2011). Mapping patient flow in a regional Australian emergency department: A model driven approach. *International Emergency Nursing, 19*(2), 75–85. doi:10.1016/j.ienj.2010.03.003 PMID:21459349

Maryland Healthcare Commission. (2007). *Use of Maryland Hospital Emergency Departments: An Update and Recommended Strategies to Address Crowding.* Author.

McCarthy, M. L., Aronsky, D., Jones, I. D., Miner, J. R., Band, R. A., Baren, J. M., & Shesser, R. et al. (2008). The emergency department occupancy rate: A simple measure of emergency department crowding? *Annals of Emergency Medicine, 51*(1), 15–24. doi:10.1016/j.annemergmed.2007.09.003 PMID:17980458

McCarthy, M. L., Zeger, S. L., Ding, R., Levin, S. R., Desmond, J. S., Lee, J., & Aronsky, D. (2009). Crowding delays treatment and lengthens emergency department length of stay, even among high-acuity patients. *Annals of Emergency Medicine, 54*(4), 492–503. doi:10.1016/j.annemergmed.2009.03.006 PMID:19423188

Medeiros, D. J., Swenson, E., & DeFlitch, C. (2008, December). Improving patient flow in a hospital emergency department. *Proceedings of the 40th Conference on Winter Simulation*, 1526-1531. doi:10.1109/WSC.2008.4736233

Miele, V., Andreoli, C., & Grassi, R. (2006). The management of emergency radiology: Key facts. *European Journal of Radiology, 59*(3), 311–314. doi:10.1016/j.ejrad.2006.04.020 PMID:16806785

Miller, M. J., Ferrin, D. M., & Messer, M. G. (2004, December). Fixing the emergency department: A transformational journey with EDSIM. In *Simulation Conference, 2004. Proceedings of the 2004* (Vol. 2, pp. 1988-1993). IEEE. doi:10.1109/WSC.2004.1371560

Miro, O., Sanchez, M., Espinosa, G., Coll-Vinent, B., Bragulat, E., & Milla, J. (2003). Analysis of patient flow in the emergency department and the effect of an extensive reorganisation. *Emergency Medicine Journal, 20*(2), 143–148. doi:10.1136/emj.20.2.143 PMID:12642527

Morgareidge, D., Hui, C. A. I., & Jun, J. I. A. (2014). Performance-driven design with the support of digital tools: Applying discrete event simulation and space syntax on the design of the emergency department. *Frontiers of Architectural Research, 3*(3), 250–264. doi:10.1016/j.foar.2014.04.006

Moskop, J. C., Sklar, D. P., Geiderman, J. M., Schears, R. M., & Bookman, K. J. (2009). Emergency department crowding, part 2—barriers to reform and strategies to overcome them. *Annals of Emergency Medicine, 53*(5), 612–617. doi:10.1016/j.annemergmed.2008.09.024 PMID:19027194

Mould, G., Bowers, J., Dewar, C., & McGugan, E. (2013). Assessing the impact of systems modeling in the redesign of an Emergency Department. *Health Systems, 2*(1), 3–10. doi:10.1057/hs.2012.15

Munro, J., Mason, S., & Nicholl, J. (2006). Effectiveness of measures to reduce emergency department waiting times: A natural experiment. *Emergency Medicine Journal, 23*(1), 35–39. doi:10.1136/emj.2005.023788 PMID:16373801

Nelson, R., & Millet, I. (2004). *Data Flow Diagrams Versus Use Cases – Student Reactions.* Paper presented at the Tenth Americas Conference on Information Systems, New York, NY.

O'Shea, J. S. (2007). *The Crisis in America's Emergency Rooms and What Can Be Done.* Heritage Foundation.

Oh, C., Novotny, A. M., Carter, P. L., Ready, R. K., Campbell, D. D., & Leckie, M. C. (2016). Use of a simulation-based decision support tool to improve emergency department throughput. *Operations Research for Health Care, 9,* 29–39. doi:10.1016/j.orhc.2016.03.002

Palmer, G. (1996). Casemix Funding of Hospitals: Objectives and Objections. *Health Care Analysis, 4*(3), 185–193. doi:10.1007/BF02252878 PMID:10162141

Park, E. H., Park, J., Ntuen, C., Kim, D., & Johnson, K.Cone Memorial Hospital. (2008). Forecast driven simulation model for service quality improvement of the emergency department in the Moses H. Cone Memorial Hospital. *Asian Journal on Quality, 9*(3), 1–14. doi:10.1108/15982688200800024

Patvivatsiri, L. (2006, December). A simulation model for bioterrorism preparedness in an emergency room. *Proceedings of the 38th conference on Winter simulation,* 501-508. doi:10.1109/WSC.2006.323122

Paul, J. A., & Hariharan, G. (2007, December). Hospital capacity planning for efficient disaster mitigation during a bioterrorist attack. In *Proceedings of the 39th conference on Winter simulation: 40 years! The best is yet to come* (pp. 1139-1147). IEEE Press.

Paul, J. A., & Lin, L. (2012). Models for improving patient throughput and waiting at hospital emergency departments. *The Journal of Emergency Medicine, 43*(6), 1119–1126. doi:10.1016/j.jemermed.2012.01.063 PMID:22902245

Paul, S. A., Reddy, M. C., & DeFlitch, C. J. (2010). A Systematic Review of Simulation Studies Investigating Emergency Department Overcrowding. *Simulation, 86*(8-9), 559–571.

Paul, S. A., Reddy, M. C., & DeFlitch, C. J. (2010). A systematic review of simulation studies investigating emergency department overcrowding. *Simulation, 86*(8-9), 559–571.

Preater, J. (2002). A Bibliography of Queues in Health and Medicine. *Health Care Management Science, 5*(4), 283. doi:10.1023/A:1020334207282

Rado, O., Lupia, B., Leung, J. M., Kuo, Y. H., & Graham, C. A. (2014). Using simulation to analyze patient flows in a hospital emergency department in Hong Kong. In *Proceedings of the International Conference on Health Care Systems Engineering* (pp. 289-301). Springer International Publishing. doi:10.1007/978-3-319-01848-5_23

Richardson, D. B. (2006). Increase in patient mortality at 10 days associated with emergency department overcrowding. *The Medical Journal of Australia, 184*(5), 213. PMID:16515430

Richmond, B. M., Vescuso, P., & Peterson, S. (1990). *iThink™ Software Manuals.* Academic Press.

Rico, F., Salari, E., & Centeno, G. (2007, December). Emergency departments nurse allocation to face a pandemic influenza outbreak. In *Simulation Conference* (pp. 1292-1298). IEEE. doi:10.1109/WSC.2007.4419734

Rieffe, C., Oosterveld, P., Wijkel, D., & Wiefferink, C. (1999). Reasons why patients bypass their GP to visit a hospital emergency department. *Accident and Emergency Nursing, 7*(4), 217–225. doi:10.1016/S0965-2302(99)80054-X PMID:10808762

Robertson-Steel, I. (2006). Evolution of triage systems. *Emergency Medicine Journal, 23*(2), 154–155. doi:10.1136/emj.2005.030270 PMID:16439754

Rowe, B. H., Bond, K., Ospina, M. B., Blitz, S., Friesen, C., & Schull, M. (2006). *Emergency department overcrowding in Canada: what are the issues and what can be done?* [Technology overview no 21]. Ottawa: Canadian Agency for Drugs and Technologies in Health.

Ruohonen, T., Neittaanmaki, P., & Teittinen, J. (2006, December). Simulation model for improving the operation of the emergency department of special health care. *In Simulation Conference, 2006. WSC 06. Proceedings of the Winter* (pp. 453-458). IEEE. doi:10.1109/WSC.2006.323115

Samaha, S., Armel, W. S., & Starks, D. W. (2003, December). Emergency departments I: the use of simulation to reduce the length of stay in an emergency department. *Proceedings of the 35th conference on winter simulation: driving innovation*, 1907-1911.

Satterthwaite, P. S., & Atkinson, C. J. (2012). Using reverse triage to create hospital surge capacity: Royal Darwin Hospitals response to the Ashmore Reef disaster. *Emergency Medicine Journal, 29*(2), 160–162. doi:10.1136/emj.2010.098087 PMID:21030549

Saunders, C. E., Makens, P. K., & Leblanc, L. J. (1989). Modeling emergency department operations using advanced computer simulation systems. *Annals of Emergency Medicine, 18*(2), 134–140. doi:10.1016/S0196-0644(89)80101-5 PMID:2916776

Schneider, S. M., Gallery, M. E., Schafermeyer, R., & Zwemer, F. L. (2003). Emergency department crowding: A point in time. *Annals of Emergency Medicine, 42*(2), 167–172. doi:10.1067/mem.2003.258 PMID:12883503

Schull, M. J., Szalai, J. P., Schwartz, B., & Redelmeier, D. A. (2001). Emergency department overcrowding following systematic hospital restructuring trends at twenty hospitals over ten years. *Academic Emergency Medicine, 8*(11), 1037–1043. doi:10.1111/j.1553-2712.2001.tb01112.x PMID:11691665

Schull, M. J., Vermeulen, M., Slaughter, G., Morrison, L., & Daly, P. (2004). Emergency department crowding and thrombolysis delays in acute myocardial infarction. *Annals of Emergency Medicine, 44*(6), 577–585. doi:10.1016/j.annemergmed.2004.05.004 PMID:15573032

Schull, M. J., Vermeulen, M. J., Stukel, T. A., Guttmann, A., Leaver, C. A., Rowe, B. H., & Sales, A. (2012). Evaluating the effect of clinical decision units on patient flow in seven Canadian emergency departments. *Academic Emergency Medicine, 19*(7), 828–836. doi:10.1111/j.1553-2712.2012.01396.x PMID:22805630

Siddharthan, K., Jones, W. J., & Johnson, J. A. (1996). A priority queuing model to reduce waiting times in emergency care. *International Journal of Health Care Quality Assurance, 9*(5), 10–16. doi:10.1108/09526869610124993 PMID:10162117

Sinreich, D., & Jabali, O. (2007). Staggered work shifts: A way to downsize and restructure an emergency department workforce yet maintain current operational performance. *Health Care Management Science, 10*(3), 293–308. doi:10.1007/s10729-007-9021-z PMID:17695139

Sinreich, D., & Marmor, Y. (2005). Emergency department operations: The basis for developing a simulation tool. *IIE Transactions, 37*(3), 233–245. doi:10.1080/07408170590899625

Strunk, B. C., & Cunningham, P. J. (2002). *Treading water: Americans' access to needed medical care, 1997-2001.* Academic Press.

Subash, F., Dunn, F., McNicholl, B., & Marlow, J. (2004). Team triage improves emergency department efficiency. *Emergency Medicine Journal, 21*(5), 542–544. doi:10.1136/emj.2002.003665 PMID:15333524

Sun, B. C., Hsia, R. Y., Weiss, R. E., Zingmond, D., Liang, L.-J., Han, W., & Asch, S. M. et al. (2013). Effect of emergency department crowding on outcomes of admitted patients. *Annals of Emergency Medicine, 61*(6), 605–611. doi:10.1016/j.annemergmed.2012.10.026 PMID:23218508

Swisher, J. R., Jacobson, S. H., Jun, J. B., & Balci, O. (2001). Modeling and analyzing a physician clinic environment using discrete-event (visual) simulation. *Computers & Operations Research, 28*(2), 105–125. doi:10.1016/S0305-0548(99)00093-3

Van Uden, C. J. T., Winkens, R. A. G., Wesseling, G. J., Crebolder, H. F. J. M., & Van Schayck, C. P. (2003). Use of out of hours services: A comparison between two organisations. *Emergency Medicine Journal, 20*(2), 184–187. doi:10.1136/emj.20.2.184 PMID:12642541

Wang, T., Guinet, A., Belaidi, A., & Besombes, B. (2009). Modelling and simulation of emergency services with ARIS and Arena. Case study: The emergency department of Saint Joseph and Saint Luc Hospital. *Production Planning and Control, 20*(6), 484–495. doi:10.1080/09537280902938605

Weil, G., Heus, K., Francois, P., & Poujade, M. (1995). Constraint programming for nurse scheduling. *Engineering in Medicine and Biology Magazine, IEEE, 14*(4), 417–422. doi:10.1109/51.395324

Weng, S. J., Cheng, B. C., Kwong, S. T., Wang, L. M., & Chang, C. Y. (2011, December). Simulation optimization for emergency department resources allocation. *Simulation Conference (WSC) Proceedings*, 1231–1238.

Wiinamaki, A., & Dronzek, R. (2003, December). Emergency departments I: using simulation in the architectural concept phase of an emergency department design. *Proceedings of the 35th conference on Winter simulation: driving innovation*, 1912-1916.

Xiao, N., Sharman, R., Rao, H. R., & Dutta, S. (2012). A simulation-based study for managing hospital emergency departments capacity in extreme events. *International Journal of Business Excellence, 5*(1-2), 140–154. doi:10.1504/IJBEX.2012.044578

Yi, P., George, S. K., Paul, J. A., & Lin, L. (2010). Hospital capacity planning for disaster emergency management. *Socio-Economic Planning Sciences, 44*(3), 151–160. doi:10.1016/j.seps.2009.11.002

Yoon, P., Steiner, I., & Reinhardt, G. (2003). Analysis of factors influencing length of stay in the emergency department. *Canadian Journal of Emergency Medical Care, 5*(03), 155–161. doi:10.1017/S1481803500006539 PMID:17472779

KEY TERMS AND DEFINITIONS

Arena: A discrete event simulation software which helps the modeler in building an experiment model that is similar to the real system and perform experimentation where improvements can be suggested without any interruption of the currently working system.

Data Mining: The fact of dealing with big data where new information can be generated from pre-existing databases.

Experimentation: The process of improving the system by applying new rules and suggesting new operations.

Overcrowding: The fact of having excessive numbers of patients needing or receiving care.

Patient Flow: The process that a patient follows, from the time he enters the system until he is discharged. Patient flow includes both medical and administrative processes.

Patient LoS: The length of stay of a patient spends in the system.

Queuing Analysis: A method used in order to improve patient throughput.

Simulation Modeling: A model designed using a simulation software for a process or system over a period of time.

Waste: A non-added value activity that a certain process may encounter. Customers usually are not willing to pay for wasted activities.

What-If-Analysis: The simulation of several scenarios by applying some changes to the inputs and analyzing the outcome of the outputs.

Chapter 6
Analyzing Interval Systems of Human T–Cell Lymphotropic Virus Type I Infection of CD4⁺ T–Cells

Zohreh Dadi
University of Bojnord, Iran

ABSTRACT

Human T-cell lymphotropic virus type I (HTLV-I) infects a type of white blood cell called a T lymphocyte. HTLV-I infection is seen in diverse region of the world such as the Caribbean Islands, southwestern Japan, southeastern United States, and Mashhad (Iran). This virus is the etiological agent of two main types of disease: HTLV-I-associated myelopathy/tropical spastic paraparesis and adult T cell leukemia. Also, the role of HTLV-I in the pathogenesis of autoimmune diseases such as HTLV-I associated arthropathy and systemic lupus erythematosus is under investigation. In this chapter, the author considers an ODE model of T-cell dynamics in HTLV-I infection which was proposed by Stilianakis and Seydel in 1999. Mathematical analysis of the model with fixed parameters has been done by many researchers. The author studies dynamical behavior (local stability) of this model with interval uncertainties, called interval system. Also, effective parameters in the local dynamics of model are found. For this study, interval analysis and particularly of Kharitonov's stability theorem are used.

INTRODUCTION

Recently, attention of many researchers has been attracted to the study of population dynamics of infectious diseases, such as human immunodeficiency virus (HIV), hepatitis B virus (HBV), and human T cell lymphotropic virus type I (HTLV-I) (Arafa, Rida, & Khalil, 2011; Asquith & Bangham, 2008; Asquith et al., 2005; Atay, Başbük, & Eryılmaz, 2016; Bangham, 2000; Bangham & Osame, 2005; Bangham et al., 2009; Blattner et al., 1982; Blattner et al., 1983; Bofill et al., 1992; Cai, Li, & Ghosh, 2011; Cann & Chen, 1996; Chiavetta et al., 2003; Dadi & Alizade, 2016; DeBoer & Perelson, 1998; Elaiw, 2010; Eshima

DOI: 10.4018/978-1-5225-2515-8.ch006

et al., 2009; Eshima, Tabata, Okada, & Karukaya, 2003; Gokdogan & Merdan, 2011; Gómez-Acevedo & Li, 2005; Katri & Ruan, 2004; Lang, 2009; Lang & Li, 2012; Lim & Maini, 2014; Mortreux, Gabet, & Wattel, 2003; Mortreux, Kazanji, Gabet, de Thoisy, & Wattel, 2001; Murphy et al., 1991; Nelson, Murray, & Perelson, 2000; Nowak & Bangham, 1996; Oguma, 1990; Olavarria, Gomes, Kruschewsky, Galvão-Castro & Grassi, 2012; Perelson & Nelson, 1999; Poiesz, 1980; Ramirez, Cartier, Torres, & Barria, 2007; Ribeiro, Mohri, Ho, & Perelson, 2002; Richardson et al., 1997; Richardson, Edwards, Cruickshank, Rudge, & Dalgleish, 1990; Robbins, 2010; Seigel, Nash, Poiesz, Moore, & O'Brien, 1986; Seydel, & Kramer, 1996; Seydel & Stilianakis, 2000; Shirdel et al., 2013; Song & Li, 2006; Stilianakis & Seydel, 1999; Sun & Wei, 2013; Tortevoye, Tuppin, Carles, Peneau, & Gessain, 2005; Vieira, Cheng, Harper, & Senna, 2010; Wang, Fan, & Torres, 2010; Wang, Li, & Kirschner, 2002; Wattel, Vartanian, Pannetier, &Wain-Hobson, 1995; Williams, Fang, & Slamon, 1988; Yamamoto, Okada, Koyanagi, Kannagi, & Hinuma, 1982; Yu, Nieto, Torres, & Wang, 2009).

The discovery of HTLV-I as the first human retrovirus in 1980 has had several notable implications, (Poiesz et al., 1980). First, clear proof of existence a relationship between viruses and cancer. Second, making an opportunity to investigate the mechanisms what lead to chronic demyelinating disease. There exists an obvious association of HTLV-I with a neurologic disease similar to multiple sclerosis (MS). Finally, the discovery and isolation of human immunodeficiency virus (HIV) was facilitated. HIV has caused a global epidemic of a rapidly progressive fatal illness: acquired immune deficiency syndrome, AIDS.

In fact, HTLV-I as a C-type retrovirus is the etiological agent of two main types of disease (Cann & Chen, 1996);

- HTLV-I associated myelopathy/tropical spastic paraparesis (HAM/TSP) and
- Adult T cell leukemia (ATL).

The virus not only induces HAM/TSP in a small proportion of HTLV-I carriers, but also is associated with other autoimmune diseases such as HTLV-I associated arthropathy (HAAP). In addition, the role of HTLV-I in the pathogenesis of systemic lupus erythematosus (SLE) has been discussed extensively, (Shirdel et al., 2013). The infection is also associated with an increasing occurrence of infectious diseases such as infective dermatitis in children, tuberculosis, disseminated strongyloidiasis, and scabies (Olavarria, Gomes, Kruschewsky, Galvão-Castro, & Grassi, 2012).

Infection with this virus is now a global epidemic, affecting 20 million to 40 million people. In the areas where HTLV-I is endemic, significant causes of mortality and morbidity are HAM/TSP and ATL. The highest prevalence of this infection is found mainly in the tropics and subtropics: the Caribbean Islands, southwestern Japan, Central and South Africa, South America and the Middle East. The virus is also present in USA, especially in southeastern United States, and Mashhad in the northeast of Iran which the prevalence of HTLV-I infection is estimated to be 2-3% in the whole population, (Shirdel et al., 2013).

HTLV-I is transmitted by four major routes:

- Sexual transmission,
- Vertical transmission from mother to child,
- Infection by blood transfusion,
- Needle-sharing among drug users.

It is interesting to know that HTLV-I infection cannot be transmitted from person to person by coughing, kissing, cuddling, sneezing or daily social contacts. Although primary infection leads to a chronic infection that seems to last life-long, a small minority of persons infected with HTLV-I will develop disease due to HTLV-I. About 3% of infected people develop symptoms of ATL and another 3% develop symptoms of HAM/TSP, (Katri & Ruan, 2004). In the other words, the virus appears to remain in the body throughout life without causing any harm at all. Also, these diseases will be developed after 20 - 30 years. This leads to two important and unresolved questions:

1. Why is it that only a few people infected with HTLV-I develop either ATL or HAM/TSP?, and
2. Why do these diseases develop after such a long time?

Understanding of mechanism which HTLV-I infection causes ATL, HAM/TSP or other disease is not easy, but mathematical modeling can help researchers for exploring complex mechanisms of HTLV-I infection and insight to treatment. Unfortunately, at present there is no cure or neutralizing vaccine for the chronic infection. Mathematical model of this infection is an excellent candidate because of

- The relatively simple nature of the HTLV-I virus,
- Lay a firm foundation for the modeling of the closely related, but more complicated, HIV virus,
- And contribute significant insights for answering to the above questions.

Aim of this chapter is studying dynamics of a mathematical model of human T cell lymphotropic virus type I infection of CD4$^+$ T cells with interval uncertainties, also called interval system. To the best of the author's knowledge, it is the first time to deal with the dynamical properties of interval systems of HTLV-I infection of CD4$^+$ T cells. The chapter proposes the use of interval analysis and particularly of Kharitonov's stability theorem for the study of the model with interval parameters and obtaining stability region of the uninfected steady state and the (positive) infected steady states.

This chapter is organized as follows. In the second section, studies on HTLV-I infection model are reviewed. In the third section, the author presents mathematical model of HTLV-I infection with interval parameters. Also, some basic definition and theorems are stated. In next section, the author obtains some conditions on interval parameters for existence and stability of equilibrium points of the model. Also, based on data of studies 1999 to 2016, the author presents numerical results of the model for a time span of 30 years with interval parameters. Existence of long chronic infection with low levels of infected CD4$^+$ T cells is represented by the numerical simulations. Finally, a discussion is given to review the results of the chapter and state further works for future.

BACKGROUND

There is a great deal of literature about human T cell lymphotropic virus type I. It should be noted that first studies on the dynamics of human T cell lymphotropic virus type I were done by Seigel et al. (1986), and Oguma (1990). Works of them completely were different. Also, Blattner et al. (1982, 1983), Yamamoto et al. (1982), Williams et al. (1988), Cann and Chen (1996) did first investigations on this infection from the point of view epidemiology.

Seigel et al. (1986) examined the progress of HTLV-I proviral integration over a 3-period of in vitro culture in two human lymphoma line, Hut 102 and MJ. Oguma (1990) focused on three major routes of transmittance of this infection in various areas of Japan; breast milk, semen, or blood transfusion. After that, Seydel and Kramer (1996) presented a modeling approach for transmission and population dynamics of human T cell lymphotropic virus type I (HTLV-I) infection. This presented model of HTLV-I transmission dynamics included various pieces of information on population and transmission patterns. The model defined the dynamics between subpopulations (susceptible, infected and diseased individuals) with certain transmission routes; mother-to-child and heterosexual transmission. The simple structure of their model helped researchers to study the dynamics of this infection. Among the forms of horizontal transmission, they only took heterosexual transmission into account, since there was some evidence that this transmission route played the major role in horizontal HTLV-I transmission in the Jamaican population (Murphy et al., 1991). According to Seydel and Kramer (1996)," Homosexual contacts, needle-sharing among i.v. drug users, also blood-borne infections, seem to account for only few cases of HTLV-I infected individuals. In addition, only blood products which contain cellular components are known to transmit the infection to recipients, whereas eg., plasma-factor concentrates for patients with hemophilia are not sufficient." Furthermore, they used a steady-state analysis of their model to estimate transmission rates for males and females. Their studies showed that the rate of heterosexual transmission was 2.7 times higher if the carrier was male. At the same time, Nowak and Bangham (1996) modeled the dynamics of immune responses to persistent viruses. On the other hand, Yamamoto et al.(1982), Williams et al.(1988), and Richardson et al. (1990, 1997) had shown that infection by HTLV-I is characterized by cell-to-cell infection of CD4$^+$ T cells which HTLV-I preferentially infects. These researches showed that primary infection leads to a chronic infection that seems to last life-long.

Some years later, Stilianakis and Seydel in 1999, developed a simple model of CD4+ T cell dynamics in HTLV-I infection. Their model suggested a possible pathogenic mechanism of HTLV-I infection. According to Stilianakis and Seydel (1999) "only a small fraction of infected individuals progress to disease and about 2–5% of HTLV-I carriers develop symptoms of ATL and about 2% of HTLV-I carriers develop symptoms of ATL." They explained T cell dynamics after HTLV-I infection can be described in a mathematical model with coupled differential equations. They modeled the infection process with assumption cell-to-cell infection of CD4$^+$ T cells. Their model allowed for CD4$^+$ T cell subsets of susceptible, latently infected and actively infected cells as well as for leukemia cells. They showed that "a simple mechanism of virus-harboring by latently infected T cells followed by activation and transmission can be expressed dynamically and account for the long chronic phase observed in HTLV-I infection." They used the parameter values which came from immunological estimates about the lifespan of uninfected, latently infected or actively infected T cells. These values are based on the studies of process of HIV infection because the viral transmission mechanism of HTLV-I infection was not precisely known. Therefore, due to the lack of data and HTLV-I associated estimates, they had made some reasonable assumptions based on estimates from the thoroughly investigated HIV-I infection taking into account the specific characteristics of HTLV-I infection. They assumed that ATL cells were not infectious. In fact, their work was to show that a quantitative description of HTLV-I infection as a persistent infection can be provided by some basic processes. Seydel and Stilianakis (2000) explored the T cell dynamics after infection with HTLV-I and analyzed the relation between transmission mode, virulence pattern, viral load, and latency period with a mathematical model. They found that "the initial viral doses may be an important factor contributing to the variation in latency period in interaction with the virulence pattern. In addition, the results give insight into population dynamics of a retrovirus infection with less genetic diversity, lower cytopathogenicity, but higher viral load than HIV." Wang et al. (2002) completely determined the global dynamics of this model.

In the next year, Eshima et al. (2003) generalized their previous work in 2001 that was a continuous time HTLV-I model with no age structure in the population. In 2003, they considered the population dynamics of HTLV-I infection in a discrete-time mathematical model incorporating an age structure based on the life style of Japan. They showed that HTLV-I in Japan will almost die out within one hundred years. It should be noted that life styles vary from country to country. Hence, this HTLV-I model needs to be modified to fit the life style of the reproductive population if the country has a life style different from that of Japan.

For distinguishing between contact and infectivity rates, Katri and Ruan (2004) modified the parameters of the model of Wang et al. (2002). Then, they introduced a discrete time delay to describe the time between emission of contagious particles by active CD4$^+$ T cells and infection of pure cells. They studied the effect of time delay on the stability of endemically infected equilibrium. As mentioned, HTLV-I causes disabling inflammatory disease HAM/TSP and adult T cell leukemia. Therefore, many researchers studied on modeling the virus-host immunology interaction in diseases like many immunopathological diseases, Asquith et al. (2005). Their results introduced some important factors might play role in HAM/TSP pathogenesis. In another study which is done by Tortevoye et al. (2005), they compared the seroprevalence and seroincidence rates of human T cell lymphotropic virus type I and human immunodeficiency virus I in pregnant women in several ethnic groups in French Guiana between July 1, 1991 and June 30, 2001. Tortevoye et al. (2005) found a slight decrease over time for HTLV-I infection which is highly endemic in groups of African origin while HIVI spread rapidly in an epidemic mode, especially in the groups of the lowest socioeconomic levels.

A mathematical model for the infection of CD4$^+$ T cells by HTLV-I is proposed and analyzed by Gómez-Acevedo and Li (2005) via the following theory, "the HTLV-I infection consists of two steps: a transient phase of reverse transcription and a phase of persistent multiplication of infected CD4$^+$ T cells. When an infected T cell multiplies, proviruses can be passed to the genome of the daughter cells, as a form of vertical transmission. This two-step process can explain the observed high proviral load and low genetic variability in HTLV-I infected T cells." This theory is based on clinical researches which are done by Wattel et al. (1995), Bangham (2000), Mortreux et al. (2001), and Mortreux et al. (2003). One of interesting results of Gómez-Acevedo and Li (2005) was backward bifurcation which raised many new challenges to effective infection control. Moreover, studying cellular immune response to HTLV-I has attracted the attention of researchers. There is strong evidence on the decrease of proviral load and the risk of associated inflammatory diseases such as HAM/TSP when an efficient cytotoxic T lymphocyte (CTL) responses to HTLV-I at the individual level and the population level, (Bangham & Osame, 2005). In HTLV-I infection, actively infected T cells can infect other T cells and can be converted to ATL cells. Song and Li, (2006) considered the classical mathematical model with the saturation response of infection rate. Their analysis on dynamics of infection of CD4+ T cells by HTLV-I virus and progression of ATL was complete. They obtained the condition for infected T cells die out and the condition for HTLV-I infection becomes chronic. Also, Ramirez et al. (2007) studied on the dynamic patterns of proviral load and mRNA Tax expression and showed that they related to the development of HAM/TSP.

One of important question in study of HTLV-I infection is "How does HTLV-I persist despite a strong cell-mediated immune response?" This question is the title of a paper which is done by Asquith and Bangham, (2008). They applied a combination of mathematical methods and experimental techniques to find important factors on both sides of the in vivo host-virus interaction that they play a significant role to determine HTLV-I proviral load and disease risk. In addition, Asquith and Bangham (2008) explained how these key factors interact to enable viral persistence. Also, their work raised three important questions as follows which can be the subject of future studies:

1. What factors other than HLA genotype determine the efficiency of the antiviral CTL response?
2. What determines the rate of expression of the HTLV-I provirus?
3. How can we reconcile low-level viral expression with a large contribution of CTL in controlling proviral load?

Another work on the immune control of HTLV-I infection is done by Bangham et al. (2009). They considered two important questions. "First, what determines the strength of an individual's HTLV-I specific CTL response? Second, what controls the rate of expression of HTLV-I in vivo, which is greater in patients with HAM/TSP than in asymptomatic carriers with the same proviral load?" They obtained a relationship between the frequencies of HTLV-I infected T cell clones in vivo and dynamic balance between positive and negative selection forces that differ among the clones.

One of significant questions on HTLV-I infection modeling is about the relationship between age and gender and the HTLV-I prevalence rate. This question was answered by Eshima et al. (2009). Another question in modeling for HTLV-I infection of CD4$^+$ T cells is what type functions can be assumed to introduce the force of infection. Cai et al. (2011) introduced a function in general form such that the resulting incidence term contains, as special cases, the bilinear and the saturation incidences. This model was an extension of the model of Katri and Ruan (2004), Wang et al. (2002) and Song and Li (2006). Furthermore, Arafa et al. (2011) introduced fractional-order into a model of HTLV-I infection of CD4$^+$T cells which was used by Katri and Ruan (2004). They applied generalized Euler method (GEM) to obtain approximate and analytical solutions of this problem. They focused on two rates in the model; the rate at which uninfected cells are contacted by actively infected cells and the rate of infection of T cells with virus from actively infected cells. From their obtained results in this study, it was clear that varying the values of these two rates will alter the number of uninfected CD4$^+$ T cells, infected cells, and leukemic cells. In this year (2011), Gokdogan and Merdan considered the model of Katri and Ruan (2004) and used a multistage homotopy perturbation method for solving the problem. They compared the multistage homotopy perturbation solution and classical Runge-Kutta solution. They obtained higher accuracy solution via the multistage homotopy perturbation algorithm. After that, Atay et al. (2016) used a numerical algorithm based on the Magnus series expansion to solve the model of HTLV-I infection of CD4$^+$T cells which was used by Katri and Ruan (2004). They applied the fourth order explicit Runge-Kutta and algorithms for third and fourth order Magnus expansion method to the HTLV-I infection of CD4$^+$T cells model. Then they compared these results and found that the numerical solutions of the fourth order Magnus expansion method are in excellent agreement with respect to the fourth order explicit Runge-Kutta solutions. According to Atay et al. (2016), "Magnus expansion method is an efficient and accurate tool for human T cell lymphotropic virus I (HTLV-I) infection of CD4$^+$T cells model."

The author would like to point out that there is no study related to the model of HTLV-I infection CD4$^+$ T cells with interval parameters. In the next sections, this model will be proposed and analyzed.

HUMAN T CELL LYMPHOTROPIC VIRUS I INFECTION OF
CD4⁺ T CELLS MODEL WITH INTERVAL PARAMETERS

The author has studied almost all mathematical models of HTLV-I infection up to now. In this chapter, the proposed model in Stilianakis and Seydel (1999), Wang and Kirschner (2002), Katri and Ruan (2004), Gokdogan and Merdan (2011), Arafa et al. (2011), and Atay et al. (2016) is extended by using interval analysis.

As mentioned in the previous section, HTLV-I is the first human retrovirus in the genus Delta retrovirus. Retroviruses are RNA viruses that produce DNA from RNA by using an enzyme called reverse transcriptase. The DNA is subsequently incorporated into the host's genome. Note that the latency period can persist for a long period of time. Although latently infected cells contain the virus, they do not produce DNA and are incapable of contagion. These cells can become active and infect healthy cells if they are stimulated by antigen. Actively infected cells may also be converted to ATL cells, (Wang and Kirschner, 2002). According to Lang (2009), "The primary target of HTLV-I are CD4⁺ T cells. Indeed, HTLV-I virions do not exist as cell-free viral particles and are confined to CD4⁺ T cells. A CD4⁺ T cell which has been infected by the HTLV-I virus is referred to as a proviral cell. This leads to two different modes of viral replication. First, direct contact between a proviral cell and a healthy CD4⁺ T cell may result in a transmission of HTLV-I. Second, since HTLV-I is a retrovirus, mitosis of a proviral cell produces two new proviral cells. In the case of direct contact it is clear that HTLV-I genes must be active in order for there to be virions present to transfer between cells. In the second case it is possible for mitosis to occur either as a result of HTLV-I expression or as a result of the normal cell cycle."

To the best of the author's knowledge, the first mathematical model of HTLV-I infection as an ordinary differential equations (ODEs) system is presented by Seydel and Karmer (1996). But Stilianakis and Seydel (1999) proposed a model that formulates a system of nonlinear differential equations that divides CD4⁺ T cells into four compartments: uninfected CD4⁺ T cells, latently infected cells, actively infected cells, and leukemia cells. The dynamical behavior of this model with fixed parameters has been investigated by Wang and Kirschner (2002). After these studies, Katri and Ruan (2004) modified the parameters of the model to distinguish between contact and infectivity rates. They did this modification "in order to take into account the probabilistic nature of infection (though stochastic modeling of HTLV-I infection, given the unusually high proviral load, has and should be pursued further)." Moreover, Katri and Ruan (2004) introduced a discrete time delay to the model for describing the time between the emission of contagious particles by active CD4⁺ T cells and the infection of pure cells. The model of Katri and Ruan (2004) studied by Arafa et al. (2011). They introduced fractional-order into the model and gave approximate and analytical solutions by generalized Euler method. Moreover, some numerical algorithms for solving the model of Katri and Ruan (2004) presented by Gokdogan and Merdan (2011), and Atay et al. (2016).

Motivated by the above, the author considers the ODE model of T cell dynamics in human T cell lymphotropic virus-I infection was proposed by Katri and Ruan (2004) as follows

$$\begin{cases} \dfrac{dT}{dt} = \lambda - \mu_T T - \kappa T_A T, \\[2mm] \dfrac{dT_L}{dt} = \kappa_1 T_A T - (\mu_L + \alpha)T_L, \\[2mm] \dfrac{dT_A}{dt} = \alpha T_L - (\mu_A + \rho)T_A, \\[2mm] \dfrac{dT_M}{dt} = \rho T_A + \beta T_M (1 - \dfrac{T_M}{T_{M_{max}}}) - \mu_M T_M, \end{cases} \qquad (1)$$

where "$T(t)$ represents the concentration of healthy CD4+ T cells at time t, $T_L(t)$ represents the concentration of latently infected CD4+ T cells, $T_A(t)$ the concentration of actively infected CD4+ T cells, and $T_M(t)$ the concentration of leukemic cells at time t. To explain the parameters, note that λ is the source of CD4+ T cells from precursors μ_T is the natural death rate of CD4+ T cells, κ is the rate at which uninfected cells are contacted by actively infected cells. The parameter κ_1 represents the rate of infection of T cells with virus from actively infected cells. μ_L, μ_A and μ_M are blanket death terms for latently infected, actively infected and leukemic cells, to reflect the assumption that we do not initially know whether the cells die naturally or by bursting. In addition, α and ρ represent the rates at which latently infected and actively infected cells become actively infected and leukemic, respectively. ATL cells grow at a rate β of a classical logistic growth function. $T_{M_{max}}$ is the maximal number that ATL cells proliferate."

Now, with a sufficient motivation and introduction, the author studies model (1). First, the author presents some background related to interval polynomials. Then, the author obtains some results on the stability of model (1) with interval parameters κ and κ_1.

Preliminaries

The author states some definition and theorems which is used in next section, (Bhattacharyya, Chapellat, & Keel, 1995; Kharitonov, 1978). An interval matrix which is denoted by:

$$\mathcal{A} = (I_{ij})_{i,j=1}^n = \{A \mid A_{ij} \in I_{ij}, i, j = 1, \dots, n\}, \qquad (2)$$

is the set of all matrices with interval entries. Similarly, an interval polynomial is a set of polynomials with interval coefficients as follows:

$$\mathcal{S} = I_0 + I_1\lambda + \dots + I_{n-1}\lambda^{n-1} + I_n\lambda^n = \{P = a_0 + a_1\lambda + \dots + a_n\lambda^n \mid a_j \in I_j, j = 1, \dots, n\}. \qquad (3)$$

Note that:

$$\mathcal{S}_1 + \mathcal{S}_2 = \{P_1 + P_2 \mid P_1 \in \mathcal{S}_1, P_2 \in \mathcal{S}_2\},$$

and

$$\mathcal{S}_1.\mathcal{S}_2 = \{P_1.P_2 | P_1 \in \mathcal{S}_1, P_2 \in \mathcal{S}_2\}.$$

Consider an interval polynomial

$$\mathcal{S} = I_0 + I_1\lambda + \ldots + I_{n-1}\lambda^{n-1} + \lambda^n, \qquad I_j = [a_j, b_j], \tag{4}$$

and define:

$$\begin{cases} g_1(\mathcal{S}, \lambda) = a_0 + b_2\lambda^2 + a_4\lambda^4 + \ldots, \\ g_2(\mathcal{S}, \lambda) = b_0 + a_2\lambda^2 + b_4\lambda^4 + \ldots, \\ h_1(\mathcal{S}, \lambda) = a_1\lambda + b_3\lambda^3 + a_5\lambda^5 + \ldots, \\ h_2(\mathcal{S}, \lambda) = b_1\lambda + a_3\lambda^3 + b_5\lambda^5 + \ldots. \end{cases} \tag{5}$$

Theorem (Kharitonov)

The interval polynomial (4) is Hurwitz stable if and only if the following polynomials are Hurwitz stable:

$$\begin{cases} g_1\left(\mathcal{S},.\right) + h_1\left(\mathcal{S},.\right), \\ g_2\left(\mathcal{S},.\right) + h_1\left(\mathcal{S},.\right), \\ g_1\left(\mathcal{S},.\right) + h_2\left(\mathcal{S},.\right), \\ g_2\left(\mathcal{S},.\right) + h_2\left(\mathcal{S},.\right). \end{cases}$$

Descartes' Criterion

If the terms of a single-variable polynomial with real coefficients are ordered by descending variable exponent, then the number of positive roots of the polynomial is less than or equal to the number of sign differences between consecutive nonzero coefficients.

MAIN RESULTS

Consider system (1) with interval parameters $\kappa = [\kappa^{\min}, \kappa^{Max}]$ and $\kappa_1 = [\kappa_1^{\min}, \kappa_1^{Max}]$. This system has non-negative three equilibrium points which are called infection-free, leukemic and infection equilibrium points as follows

$$P_1 = (\frac{\lambda}{\mu_T}, 0, 0, 0)$$

$$P_2 = (\frac{\lambda}{\mu_T}, 0, 0, (1 - \frac{\mu_M}{\beta})T_{M_{max}})$$

$$P_3 = (\bar{T}, \bar{T}_L, \bar{T}_A, \bar{T}_M)$$

where

$$\bar{T} = \frac{\mu_A^\rho \mu_L^\alpha}{\kappa_1 \alpha}, \bar{T}_A = \frac{\lambda \kappa_1 \alpha - \mu_T \mu_A^\rho \mu_L^\alpha}{\kappa \mu_A^\rho \mu_L^\alpha}, \bar{T}_L = \frac{\lambda \kappa_1 \alpha - \mu_T \mu_A^\rho \mu_L^\alpha}{\kappa \alpha \mu_L^\alpha},$$

$$\mu_A^\rho := \mu_A + \rho, \mu_L^\alpha := \mu_L + \alpha$$

and $\bar{T}_M$ is positive root of the following polynomial

$$\bar{T}_M^2 - (\frac{\beta - \mu_M}{\beta} T_{M_{Max}})\bar{T}_M - \frac{\lambda \kappa_1 \alpha - \mu_T \mu_A^\rho \mu_L^\alpha}{\beta \kappa \mu_A^\rho \mu_L^\alpha} \rho T_{M_{Max}} = 0. \tag{6}$$

It is easy to prove equation (6) has only one positive root

$$\bar{T}_M = \frac{1}{2}\{(\frac{\beta - \mu_M}{\beta} T_{M_{Max}}) + \sqrt{(\frac{\beta - \mu_M}{\beta} T_{M_{Max}})^2 + 4\frac{\lambda \kappa_1 \alpha - \mu_T \mu_A^\rho \mu_L^\alpha}{\beta \kappa \mu_A^\rho \mu_L^\alpha} \rho T_{M_{Max}}}\}.$$

Following the line in Katri and Ruan (2004), behavior of the system (1) depends on the basic reproduction number:

$$R_0 = \frac{\alpha \kappa_1 T_0}{\mu_A^\rho \mu_L^\alpha}, \tag{7}$$

where $T_0 = \frac{\lambda}{\mu_T}$. The author should be noted that Katri and Ruan (2004) and other researchers did not obtain P_2. Moreover, note that P_2 ($\neq P_1$) exists if and only if $\beta - \mu_M$ is positive, since all T cell sub-populations at an equilibrium point must be non-negative. Therefore, one can state the following proposition.

Proposition 1

There are four cases:

- If $R_0 \leq 1$ and $\beta - \mu_M$ are non-positive, then there is only equilibrium point P_1, infection-free equilibrium.

- If $R_0 \leq 1$ and $\beta - \mu_M$ are positive, then there are two equilibrium points P_1 and P_2, infection-free and leukemic equilibrium points.
- If $R_0 > 1$ and $\beta - \mu_M$ are non-positive, then there are two equilibrium points P_1 and P_3, infection-free and infection equilibrium points.
- If $R_0 > 1$ and $\beta - \mu_M$ are positive, then there are three equilibrium points P_1, P_2 and P_3, infection-free, leukemic and infection equilibrium points.

The Jacobian matrix of system (1) at P =(T, T_L, T_A, T_M) can be computed as follows:

$$
A_P = \begin{pmatrix}
-(\mu_T + \kappa T_A) & 0 & -\kappa T & 0 \\
\kappa_1 T_A & -\mu_L^\alpha & \kappa_1 T & 0 \\
0 & \alpha & -\mu_A^\rho & 0 \\
0 & 0 & \rho & \beta(1 - 2\dfrac{T_M}{T_{M_{Max}}}) - \mu_M
\end{pmatrix}. \tag{8}
$$

It is not hard to see that

$$
S_{P_1} = (\beta - \mu_M - \sigma)(-\mu_T - \sigma)(S_2^\sigma)
$$
$$
S_{P_2} = (\mu_M - \beta - \sigma)(-\mu_T - \sigma)(S_2^\sigma)
$$

where $S_{P_i} = \det(\sigma I_4 - A_{P_i})$ for $i = 1, 2$ are characteristic equations of P_1 and P_2 and

$$
S_2^\sigma = \sigma^2 + (\mu_L^\alpha + \mu_A^\rho)\sigma - \frac{\lambda \kappa_1 \alpha - \mu_T \mu_A^\rho \mu_L^\alpha}{\mu_T}.
$$

First, we can state the following lemma then one can discuss on stability of P_1 and P_2.

Lemma 2

S_2^σ is Hurwitz stable if and only if

H1: $\kappa_1^{Max} < \dfrac{\mu_T \mu_A^\rho \mu_L^\alpha}{\lambda \alpha}$.

Proof

Rewrite S_2^σ as follows:

$$S_2^\sigma = \sigma^2 + C_1\sigma + C_2 \qquad\qquad (9)$$

where

$$C_1 := (\mu_L^\alpha + \mu_A^\rho), \quad C_2 := -\frac{\lambda\kappa_1\alpha - \mu_T\mu_A^\rho\mu_L^\alpha}{\mu_T}.$$

First, we assume that κ and κ_1 are interval parameters and others are fixed parameters. Thus, C_1 is a fixed parameter and C_2 is an interval parameter, $C_2 = [C_2^{\min}, C_2^{Max}]$. By Kharitonov's theorem S_2^σ is Hurwitz stable if and only if

$$S_2^{\sigma,\min} = \sigma^2 + C_1\sigma + C_2^{\min}$$

and

$$S_2^{\sigma,Max} = \sigma^2 + C_1\sigma + C_2^{Max}$$

are Hurwitz stable. Therefore, by Descartes' criterion, it is sufficient that $C_2^{\min}$ and C_2^{Max} are positive since fixed parameter C_1 is positive. On the other hand, by interval analysis

$$C_2 = [C_2^{\min}, C_2^{Max}] = [\frac{\mu_T\mu_A^\rho\mu_L^\alpha - \lambda\kappa_1^{Max}\alpha}{\mu_T}, \frac{\mu_T\mu_A^\rho\mu_L^\alpha - \lambda\kappa_1^{\min}\alpha}{\mu_T}].$$

The proof is complete.

Result

S_{P_1} is Hurwitz stable if and only if $\kappa_1^{Max} < \dfrac{\mu_T\mu_A^\rho\mu_L^\alpha}{\lambda\alpha}$ and $\beta - \mu_M < 0$. Also, S_{P_2} is Hurwitz stable if and only if $\kappa_1^{Max} < \dfrac{\mu_T\mu_A^\rho\mu_L^\alpha}{\lambda\alpha}$ and $\beta - \mu_M > 0$.

The above discussion yields the following proposition.

Proposition 3

If $\kappa_1^{Max} < \dfrac{\mu_T\mu_A^\rho\mu_L^\alpha}{\lambda\alpha}$, then there are two cases:

- If $\beta - \mu_M < 0$ then P_1 is a stable equilibrium point and there is no another equilibrium point.
- If $\beta - \mu_M > 0$ then P_1 is a saddle equilibrium point and P_2 is a stable equilibrium point.

Similarly, characteristic equation of P_3 can be obtained by using matrix (8). Indeed,

$$S_{P_3} = (M' - \sigma)(S_3^{\sigma})$$

(10)

such that

$$M' = \beta(1 - 2\frac{\bar{T}_M}{T_{M_{Max}}}) - \mu_M$$

(11)

$$S_3^{\sigma} = \sigma^3 + D_1\sigma^2 + D_2\sigma + D_3$$

(12)

where,

$$D_1 = \kappa\bar{T}_A + \mu_L^{\alpha} + \mu_A^{\rho} + \mu_T,$$

$$D_2 = (\kappa\bar{T}_A + \mu_T)(\mu_L^{\alpha} + \mu_A^{\rho}) + \mu_A^{\rho}\mu_L^{\alpha} - \alpha\kappa_1\bar{T},$$

$$D_3 = (\kappa\bar{T}_A + \mu_T)(\mu_A^{\rho}\mu_L^{\alpha} - \alpha\kappa_1\bar{T}) + \alpha\kappa\kappa_1\bar{T}\bar{T}_A.$$

Interval parameters $D_1 = [D_1^{\min}, D_1^{Max}]$, $D_2 = [D_2^{\min}, D_2^{Max}]$, $D_3 = [D_3^{\min}, D_3^{Max}]$ can be computed by interval analysis:

$$D_1 = \frac{\lambda\kappa_1\alpha}{\mu_A^{\rho}\mu_L^{\alpha}} + \mu_L^{\alpha} + \mu_A^{\rho} = [\frac{\lambda\kappa_1^{min}\alpha}{\mu_A^{\rho}\mu_L^{\alpha}} + \mu_L^{\alpha} + \mu_A^{\rho}, \frac{\lambda\kappa_1^{Max}\alpha}{\mu_A^{\rho}\mu_L^{\alpha}} + \mu_L^{\alpha} + \mu_A^{\rho}],$$

$$D_2 = \frac{\lambda\kappa_1\alpha}{\mu_A^{\rho}\mu_L^{\alpha}}(\mu_L^{\alpha} + \mu_A^{\rho}) = [\frac{\lambda\kappa_1^{min}\alpha}{\mu_A^{\rho}\mu_L^{\alpha}}(\mu_L^{\alpha} + \mu_A^{\rho}), \frac{\lambda\kappa_1^{Max}\alpha}{\mu_A^{\rho}\mu_L^{\alpha}}(\mu_L^{\alpha} + \mu_A^{\rho})],$$

$$D_3 = \lambda\kappa_1\alpha - \mu_T\mu_A^{\rho}\mu_L^{\alpha} = [\lambda\kappa_1^{min}\alpha - \mu_T\mu_A^{\rho}\mu_L^{\alpha}, \lambda\kappa_1^{Max}\alpha - \mu_T\mu_A^{\rho}\mu_L^{\alpha}].$$

By Kharitonov's theorem, S_3^{σ} is Hurwitz stable if and only if:

$$S_3^{\sigma,1} = \sigma^3 + D_1^{\min}\sigma^2 + D_2^{Max}\sigma + D_3^{Max},$$
$$S_3^{\sigma,2} = \sigma^3 + D_1^{Max}\sigma^2 + D_2^{\min}\sigma + D_3^{\min},$$
$$S_3^{\sigma,3} = \sigma^3 + D_1^{Max}\sigma^2 + D_2^{Max}\sigma + D_3^{\min},$$
$$S_3^{\sigma,4} = \sigma^3 + D_1^{\min}\sigma^2 + D_2^{\min}\sigma + D_3^{Max},$$

are Hurwitz stable. Stability of them is equivalent to the following conditions:

$$D_1^{\min} > 0, D_3^{Max} > 0, D_1^{\min} D_2^{Max} - D_3^{Max} > 0,$$
$$D_1^{Max} > 0, D_3^{\min} > 0, D_1^{Max} D_2^{\min} - D_3^{\min} > 0,$$
$$D_1^{Max} > 0, D_3^{\min} > 0, D_1^{Max} D_2^{Max} - D_3^{\min} > 0,$$
$$D_1^{\min} > 0, D_3^{Max} > 0, D_1^{\min} D_2^{\min} - D_3^{Max} > 0.$$

Furthermore, $D_1^{\min} > 0$. Hence, these conditions hold if and only if:

$$D_3^{\min} > 0, \ D_1^{\min} D_2^{\min} - D_3^{Max} > 0. \tag{13}$$

Therefore, S_3^σ is Hurwitz stable if and only if

H2: $\kappa_1^{min} > \dfrac{\mu_T \mu_A^\rho \mu_L^\alpha}{\lambda \alpha}$, $\tag{14}$

H3: $(\kappa_1^{min})^2 \dfrac{(\mu_L^\alpha + \mu_A^\rho)\lambda^2 \alpha^2}{(\mu_L^\alpha \mu_A^\rho)^2} + \kappa_1^{min} \dfrac{(\mu_L^\alpha + \mu_A^\rho)^2 \lambda \alpha}{\mu_L^\alpha \mu_A^\rho} - \kappa_1^{Max} \lambda \alpha + \mu_T \mu_A^\rho \mu_L^\alpha > 0.$ $\tag{15}$

Now, the following proposition can be stated.

Proposition 4

If 14 and 15 hold, then there are two cases:

- If $M' > 0$, then P_3 is a saddle equilibrium point,
- If $M' < 0$, then P_3 is a stable equilibrium point.

Now, one completely understands the local stability of all equilibria of system (1) with interval parameters $\kappa = [\kappa^{\min}, \kappa^{Max}]$ and $\kappa_1 = [\kappa_1^{\min}, \kappa_1^{Max}]$. Also, it is seen that one of interval parameters, $\kappa = [\kappa^{\min}, \kappa^{Max}]$, is not effective on the stability of equilibria.

Remark 5

It is clear that (9) and (12), S_2^σ and S_3^σ, do not have zero as a root if

H4: $0 \notin \kappa_1 = [\kappa_1^{\min}, \kappa_1^{Max}].$ $\tag{16}$

Remark 6

Note that $M' > 0$ is equivalent to

H5: $\bar{T}_M > \dfrac{1}{2} T_{M_{Max}} \left(\dfrac{\beta - \mu_M}{\beta} \right)$.   (17)

All results can be summarized as follows:

- If $(H1)$ holds, $R_0 \leq 1$ and $\beta - \mu_M < 0$, then P_1 is an asymptotically stable equilibrium point.
- If $(\sim H1)$ and $(H4)$ hold, $R_0 \leq 1$ and $\beta - \mu_M < 0$, then there is P_1 as a saddle equilibrium point.
- If $(H1)$ holds, $R_0 \leq 1$ and $\beta - \mu_M > 0$, then P_1 is a saddle equilibrium point and P_2 is an asymptotically stable equilibrium point.
- If $(\sim H1)$ and $(H4)$ hold, $R_0 \leq 1$ and $\beta - \mu_M > 0$, then P_1 and P_2 are saddle equilibrium points.
- If $(H1)$ holds, $R_0 > 1$ and $\beta - \mu_M < 0$, then there is P_1 as an asymptotically stable equilibrium point and there is no another equilibrium point.
- If $(\sim H1)$, $(H2)$, $(H3)$, $(H4)$ and $(H5)$ hold, $R_0 > 1$ and $\beta - \mu_M < 0$, then P_1 is a saddle equilibrium point and P_3 is an asymptotically stable equilibrium point.
- If $(\sim H1)$, $((\sim H2)$ or $(\sim H3)$ or $(\sim H5))$, and $(H4)$ hold, $R_0 > 1$ and $\beta - \mu_M < 0$ then P_1 and P_3 are saddle equilibrium points.
- If $(H1)$ holds, $R_0 > 1$ and $\beta - \mu_M > 0$, then P_1 is a saddle equilibrium point and P_2 is an asymptotically stable equilibrium point.
- If $(\sim H1)$ and $(H2)$, $(H3)$, $(H4)$ and $(H5)$ hold, $R_0 > 1$ and $\beta - \mu_M > 0$, then P_1 and P_2 are saddle equilibrium points and P_3 is an asymptotically stable equilibrium point.
- If $(\sim H1)$, $((\sim H2)$ or $(\sim H3)$ or $(\sim H5))$, and $(H4)$ hold, $R_0 > 1$ and $\beta - \mu_M > 0$, then two cases occur:
  - P_1, P_2 and P_3 are saddle equilibrium points, or
  - P_1 and P_2 are saddle equilibrium points and P_3 is an unstable equilibrium point.

NUMERICAL SIMULATION

There is some data based on studies of Stilianakis and Seydel (1999), Wang and Kirschner (2002), Katri and Ruan (2004), Gokdogan and Merdan (2011), Arafa et al. (2011), and Atay et al. (2016). As mentioned in the second section, the parameter values of HTLV-I infection are not available. According to Stilianakis and Seydel (1999), "Estimates for most of the parameters are not available and have been made on the basis of reasonable assumptions. Some of these assumptions are parameter estimates known from the HIV-I infection process, which were modified taking into account the specific differences between HIV-I and HTLV-I infection."

In this chapter, the author assumes that the source of CD4+ T cells from precursors λ is 4/day, CD4+ T cells die naturally at a rate of $\mu_T = 0.006$/day. Uninfected cells are contacted by actively infected cells with the rate $\kappa = 0.001$. The blanket death terms for latently infected μ_L, actively infected μ_A and leukemic cells μ_M are assumed 0.006/day, 0.05/day, and 0.0005/day, respectively. In addition, latently infected and actively infected cells become actively infected and leukemic, with rates $\alpha = 0.0004$/day and

$\rho = 0.00004$/day. Rate of growing ATL cells is considered $\beta = 0.0003$/day. Finally, the maximal number that ATL cells proliferate is $T_{M_{max}} = 2200$/mm^3. Also, the following initial values for variables are considered:

- The initial value of healthy CD4$^+$ T cells $T(0)=1000$/mm^3,
- The initial value of latently infected CD4$^+$ T cells $T_L(0)= 250$/mm^3,
- The initial value of actively infected CD4$^+$ T cells $T_A(0)= 1.5$/mm^3,
- The initial value of leukemic cells CD4$^+$ T cells $T_M(0)=0$/mm^3.

According to the forth section, one can compute for $\kappa_1 \in [0.3, 3.5]$, infection equilibrium point is asymptotically stable point, $P_3 = (778, 1.68, 204.36, 0.0141)$. The interval of κ_1 is obtained by using ($H2$) and ($H3$):

$$\kappa_1^{min} > 0.285,$$

$$\kappa_1^{max} < 3.58.$$

Numerical results of model (1) for a time span of 30 years with the above parameter and variable values are shown in Figure 1. This figure represents existence of long chronic infection with low levels of infected CD4$^+$ T cells. The above computation shows all infected CD4$^+$ T cells after 30 years of chronic infection are about 20.6% of the initial total T cell number. Moreover, actively infected CD4$^+$ T cells and leukemic cells CD4$^+$ T cells remain at a very low level. Actively infected CD4$^+$ T cells are 0.8% and leukemic cells CD4$^+$ T cells are almost 0.01% of the total of all infected CD4$^+$ T cells. These results show a minor proportion of leukemia cells in asymptomatic carriers of HTLV-I.

FUTURE RESEARCH DIRECTIONS

Local stability of all the equilibria of this model is fully understood. The author would like to identify necessary conditions for the global stability of them. Moreover, the author would like to have a better understanding of the bifurcations occur in this model.

CONCLUSION

In this Chapter, a model of human T cell lymphotropic virus type I infection is considered. The model formulates a system of nonlinear differential equations that divides CD4$^+$ T cells into four compartments: uninfected CD4$^+$ T cells, latently infected cells, actively infected cells, and leukemia cells. Taking place the infection through a cell-to-cell interaction between actively infected and uninfected T cells was the main assumption in this model.

Investigating dynamical behavior of this system with interval parameters was the main aim of this study. The author considered the rate at which uninfected cells are contacted by actively infected cells

Figure 1. Prediction of HTLV-I infection by the model

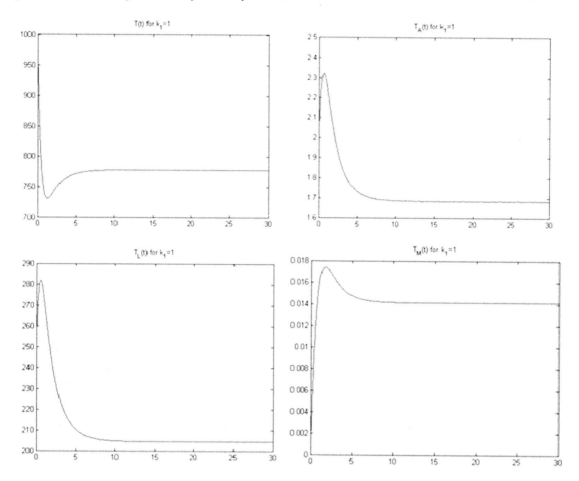

and therate of infection of T cells with virus from actively infected cells as interval parameters. Interval analysis and particularly of Kharitonov's stability theorem was used for the study of the model. The author obtained stability region of the uninfected steady state and the (positive) infected steady states. These regions showed each of equilibria (infection-free, leukemic and infection equilibrium points) where can be stable. Also, it is seen that the rate at which uninfected cells are contacted by actively infected cells as an interval parameter was not effective on stability of equilibria. Local stability of all the equilibria of this model is fully found. Furthermore, the validity of the main results is illustrated by numerical simulations.

ACKNOWLEDGMENT

The author would like to thank referees for careful reading and helpful comments on this chapter and IGI Global for giving the opportunity to consider this work.

REFERENCES

Arafa, A. A. M., Rida, S. Z., & Khalil, M. (2011). Fractional order model of human T-cell lymphotropic virus I (HTLV-I) infection of CD4+ T-cells lymphotropic virus type 1 (HTLV-I). *Advanced Studies in Biology*, *3*(7), 347–353.

Asquith, B., & Bangham, C. R. M. (2008). How does HTLV-I persist despite a strong cell-mediated immune response? *Trends in Immunology*, *29*(1), 4–11. doi:10.1016/j.it.2007.09.006 PMID:18042431

Asquith, B., Mosley, A. J., Heaps, A., Tanaka, Y., Taylor, G. P., McLean, A. R., & Bangham, C. R. M. (2005). Quantification of the virus-host interaction in human T lymphotropic virus I infection. *Retrovirology*, *2*(75), 1–9. PMID:16336683

Atay, M. T., Başbük, M., & Eryılmaz, A. (2016). A geometric integration based on magnus series expansion for human T cell lymphotropic virus I (HTLV-I) infection of CD4+T cells model. *Journal of Advances in Applied Mathematics*, *1*(2), 98–106. doi:10.22606/jaam.2016.12002

Bangham, C. R., Meekings, K., Toulza, F., Nejmeddine, M., Majorovits, E., Asquith, B., & Taylor, G. P. (2009). The immune control of HTLV-I infection: Selection forces and dynamics. *Frontiers in Bioscience (Landmark Edition)*, *14*, 28892903. PMID:19273242

Bangham, C. R., & Osame, M. (2005). Cellular immune response to HTLV-I. *Oncogene*, *24*(39), 6035–6046. doi:10.1038/sj.onc.1208970 PMID:16155610

Bangham, C. R. M. (2000). The immune response to HTLV-I. *Current Opinion in Immunology*, *12*(4), 397–402. doi:10.1016/S0952-7915(00)00107-2 PMID:10899027

Bhattacharyya, S. P., Chapellat, H., & Keel, L. H. (1995). *Robust Control: The Parametric Approach*. Prentice Hall.

Blattner, W. A., Blayney, D. W., Robert-Guroff, M., Sarngadharan, M. G., Kalyanaraman, V. S., Sarin, P. S., & Gallo, R. C. et al. (1983). Epidemiology of human T cell leukemia/lymphoma virus. *The Journal of Infectious Diseases*, *147*(3), 406–416. doi:10.1093/infdis/147.3.406 PMID:6300254

Blattner, W. A., Kalyanaraman, V. S., Robert-Guroff, M., Lister, T. A., Galton, D. A. G., Sarin, P. S., & Gallo, R. C. et al. (1982). The human type-C retrovirus, HTLV, in Blacks from the Caribbean region, and relationship to adult T cell leukemia/lymphoma. *International Journal of Cancer*, *30*(3), 257–264. doi:10.1002/ijc.2910300302 PMID:6290401

Bofill, M., Janossy, G., Lee, C. A., MacDonald-Burns, D., Phillips, A. N., Sabin, C., & Kernoff, P. B. A. et al. (1992). Laboratory control values for CD4 and CD8 T lymphocytes. Implications for HIV-1 diagnosis. *Clinical and Experimental Immunology*, *88*(2), 243–252. doi:10.1111/j.1365-2249.1992.tb03068.x PMID:1349272

Cai, L., Li, X., & Ghosh, M. (2011). Global dynamics of a mathematical model for HTLV-I infection of CD4+T cells. *Applied Mathematical Modelling*, *35*(7), 3587–3595. doi:10.1016/j.apm.2011.01.033

Cann, A. J., & Chen, I. S. Y. (1996). Human T cell leukemia virus types I and II. Philadelphia: Lippincott-Raven Publishers.

Chiavetta, J. A., Escobar, M., Newman, A., He, Y., Driezen, P., Deeks, S., & Sher, G. et al. (2003). Incidence and estimated rates of residual risk for HIV, hepatitis C, hepatitis B and human T-cell lymphotropic viruses in blood donors in Canada 1990-2000. *Canadian Medical Association Journal, 169*(8), 767–773. PMID:14557314

Dadi, Z., & Alizade, S. (2016). Codimension-one bifurcation and stability analysis in an immunosuppressive infection model. SpringerPlus, 5, 106-121.

DeBoer, R. J., & Perelson, A. S. (1998). Target cell limited and immune control models of HIV infection: A comparison. *Journal of Theoretical Biology, 190*(3), 201–214. doi:10.1006/jtbi.1997.0548 PMID:9514649

Elaiw, A. M. (2010). Global properties of a class of HIV models. *Nonlinear Analysis Real World Applications, 11*(4), 2253–2263. doi:10.1016/j.nonrwa.2009.07.001

Eshima, N., Iwata, O., Iwata, S., Tabata, M., Higuchi, Y., Matsuishi, T., & Karukaya, S. (2009). Age and gender specific prevalence of HTLV-I. *Journal of Clinical Virology, 45*(2), 135–138. doi:10.1016/j.jcv.2009.03.012 PMID:19386541

Eshima, N., Tabata, M., Okada, T., & Karukaya, S. (2003). Population dynamics of HTLV-I infection: A discrete-time mathematical epidemic model approach. *Mathematical Medicine and Biology, 20*(1), 29–45. doi:10.1093/imammb/20.1.29 PMID:12974497

Gokdogan, A., & Merdan, M. (2011). A multistage homotopy perturbation method for solving human T cell lymphotropic virus I (HTLV-I) infection of CD4$^+$T cells model. *Middle-East Journal of Scientific Research, 9*(4), 503–509.

Gómez-Acevedo, H., & Li, Y. M. (2005). Backward bifurcation in a model for HTLV-I infection of CD4$^+$ T Cells. *Bulletin of Mathematical Biology, 67*(1), 101–114. doi:10.1016/j.bulm.2004.06.004 PMID:15691541

Katri, P., & Ruan, S. (2004). Dynamics of human T cell lymphotropic virus I (HTLV-I) infection of CD4$^+$ T cells. *Comptes Rendus Biologies, 327*(11), 1009–1016. doi:10.1016/j.crvi.2004.05.011 PMID:15628223

Kharitonov, V. L. (1978). Asymptotic stability of an equilibrium position of a family of systems of linear differential equations. *Differensial'nye Uravnenya, 14*, 2086–2088.

Lang, J. (2009). *Periodic Solutions and Bistability in a Model for Cytotoxic T-Lymphocyte (CTL) Response to Human T-Cell* (M.Sc. dissertation). University of Alberta, Canada.

Lang, J., & Li, M. Y. (2012). Stable and transient periodic oscillations in a mathematical model for CTL response to HTLV-I infection. *Journal of Mathematical Biology, 65*(1), 181–199. doi:10.1007/s00285-011-0455-z PMID:21792554

Lim, A. G., & Maini, P. K. (2014). HTLV-I infection: A dynamic struggle between viral persistence and host immunity. *Journal of Theoretical Biology, 352*, 92–108. doi:10.1016/j.jtbi.2014.02.022 PMID:24583256

Mortreux, F., Gabet, A. S., & Wattel, E. (2003). Molecular and cellular aspects of HTLV-I associated leukemogenesis in vivo. *Leukemia, 17*(1), 26–38. doi:10.1038/sj.leu.2402777 PMID:12529656

Mortreux, F., Kazanji, M., Gabet, A. S., de Thoisy, B., & Wattel, E. (2001). Two-step nature of human T-cell leukemia virus type1 replication in experimentally infected squirrel monkeys (Saimiri sciureus). *Journal of Virology, 75*(2), 1083–1089. doi:10.1128/JVI.75.2.1083-1089.2001 PMID:11134325

Murphy, E. L., Figueroa, J. P., Gibbs, W. N., Holding-Cobham, M., Cranston, B., Malley, K., & Blattner, W. A. et al. (1991). Human T lymphotropic virus type I (HTLV-I) seroprevalence in Jamaica: I.demographic determinants. *American Journal of Epidemiology, 33*(11), 1114–1124. doi:10.1093/oxfordjournals.aje. a115824 PMID:2035515

Nelson, P. W., Murray, J. D., & Perelson, A. S. (2000). A model of HIV-1 pathogenesis that includes an intracellular delay. *Mathematical Biosciences, 163*(2), 201–215. doi:10.1016/S0025-5564(99)00055-3 PMID:10701304

Nowak, M. A., & Bangham, C. R. M. (1996). Population dynamics of immune responses to persistence viruses. *Science, 272*(5258), 74–79. doi:10.1126/science.272.5258.74 PMID:8600540

Oguma, S. (1990). Simulation of dynamic changes of human T cell leukemia virus type I carriage rates. *Japanese Journal of Cancer Research, 81*(1), 1521. doi:10.1111/j.1349-7006.1990.tb02501.x PMID:2108943

Olavarria, E. N., Gomes, A. N., Kruschewsky, R. A., Galvão-Castro, B., & Grassi, M. F. R. (2012). Evolution of HTLV-1 proviral load in patients from Salvador, Brazil. *The Brazilian Journal of Infectious Diseases, 16*(4), 357–360. doi:10.1016/j.bjid.2012.06.022 PMID:22846124

Perelson, A. S., & Nelson, P. W. (1999). Mathematical analysis of HIV-I dynamics in vivo. *SIAM Review, 41*(1), 3–44. doi:10.1137/S0036144598335107

Poiesz, B. J., Ruscetti, F. W., Gazdar, A. F., Bunn, P. A., Minna, J. D., & Gallo, R. C. (1980). Detection and isolation of type C retrovirus particles from fresh and cultured lymphocytes of a patient with cutaneous T-cell lymphoma. *Proceedings of the National Academy of Sciences of the United States of America, 77*(12), 7415–7419. doi:10.1073/pnas.77.12.7415 PMID:6261256

Ramirez, E., Cartier, L., Torres, M., & Barria, M. (2007). Temporal dynamics of human T lymphotropic virus type I tax mRNA and proviral DNA load in peripheral blood mononuclear cells of human Tlymphotropic virus type Iassociated myelopathy patients. *Journal of Medical Virology, 79*(6), 782–790. doi:10.1002/jmv.20844 PMID:17457906

Ribeiro, R. M., Mohri, H., Ho, D. D., & Perelson, A. S. (2002). In vivo dynamics of T cell activation, proliferation, and death in HIV-1 infection: Why are CD4$^+$ but not CD8$^+$ T cells depleted? *Proceedings of the National Academy of Sciences of the United States of America, 99*(24), 15572–15577. doi:10.1073/pnas.242358099 PMID:12434018

Richardson, J. H., Edwards, A. J., Cruickshank, J. K., Rudge, P., & Dalgleish, A. G. (1990). In vivo cellular tropism of human T cell leukemia virus type I. *Journal of Virology, 64*, 5682–5687. PMID:1976827

Richardson, J. H., Hollsberg, P., Windhagen, A., Child, L. A., Hafler, D. A., & Lever, A. M. (1997). Variable immortalizing potential and frequent virus latency in blood-derived T-cell clones infected with human T-cell leukemia virus type I. *Blood, 89*, 3303–3314. PMID:9129036

Robbins, F. W. A. (2010). Mathematical model of HIV infection: Simulating T4, T8, macrophages, antibody, and virus via specific anti-HIV response in the Presence of adaptation and tropism. *Bulletin of Mathematical Biology, 72*(5), 1208–1253. doi:10.1007/s11538-009-9488-5 PMID:20151219

Seigel, L. J., Nash, W. G., Poiesz, B. J., Moore, J. L., & OBrien, S. J. (1986). Dynamic and nonspecific dispersal of human Tcell leukemia/lymphoma virus type I integration in cultured lymphoma cells. *Virology, 154*(1), 6775. doi:10.1016/0042-6822(86)90430-7 PMID:3019009

Seydel, J., & Kramer, A. (1996). Transmission and population dynamics of HTLV-I infection. *International Journal of Cancer, 66*(2), 197–200. doi:10.1002/(SICI)1097-0215(19960410)66:2<197::AID-IJC10>3.0.CO;2-A PMID:8603811

Seydel, J., & Stilianakis, N. I. (2000). HTLV-I Dynamics: A mathematical model. *Sexually Transmitted Diseases, 27*(10), 652–653. doi:10.1097/00007435-200011000-00031

Shirdel, A., Hashemzadeh, K., Sahebari, M., Rafatpanah, H., Hatef, M. R., Rezaieyazdi, Z., & Farid-Hosseini, R. et al. (2013). Is there any association between human lymphotropic virus type I (HTLV-I) infection and systemic lupus erythematosus? An Original Research and Literature Review. *Iranian Journal of Basic Medical Sciences., 16*, 252–257. PMID:24470872

Song, X., & Li, Y. (2006). Global stability and periodic solution of a model for HTLV-I infection and ATL progression. *Applied Mathematics and Computation, 180*(1), 401–410. doi:10.1016/j.amc.2005.12.022

Stilianakis, N. I., & Seydel, J. (1999). Modeling the T-cell dynamics and pathogenesis of HTLV-I infection. *Bulletin of Mathematical Biology, 61*(5), 935–947. doi:10.1006/bulm.1999.0117 PMID:17886750

Sun, X., & Wei, J. (2013). Global dynamics of a HTLV-I infection model with CTL response. *Electronic Journal of Qualitative Theory of Differential Equations, 40*(40), 1–15. doi:10.14232/ejqtde.2013.1.40

Tortevoye, P., Tuppin, P., Carles, G., Peneau, C., & Gessain, A. (2005). Comparative trends of seroprevalence and seroincidence rates of human T cell lymphotropic virus type I and human immunodeficiency virus 1 in pregnant women of various ethnic groups sharing the same environment in French Guiana. *The American Journal of Tropical Medicine and Hygiene, 73*(3), 560565. PMID:16172481

Vieira, I. T., Cheng, R. C. H., Harper, P. R., & Senna, V. (2010). Small world network models of the dynamics of HIV infection. *Annals of Operations Research, 178*(1), 173–200. doi:10.1007/s10479-009-0571-y

Wang, K., Fan, A., & Torres, A. (2010). Global properties of an improved hepatitis B virus model. *Nonlinear Analysis Real World Applications, 11*(4), 3131–3138. doi:10.1016/j.nonrwa.2009.11.008

Wang, L., Li, M. Y., & Kirschner, D. (2002). Mathematical analysis of the global dynamics of a model for HTLV-I infection and ATL progression. *Mathematical Biosciences, 179*(2), 207–217. doi:10.1016/S0025-5564(02)00103-7 PMID:12208616

Wattel, E., Vartanian, J. P., Pannetier, C., & Wain-Hobson, S. (1995). Clonal expansion of human T cell leukemia virus type I-infected cells in asymptomatic and symptomatic carriers without malignancy. *Journal of Virology, 69*, 2863–2868. PMID:7707509

Williams, A. E., Fang, C. T., Slamon, D. J., Poiesz, B., Sandler, S., Darr, W., & et, et al.. (1988). Seroprevalence and epidemiological correlates of HTLV–I infection in U. S. blood donors. *Science, 240*(4852), 643–646. doi:10.1126/science.2896386 PMID:2896386

Yamamoto, N., Okada, M., Koyanagi, Y., Kannagi, M., & Hinuma, Y. (1982). Transformation of human leukocytes by cocultivation with an adult T cell leukemia virus producer cell line. *Science, 217*(4561), 737–739. doi:10.1126/science.6980467 PMID:6980467

Yu, Y., Nieto, J. J., Torres, A., & Wang, K. (2009). A viral infection model with a nonlinear infection rate. Boundary Value Problems, ArticleID 958016.

KEY TERMS AND DEFINITIONS

Equilibrium Point: Let $\dot{x} = f(x)$, $x \in \mathbb{R}^n$ be an autonomous differential equation. If $f(x_0) = 0$, then x_0 is called an equilibrium point. This means that there is a constant function $\phi : \mathbb{R} \to \mathbb{R}^n$ which $\phi(t) \equiv x_0$.

Human T-Cell Lymphotropic Virus Type I: Human T-Cell Lymphotropic Virus Type I is the first human retrovirus and the etiological agent of HTLV-I associated myelopathy/tropical spastic paraparesis and adult cell leukemia.

Infection Equilibrium Point: An equilibrium point is called infection equilibrium point if the population of four subsets of CD4+ T cells (susceptible, latently infected, actively infected and leukemia cells) is not zero.

Infection-Free Equilibrium Point: An equilibrium point is called infection-free equilibrium point if the number of latently infected cells, actively infected cells and leukemia cells are zero.

Interval System: A dynamical system with interval parameters is called interval system.

Kharitonov's Stability Theorem: Kharitonov's stability theorem discusses on Hurwitz stability of an interval polynomial by using interval analysis. This theorem shows that Hurwitz stability of an interval polynomial is equivalent to Hurwitz stability of four polynomials with fixed coefficients.

Leukemic Equilibrium Point: An equilibrium point is called leukemic equilibrium point if the number of latently infected cells and actively infected cells are zero, but the population of leukemia cells is not zero.

Modeling: The modeling of HTLV-I infection is based on the assumption cell-to-cell infection of CD4+ T cells. The model of HTLV-I infection introduces the dynamics between four subsets of CD4+ T cells; susceptible, latently infected, actively infected and leukemia cells.

Chapter 7
Global Dynamics of an Immunosuppressive Infection Model Based on a Geometric Approach

Zohreh Dadi
University of Bojnord, Iran

ABSTRACT

By clinical data, drug treatment sometimes is ineffective to eradicate the infection completely from the host in some human pathogens such as human immunodeficiency virus (HIV), hepatitis B virus (HBV), hepatitis C virus (HCV), and human T cell lymphotropic virus type I. Therefore, mathematical modeling can play a significant role to understand the interactions between viral replication and immune response. In this chapter, the author investigates the global dynamics of antiviral immune response in an immunosuppressive infection model which was studied by Dadi and Alizade (2016). In this model, the global asymptotic stability of an immune control equilibrium point is proved by using the Poincare–Bendixson property, Volterra–Lyapunov stable matrices, properties of monotone dynamical systems and geometric approach. The analysis and results which are presented in this chapter make building blocks towards a comprehensive study and deeper understanding of the dynamics of immunosuppressive infection model.

INTRODUCTION

In mathematical modeling of biological phenomena, one of complex systems is the immune system. The immune system is human body primary defense against pathogenic organisms and cells that have become malignantly transformed. Also, it involves multiple cell types and hundreds of soluble mediators and different receptor ligand interactions. The immune system can produce different types and intensity of responses, learn from experience and exhibit memory. Therefore, the modeling of immune system needs the knowledge about cells, molecules, and genes that make up that. This knowledge is based on the Human Genome Project progresses which uncover the genes and molecules that influence the behavior of single lymphocytes.

DOI: 10.4018/978-1-5225-2515-8.ch007

It is important to understand the behavior of the cells of immune system and how every cell of immune system interacts with other cells to generate an immune response. Furthermore, it should be noted that modeling in immunology is in contrast to the field of neurophysiology. In fact, the behavior of a single cell of immune system is not described in immunology. This means that the equivalents of the Hodgkin-Huxley (1952) equations do not exist in immunology. Hence, understanding interactions among the elementary components of a system in immunology is the major part in modeling. Quantitative results which are obtained by mathematical modeling can help researchers to modify and complete their understanding of immunological phenomena, (Barnes et al., 2002; Bekkering, Stalgis, McHutchison, Brouwer, & Perelson, 2001; Borghans, De Boer, Sercarz, & Kumar, 1998; Borghans, Noest, & De Boer, 1999; Borghans, Taams, Wauben, & De Boer, 1999; Butler & Waltman, 1986; Canabarro, Gléeria, & Lyra, 2004; Celada & Seiden, 1992; Celada & Seiden, 1996; Chun et al. 1997; Coppel,1965; Dadi & Alizade, 2016; De Boer & Perelson,1993; Detours & Perelson, 1999; Detours & Perelson, 2000; Diepolder et al. 1998; Fenton, Lello, & Bonsall, 2006; Hlavacek, Redondo, Metzger, Wofsy, & Goldstein, 2001; Kalams & Walker, 1998; Kepler & Perelson, 1993; Kesmir & De Boer, 1999; Komarova, Barnes, Klenerman, & Wodarz, 2003; Lang & Li, 2012; Lechner et al., 2000; Lechner et al., 2000b; Lewin et al. 2001; Li & Shu, 2010a, 2010b, 2011, 2012; Lifson et al., 2000, 2001; Liu & Wang, 2010; Lohr et al., 1998; Maini, & Bertoletti, 2000; McKeithan, 1995; McLean, Rosado, Agenes, Vasconcellos, & Freitas, 1997; Mukandavire, Garira, & Chiyaka, 2007; Nelson, Murray, & Perelson, 2000; Nelson & Perelson, 2002; Neumann et al., 1998; Ortiz et al. 2002; Percus, J.K., Percus, O.E. & Perelson, 1993; Perelson, 2002; Perelson, & Oster, 1979; Perelson & Weisbuch, 1997; Pugliese & Gandolfi, 2008; Rosenberg et al., 2000; Segel & BarOr, 1999; Shamsara, Mostolizadeh, & Afsharnezhad, 2016; Shu, Wang, &Watmough, 2014; Smith, Forrest, Ackley, & Perelson, 1999; Tam, 1999; Wang, Wang, Pang, & Liu, 2007; Whalley et al., 2001; Wodarz et al., 2000; Wodarz & Nowak, 1999; Zhu & Zou, 2008).

On the other hand, the interactions between the cells of immune system are very complicated. Therefore, the improvement of immunological models is a significant subject to study in recent decades.

The immune system has more than 10^7 different clones of cells that communicate via cell-cell contact and the secretion of molecules. It carries out pattern recognition tasks, learns, and preserves a memory of the antigens that it has fought. Like nervous system, cooperation among large numbers of the components of immune system for performing complex tasks such as learning and memory has attracted attention of many researchers who study on immunology, dynamical systems and statistical physics. Researchers believe that applying methods and concepts from statistical physics is especially suited to theoretical immunology, because there is not enough knowledge about the detail of mechanisms which are responsible for the observed behaviors in immune system. Moreover, dynamical systems help them to describe the time evolution of immune response. Researchers generally look for generic properties among the models of immune system, since these properties just depend on the general features of the model, and not on its details. According to Perelson and Weisbuch (1997), dynamical systems answer some of the questions about generic properties of the immune system such as: "Are the attractors limit points, limit cycles, or chaotic? What is their number? What are their basins of attraction? How do these properties relate to the parameters of the differential system? How can one force transitions among the different dynamical regimes? If our hypotheses about the universality of a model are true, the generic properties, qualitative classification of the attractors, and scaling laws should be evident in the phenomenology of the mammalian immune system." Indeed, theories and techniques of theoretical physics and mathematics play an important role to make towards increasing understanding of complex systems such as nervous system and immune system.

These views cause two forms of theory in immunology: verbal or nonmathematical and mathematical. As Perelson and Weisbuch (1997) mentioned, "nonmathematical theories have been pioneered by experimental immunologists, such as MacFarlane Burnet, the inventor of clonal selection theory, and Neils Jerne, the inventor of idiotypic network theory. These theories, while not originally formulated in a quantitative way, have been developed into quantitative theories. The other class of theories has been formulated mathematically." In the studying of immune response model, these classes have a momentous role in the development of immunology. Answering to the questions about dynamical properties of immune systems is both important and hard. Because collecting data from one animal at many time points is very difficult work, researchers rarely do dynamic experiments. Even if these experiments are sometimes done, there is no enough data which has obtained at more than a few time points. Therefore, mathematical view in immunology has attracted attention of researchers. Mathematical modeling can be used for dynamic analysis of immunological phenomena without doing expensive dynamic experiments. Segel (1995) has pointed that one of the hallmarks of a complex system is that it is a system which cannot be described by a single model. He well illustrated that there are different models for a phenomenon because of different individuals and different groups. According to Perelson and Weisbuch (1997), "The payoffs for developing successful models will be increased understanding of the operation of the immune system, the generation of new ideas, and new experiments to test them, as well as the eventual possibility of conducting immunological experiments in *machina* rather than in *vitro* or in *vivo* (Celada and Seiden, 1992, 1996)." One of the interesting areas in the study of the dynamical behaviors of a complex system in immunology and brain research is its local and global behavior. Development the principles and ideas in complex systems, nonlinear science, and the tools of computer simulation help to uncover the remaining mysteries of these systems.

In this chapter, the author would like to investigate global dynamics of antiviral immune response in an immunosuppressive infection model. Immunosuppressive infection in immunology studies has attracted much attention, (Bekkering et al. 2001; Canabarro et al., 2004; Chun et al. 1997; Dadi & Alizade, 2016; Diepolder et al. 1998; Fenton et al. 2006; Jacquez & Simon 2002; Komarova et al. 2003; Lang & Li, 2012; Lewin et al. 2001; Li & Shu 2010a, 2010b, 2011, 2012; Lifson et al. 2000, 2001; Lohr et al. 1998; Maini & Bertoletti 2000; Mukandavire et al. 2007; Nelson et al. 2000; Nelson & Perelson 2002; Neumann et al. 1998; Ortiz et al. 2002; Perelson 2002; Pugliese & Gandolfi, 2008; Rosenberg et al. 2000; Shamsara et al., 2016; Shu et al., 2014; Tam, 1999; Wang et al., 2007; Whalley et al. 2001; Zhu & Zou 2008).

Almost all of the researchers studied locally and globally stability of immunosuppressive infection model by means of Lyapunov function method. In this procedure, there is no systematic way to construct Lyapunov function. In this chapter, in order to obtain more nonlinear dynamic characteristics of the immunosuppressive infection model, the author considers introduced model in Dadi and Alizade (2016) and studies its global dynamics. For this aim, the author uses the properties of monotone dynamical systems and geometric approach.

The chapter is organized as follows. The focus of the second section is on the literature review of the immunosuppressive infection. In the third section, an immunosuppressive infection model is proposed where it shows the dynamics between an immunosuppressive infection and antiviral immune responses at various degrees of complexity. In this section, the author states some necessary definitions and theorems. In next section, the author states some conditions to the existence of equilibrium points of this model. The author proves Volterra-Lyapunov stability and global stability of its equilibrium points by using the Poincare-Bendixson property, Volterra–Lyapunov stable matrices, properties of monotone dynamical systems, and geometric approach. Finally, a brief discussion will be given in the last section.

BACKGROUND

According to recent studies, there are successes in the analyzing of immunological models such as dynamic and interactions of immune system with human immunodeficiency virus (HIV), human T cell lymphotropic virus type I (HTLV-I), hepatitis C virus (HCV), hepatitis B virus (HBV), cytomegalovirus (CMV) and lymphocytic choriomeningitis virus (LCMV), (Bekkering et al., 2001; Borghans et al., 1998; Borghans et al., 1999; Borghans et al., 1999; Chun et al. 1997; Dadi & Alizade, 2016; De Boer & Perelson, 1993; Detour & Perelson, 1999; Detours & Perelson, 2000; Hlavacek et al., 2001; Kepler & Perelson, 1993; Kesmir & De Boer, 1999; Komarova et al., 2003; Lewin et al. 2001; McKeithan, 1995; McLean et al.,1997; Neumann et al., 1998; Percus et al., 1993; Perelson, 2002; Perelson & Oster, 1979; Perelson & Weisbuch, 1997; Segel & BarOr, 1999; Shu et al., 2014; Shamsara et al., 2016; Smith et al.,1999; Whalley et al., 2001). This chapter focuses on immunosuppressive infection model because of clinical reports which have shown ineffective of drug treatment on some human pathogens such as human immunodeficiency virus (HIV), hepatitis B virus (HBV), and hepatitis C virus (HCV), (Barnes et al., 2002; Bekkering et al., 2001; Chun et al. 1997; Diepolder et al. 1998; Kalams & Walker, 1998; Lechner et al., 2000; Lechner et al., 2000; Lewin et al. 2001; Lifson et al., 2000, 2001; Lohr et al., 1998; Maini & Bertoletti, 2000; Neumann et al., 1998; Perelson, 2002; Rosenberg et al., 2000; Whalley et al., 2001; Wodarz et al., 2000). Based on these studies (Bekkering et al. 2001; Chun et al. 1997; Lewin et al. 2001; Neumann et al. 1998; Perelson 2002; Whalley et al. 2001), the infection can not sometimes completely be eradicated from the host by drug treatment for these diseases. These human pathogens are able to suppress immune responses and establish a persistent and productive infection that eventually results in pathology. The central component orchestrating antiviral effectors mechanisms are, directly or indirectly, virus-specific CD4 T helper cell responses. Therefore, one of intense potent strategies is to impair them. As mentioned in Komarova et al. (2003), the most prominent examples of this are HIV, hepatitis C virus (HCV), and hepatitis B virus (HBV) infection (Diepolder et al. 1998; Kalams & Walker, 1998; Lechner et al., 2000; Lechner et al., 2000; Lohr et al., 1998; Maini & Bertoletti, 2000; Rosenberg et al., 2000) pursuant to clinical data. Also, Komarova et al. (2003) has noted that drug treatment is ineffective in all cases, and lifelong therapy is generally necessary to control viral replication in HIV, (Bekkering et al., 2001; Chun et al. 1997; Lewin et al. 2001; Neumann et al., 1998; Perelson, 2002; Whalley et al., 2001). The drug treatment to boost virus-specific immunity is an alternative strategy which concludes sustained viral suppression in the absence of drugs. In the study of human immunodeficiency virus, this has been found (Lifson et al., 2000; Lifson et al., 2001; Rosenberg et al., 2000).

In researches, the impairment of specific helper cell responses has been observed in human immunodeficiency virus, hepatitis C virus and hepatitis B virus. Furthermore, human immunodeficiency virus induces the destruction of specific immune cells during the chronic phase of the infection while both hepatitis C virus and hepatitis B virus are not able to induce the destruction of specific immune cells, (Barnes et al., 2002; Diepolder et al. 1998; Maini & Bertoletti, 2000). Komarova et al. (2003) has used mathematical modeling to show that a single phase of drug therapy can result in the establishment of sustained immunity. Their studies were on immune response dynamics during therapy in the context of immunosuppressive infections. The general mathematical framework which was presented by them is based on a simple relationship between the timing of therapy and the efficacy of the drugs required for success. The significant suggestion of this study was that a single phase of treatment can result in long term immune mediated control of an immunosuppressive infection. According to Komarova et al. (2003), "In the presence of strong viral suppression, the model suggests that therapy should be stopped relatively early and that a longer duration of treatment can lead to failure. In contrast, with weaker viral suppression, stopping treatment too early is detrimental. Instead, therapy should be continued beyond a time threshold. The model further suggests that interruption therapy can be helpful in a restricted parameter region."

Komarova et al. (2003) has shown bistability for a virus dominant equilibrium (no sustained immunity) and an immune control equilibrium (with sustained immunity). Therefore, a solution from the basin of the attraction of the virus dominant equilibrium can be lifted to that of the immune control equilibrium via a single phase of therapy. This was equivalent to sustained immunity when the treatment is stopped. The model of Komarova et al. (2003) was a two dimensional ordinary differential equations system and immune response was assumed to be instantaneous. On the other hand, the process of immune response is a sequence of events such as antigenic activation, selection, and proliferation of immune cells. Therefore, the time lag between these events was taken into consideration in modeling, (Canabarro et al., 2004; Dadi & Alizade, 2016; Fenton et al. 2006; Jacquez & Simon, 2002; Lang & Li, 2012; Li & Shu, 2010 a, 2010b, 2011, 2012; Liu & Wang, 2010; Mukandavire et al., 2007; Nelson et al., 2000; Nelson & Perelson, 2002; Ortiz et al., 2002; Pugliese & Gandolfi, 2008; Shu et al., 2014; Tam, 1999; Wang et al., 2007; Zhu & Zou, 2008) and reference therein.

Tam (1999) considered a model which describes the interaction between a replicating virus and host cells. He has investigated effect of delay in that model. Also, Nelson et al. (2000), Nelson and Perelson (2002) studied on delay models of HIV-I infection. In 2002, Ortiz et al. studied the effect of highly active antiretroviral therapy on the frequency of HIV-I-specific CD8+ T cells in patients. They have observed oscillatory viral loads and immune cells during drug therapies. According to Fenton et al. (2006), "first, there may be an explicit time delay between infection and immune initiation, second, there may be a gradual build-up in immune efficacy during which the immune response develops, before reaching maximal specificity to the pathogen." These points help researchers to develop their models and obtain real results, (Wang et al., 2007; Mukandavire et al., 2007). Zhu and Zou (2008) studied a mathematical model for HIV-I infection with two different delays, "for (i) a latent period between the time target cells are contacted by the virus particles and the time the virions enter the cells and (ii) a virus production period for new virions to be produced within and released from the infected cells." Liu and Wang (2010) analyzed the global stability of the mathematical model of HIVI pathogenesis which was proposed by Nelson and Perelson. In this year, Li and Shu (2010a) investigated the dynamics of an in-host model with general form of target-cell dynamics, nonlinear incidence, and distributed delay. Their model can be used for the in vivo infection dynamics of many viruses such as HIV-I, HCV, and HBV. Also, they (2010b) studied the global dynamics of an in-host viral model with intracellular delay in another work. In next year, Li and Shu (2011) proved the phenomenon of stability switch in mathematical models for the cytotoxic T lymphocyte (CTL) response to HTLV-I infection by considering time lag in their model. Lang and Li (2012) investigated the consequences of a more general CTL response and obtained complex behaviors which have not been observed previously.

Shu et al. (2014) considered the general model of Komarova et al. (2003). They assumed "when the virus load is low, the level of immune response is simply proportional to both the viral load, and the immune response, but that the immune response saturates when the virus load is sufficiently high."

By means of this assumption and works of Fenton et al. (2006), they presented an immunosuppressive infection model with delay. Also, they considered some conditions on parameters of their model. Then, they showed the existence of four equilibrium points and investigated stability of all equilibrium points. Dadi and Alizade (2016) considered the model of Shu et al. (2014), but they assumed other conditions on parameters of that model. They obtained new equilibrium point and proved that saddle-node bifurcation and transcritical bifurcation can be occurred when delay parameter is absent. Also, they showed that the delay model has a saddle-node bifurcation by using center manifold theory. But, they did not study the global dynamics of equilibrium points of their model.

IMMUNOSUPPRESSIVE INFECTION MODEL

In this chapter, the model of Komarova et al. (2003) is considered and its global dynamics is studied by using classical Poincaré-Bendixson theory, the properties of monotone dynamical systems, and geometric approach.

Komarova et al. (2003) introduced the following system

$$
\begin{cases}
\dot{y} = yg_r(y) - yz, \\
\dot{z} = zf(y),
\end{cases}
\tag{1}
$$

where shows the dynamics between an immunosuppressive infection and antiviral immune responses at various degrees of complexity. The model contains two variables: virus population, y and a population of immune cells, z. The exact identity of immune cells is left open. Komarova et al. (2003) has assumed that the degree of immune expansion depends on virus load, and that the response inhibits virus growth. Thus, it could correspond to any branch of adaptive immune system such as CD8 T cells, antibodies, or CD4 T cells. In their model, virus population grows at a rate described by function $g_r(y)$ that depends on the amount of virus, y, and viral replication rate, r. The inhibition of virus population by immune response is at a rate yz. Immune expansion which is determined by virus load is described by function $f(y)$. Growth and decay in population is shown with positive and negative values. According to Komarova et al. (2003), they made the assumption on the virus growth function that the higher the replication rate of the virus, r, the higher the viral growth rate. Another their assumption was that virus growth is density dependent: "growth slows down at higher virus loads; when virus load crosses a threshold, growth stops and the virus population declines, corresponding to target cell limitation where the virus runs out of cells to infect." The assumption on the immune expansion function was that the presence of virus can both stimulate and impair immunity, depending on virus load, "If virus load lies below a threshold, the rate of immune expansion is negative. That is, levels of antigen are too low to induce a response. If virus load lies above a threshold, the rate of immune expansion is also negative, because immune impairment out-weighs antigenic stimulation. Thus, high virus loads inhibit immunity. Immune expansion is positive for intermediate virus loads, because antigenic stimulation is strong relative to immune impairment."

Komarova et al. (2003) presented the following functions in the appendix of their study

$$g_r(y) = ry(1 - \frac{y}{k}) - ay,$$

$$f(y) = \frac{cy}{1 + dy} - qy - b.$$

Shu et al. (2014), Dadi and Alizade (2016) and Shamsara et al. (2016) considered the following system and obtained its stability with different conditions

$$\begin{cases} \dot{y} = y(r(1 - \frac{y}{k}) - a - pz), \\ \dot{z} = z(\frac{cy}{1 + dy} - qy - b). \end{cases} \tag{2}$$

Shu et al. (2014) assumed that $(c - q - bd)^2 - 4bdq > 0$ They obtained four equilibrium points and studied stability of them. Also, they considered this model with delay as follows and showed interesting and important results on its dynamical behaviors

$$\begin{cases} \dot{y} = ry(1 - \frac{y}{k}) - ay - pyz, \\ \dot{z} = \frac{cz(t - \tau)y(t - \tau)}{1 + dy(t - \tau)} + z(-qy - b). \end{cases}$$

Dadi and Alizade (2016) and Shamsara et al. (2016) studied system (2) with the following assumption, simultaneously:

$$(c - q - bd)^2 - 4bdq = 0.$$

It should be noted that Dadi and Alizade (2016) studied system (2) with delay and without delay. Dadi and Alizade (2016) obtained significant results on this model from the stability and codimension-one bifurcation point of view. They proved that this model without delay parameter has saddle-node bifurcation and transcritical bifurcation. Also, they showed that the delay model has a saddle-node bifurcation. They used Sotomayor theorem and center manifold theory in their study. In this year, Shamsara et al. (2016) also considered system (2) and proved the existence of transcritical bifurcation in system (2).

The author would like to point out that the techniques which are used in most papers are similar. To the best of the author's knowledge, it is the first time to deal with the dynamical properties of system (2) based on the Poincare–Bendixson property, Volterra–Lyapunov stable matrices, properties of monotone dynamical systems, and geometric approach. In this chapter, the author investigates the global dynamics of system (2) by using these methods.

Preliminaries

Some necessary concepts and notations are introduced in the following that they will facilitate global stability analysis. Also, several known results on stable matrices are presented which they build the theoretical foundation of this chapter.

Definition 1

(Redheffer, 1985) A nonsingular matrix A is Volterra–Lyapunov stable if there is a positive diagonal matrix M such that $MA + A^T M^T < 0$, i.e., $MA + A^T M^T$ is symmetric negative definite.

The following lemma determines all 2×2 Volterra–Lyapunov stable matrices.

Lemma 2

(Redheffer, 1985) Let $D = \begin{bmatrix} a & b \\ c & d \end{bmatrix}$ be a 2×2 matrix. Then D is Volterra–Lyapunov stable if and only if $a < 0$, $d < 0$, $\det(D) > 0$.

Consider a bounded convex open set $D \subset \mathbb{R}^n$ and a C^1-function $x \mapsto F(x) \in \mathbb{R}^n$ for $x \in D$. Define the following differential equation:

$$\frac{dx}{dt} = F(x). \tag{3}$$

Let $x(t, x_0)$ be the solution of equation (3) such that $x(0, x_0) = x_0$. A subset K is said to be absorbing in D if the following relation holds for sufficiently large t and any compact subset $K_1 \subset D$

$$x(t, K_1) \subset K.$$

If equilibrium point $\bar{x}$ is locally stable and all trajectories in D converge to $\bar{x}$, then $\bar{x}$ is said to be globally stable in D. To study the global stability of equilibrium solution $\bar{x}$, we assume:

(H1) there exists a compact absorbing set $K \subset D$,
(H2) the system has an unique equilibrium point $\bar{x}$ in D.

Definition 3

(Butler & Waltman, 1986) System (3) is said to be uniformly persistent if there exists a constant $c>0$ such that each component of any solution $x(t)$ with $x(0) = x_0 \in D$ satisfies for $i = 1,\ldots, n$

$$\liminf_{t \to \infty} x_i(t) > c.$$

The boundedness of D and uniform persistence imply system (3) has a compact absorbing subset of D.

Definition 4

(Hale, 1969) System (3) is said to satisfy the Poincare-Bendixson property if any nonempty compact omega limit set of that contains no equilibria is a closed orbit.

Definition 5

(Coopel, 1965) Suppose system (3) has a periodic solution $x = p (t)$ with the least period $\omega > 0$ and orbit $\gamma = \{p (t) \mid 0 \le t \le \omega\}$. This orbit is orbitally stable if for each $\varepsilon > 0$ there exists a $\delta > 0$ such that any solution $x (t)$, for which the distance of $x (0)$ from γ is less than δ, remains at a distance less than ε from γ for all $t \ge 0$.

It is asymptotically orbitally stable if the distance of $x (t)$ from γ also tends to zero as $t \to \infty$.

The orbit γ is asymptotically orbitally stable with asymptotic phase if it is asymptotically orbitally stable and there is an $\eta > 0$ such that any solution $x (t)$, for which the distance of $x (0)$ from γ is less than η, satisfies $\mid x (t) - p (t - \tau) \mid \to 0$ as $t \to \infty$ for some τ which may depend on $x (0)$.

Now, a criterion given in Muldowney (1990) can be stated for the asymptotic orbital stability of a periodic orbit of system (3).

Theorem 6

A sufficient condition for a periodic orbit $\gamma = \{p (t) \mid 0 \le t \le \omega\}$ of system (3) to be asymptotically orbitally stable with asymptotic phase is that the following linear system is asymptotically stable, where $\dfrac{\partial F^{[2]}}{\partial x}$ is the second compound matrix of the Jacobian $\dfrac{\partial F}{\partial x}$,

$$\frac{dz}{dt} = (\frac{\partial F^{[2]}}{\partial x} (p(t))z.$$

Now, consider the following theorem which was given in Li and Muldowney (1996).

Theorem 7

Assume that:

1. conditions (H1) and (H2) hold,
2. $\bar{x}$ is locally asymptotically stable equilibrium point of system (3),
3. system (3) satisfies the Poincare–Bendixson property,
4. each periodic orbit of (3) in D is orbitally asymptotically stable.

Then the unique equilibrium point $\bar{x}$ is globally asymptotically stable in D.

MAIN RESULTS

Consider system (2). Let $\mathbb{R}^2_+$ denote the positive region of $\mathbb{R}^2$. Define

$$\Delta = \{(y,z) \in R^2_+ \mid y \leq k, y + \frac{p}{c}z \leq \frac{rk}{\mu}, \mu = \min\{a,b\}\}.$$

First, it is shown that Δ is the feasible region of system (2). It is not hard to verify from system (2) that $\mathbb{R}^2_+$ is positively invariant. Restrict any further analysis of this system to $\mathbb{R}^2_+$, since variables are non-negative quantities. From system (2), one gets

$$\dot{y} \leq (r - a)y(t) - \frac{r}{k}y(t)^2 \Rightarrow y(t) \leq \frac{k}{1 + ce^{(r-a)t}}$$

then

$$\limsup_{t \to \infty} y(t) = \begin{cases} 0 & r - a < 0 \\ k & r - a > 0 \end{cases}$$
$$\Rightarrow \forall t > 0, \quad y(t) \leq k \qquad if \qquad y(0) \leq k.$$

Also,

$$\dot{y} + \frac{p}{c}\dot{z} \leq ry(t) - \mu(y + \frac{p}{c}z)$$

where $\mu = \min\{a, b\}$, therefore

$$\limsup_{t \to \infty} (y(t) + \frac{p}{c}z(t)) \leq \frac{rk}{\mu},$$

this means

$$\forall t > 0, \quad (y(t) + \frac{p}{c}z(t)) \leq \frac{rk}{\mu} \qquad if \qquad (y(0) + \frac{p}{c}z(0)) \leq \frac{rk}{\mu}.$$

Now, restrict all further analysis to the feasible region Δ. In next sections, the author will have studied the existence and the stability properties of equilibrium points of system (2) in the feasible region.

Existence

It is not complicated to show that system (2) has between one and four equilibrium points. First, define some useful quantities:

$(Q1)$ $\qquad g(y) = qdy^2 - (c - q - bd)y + b,$

$(Q2)$ $\qquad y = \dfrac{c - q - bd}{2qd},$

$(Q3)$ $\qquad \delta = (c - q - bd)^2 - 4bqd,$

$(Q4)$ $\qquad y^{\pm} = \dfrac{c - q - bd \pm \sqrt{\delta}}{2qd}.$

Equilibrium points of system (2) are obtained from the following system

$$\begin{cases} ry(1 - \dfrac{y}{k}) - ay - pyz = 0, \\ z(\dfrac{cy}{1 + dy} - qy - b) = 0. \end{cases}$$

In order to identify all the possible equilibria of system (2), break our discussion into several cases.

Case 1: Consider (Q2). Let $\dfrac{c - q - bd}{2qd} \leq 0$. Therefore, there are at most two equilibrium points since

the quadratic polynomial Q1 has not positive zero. If $z = 0$, then $y = 0$ or $y = \dfrac{k(r - a)}{r}$. Hence,

there always exists a trivial equilibrium point $E_0 = (y_0, z_0) = (0, 0)$. If $r > a$, then there exists an-

other equilibrium point $E_1 = (y_1, z_1) = (\dfrac{k(r - a)}{r}, 0)$. This point is called the virus dominant

equilibrium (VDE).

Case 2: Consider (Q3). Let $\dfrac{c - q - bd}{2qd} > 0$ and $\delta > 0$. In this case, the quadratic polynomial Q1 has

other two positive roots as presented at Q4. Hence, there exist $E_1^* = (y^-, z^-)$ and $E_2^* = (y^+, z^+)$

where $z^{\pm} = \dfrac{r(k - y^{\pm}) - ak}{kp}$. These equilibria are called the immune control equilibrium points.

See the detail of the proof in Shu et al. (2014).

Case 3: Consider (Q3). Let $\dfrac{c - q - bd}{2qd} > 0$ and $\delta = 0$. In this case, Dadi and Alizade (2016) proved that

the quadratic polynomial Q1 has another positive root. They obtained immune control equilibrium point $E* = (y*, z*)$ where $y^* = \dfrac{c - q - bd}{2qd}$ and $z^* = \dfrac{r(k - y^*) - ak}{kp}$. Also, Shamsara et al. (2016)

proved the existence of $E* = (y*, z*)$ such that $y^* = \sqrt{\dfrac{b}{qd}}$ and was equivalent to $y^* = \dfrac{c - q - bd}{2qd}$.

Volterra–Lyapunov Stability

Locally stability of all above cases is studied by Dadi and Alizade (2016), Shamsara et al. (2016) and Shu et al. (2014). In this section, the author investigates Volterra–Lyapunov stability of system (2).

The Jacobian matrix of system (2) at an arbitrary equilibrium point is as follows

$$J = \begin{bmatrix} r - \dfrac{2r}{k}y - a - pz & -py \\ \dfrac{cz}{(1 + dy)^2} - qz & \dfrac{-g(y)}{1 + dy} \end{bmatrix} \tag{4}$$

where $g(y)$ is defined at Q1.

Case 1: Let $\dfrac{c - q - bd}{2qd} \leq 0$. Hence, $g(y)$ is positive for all y since all parameters is assumed positive.

In this case, there are two equilibrium points E_0 and E_1. It is easy to obtain

$$J\big|_{E_0} = \begin{bmatrix} r - a & 0 \\ 0 & -b \end{bmatrix} \qquad and \qquad J\big|_{E_1} = \begin{bmatrix} -r + a & -p\dfrac{k(r - a)}{r} \\ 0 & \dfrac{-g(y_1)}{1 + dy_1} \end{bmatrix}.$$

Thus

- E_0 is Volterra–Lyapunov stable iff $r < a$,
- E_1 is Volterra–Lyapunov stable iff $r > a$.

Case 2: Let $\dfrac{c - q - bd}{2qd} > 0$ and $\delta > 0$. In this case, $g(y)$ is equal zero for $y^{\pm}$. Also, Shu et al. (2014) showed that $y^{\pm} < y_1$. It is obvious that $g(y)$ is an increasing function on interval (y^+, ∞). This means that the sign of $g(y_1)$ is positive. Thus, it is not hard to see

- E_0 is Volterra–Lyapunov stable iff $r < a$,
- E_1 is Volterra–Lyapunov stable iff $r > a$,
- E_1 and E_2* is not Volterra–Lyapunov stable.

Case 3: Let $\dfrac{c - q - bd}{2qd} > 0$ and $\delta = 0$. Similar to case 2, $g(y_1)$ is positive and $g(y*) = 0$. The following results are obtained.

○ E_0 is Volterra–Lyapunov stable iff $r < a$,
○ E_1 is Volterra–Lyapunov stable iff $r > a$,
○ E^* is not Volterra–Lyapunov stable.

Global Stability

Stability of equilibrium points E_0, E_1, E_1^* and E_2^*, case 2, is analyzed by Shu et al. (2014). Dadi and Alizade (2016) investigated the stability, saddle-node bifurcation and transcritical bifurcation of system (2) in case 3. Also, Shamsara et al. (2016) studied the stability and transcritical bifurcation of system (2) in this case, simultaneously. Dadi and Alizade (2016) showed that "with increasing r, equilibrium point E_1 occurs. In this case the system has a branch of stable equilibrium point E_1 and a branch of unstable equilibrium point E_0 that express transcritical bifurcation. In the branch of stable equilibrium point E_1, the patient has viral cells without any immune response. Therefore as shown if the viral replication rate r, is greater than the threshold value of r_t where

$$
r_t = \begin{cases} \dfrac{ak}{k - y^*} & y^* < k \\ \infty & y^* \geq k \end{cases}
$$

then two equilibrium points E_1 and E^* at the same time are stable." The global stability of equilibrium points E_0, E_1 is done at the same way in Shu et al. (2014). Hence, the author just investigates the global stability of equilibrium point E^*, by different way. This aim is performed in three steps.

First Step

First, the author would like to prove that system (2) is persistent. For this goal, two following lemmas are useful. In the first lemma, omega limit points of system (2) on boundary of feasible region Δ are found. Then the future of any orbit starting in the interior of feasible region Δ studies.

Lemma 8

The trivial equilibrium point, E_0, is the only omega limit point of system (2) on the boundary of Δ, $\partial\Delta$.
   Proof. The boundary of Δ has three edges if $r \leq \mu$ and four edges if $r > \mu$ as follows

$$
e_1 = \{(y,z) \in \Delta \mid y = 0, 0 \leq z \leq \frac{rkc}{p\mu}\}
$$

$$
e_2 = \{(y,z) \in \Delta \mid y + \frac{p}{c}z = \frac{rk}{\mu}\}
$$

$$
e_3 = \{(y,z) \in \Delta \mid z = 0, 0 \leq y \leq \min\{\frac{rk}{\mu}, k\}\}
$$

$$
e_4 = \{(y,z) \in \Delta \mid y = k, 0 \leq z \leq \frac{c}{p}(\frac{rk}{\mu} - k), r > \mu\}.
$$

On the z-axis, system (2) reduces to

$$\begin{cases} \dot{y} = 0, \\ \dot{z} = -bz. \end{cases}$$

It is obvious that $z(t) \to 0$ as $t \to \infty$. Similarly, the reduced system on y-axis is

$$\begin{cases} \dot{y} = (r-a)y - \dfrac{r}{k}y^2, \\ \dot{z} = 0. \end{cases}$$

Then $y(t) \to 0$ as $t \to \infty$. For other edges, vector fields are transversal to them. Thus E_0 is the only omega limit point of system (2) on the boundary of Δ.

Lemma 9

The omega limit point of any orbit starting in the interior of Δ, Δ^0, is not E_0.

Proof. Let initial value $(\bar{y}, \bar{z})$ be close to E_0. If $\dot{y} > 0$, then $y(t) > 0$ for each $t > 0$ since $\bar{y} > 0$. This means $y(t)$ is increasing and moving away from E_0. Now, assume that $\dot{y} < 0$, then one can obtain

$$r(1 - \frac{y}{k}) - a - pz < 0.$$

Therefore, the following inequality is satisfied since $y(t) \leq k$

$$\dot{z} = z(\frac{cy}{1+dy} - qy - b)$$
$$> \frac{a\,g(y)}{p(1+dy)}.$$

It is clear that $\dot{z} > 0$ as long as y is close to zero. Hence, trajectory $z(t)$ always moves away from zero. The proof is complete.

Now, the following theorem can be stated by combining lemma 8, lemma 9 and definition 3.

Theorem 10

System (2) is uniformly persistent.

Proof. By lemma 8 and lemma 9, each component of solution $(y(t), z(t))$ with initial value in interior of Δ does not tend to E_0. Thus, there is a positive number $c > 0$ such that

$$\liminf_{t \to \infty} y(t) > c, \quad \liminf_{t \to \infty} z(t) > c.$$

The boundedness of Δ and uniform persistence imply the existence of a compact absorbing subset of Δ. Hence, below corollary immediately is obtained.

Corollary 11

System (2) satisfies assumptions H1 and H2.

Second Step

In this step, it is proved that each periodic orbit of system (2) in Δ is orbitally asymptotically stable.

Consider system (2). The second compound matrix of system (2) is given by

$$J^{[2]} = r(1 - \frac{2y}{k}) - a - pz + \frac{cy}{1 + dy} - qy - b.$$

Define the following second compound system along periodic solution $\gamma(t) = (y(t), z(t))$ of system (2)

$$X' = J^{[2]}X. \tag{5}$$

By theorem 6, this periodic solution is asymptotically orbitally stable with asymptotic phase if one can prove the asymptotically stability of system (5). In order to prove this aim, define a Lyapunov function (is a positive function) as follows

$$V(X) = |X|.$$

In the previous step, the persistence of system (2) was proved. Hence, the distance of periodic solution $\gamma(t)$ from the boundary of Δ is positive. This means that there is a positive constant $\varepsilon_\gamma > 0$ such that $\varepsilon_\gamma \le y(t) \le k$. Estimate the right derivative of $V(X)$ along a solution X of system (5) and periodic solution $\gamma(t) = (y(t), z(t))$ of system (2)

$$D_+ |X| \le J^{[2]}|X|.$$

Consider T as the period of periodic solution $\gamma(t)$. It is not hard to show that

$$
\begin{aligned}
\int_0^T J^{[2]} dt &= \int_0^T (r(1 - \frac{2y}{k}) - a - pz + \frac{cy}{1 + dy} - qy - b)dt \\
&= \int_0^T (\frac{\dot{z}}{z} + \frac{\dot{y}}{y} - \frac{r}{k}y)dt \\
&\le -\frac{r}{k}\varepsilon_\gamma T < 0.
\end{aligned}
$$

Therefore,

$$D_+ V(X) \le J^{[2]}V$$
$$\le -\frac{r}{k}\varepsilon_\gamma TV < 0.$$

Thus, system (2) is asymptotically stable and the following result is satisfied.

Theorem 12

Any non constant periodic solution of system (2), if it exists, is asymptotically orbitally stable with asymptotic phase.

Third Step

Finally, this is investigated that system (2) satisfies the Poincare-Bendixon property or not. System (2) is said to satisfy the Poincare Bendixon property if it satisfies in definition 4.

Let Ω be an omega limit set of system (2) in the interior of Δ. It is obvious that the only interior equilibrium point is E^*. Therefore, if Ω does not contain E^* then it contains no other equilibrium point. This implies that Ω is a closed orbit. If Ω contains E^*, then E^* attracts any orbit that gets arbitrarily close to it due to asymptotically stability of E^*. Then $\Omega = \{E^*\}$.

Summing up three steps together yields the following theorem.

Theorem 13

The immune control equilibrium point E^* of system (2) is globally asymptotically stable in Δ.

FUTURE RESEARCH DIRECTIONS

The author would like to identify necessary conditions for stability of the equilibria of this model with delayed antiviral immune response and classical diffusion. Also, the author would like to study the bifurcations occur in this model.

CONCLUSION

The main aim of this chapter was the study of the global asymptotic stability of immune control equilibrium point for an immunosuppressive infection model in the feasible region of the model. The methods of monotone dynamical systems, Volterra-Lyapunov stability, and geometric approach were used in this study. This model represented biologically important cases in the study of immunosuppressive infection dynamics. The results of this chapter build a solid base for future study on the dynamical behavior of general immunosuppressive infection model and for deeper understanding of the fundamental immunosuppressive infection mechanism. The geometric approach which is used in this study has gained some popularity since it has less constraint on models. But the implementation of this approach involves many nontrivial technical details such as the estimation of Lozinskii measure.

ACKNOWLEDGMENT

The author thanks referees for their suggestions that improved this chapter and IGI Global for giving the opportunity to consider this work.

REFERENCES

Barnes, E., Harcourt, G., Brown, D., Lucas, M., Phillips, R., Dusheiko, G., & Klenerman, P. (2002). The dynamics of T-lymphocyte responses during combination therapy for chronic hepatitis C virus infection. *Hepatology (Baltimore, Md.)*, *36*(3), 743–754. doi:10.1053/jhep.2002.35344 PMID:12198669

Bekkering, F. C., Stalgis, C., McHutchison, J. G., Brouwer, J. T., & Perelson, A. S. (2001). Estimation of early hepatitis C viral clearance in patients receiving daily interferon and ribavirin therapy using a mathematical model. *Hepatology (Baltimore, Md.)*, *33*(2), 419–423. doi:10.1053/jhep.2001.21552 PMID:11172344

Borghans, J. A., De Boer, R. J., Sercarz, E., & Kumar, V. (1998). T cell vaccination in experimental autoimmune encephalomyelitis: A mathematical model. *Journal of Immunology (Baltimore, MD.: 1950)*, *161*, 1087–1093. PMID:9686566

Borghans, J. A., Noest, A. J., & De Boer, R. J. (1999). How specific should immunological memory be? *Journal of Immunology (Baltimore, MD.: 1950)*, *163*, 569–575. PMID:10395642

Borghans, J. A., Taams, L. S., Wauben, M. H., & De Boer, R. J. (1999). Competition for antigenic sites during T cell proliferation: A mathematical interpretation of in vitro data. *Proceedings of the National Academy of Sciences of the United States of America*, *96*(19), 10782–10787. doi:10.1073/pnas.96.19.10782 PMID:10485903

Butler, G. J., & Waltman, P. (1986). Persistence in dynamical systems. *Proceedings of the American Mathematical Society*, *96*, 425–428. doi:10.1090/S0002-9939-1986-0822433-4

Canabarro, A. A., Gléeria, I. M., & Lyra, M. L. (2004). Periodic solutions and chaos in a nonlinear model for the delayed cellular immune response. *Physica A*, *342*(1-2), 234–241. doi:10.1016/j.physa.2004.04.083

Celada, F., & Seiden, P. E. (1992). A computer model of cellular interactions in the immune system. *Immunology Today*, *13*(2), 56–62. doi:10.1016/0167-5699(92)90135-T PMID:1575893

Celada, F., & Seiden, P. E. (1996). Affinity maturation and hypermutation in a simulation of the humoral immune response. *European Journal of Immunology*, *26*(6), 1350–1358. doi:10.1002/eji.1830260626 PMID:8647216

Chun, T. W., Stuyver, L., Mizell, S. B., Ehler, L. A., Mican, J. A., Baseler, … Fauci, A.S. (1997). Presence of an inducible HIV-1 latent reservoir during highly active antiretroviral therapy. *Proceedings of the National Academy of Sciences USA*, *94*, 13193–13197. doi:10.1073/pnas.94.24.13193

Coppel, W. A. (1965). *Stability and asymptotical behavior of differential equations, Heath Mathematical Monographs*. Boston: D.C. Heath and Company.

Dadi, Z., & Alizade, S. (2016). Codimension-one bifurcation and stability analysis in an immunosuppressive infection model. SpringerPlus, 5, 106-121.

De Boer, R. J., & Perelson, A. S. (1993). How diverse should the immune system be? *Proceedings. Biological Sciences, 252*(1335), 171–175. doi:10.1098/rspb.1993.0062 PMID:8394577

Detours, V., & Perelson, A. S. (1999). Explaining high alloreactivity as a quantitative consequence of affinity-driven thymocyte selection. *Proceedings of the National Academy of Sciences of the United States of America, 96*(9), 5153–5158. doi:10.1073/pnas.96.9.5153 PMID:10220434

Detours, V., & Perelson, A. S. (2000). The paradox of alloreactivity and self MHC restriction: Quantitative analysis and statistics. *Proceedings of the National Academy of Sciences of the United States of America, 97*(15), 8479–8483. doi:10.1073/pnas.97.15.8479 PMID:10900009

Diepolder, H. M., Jung, M. C., Keller, E., Schraut, W., Gerlach, J. T., Gruner, N., & Pape, G. R. et al. (1998). A vigorous virus specific CD4+ T cell response may contribute to the association of HLA-DR13 with viral clearance in hepatitis B. *Clinical and Experimental Immunology, 113*(2), 244–251. doi:10.1046/j.1365-2249.1998.00665.x PMID:9717974

Fenton, A., Lello, J., & Bonsall, M. B. (2006). Pathogen responses to host immunity: The impact of time delays and memory on the evolution of virulence. *Proceedings. Biological Sciences, 273*(1597), 2083–2090. doi:10.1098/rspb.2006.3552 PMID:16846917

Hale, J. K. (1969). *Ordinary differential equations.* New York: Wiley Interscience.

Hlavacek, W. S., Redondo, A., Metzger, H., Wofsy, C., & Goldstein, B. (2001). Kinetic proofreading models for cell signaling predict ways to escape kinetic proofreading. *Proceedings of the National Academy of Sciences of the United States of America, 98*(13), 7295–7300. doi:10.1073/pnas.121172298 PMID:11390967

Jacquez, J., & Simon, C. (2002). Qualitative theory of compartmental systems with lags. *Mathematical Biosciences, 180*(1-2), 329–362. doi:10.1016/S0025-5564(02)00131-1 PMID:12387931

Kalams, S. A., & Walker, B. D. (1998). The critical need for CD4 help in maintaining effective cytotoxic T lymphocyte responses. *The Journal of Experimental Medicine, 188*(12), 2199–2204. doi:10.1084/jem.188.12.2199 PMID:9858506

Kepler, T. B., & Perelson, A. S. (1993). Cyclic re-entry of germinal center B cells and the efficiency of affinity maturation. *Immunology Today, 14*(8), 412–415. doi:10.1016/0167-5699(93)90145-B PMID:8397781

Kesmir, C., & De Boer, R. J. (1999). A mathematical model on germinal center kinetics and termination. *Journal of Immunology (Baltimore, MD.: 1950), 163*, 2463–2469. PMID:10452981

Komarova, N. L., Barnes, E., Klenerman, P., & Wodarz, D. (2003). Boosting immunity by antiviral d rug therapy: A simple relationship among timing, efficacy, and success. *Proceedings of the National Academy of Sciences of the United States of America, 100*(4), 1855–1860. doi:10.1073/pnas.0337483100 PMID:12574516

Lang, J., & Li, M. Y. (2012). Stable and transient periodic oscillations in a mathematical model for CTL response to HTLV-I infection. *Journal of Mathematical Biology, 65*(1), 181–199. doi:10.1007/s00285-011-0455-z PMID:21792554

Lechner, F., Sullivan, J., Spiegel, H., Nixon, D. F., & Ferrari, B., Davis,… Klenerman, P. (. (2000). Why do cytotoxic T lymphocytes fail to eliminate HCV? Lessons from studies using MHC class I tetramers. *Philosophical Transactions of the Royal Society of London. Series B, Biological Sciences, 355*, 1085–1092. doi:10.1098/rstb.2000.0646 PMID:11186310

Lechner, F., Wong, D. K., Dunbar, P. R., Chapman, R., Chung, R. T., Dohrenwend, P., & Walker, B. D. et al. (2000). Analysis of Successful Immune Responses in Persons Infected with Hepatitis C Virus. *The Journal of Experimental Medicine, 191*(9), 1499–1512. doi:10.1084/jem.191.9.1499 PMID:10790425

Lewin, S. R., Ribeiro, R. M., Walters, T., Lau, G. K., Bowden, S., Locarnini, S., & Perelson, A. S. (2001). Analysis of hepatitis B viral load decline under potent therapy: Complex decay profiles observed. *Hepatology (Baltimore, Md.), 34*(5), 1012–1020. doi:10.1053/jhep.2001.28509 PMID:11679973

Li, M. Y., & Muldowney, J. S. (1996). A geometric approach to the global-stability problems. *SIAM Journal on Mathematical Analysis, 27*(4), 1070–1083. doi:10.1137/S0036141094266449

Li, M. Y., & Shu, H. (2010a). Impact of intracellular delays and target-cell dynamics on in vivo viral infections. *SIAM Journal on Applied Mathematics, 70*(7), 2434–2448. doi:10.1137/090779322

Li, M. Y., & Shu, H. (2010b). Global dynamics of an in-host viral model with intracellular delay. *Bulletin of Mathematical Biology, 72*(6), 1492–1505. doi:10.1007/s11538-010-9503-x PMID:20087671

Li, M. Y., & Shu, H. (2011). Multiple stable periodic oscillations in a mathematical model of CTL response to HTLV-I infection. *Bulletin of Mathematical Biology, 73*(8), 1774–1793. doi:10.1007/s11538-010-9591-7 PMID:20976566

Li, M. Y., & Shu, H. (2012). Joint effects of mitosis and intracellular delay on viral dynamics: Two parameter bifurcation analysis. *Journal of Mathematical Biology, 64*(6), 1005–1020. doi:10.1007/s00285-011-0436-2 PMID:21671033

Lifson, J. D., Rossio, J. L., Arnaout, R., Li, L., Parks, T. L., Schneider, D. K., & Wodarz, D. et al. (2000). Containment of simian immunodeficiency virus: Cellular immune responses and protection from rechallenge following transient postinoculation antiretroviral treatment. *Journal of Virology, 74*(6), 2584–2593. doi:10.1128/JVI.74.6.2584-2593.2000 PMID:10684272

Lifson, J. D., Rossio, J. L., Piatak, M., Parks, T., Li, L., Kiser, R., & Wodarz, D. et al. (2001). Role of CD8(+) lymphocytes in control of simian immunodeficiency virus infection and resistance to rechallenge after transient early antiretroviral treatment. *Journal of Virology, 75*(21), 10187–10199. doi:10.1128/JVI.75.21.10187-10199.2001 PMID:11581387

Liu, S., & Wang, L. (2010). Global stability of an HIV-1 model with distributed intracellular delays and a combination therapy. *Mathematical Biosciences and Engineering, 7*(3), 675–685. doi:10.3934/mbe.2010.7.675 PMID:20578792

Lohr, H. F., Krug, S., Herr, W., Weyer, S., Schlaak, J., Wolfel, T., & Meyer zum Buschenfelde, K. H. et al. (1998). Quantitative and functional analysis of core-specific T helper cell and CTL activities in acute and chronic hepatitis B. *Liver, 18*(6), 405–413. doi:10.1111/j.1600-0676.1998.tb00825.x PMID:9869395

Maini, M. K., & Bertoletti, A. (2000). How Can the Cellular Immune Response Control Hepatitis B Virus Replication? *Journal of Viral Hepatitis, 7*(5), 321–326. doi:10.1046/j.1365-2893.2000.00234.x PMID:10971819

McKeithan, T. W. (1995). Kinetic proofreading in T-cell receptor signal transduction. *Proceedings of the National Academy of Sciences of the United States of America, 92*(11), 5042–5046. doi:10.1073/pnas.92.11.5042 PMID:7761445

McLean, A. R., Rosado, M. M., Agenes, F., Vasconcellos, R., & Freitas, A. A. (1997). Resource competition as a mechanism for B cell homeostasis. *Proceedings of the National Academy of Sciences of the United States of America, 94*(11), 5792–5797. doi:10.1073/pnas.94.11.5792 PMID:9159153

Mukandavire, Z., Garira, W., & Chiyaka, C. (2007). Asymptotic properties of an HIV/AIDS model with a time delay. *Journal of Mathematical Analysis and Applications, 330*(2), 916–933. doi:10.1016/j.jmaa.2006.07.102

Muldowney, J. S. (1990). Compound matrices and ordinary differential equations. *The Rocky Mountain Journal of Mathematics, 20*(4), 857–872. doi:10.1216/rmjm/1181073047

Nelson, P., Murray, J., & Perelson, A. (2000). A model o f HIV-1 pathogenesis that includes an intracellular delay. *Mathematical Biosciences, 163*(2), 201–215. doi:10.1016/S0025-5564(99)00055-3 PMID:10701304

Nelson, P., & Perelson, A. (2002). A Mathematical analysis of delay differential equation models of HIV- 1 infection. *Mathematical Biosciences, 179*(1), 73–94. doi:10.1016/S0025-5564(02)00099-8 PMID:12047922

Neumann, A. U., Lam, N. P., Dahari, H., Gretch, D. R., Wiley, T. E., Layden, T. J., & Perelson, A. S. (1998). Hepatitis C viral dynamics in vivo and the antiviral efficacy of interferon-α therapy. *Science, 282*(5386), 103–107. doi:10.1126/science.282.5386.103 PMID:9756471

Ortiz, G. M., Hu, J., Goldwitz, J. A., Chandwani, R., Larsson, M., Bhardwaj, N., & Nixon, D. F. et al. (2002). Residual viral replication during antiretroviral therapy boosts human immunodeficiency virus type 1-specific CD8+ T- cell responses in subjects treated early after infection. *Journal of Virology, 76*(1), 411–415. doi:10.1128/JVI.76.1.411-415.2002 PMID:11739706

Percus, J. K., Percus, O. E., & Perelson, A. S. (1993). Predicting the size of the T-cell receptor and antibody combining region from consideration of efficient self-non-self discrimination. *Proceedings of the National Academy of Sciences of the United States of America, 90*(5), 1691–1695. doi:10.1073/pnas.90.5.1691 PMID:7680474

Perelson, A. S. (2002). Modelling viral and immune system dynamics. *Nature Reviews. Immunology, 2*(1), 28–36. doi:10.1038/nri700 PMID:11905835

Perelson, A. S., & Oster, G. F. (1979). Theoretical studies of clonal selection: Minimal antibody repertoire size and reliability of self–non-self discrimination. *Journal of Theoretical Biology, 81*(4), 645–670. doi:10.1016/0022-5193(79)90275-3 PMID:94141

Perelson, A. S., & Weisbuch, G. (1997). Immunology for physicists. *Reviews of Modern Physics, 69*(4), 1219–1267. doi:10.1103/RevModPhys.69.1219

Pugliese, A., & Gandolfi, A. (2008). A simple model o f pathogen-immune dynamics including specific and non-specific immunity. *Mathematical Biosciences, 214*(1-2), 73–80. doi:10.1016/j.mbs.2008.04.004 PMID:18547594

Redheffer, R. (1985). Volterra multipliers I. *SIAM Journal on Algebraic and Discrete Methods, 6*, 592–611.

Rosenberg, E. S., Altfeld, M., Poon, S. H., Phillips, M. N., & Wilkes, B. M. (2000). Immune control of HIV-1 after early treatment of acute infection. *Nature, 407*(6803), 523–526. doi:10.1038/35035103 PMID:11029005

Segel, L. A. (1995). Grappling with *complexity*. *Complexity, 1*(2), 18–25. doi:10.1002/cplx.6130010207

Segel, L.A., & Baror, R. L. (1999). On the role of feedback in promoting conflicting goals of the adaptive immune system. *Journal of Immunology (Baltimore, MD.: 1950), 163*, 1342–1349. PMID:10415033

Shamsara, E., Mostolizadeh, R., & Afsharnezhad, Z. (2016). Transcritical bifurcation of an immunosuppressive infection model. *Iranian Journal of Numerical Analysis and Optimization, 6*(2), 1–15.

Shu, H., Wang, L., & Watmough, J. (2014). Sustained and transient oscillation and chaos induced by delayed antiviral immune response in an immunosuppressive infection model. *Journal of Mathematical Biology, 68*(1-2), 477–503. doi:10.1007/s00285-012-0639-1 PMID:23306425

Smith, D. J., Forrest, S., Ackley, D. H., & Perelson, A. S. (1999). Variable efficacy of repeated annual influenza vaccination. *Proceedings of the National Academy of Sciences of the United States of America, 96*(24), 14001–14006. doi:10.1073/pnas.96.24.14001 PMID:10570188

Tam, J. (1999). Delay effect in a model for virus replication. *IMA Journal of Mathematics Applied in Medicine and Biology, 16*(1), 29–37. doi:10.1093/imammb/16.1.29 PMID:10335599

Wang, K., Wang, W., Pang, H., & Liu, X. (2007). Complex dynamic behavior in a viral model with delayed immune response. *Physica D. Nonlinear Phenomena, 226*(2), 197–208. doi:10.1016/j.physd.2006.12.001

Whalley, S. A., Murray, J. M., Brown, D., Webster, G. J., Emery, V. C., Dusheiko, G. M., & Perelson, A. S. (2001). Kinetics of acute hepatitis B virus infection in humans. *The Journal of Experimental Medicine, 193*(7), 847–854. doi:10.1084/jem.193.7.847 PMID:11283157

Wodarz, D., & Nowak, M. A. (1999). Specific therapy regimes could lead to long-term control of HIV. *Proceedings of the National Academy of Sciences of the United States of America, 96*(25), 14464–14469. doi:10.1073/pnas.96.25.14464 PMID:10588728

Wodarz, D., Page, K. M., Arnaout, R. A., Thomsen, A. R., Lifson, J. D., & Nowak, M. A. (2000). A new theory of cytotoxic T-lymphocyte memory: Implications for HIV treatment. *Philosophical Transactions of the Royal Society of London. Series B, Biological Sciences*, *355*(1395), 329–343. doi:10.1098/rstb.2000.0570 PMID:10794051

Zhu, H., & Zou, X. (2008). Impact of delays in cell infection and virus production o n HIV-1 dynamics. *Mathematical Medicine and Biology*, *25*(2), 99–112. doi:10.1093/imammb/dqm010 PMID:18504248

KEY TERMS AND DEFINITIONS

Equilibrium Point: Let $\dot{x} = f(x)$, $x \in \mathbb{R}^n$ be an autonomous differential equation. If $f(x_0) = 0$, then x_0 is called an equilibrium point. This means that there is a constant function $\phi : \mathbb{R} \to \mathbb{R}^n$ which $\phi(t) \equiv x_0$.

Geometric Approach: Geometric approach is the approach which is based on Poincare-Bendixson property for studying the global stability of equilibrium points in a nonlinear autonomous differential equation.

Global Stability: Let $\dot{x} = f(x)$, $x \in D \subset \mathbb{R}^n$ where D is the feasible region of this system. Also, consider x_0 as an equilibrium point. This point is globally stable if the omega limit set of every point of D is x_0 .

Immune Control Equilibrium Point: An equilibrium point of immunosuppressive infection model is called immune control equilibrium point if the number of antiviral immune responses is not zero.

Immunosuppressive Infection Model: An ordinary differential equations system which shows the dynamics between immunosuppressive infection and antiviral immune responses is called immunosuppressive infection model.

Monotone Dynamical Systems: Let X be a metric space with an ordering $x \geq y$. A dynamical system with flow ϕ on X is called monotone if this order is preserved by the flow: $\phi_t(x) \geq \phi_t(y)$ for each $t \in \mathbb{R}^{>0}$.

Poincare-Bendixson Property: Let $\dot{x} = f(x)$, $x \in D \subset \mathbb{R}^n$ be an autonomous differential equation, f be a C^1 function on D, and D be an open set. If any nonempty compact omega limit set of this system which does not contain any equilibrium points is a closed orbit, then this system satisfies the Poincare-Bendixson property. This property is used to determine the global behavior of bounded trajectories of the system.

Volterra-Lyapunov Stable: A square matrix A is Volterra-Lyapunov stable if there exists a positive diagonal matrix M such that $MA + A^T M^T$ is symmetric negative definite. Volterra-Lyapunov matrix properties can be used for the studying dynamical behavior of nonlinear models.

Section 2
Statistical Analysis Techniques

Chapter 8
Strategic Analytics to Drive Provincial Dialysis Capacity Planning:
The Case of Ontario Renal Network

Neal Kaw
University of Toronto, Canada

Somayeh Sadat
Tarbiat Modares University, Iran

Ali Vahit Esensoy
Cancer Care Ontario, Canada

Zhihui (Amy) Liu
Cancer Care Ontario, Canada

Sarah Jane Bastedo
Ontario Renal Network, Canada

Gihad Nesrallah
St. Michael's Hospital, Canada

ABSTRACT

This chapter discusses applications of analytics at the strategic level of health system planning in the province of Ontario, Canada. To supplement the strategic priorities of the Ontario Renal Plan I, a roadmap developed by the Ontario Renal Network to guide its directions in coordinating renal care province-wide, an interactive user-friendly analytical capacity planning model was developed to forecast the growth of the prevalent chronic dialysis patient population and estimate consequent future need for hemodialysis stations at Ontario's dialysis facilities. The model also projects operational funding to care for dialysis patients, vascular surgeries to achieve arteriovenous fistula targets, peritoneal dialysis catheter insertions to achieve peritoneal dialysis prevalence targets, and incident dialysis patients to be sent home to achieve prevalent home dialysis targets. The model uses a variety of analytical methods, including time series analysis, mathematical optimization, geo-spatial analysis and Monte Carlo simulation.

DOI: 10.4018/978-1-5225-2515-8.ch008

INTRODUCTION

Chronic Kidney Disease (CKD)

A diagnosis of CKD generally means that the kidneys have not been working properly in eliminating wastes and excess fluids from the body for at least 3 months. CKD is divided into five stages that depend on severity. If detected in early stages of the disease, it may be possible to slow the progression of kidney failure through lifestyle changes and medication. Once the kidneys fail (in stage 5 of CKD, which is also known as End-Stage-Renal-Disease or ESRD), patients may receive renal replacement therapies (dialysis or transplant) or opt for palliative care. A transplanted kidney may fail at any point and the patient be put on dialysis or opt to receive palliative care. While it is ideal to detect CKD as early as possible, the disease may go undetected up to the point when the patient needs dialysis. In fact, such "crash start" patients comprised about a quarter of new dialysis patients in Ontario in 2014 (Ontario Renal Network, 2015).

There are two main dialysis modalities: hemodialysis and peritoneal dialysis. Hemodialysis draws the patient's blood through a filter to remove waste products and excess water, and normalize blood chemistry. Hemodialysis requires a vascular access. Arteriovenous (AV) fistula and the AV grafts are vascular access designed for long-term use, with AV fistula deemed to be the superior vascular access type. Both AV fistulae and AV grafts are established by surgical procedures. However, these procedures are technically challenging, and many patients have suboptimal anatomy that precludes successful fistula or graft creation. Consequently, while AV access are associated with better patient outcomes, many patients require a central venous catheter for long-term hemodialysis access. Peritoneal dialysis utilizes the peritoneum, a membrane that lines the abdominal cavity as the filter and a catheter implanted in the abdominal wall to instill and withdraw dialysis fluid.

Hemodialysis patients may receive dialysis care in a facility or at home, while peritoneal dialysis is generally performed at home. In-facility patients generally receive dialysis 3-5 times per week, while home dialysis patients are able to dialyze more frequently. Patients receiving home hemodialysis often dialyze overnight (nocturnal hemodialysis) to maximize hours of treatment while minimizing the number of daytime hours impacted by the therapy. From time to time, home dialysis patients may temporarily require care at a hub facility due to complications or the need for more intensive care. Such instances are called "fall backs".

A simplified CKD disease progression pathway is shown in Figure 1. At each transition point, a minority of patients progress to the next state. Other potential states include death, relocation, and non-dialytic management of kidney failure (conservative care with palliation).

CKD Worldwide

CKD is a growing problem worldwide, with an estimated prevalence of 200 million people worldwide and a growing burden especially in low to middle income countries undergoing epidemiologic transition towards non-communicable chronic diseases (Ojo, 2014). Other studies have estimated the prevalence of CKD to be around 8-16% (Jha et al., 2013) and 13.4% (Hill et al., 2016). The 2015 Global Burden of Disease study found all-age Disability-Adjusted-Life-Years or DALYs (in thousands) of 35259.7 (up from 29488.3 in 2005) or in other words 19.6 percentage of change between 2005 and 2015, moving up from the 22nd leading cause of global DALYs for both sexes in 2005 to the 20th (Kassebaum et al., 2016).

Figure 1. Typical CKD Disease Progression Pathway is shown in the figure

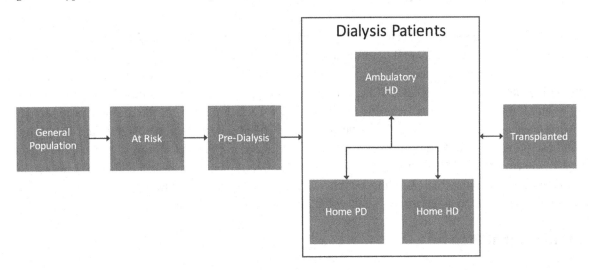

All age deaths (in thousands) were found to be 417.8 (up from 299.4 in 2005) or a 39.5% increase in the 2015 Global Burden of Disease Study (Wang et al., 2016).

While currently developed geographies of Europe, USA, Canada, and Australia generally have higher prevalence of CKD compared to growing economies such as sub-Saharan Africa and India (Hill et al., 2016), CKD is projected to grow fastest in the poorest parts of the world which unfortunately have reduced availability of renal replacement therapy (Jha, 2014). In fact, over 100 countries of combined population of over a billion people have no provision of chronic maintenance dialysis or kidney transplantation (Ojo, 2014). As such, ensuring provision of dialysis or kidney transplantation is a priority worldwide.

About ORN

Established in 2009, the Ontario Renal Network (ORN), a division of Cancer Care Ontario (CCO) and an agency of the provincial government, coordinates and manages the delivery of Chronic Kidney Disease (CKD) services in the province of Ontario, Canada. Prior to its establishment, the Ontario Ministry of Health and Long Term Care (MOHLTC) managed the delivery of CKD services throughout the province. To increase coordination and integration in system planning, provincial oversight and coordination of CKD was transferred from the MOHLTC to the ORN under the auspices of CCO. The MOHLTC-CCO-ORN Accountability Agreement established specific areas of accountability for ORN including provincial and regional program management, performance measurement and management, information technology, and communications and stakeholder relations. (Woodward et al., 2014)

About Ontario

Ontario is a large province in the east central Canada with a total area of 1,076,395 square meters comprising of land and water. As of July 1, 2016, it had a population of 13,982,884 people (38.5% of the population of Canada). Its nominal GDP was 763,276 million$ (38.4% of Canada) in 2015. (Ontario Ministry of Finance, 2016)

Organization of CKD Care in Ontario

ORN provides overall leadership and direction to effectively organize and manage the delivery of CKD services for approximately 12,000 Ontarians with CKD requiring pre-dialysis care, and an additional 10,500 Ontarians with advanced CKD that require dialysis. CKD services in Ontario are organized in a hub and spoke model of care with 26 Regional Renal Programs, each consisting of a regional hospital as the hub linked with affiliated satellite facilities. ORN works closely with the regional programs that provide dialysis and other kidney care services within 105 facilities, including hospitals and community-based facilities (Ontario Renal Network, 2015). The 26 Regional Renal Programs each fall into one of the 14 Ontario's Local Health Integration Networks (LHINs), which are health authorities responsible for planning, integrating, and funding healthcare services based on community needs. For planning purposes, each LHIN may be further subdivided into a number of sub-LHINs.

Ontario Renal Plan I

The ORN launched the first Ontario Renal Plan in 2012, which was a roadmap to guide its directions in coordinating renal care province-wide. ORP I set seven strategic priorities with specific targets for 2012-2015 as follows: 1) Strengthening accountability to patients; 2) Reducing the impact of CKD by improving early detection and prevention of progression; 3) Improving peritoneal and vascular access for dialysis patients; 4) Improving uptake of independent dialysis; 5) Ensuring Ontario has the necessary infrastructure to care for CKD patients; 6) Strengthening Ontario CKD care through research and innovation; and 7) Aligning funding to high quality patient-focused care (Ontario Renal Plan, 2012).

Specific targets were set for a number of strategic priorities to be achieved by 2015. For the strategic priority of improving peritoneal and vascular access for dialysis patients, the target was specified as a 2% absolute decrease per year in prevalent hemodialysis catheter use. For independent dialysis (referred to as home dialysis throughout this chapter), the target was that 40% of all new dialysis patients will be on an independent dialysis option within 6 months of initiating dialysis. (Ontario Renal Plan, 2012)

Development of a funding framework to align funding to high quality patient-focused care, now part of the MOHLTC's Health System Funding Reform, was completed in 2014 based on "clinical and financial data; advised by clinicians, administrators and policymakers at both a provincial and regional level; and CCO's experience with case-based funding" (Woodward et al, 2014). In particular, a number of patient-based funding bundles were developed to ensure CKD care is funded based on the types and volumes of patients treated. Work is in progress to expand and refine the funding bundles over time.

Objective of the Chapter

This chapter reports on a strategic analytics project that developed an interactive strategic regional capacity planning tool of the CKD health system. The tool encompassed a mathematical model derived from historical data captured in ORRS, OHIP CHDB, and WTIS. The project aimed to inform a number of planning considerations at the local and provincial level, specifically around the demand for chronic dialysis services and required resources (dialysis stations, bundled patient-based funding, AV fistula surgeries and PD catheter insertions), and incident dialysis patients to be sent home to achieve target prevalent home dialysis rates from FY2013/14 to FY2024/25.

BACKGROUND

By 2013, when the project described in this chapter began, CCO had already implemented numerous information technology solutions to collect, manage, and report on health system data and support its programs. Within CCO, there were over 170 data holdings, which included data collected from external partners such as the MOHLTC, the Canadian Institute for Health Information (CIHI), and the Institute for Clinical Evaluative Sciences (ICES) (Garay et al., 2014). In particular, the Ontario Renal Reporting System (ORRS) was launched in 2010 to collect patient-level data on dialysis and pre-dialysis care provided in Ontario using a web-based application. The dataset is used to support health professionals, policy-makers, and researchers in planning, funding, and performance and quality reporting in a timely manner (Garay et al., 2014; Woodward et al., 2014). The ORRS is a province wide registry that collects patient-level data from all chronic kidney disease providers in Ontario (Ontario Renal Network, 2016). The dataset is robust and accurate enough to fully support funding allocations in a patient-based, bundled dispersant model for chronic kidney disease services (Ministry of Health and Long-term Care, 2016).

Another web-based tool used to collect data is the Wait Time Information System (WTIS) that collects and reports wait time information for over 190 procedures in 13 key surgical areas and diagnostic imaging cases (Garay et al., 2014). Among datasets collected from external partners is the Ontario Health Insurance Plan Claims History Database (OHIP CHDB) that captures all claims made by physicians for insured services provided to Ontario residents, as well as the Registered Persons Database (RPDB), which is a population-based registry maintained by the MOHLTC and includes a historical listing of the unique health numbers issued in Ontario along with some demographic information.

For many years, CCO had successfully applied the data for operational planning and reporting. In 2012, the intersection of increasing resource constraints on health systems across Canada driving the need for improving efficiency and effectiveness and the breadth and volume of data at CCO led to establishing a Strategic Analytics (SA) practice. The practice aims to provide data-driven insights to CCO programs by performing advanced end-to-end analytics. In particular, the practice applies an array of descriptive, predictive, and prescriptive analytics modeling to enhance current and future state system management and planning, with a vision of fully embedding evidence into healthcare decision-making. Using the data to predict and model the future state compared to routine operational planning and reporting was in its infancy when the Strategic Analytics practice was launched. (Garay et al., 2014)

Since its inception, SA has led a number of successful projects in close collaboration with CCO's programs. This chapter reports on a project started in 2013 that developed an interactive strategic regional capacity planning tool of the CKD health system. This project was a continuation of ORN's efforts to gain an evidence-based understanding of the supply and demand for dialysis services at the provincial and local levels to guide its future capital investments, including Provincial Dialysis Assessments conducted in 2010 and 2012 in collaboration with the ICES, the Centre for Research in Healthcare Engineering, and CKD programs (Woodward et al., 2014).

The project explained in this chapter has a much broader scope than the previous assessments and aims to inform a number of planning considerations at the local and provincial level, specifically around the demand for chronic dialysis services and required resources (dialysis stations, bundled patient-based funding, AV fistula surgeries and PD catheter insertions), and incident dialysis patients to be sent home to achieve target prevalent home dialysis rates from FY2013/14 to FY2024/25. Model's projections of chronic dialysis patients, required dialysis stations, and funding are actively used by ORN in their planning efforts, while the rest of the model outputs are useful supplemental information available as required to ORN.

SA was engaged in April 2013 to define the scope of the model. A working group, composed of SA, the ORN planning Analyst, and ORN informatics staff, was formed to deliver the project. A steering committee was also created to provide strategic guidance from the perspective of both the ORN and regional renal programs. Model development officially started in May 2013, and during the course of the project (May 2013 to February 2014) seven steering committee meetings were held that helped monitor the project's progress against timelines, refine and validate the components of the model, and revise the documents and outputs from the project in accordance with project timelines.

An intermediate model was created by October 2013 and produced outputs on required dialysis stations that were used as part of the planning process for FY2014/15 by the ORN and the regional renal programs. Representatives from SA were engaged to help communicate model assumptions and output to regional medical and administrative leadership, and incorporate feedback into the model. This feedback was critical to the model's development, ensuring that the model had face validity and best accounted for local program and population characteristics that were not apparent at the provincial level. The complete model, which also includes bundled patient-based funding, vascular surgery and PD catheter insertion projections, and incident dialysis patients to be sent home to achieve prevalent home dialysis targets, was used as of February 2014 to further support the ORN and regional renal programs in their planning and can be refreshed in one-year increments to support future planning.

This study is by no means the first study that applies analytics to strategic issues in Canada. Strategic analytics of mixed methodologies have been applied to predict various trends using administrative datasets that were used in this project as well as additional data sources. Examples include predicting trends in cardiovascular complications (Booth et al., 2006), laboratory testing for diabetes (Wilson et al., 2009), rectal cancer surgery (Musselman et al., 2012), utilization of echocardiography (Blecker et al., 2013), age of diagnosis of childhood asthma (Radhakrishnan et al., 2014), asthma prevalence and incidence (Gershon et al., 2010a), chronic obstructive pulmonary disease prevalence, incidence, and mortality (Gershon et al., 2010b), use of antidepressants among elderly (Mamdani et al., 2000), prescribing of antidepressants following acute myocardial infarction (Benazon et al., 2005), nurse practitioners' prescribing to older adults (Tranmer, 2015), IUD insertion (Dunn et al., 2009), and 1-year survival of people admitted to hospital (van Walraven, 2013).

However, to the best of our knowledge, this is the first study that presents a data-driven strategic decision support tool used by stakeholders in an interactive manner to support multiple strategic priorities specified in the organization's strategic roadmap.

MAIN FOCUS OF THE CHAPTER

The section provides an overview of the model structure, followed by high level descriptions of the eight major modules of the model, complete with the data sources and methods used in each module, as well as a snapshot of the user-friendly model interface.

Overview of the Model Structure

The model has eight modules. Time series analysis was performed to project the prevalent chronic dialysis patient population at the sub-LHIN level (Module 1). The projected numbers of patients are allocated to each CKD program, dialysis facility, and modality (Module 2), taking into account the fall back rates at each facility (Module 3). This data is then translated into the number of required dialysis stations at each facility (Module 4) and the number of incident dialysis patients to be sent home to achieve the prevalent home dialysis rates (Module 5). Finally for each facility, we forecast the total bundled patient-based funding required (Module 6) and the number of vascular surgeries and PD catheter insertions needed to achieve AV fistula and PD prevalence targets respectively (Module 7). Each module is a mathematical model that turns a number of input variables, based in various data sources or as outputted by preceding modules, into output variables of interest. A schematic diagram of how the modules are interrelated is presented in Figure 2. A final module, not depicted in the figure, deals with estimating confidence intervals for the chronic dialysis projections (Module 8). Module 8 does not fit into Figure 2 because it re-uses much of the architecture of the preceding modules.

This chapter reviews the analytical foundations of all the modules and presents some high level results. More detailed results and their implications on CKD care system performance are discussed in Kaw et al. (2016).

1. **Module 1: Chronic Dialysis Patients Forecast:** This module forecasts the number of chronic dialysis patients at the sub-LHIN level from FY2013/14 to FY2024/25.
   a. **Module 1: Data Sources and Other Input Parameters:**
      i. CKD patients who received dialysis in Ontario from FY1999/00Q1 to FY2012/13Q2 from OHIP CHDB, and their residence postal code from RPDB
      ii. Chronic dialysis patients from FY2010/11Q2 to FY2012/13Q4 from ORRS

Figure 2. An illustration of the individual modules that build the final model is provided. An 8th module, not depicted in the figure, deals with estimating confidence intervals for the chronic dialysis projections.

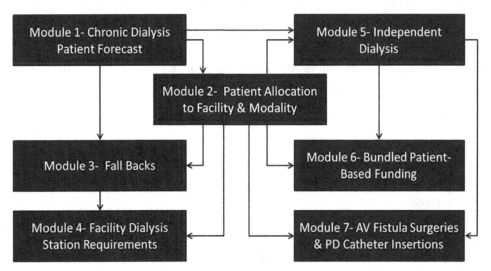

b. **Module 1: Methods:** Physician billings for dialysis therapies from January 1999 to December 2012 from OHIP CHDB were used to identify patients on dialysis. Prevalent chronic dialysis patients were defined as individuals who either had

  i.   A chronic dialysis treatment during the quarter, as well as chronic and/or any other dialysis treatment in the following quarter; or

  ii. Any dialysis treatment during the quarter, chronic and/or other dialysis treatment in the following quarter, and chronic dialysis treatment in any preceding quarter.

Appendix 1: Chronic Dialysis Billing Codes lists chronic dialysis and other dialysis treatment fee codes used to identify dialysis therapies in this module.

To assign historical patients to their sub-LHIN of residence, a sequence of steps were followed. First, historical patient postal codes were converted to latitude and longitude coordinates using the geocoding package PCCF+ version 5K. Each postal code was then assigned to the sub-LHIN within which it is located, using the geographic information system (GIS) software ArcGIS. ArcGIS Network Analyst was used to perform a drive time analysis for each historical patient to identify instances where patient resident location may be inaccurately captured., Wherever it was found that a facility-based dialysis patient's drive time from home to facility was longer than 3.5 hours, it was assumed that the postal code data was erroneous, and the patient was instead assigned to the sub-LHIN within which their treatment facility was located.

ORRS records on all chronic dialysis patients in Ontario from its inception in 2010 to 2012 along with their residence information was also used to complement the analysis. The two data sources overlapped for a period of time (from July 2010 to December 2012), but there were minor discrepancies between the two. A mathematical modeling technique, integer programming, was used to minimize the discrepancies between the two datasets, with the understanding that ORRS is a more accurate source of information on the number of chronic dialysis patients.

Specifically, the problem was formulated as an unconstrained optimization that aimed to find an integer (to add to the number of patients recorded in OHIP CHDB) that minimized the discrepancy between the two datasets over the overlapping period. Let R_{rt} be the number of patients in geographic region r at time t according to ORRS; and H_{rt} be the number according to OHIP. Let T be set of time indices at which data is available from both sources. Let v_r be the integer number of patients to add to the OHIP time series as an adjustment. The following optimization problem determines for each geographic region the adjustment that minimizes the total discrepancy over all time indices:

$$\text{minimize}_{v_r \in \mathbb{Z}} \sum_{t \in T} \left| R_{rt} - \left(H_{rt} + v_r \right) \right|$$

The results of the integer programming were used to adjust the historical time series coming from OHIP data. Readers interested to learn more about integer programming are referred to Chen et al. (2010) and Jünger et al. (2009).

Across all sub-LHINs in the province, the total adjustment was an increase of 182 patients. The two sources were then joined to form a single set of historical chronic dialysis patient volumes.

To forecast the chronic dialysis patient population in each region from FY2013/14 to FY2024/25, we used a time series analysis. This method is different from non-time series regression techniques, because it takes into account the correlation between the observations over time. In time series analysis, a statistical model of the outcome of interest (number of chronic dialysis patients) is built at regularly spaced intervals over time to describe the historical trends in the data and to forecast the future based on the trend (Quinn et al, 2009). Readers interested to learn more about time series analysis are referred to Schelter (2006), Lütkepohl (2005), and Bisgaard (2011).

To predict the number of chronic dialysis patients in each sub-LHIN, four time series forecasting models were fitted and compared, namely a simple exponential smoothing model, a linear trend with autoregressive error model, a damped trend exponential smoothing model, and a linear (holt) exponential smoothing model. Where a single sub-LHIN did not have enough patient volumes to enable a robust forecast, it was merged with its neighboring sub-LHIN(s). Sub-LHINs were merged only when their percentage shares of the merged geography's population did not seem to change much over time.

For each sub-LHIN or merged geography of neighboring sub-LHIN, the time series model with the smallest mean absolute percentage error was selected.

Two forecasts were created for certain sub-LHINs or merged geographies of neighboring sub-LHINs where chronic dialysis patient growth had plateaued in recent years. It was not clear whether the full historical chronic dialysis patient growth should be considered for the time series analysis, or if the plateauing trend in recent years is a better reflection of reality. As such, a high scenario (taking into account all 14 years of historical data) and a low scenario (taking into account only recent years with plateaued demand) for the forecasts were created. These high and low scenarios resulted in high and low estimates of required dialysis stations in the facilities affected.

2. **Module 2: Patient Allocation to Facility and Modality:** This module allocates volume of chronic dialysis patients to each regional renal program, facility, and modality.
    a. **Module 2: Data Sources and Other Input Parameters:**
        i. Output from Module 1 – Chronic Dialysis Patients Forecast.
        ii. Target Hemodialysis (HD) and Peritoneal Dialysis (PD) Home Dialysis rates for FY2013/14 to FY2024/25 as provided by CKD regional programs.
        iii. ORRS patient location data from FY2010/11Q2 to FY2012/13Q4.
    b. **Module 2: Methods:**

ORRS data was used to calculate percentage of chronic dialysis patients within each sub-LHIN or merged geography of neighboring sub-LHINs that have historically received treatment from each regional renal program. This percentage was then multiplied by the chronic dialysis patient forecasts for each sub-LHIN or merged geography of neighboring sub-LHINs to calculate the number of chronic dialysis patients in each regional renal program. The equation used for this was the following: $P_{pts} = \sum_{r} f_{rts} t_{rp}$

Target home dialysis rates provided by regional renal programs were used to assign patients to ID (HD or PD) versus in-facility dialysis. The equations used for this were the following: $M_{mpts} = P_{pts} i_{mpt}$

The historical distribution of facility-based HD patients of each regional renal program among its affiliated facilities was then used to assign patients to the regional renal program's affiliated facilities. The equation used for this was the following: $L_{fts} = \sum_{p} P_{pts} h_{pt} a_{pf}$

Table 1 lists what each variable denotes in the equations.

Table 1. Definitions of variables used in equations for modules 2 to 7

Variable	Denotes
P_{pts}	patients at regional program p at time t in demand scenario s
f_{rts}	forecasted patients living in geographic region r at time t in demand scenario s
t_{rp}	percentage of patients in geographic region r who travel for treatment to regional program p
L_{fts}	facility-based HD patients at facility f at time t in demand scenario s
M_{mpts}	ID patients using modality m at program p at time t in demand scenario s
h_{pt}	percentage of patients in regional program p at time t, who use facility-based HD (as opposed to ID)
i_{mpt}	percentage of ID patients using modality m in regional program p at time t
a_{pf}	percentage of facility-based HD patients in regional program p who receive treatment at facility f
n_f	percentage of facility-based HD patients at facility f who are treated using a non-nocturnal modality
F_{fts}	patients who require reserve capacity at facility f at time t in demand scenario s
r_{pf}	percentage of patients in regional program p for whom reserve capacity is required at facility f
S_{ftsk}	surplus of HD stations at facility f at time t in demand scenario s, under utilization rate scenario k
s_f	current number of approved HD operating stations at facility f
u_{fk}	utilization rate of HD stations at facility f under utilization scenario k, in unit of patients per station
I_{mpts}	patients in program p who are incident in the one-year period preceding time t, who have to assigned to ID modality m within six months of their day of incidence
c_{mp}	percentage of ID patients using modality m in program p who were prevalent patients using the same modality one year earlier
d_{mp}	percentage of ID patients using modality m in program p who were prevalent patients using facility-based HD one year earlier
e_{mp}	percentage of incident patients who are assigned to ID modality m at program p who would be sent home within six months of initiating dialysis (versus those who are sent home more than six months after they initiate dialysis)
A_{fbts}	annualized facility-based HD patients in bundle b at facility f in the one-year period preceding time t, in demand scenario s
B_{mpbts}	annualized ID patients in bundle b at program p in the one-year period preceding time t, in demand scenario s
y_{fb}	percentage of facility-based HD patients at facility f who are in bundle b
z_{mpb}	percentage of ID patients using modality m at program p who are in bundle b
V_{pts}	number of AV fistula surgeries program p should perform in the one-year period preceding time t, in demand scenario s
D_{pts}	number of PD catheter insertions program p should perform in the one-year period preceding time t, in demand scenario s
w_{pt}	percentage of HD patients (both home and facility-based) at program p at time t, who are using an AV fistula
x_p	ratio of the number of AV fistula surgeries performed in a one-year period at program p, to the number of patients using an AV fistula at the end of the period

3. **Module 3: Fall Backs:** This module estimates the number of fall back patients that should be planned for at each treatment facility. Fall back patients include both home dialysis patients who fall back to a facility for dialysis treatment, and satellite patients who fall back to a regional centre or a different satellite. Fall back patient volumes could increase as home dialysis targets are met, eroding the capacity gains made from changing patients from an institutional to a home treatment modality. This module captures this feedback effect.

    a. **Module 3: Data Sources and Other Input Parameters:**

        i. Output from Module 2 – Patient Allocation to Facility and Modality.

        ii. Patient treatment location data from ORRS in the year 2012.

    b. **Module 3: Methods:** Fall back rates were estimated by analysis of historical patient movements in ORRS data. The number of fall back patients present at each facility was counted daily over the course of year 2012. The 90th percentile number of fall back patients at a facility was used as the numerator for that facility's rate. The denominator was the total number of patients in the regional renal program that the facility is part of.

A fall back patient at a regional centre was defined as a patient who transfers to a regional centre either from home or a different facility, stays for a period of time not longer than 90 days, and then either transfers to home, transfers to a different facility, or has an attrition event. Fall backs were limited to a length of 90 days, because patients who transfer for a period longer than 90 days would be counted as part of the chronic patient population at both their original location and their fall back location, eliminating the need to capture their fall back episode. Attrition events include death, recovery, transfer out of region, transplant, withdrawal, and loss to follow-up. Fall back patients at satellites were defined the same way except that only patients who transferred either from home or another satellite were counted.

The calculated fall back rates were applied to the forecasted total patient volumes for each regional renal program, to estimate the 90th percentile number of fall back patients that will be present at the each facility in each quarter. The equation used for this was the following:

$$F_{fts} = \sum_p P_{pts} r_{pf} .$$

4. **Module 4: Facility Dialysis Station Requirements:** This module calculates the required dialysis stations for each facility to account for both the care of in-facility chronic dialysis patients as well as the care required for fall back patients. This module separates each facility's in-facility population between nocturnal and non-nocturnal (conventional) hemodialysis, and bases capacity requirements on the non-nocturnal population only.

    a. **Module 4: Data Sources and Other Input Parameters:**

        i. Output from Module 2 – Patient Allocation to Facility and Modality.

        ii. Output from Module 3 – Fall Backs.

        iii. Number of HD stations and station shifts per week at each facility as obtained from the Regional Renal Programs.

        iv. Maximum utilization rate of 6 patients per station as provided by the ORN.

        v. ORRS data from FY2012/13 was used to calculate ratio of nocturnal patient by facility.

    b. **Module 4: Methods:** The historical percentage of non-nocturnal (conventional) patients at each facility was multiplied by in-facility chronic dialysis patient projections from Module 2 – Patient Allocation to Facility and Modality for each facility to calculate projected number of non-nocturnal HD patients at each location. These patient volumes were used to calculate the required number of baseline dialysis stations at each facility, using the current as well as maximum utilization rates. Current utilization rates (actual number of patients per station) at each facility were calculated based on the assumption that each HD patient would require, on average, 3 shifts per week. The number of fall back patients at each facility, as outputted by Module 3 – Fall Backs, was then used to calculate the required number of reserve HD stations for fall back patients.

The total required baseline and reserved dialysis stations at each facility were then compared to the number of HD stations in that facility to calculate the projected surplus or deficit of HD stations from FY2013/14 to FY2024/25.

The steps summarized in the previous two paragraphs can be represented by the following equation:

$$S_{ftsk} = s_f - \frac{L_{fts}n_f + F_{fts}}{u_{fk}}$$

The calculation of required dialysis stations was based only on the number of non-nocturnal patients at each facility. A facility's nocturnal and non-nocturnal patients can be viewed as populations with independent capacity needs, because while they would be using the same equipment, they would never be using it during the same hours. The model used only non-nocturnal patient volumes because the percentage of patients receiving nocturnal dialysis is small enough that as long as sufficient capacity exists for a facility's non-nocturnal patients, it is certain that sufficient capacity will also exist for nocturnal patients.

In addition, a separate scenario assuming 15% reserve capacity (regardless of the historic fall back rates) was also implemented for regional dialysis centres. The 15% reserved capacity scenario is a "rule of thumb" historically used that incorporates not only fall backs but also capacity that should be reserved for acute dialysis patient crash starts. As such, the two scenarios should not be compared as equivalent scenarios, since the fall back patient numbers outputted by Module 3 – Fall Backs do not incorporate acute dialysis patients' use of dialysis stations.

Assuming 15% reserve capacity, the surplus of stations would be calculated using the following equations:

$$S_{ftsk} = s_f - \frac{L_{fts}n_f}{0.85u_{fk}}$$

5. **Module 5: Independent Dialysis:** This module calculates the number of incident chronic dialysis patients in each FY who should be sent home within six months of their day of incidence, for each regional renal program to reach its target prevalent dialysis rate. The incidence date is the first treatment date. Six months following dialysis initiation was chosen as the relevant interval of time for the ORP target, because it was thought to be a long enough interval to allow patients eligible for home dialysis to complete home dialysis selection and training.

   a. **Module 5: Data Sources and Other Input Parameters:**
      i. Output from Module 1 – Chronic Dialysis Patients Forecast.
      ii. Output from Module 2 – Patient Allocation to Facility and Modality.
      iii. ORRS data from FY2011/12 and FY2012/13.
      iv. Target HD and PD ID rates for FY2013/14 to FY2024/25 as provided by regional renal programs.

The target home HD and PD rates are prevalent rate targets for each fiscal year set by the individual regional renal programs according to their own plans. Although there is a provincial target to have 40% of prevalent patients using home dialysis, for the purposes of capacity planning the regional renal programs are asked to set targets that they believe are realistically achievable, even if these fall short of the provincial target.

b.   **Module 5: Methods:** The output from Module 2 – Patient Allocation to Facility and Modality includes the projected number of patients using home HD or PD at the end of each fiscal year. The following method was applied separately to the home HD and PD patients. While Figure 3 shows the breakdown for home HD calculation only, a similar breakdown was done for the Home PD patients to support the calculations.

For each fiscal year, historical ORRS data is used to determine how many of the home patients active at the end of the fiscal year were prevalent patients using the same home modality at the end of the previous fiscal year (Portion 3a of Figure 3). These patients are subtracted from the total population of home patients active at the end of the fiscal year for that year.

From the remaining number of home patients active at the end of the fiscal year, historical ORRS data is used to determine how many of the patients were prevalent patients using facility-based HD at the end of the previous fiscal year (Portion 3b of Figure 3). These patients are also subtracted from the total population of home patients active at the end of the fiscal year for that year.

The remaining number of home patients active at the end of the fiscal year (i.e. portion 3c of Figure 3) indicates how many incident patients in each FY should be using the home modality at the end of the year in order to achieve the target home dialysis rate.

Historical ORRS data were used to estimate the ratio of incident patients who would be sent home within six months of initiating dialysis versus those who are sent home more than six months after they initiate dialysis. Historical ORRS data was then used to determine how many incident patients in each FY have to be sent home within six months of their day of incidence (index date), in order to achieve the required number actively using home dialysis at the end of the FY and achieve regional renal program target ID rates.

Figure 3. Breakdown of a regional program's prevalent patients at the end of a fiscal year is demonstrated

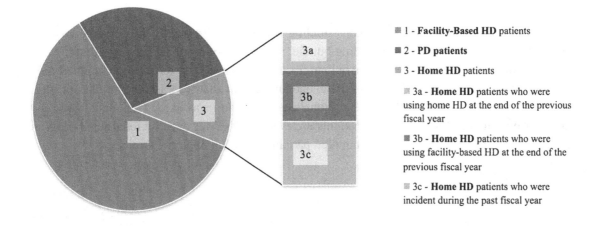

The preceding calculation steps are summarized by the following equation:

$$I_{mpts} = M_{mpts}(1 - c_{mp} - d_{mp})e_{mp}$$

6. **Module 6: Bundled Patient-Based Funding:** This module forecasts the total bundled patient-based funding required for each facility.
   a. **Module 6: Data Sources and Other Input Parameters:**
      i. Output from Module 2 – Patient Allocation to Facility and Modality.
      ii. Output from Module 5 – Independent Dialysis.
      iii. ORRS data from FY2012/13.
      iv. Patient-Based Funding definitions and reimbursement rates as listed in the 2013/14 Chronic Kidney Disease (CKD) Funding Guide.
   b. **Module 6: Methods:** Module 2 – Patient Allocation to Facility and Modality forecasts prevalent patient volumes at each regional renal program in the categories of PD and home HD, and patient volumes at each facility for facility-based HD. These patient volumes are broken down to the more specific modalities used in patient based funding bundles (e.g. CAPD and APD) where applicable, using historical ratios of these modalities in ORRS. Appendix 2 provides a mapping of patient-based funding bundles against modalities.

The quarterly projections of patients in each funding bundle at each facility are converted into annualized patient volumes. This is done using a linear interpolation between quarters to estimate the number of patients present on each day during a quarter. The assumption is that the number of patients in each bundle increases or decreases linearly throughout each quarter, rather than in peaks and troughs. The time-averaging method used applies to this module only.

The annualized patient volumes are calculated using the following equations:

$$A_{fbts} = \frac{1}{8}y_{fb}(L_{f,t-4,s} + 2L_{f,t-3,s} + 2L_{f,t-2,s} + 2L_{f,t-1,s} + L_{fts})$$

$$B_{mpbts} = \frac{1}{8}z_{mpb}(M_{mp,t-4,s} + 2M_{mp,t-3,s} + 2M_{mp,t-2,s} + 2M_{mp,t-1,s} + M_{mpts})$$

The annualized volume of patients in each funding bundle is multiplied by the corresponding reimbursement rate for each patient-based funding bundle. In the case of home HD patients (bundles C and D), a sub-bundle for initial training applies only to incident patients. To determine the bundled funding for this sub-group, output from Module 5 – Independent Dialysis that forecasts the number of incident home HD patients in each FY and at each regional renal program was used. The annualized funding amounts for both incident and prevalent patients are then summed for each regional renal program to produce the regional renal program level bundled patient-based funding projections.

7. **Module 7: AV Fistula Surgeries and PD Catheter Insertions:** This module forecasts the volume of required AV fistula surgeries for reaching AV fistula prevalence targets, and the volume of required PD catheter insertions for reaching PD prevalence targets.

    a. **Module 7: Data Sources and Other Input Parameters:**
        i.   Output from Module 2 – Patient Allocation to Facility and Modality.
        ii. Output from Module 5 – Independent Dialysis.
        iii. FY2012/13 AV fistula prevalence data from ORRS.
        iv. FY2012/13 AV fistula surgeries from the Wait Time Information System (WTIS).
        v.   PD catheter use rate (Perl et al, 2014).

    b. **Module 7: Methods:** The Ontario Renal Plan target of a 2% absolute reduction per year in the prevalence of HD catheter use was used to project target AV fistula rates that increase by 2% per year, starting from the end of FY2012/13, for each regional renal program. Using these targets, the number of prevalent AV fistula patients in each regional renal program at the end of each fiscal year was projected.

Historical data from ORRS and WTIS were combined to determine the ratio of surgeries each regional renal program performed in FY2012/13, to the number of chronic patients on AV Fistula at end of the fiscal year. This ratio was multiplied by the prevalent AV fistula patients in each regional renal program at the end of each fiscal year to calculate how many surgeries each regional renal program should perform to reach its target. The following equation was used in this calculation:

$$V_{pts} = P_{pts}\left(h_{pt} + i_{m=\text{home HD},pt}\right)w_{pt}x_p$$

Module 5 – Independent Dialysis forecasts the number of incident patients in each regional renal program and fiscal year that should begin using PD in order for the regional renal program to meet its annual PD prevalence targets. These patient volumes are inflated by applying the utilization rate for PD catheters that are implanted, which has been found to be around 83% (Perl et al, 2014). The following equation was used in this calculation:

$$D_{pts} = \frac{I_{m=\text{PD},pts}}{0.83}$$

8. **Module 8: Confidence Interval for the Chronic Dialysis Projections:** To properly account for all sources of uncertainties, such as the actual modality allocation and the actual patient travel patterns and their impact on the projected chronic prevalent dialysis patient volume, confidence intervals are needed for the projected patient volume and machines requirement at each facility. We used Monte Carlo simulation to calculate the 95% confidence intervals for these. In the Monte Carlo simulation, the inputs were repeatedly drawn 3000 times from appropriate statistical distributions, and consequently the output resulted in a distribution which reflects the uncertainty in the inputs. Based on the resulting distribution, we obtained the 2.5th and 97.5th percentiles to calculate the 95% confidence intervals for the realized patient volume and machine requirement at each facility. Readers interested to learn more about Monte Carlo simulation are referred to Thomopoulos (2012).

a. **Module 8: Data Sources and Other Input Parameters:**
   i. Sub-LHIN forecasts.
   ii. Travel matrix.
   iii. Modality allocation.
   iv. Fall back rate.
   v. Machine utilization ratio.
   vi. Machine supply.
b. **Module 8: Methods:** The simulation algorithm is as follows, and is illustrated in Figure 4.
   i. **Regional Forecast:** For each of the 97 Sub-LHINs and for the 49 FYQ's, the number of chronic dialysis patients is normally distributed.
   ii. **Program-Level Forecast:** For each of the 26 programs and at each of the 49 FYQ's, the number of patients are distributed to the programs based on the travel matrix.
   iii. **Modality Forecast:** For each of the facilities and home HD/PD dialysis modalities, the patient numbers are distributed based on the modality allocation.
   iv. **Machine Forecast:** The 15% reserve capacity for fall back in the main facility at each program was used; the facility-level patient-machine utilization ratio and the machine supply were used.

The results for selected facilities from FY2014/15 to 2024/25 illustrate that (i) the confidence intervals typically get wider over time, reflecting increasing uncertainty about future projections, and that (ii) for a facility with a larger volume, the confidence intervals are generally narrower than those for a smaller facility.

Model User Interface

A user friendly interactive model interface has been developed (a section of which is presented in Figure 5) that allows ORN staff to use it as a flexible tool to conduct various what-if scenarios through varying input parameters and policy levers to assess the impact on output variables. This interactive nature

Figure 4. Simulation steps for producing the confidence intervals for the chronic dialysis projections is demonstrated. Circles are constant inputs, the left blue box is random input distribution, and the rest of the boxes are the outputs.

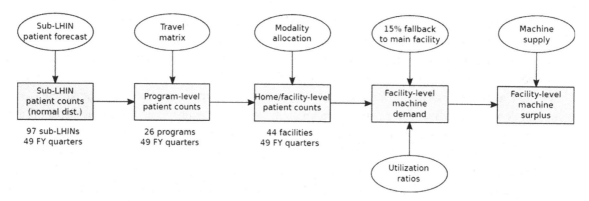

Figure 5. Partial Screenshot of the Model User Interface is demonstrated

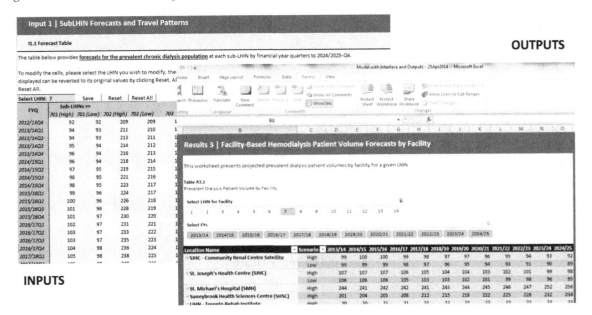

INPUTS

of the user interface facilitates ongoing conversations between ORN and local planning stakeholders, where feedback from stakeholders can rapidly be incorporated into the planning assumptions used in the model. With this approach, model results gain the face validity required to be successfully adopted by various stakeholders in their planning.

SOLUTIONS AND RECOMMENDATIONS

The model produces results at the local and provincial levels from FY 2013/14 to FY 2024/25 that can be used for planning purposes. At the local level, chronic patient projections are provided by sub-LHIN, and required dialysis stations, operational funding, AV fistula surgeries, and PD Catheter insertions are provided by facility. Incident dialysis patients to be sent home to achieve prevalent ID targets are provided for each regional renal program.

Figure 6 illustrates projected prevalent patients in a sample sub-LHIN.

As shown in Figure 7, from 2013 to 2025, the provincial prevalent chronic dialysis patient population is expected to grow between 29.6% and 35.3%.

At the sub-LHIN level, the mean absolute percent error between the predicted and observed forecasts had an average value of 3.98%, with 75% of the forecasts falling within 2.41% and 4.75%, as it can be seen in Figure 8.

Figure 9 shows Forecasted net growth in dialysis patients between 2013 and 2025, and the resulting dialysis capacity assessment for Ontario.

The model also provides all the above mentioned results at the provincial level. Figure 10 shows forecasted provincial incremental dialysis station requirements from FY2014/15 to 2024/25.

Figure 6. The model illustrates prevalent patients in a sample sub-LHIN

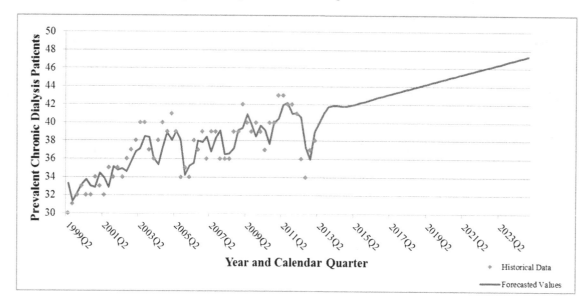

Figure 7. Forecasted provincial prevalent chronic dialysis patients is demonstrated

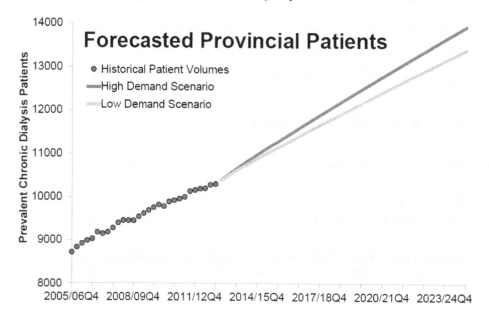

Figure 11 demonstrates provincial bundled Patient-Based Funding Projection for FY2014/15

In summary, the model is providing detailed output at the local and provincial level. It is strongly recommended that ORN uses the model output to supplement its planning processes. Model's projections of chronic dialysis patients, required dialysis stations, and funding are actively used by ORN in their planning efforts, while the rest of the model outputs are currently used as supplemental information available as required to ORN.

Figure 8. Distribution of forecast error across prevalence projections at the sub-LHIN level.

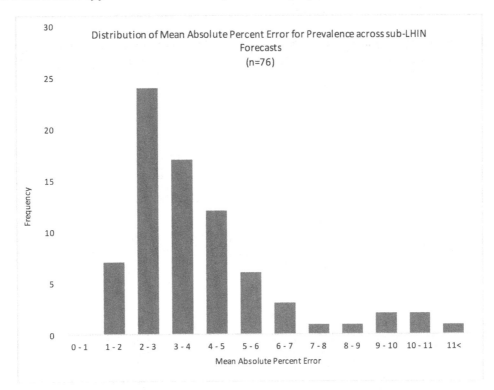

FUTURE RESEARCH DIRECTIONS

The model has some limitations that should be kept in mind when used to support local and provincial planning. In the patient volume forecasting module, the time series analysis indirectly accounts for all the risk factors that may influence the need for dialysis therapy and how they have evolved over time. This is most accurate when there are not large changes in important risk factors (Quinn et al, 2009). Older age has been suggested as a risk factor for the need for dialysis treatments, and it is possible that the rapidly changing age structures in some of the regions could make the time series analysis less accurate for these regions. As such, chronic dialysis patient projections for regions with rapidly changing age structures should be treated with caution; the performance of projection models should be assessed and when necessary these models should be refined. Moreover, historical data used for some of the modules has been limited to a few quarters due to data availability and as such the results should be interpreted with caution. To overcome these shortcomings, the ORN refreshes the model annually as more recent data becomes available. By refreshing the model frequently, changes in the underlying risk factors are gradually reflected in the time series forecasting, and as such the validity of the forecasts are enhanced. Future research could look into predicting the effects of changes in the underlying risk factors on the forecasts.

Furthermore, the patient-based funding bundles modeled are those confirmed by the end of year 2013. As the evolving funding arrangements such as the funding approach for fall back patients are confirmed, there is a need to incorporate them into the model. In the future, the organization should work closely

Figure 9. Forecasted net growth in dialysis patients between 2013 and 2025, and the resulting dialysis capacity assessment for Ontario is demonstrated

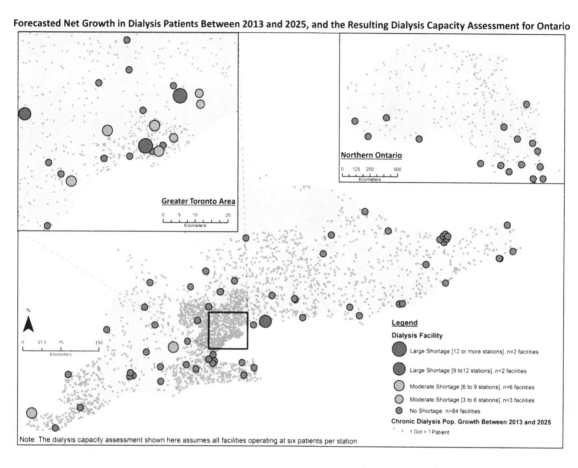

Figure 10. Forecasted Provincial Dialysis Station Shortage from FY2014/15 to 2024/25 is demonstrated

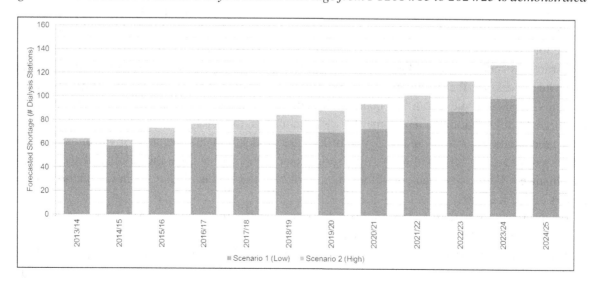

Figure 11. Provincial bundled Patient-Based Funding Projection for FY2014/15 is demonstrated

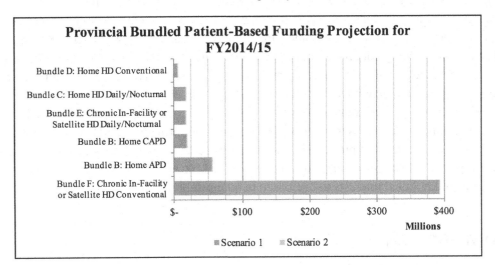

with local stakeholders to best remedy these shortcomings of the model by seeking their feedback and incorporating those into what-if analyses.

Additionally, the Ontario Renal Plan II which was released in 2015, serves as a provincial roadmap for improving the lives of those living with CKD in Ontario from 2015 to 2019. It specifies three overall goals as follows: 1) Empower and support patients and family members to be active in their care; 2) Integrate patient care throughout the kidney care journey; and 3) Improve patients' access to kidney care. For each goal, specific targets for 2019 along with strategic objectives and initiatives have been defined. (Ontario Renal Network, 2015). The organization can benefit from supporting the related planning decisions through further data-driven analytics research. Examples include 1) pre-dialysis care capacity assessment to support the target of timely access to appropriate pre-dialysis care by patients transitioning from primary care to nephrology; and 2) surgical capacity assessment to support the target of ensuring patients' timely access to vascular and peritoneal access services. Much like the example presented in the chapter, the organization can benefit by driving its strategy for the years to come through strategic analytics and move towards the vision of fully embedding evidence in healthcare decision making (Garay et al, 2014).

CONCLUSION

Administrative data, such as the ones used in this study, are a rich source of information that can be leveraged beyond their primary intended use to provide strategic insight. In fact, due to rigorous auditing and quality control mechanisms usually built into the process of producing these datasets, especially in cases where the data is used for public reporting and thus needs to be most reliable and transparent, the quality of these datasets is usually comparatively reliable for such analysis.

While this study is by no means the first study that applies analytics to strategic issues in Canada, to the best of our knowledge, this is the first study that presents a data-driven strategic decision support tool used by stakeholders in an interactive manner to support multiple strategic priorities specified in the organization's strategic roadmap. The model has benefited the organization in multiple ways. It has allowed adoption of a consistent and robust provincial approach that ensures transparency in resource allocation province-wide, while at the same time allowing local planning at each CKD program and LHIN. The model development process has been a very collaborative one, with joint governance of the project by the SA, ORN, and regional renal programs, and a repetitive process of iterative prototype development to gain incremental feedback and make improvements in every iteration.

The model is a successful example of data-driven decision making and is a step forward towards evidence-based policies to address the globally growing issue of providing CKD care. As more and more examples of models like the one presented in this chapter are developed and successfully implemented, the culture of policy making in general and health policy making in particular would gradually shift from pure advocacy and political interests to one based in quantifiable objective evidence.

ACKNOWLEDGMENT

The authors would like to sincerely thank all the sponsors of the strategic analytics project described in this chapter. In particular, the project was completed under the leadership of Graham Woodward (Director of Clinical Programs at ORN at the time) and Kiren Handa (ORN Informatics and Strategic Analytics Manager at the time). This work was not possible without their inspiration and continuous support. The authors would also like to thank all the members of the project steering committee who provided oversight and directions throughout the project, in particular Dino Villalta who, as the regional director of one of the LHINs at the time, ensured the validity and usefulness of model inputs and outputs. Many others provided invaluable support to the working group, namely Thomas Galambos, Jane Ip, Camila Iraheta, Azadeh Mostaghel, and Kelly Woltman.

REFERENCES

Benazon, N. R., Mamdani, M. M., & Coyne, J. C. (2005). Trends in the prescribing of antidepressants following acute myocardial infarction, 1993–2002. *Psychosomatic Medicine*, *67*(6), 916–920. doi:10.1097/01.psy.0000188399.80167.aa PMID:16314596

Bisgaard, S., & Kulahci, M. (2011). *Time series analysis and forecasting by example*. John Wiley & Sons. doi:10.1002/9781118056943

Blecker, S., Bhatia, R. S., You, J. J., Lee, D. S., Alter, D. A., Wang, J. T., & Tu, J. V. et al. (2013). Temporal trends in the utilization of echocardiography in Ontario, 2001 to 2009. *JACC: Cardiovascular Imaging*, *6*(4), 515–522. doi:10.1016/j.jcmg.2012.10.026 PMID:23579013

Booth, G. L., Kapral, M. K., Fung, K., & Tu, J. V. (2006). Recent trends in cardiovascular complications among men and women with and without diabetes. *Diabetes Care*, *29*(1), 32–37. doi:10.2337/diacare.29.01.06.dc05-0776 PMID:16373892

Chen, D. S., Batson, R. G., & Dang, Y. (2010). *Applied integer programming: modeling and solution*. John Wiley & Sons.

Dunn, S., Anderson, G. M., & Bierman, A. S. (2009). Temporal and regional trends in IUD insertion: A population-based study in Ontario, Canada. *Contraception, 80*(5), 469–473. doi:10.1016/j.contraception.2009.04.004 PMID:19835722

Garay, J., Cartagena, R., Esensoy, A. V., Handa, K., Kane, E., Kaw, N., & Sadat, S. (2014). Strategic analytics: towards fully embedding evidence in healthcare decision-making. *Healthcare Quarterly (Toronto, Ont.), 17*, 23-27.

Gershon, A. S., Guan, J., Wang, C., & To, T. (2010a). Trends in asthma prevalence and incidence in Ontario, Canada, 1996–2005: A population study. *American Journal of Epidemiology.* PMID:20716702

Gershon, A. S., Wang, C., Wilton, A. S., Raut, R., & To, T. (2010b). Trends in chronic obstructive pulmonary disease prevalence, incidence, and mortality in Ontario, Canada, 1996 to 2007: A population-based study. *Archives of Internal Medicine, 170*(6), 560–565. doi:10.1001/archinternmed.2010.17 PMID:20308643

Hill, N. R., Fatoba, S. T., Oke, J. L., Hirst, J. A., OCallaghan, C. A., Lasserson, D. S., & Hobbs, F. R. (2016). Global Prevalence of Chronic Kidney Disease–A Systematic Review and Meta-Analysis. *PLoS ONE, 11*(7), e0158765. doi:10.1371/journal.pone.0158765 PMID:27383068

Jha, V., Garcia-Garcia, G., Iseki, K., Li, Z., Naicker, S., Plattner, B., & Yang, C. W. et al. (2013). Chronic kidney disease: Global dimension and perspectives. *Lancet, 382*(9888), 260–272. doi:10.1016/S0140-6736(13)60687-X PMID:23727169

Jünger, M., Liebling, T. M., Naddef, D., Nemhauser, G. L., Pulleyblank, W. R., Reinelt, G., & Wolsey, L. A. (Eds.). (2009). *50 Years of integer programming 1958-2008: From the early years to the state-of-the-art.* Springer Science & Business Media.

Kassebaum, N. J., Arora, M., Barber, R. M., Bhutta, Z. A., Brown, J., Carter, A., & Cornaby, L. et al. (2016). Global, regional, and national disability-adjusted life-years (DALYs) for 315 diseases and injuries and healthy life expectancy (HALE), 1990–2015: A systematic analysis for the Global Burden of Disease Study 2015. *Lancet, 388*(10053), 1603–1658. doi:10.1016/S0140-6736(16)31460-X PMID:27733283

Kaw, N., Esensoy, A. V., Sadat, S., Liu, A., Bastedo, S., & Nesrallah, G. (2016). *Planning for dialysis capacity and bundled patient-based funding in Ontario, Canada.* Unpublished Manuscript.

Mamdani, M. M., Parikh, S. V., Austin, P. C., & Upshur, R. E. (2000). Use of antidepressants among elderly subjects: Trends and contributing factors. *The American Journal of Psychiatry, 157*(3), 360–367. doi:10.1176/appi.ajp.157.3.360 PMID:10698810

Ministry of Health and Long-term Care. (2016). *Quality-Based Procedures Clinical Handbook for Chronic Kidney Disease. January 2016.* Retried December 6, 2016, from: http://www.health.gov.on.ca/en/pro/programs/ecfa/docs/qbp_kidney.pdf

Musselman, R. P., Gomes, T., Chan, B. P., Auer, R. C., Moloo, H., Mamdani, M., & Boushey, R. P. et al. (2012). Changing trends in rectal cancer surgery in Ontario: 2002–2009. *Colorectal Disease, 14*(12), 1467–1472. doi:10.1111/j.1463-1318.2012.03044.x PMID:22487101

Ojo, A. (2014). Addressing the global burden of chronic kidney disease through clinical and translational research. *Transactions of the American Clinical and Climatological Association, 125*, 229. PMID:25125737

Ontario Ministry of Finance. (2016). *Ontario Fact Sheet. November 2016.* Retried November 30, 2016, from: http://www.fin.gov.on.ca/en/economy/ecupdates/factsheet.html

Ontario Renal Network. (2012). *Ontario Renal Plan.* Retrieved July 6, 2016, from: https://www.cancer-care.on.ca/common/pages/UserFile.aspx?fileId=253261

Ontario Renal Network. (2015). *Ontario Renal Plan II.* Retrieved July 6, 2016, from the Ontario Renal Network Website: http://www.renalnetwork.on.ca/ontario_renal_plan/#.V3wczPl97IU

Ontario Renal Network. (2016). *Ontario Renal Reporting System.* Retrieved December 6, 2016, from the Ontario Renal Network Website: http://www.renalnetwork.on.ca/hcpinfo/ontario_renal_reporting_system/#.WE2tsncZOV4

Perl, J., Pierratos, A., Kandasamy, G., McCormick, B. B., Quinn, R. R., Jain, A. K., & Oliver, M. J. et al. (2014). Peritoneal dialysis catheter implantation by nephrologists is associated with higher rates of peritoneal dialysis utilization: A population-based study. *Nephrology, Dialysis, Transplantation,* gfu359. PMID:25414373

Quinn, R. R., Laupacis, A., Hux, J. E., Moineddin, R., Paterson, M., & Oliver, M. J. (2009). Forecasting the need for dialysis services in Ontario, Canada to 2011. *Healthcare Policy, 4*(4).

Radhakrishnan, D. K., Dell, S. D., Guttmann, A., Shariff, S. Z., Liu, K., & To, T. (2014). Trends in the age of diagnosis of childhood asthma. *The Journal of Allergy and Clinical Immunology, 134*(5), 1057–1062. doi:10.1016/j.jaci.2014.05.012 PMID:24985402

Schelter, B., Winterhalder, M., & Timmer, J. (Eds.). (2006). *Handbook of time series analysis: recent theoretical developments and applications.* John Wiley & Sons. doi:10.1002/9783527609970

Thomopoulos, N. T. (2012). *Essentials of Monte Carlo simulation: Statistical methods for building simulation models.* Springer Science & Business Media.

Tranmer, J. E., Colley, L., Edge, D. S., Sears, K., VanDenKerkhof, E., & Levesque, L. (2015). Trends in nurse practitioners prescribing to older adults in Ontario, 20002010: A retrospective cohort study. *CMAJ Open, 3*(3), E299–E304. doi:10.9778/cmajo.20150029 PMID:26457291

van Walraven, C. (2013). Trends in 1-year survival of people admitted to hospital in Ontario, 1994–2009. *Canadian Medical Association Journal.*

Wang, H., Naghavi, M., Allen, C., Barber, R. M., Bhutta, Z. A., Carter, A., & Coggeshall, M. et al. (2016). Global, regional, and national life expectancy, all-cause mortality, and cause-specific mortality for 249 causes of death, 1980–2015: A systematic analysis for the Global Burden of Disease Study 2015. *Lancet, 388*(10053), 1459–1544. doi:10.1016/S0140-6736(16)31012-1 PMID:27733281

Wilson, S. E., Lipscombe, L. L., Rosella, L. C., & Manuel, D. G. (2009). Trends in laboratory testing for diabetes in Ontario, Canada 1995–2005: A population-based study. *BMC Health Services Research, 9*(1), 41. doi:10.1186/1472-6963-9-41 PMID:19250533

Woodward, G. L., Iverson, A., Harvey, R., & Blake, P. G. (2014). Implementation of an agency to improve chronic kidney disease care in Ontario: Lessons learned by the Ontario Renal Network. *Healthcare Quarterly (Toronto, Ont.), 17,* 44-47.

KEY TERMS AND DEFINITIONS

Arteriovenous (AV) Fistula: Generally considered as the optimal long-term vascular access for hemodialysis as it provides adequate blood flow, lasts a long time, and has a lower complication rate than other types of access.

Chronic Kidney Disease (CKD): The presence of kidney damage, or a decreased level of kidney function, for at least three months, divided into five stages, depending on severity.

Dialysis: A procedure that replaces the filtering capability of a failed kidney. Dialysis can further be divided into hemodialysis (HD) and peritoneal dialysis (PD).

End Stage Renal Disease (ESRD): Stage 5 CKD. ESRD Patients typically need renal replacement therapy (i.e., dialysis or transplant).

Hemodialysis (HD): A type of dialysis that filters the person's blood through a machine to remove waste products and toxins.

Independent Dialysis: Dialysis administered outside of a hospital or other dialysis facility, typically at patient's place of residence.

Peritoneal Dialysis: A type of dialysis that utilizes the peritoneum that lines the abdominal cavity as the filter. The lifeline is a catheter which is placed in the lower abdomen.

Vascular Access: A lifeline for hemodialysis that provides an access for blood to pass through the dialysis filter and delivers back "cleaned" blood.

APPENDIX 1: CHRONIC DIALYSIS BILLING CODES

To identify chronic dialysis treatments, the following fee codes in the 2013 OHIP Schedule of Benefits (SOB) were used.

Table 2.

Chronic Dialysis Codes	
G860	Chronic hemodialysis hospital location
G861	Chronic peritoneal dialysis hospital location
G862	Hospital self care Chronic hemodialysis
G863	Chronic hemodialysis IHF location
G864	Chronic Home peritoneal dialysis
G865	Chronic Home hemodialysis
G866	Intermittent hemodialysis treatment centre

Table 3.

Other Dialysis Codes	
G082	Continuous venovenous hemodialfiltration
G083	Continuous venovenous hemodialysis
G085	Continuous venovenous hemofiltration
G090	Veneovenous slow continuous ultrafiltration
G091	Continuous arteriovenous hemodialysis
G092	Continuous arteriovenous hemodiafiltration
G093	Hemodiafiltration – Contin. Init & Acute (repeatx3)
G094	Hemodiafiltration – Contin. Chronic
G095	Slow Continuous Ultra Filtration - Initial & Acute (repeat)
G096	Slow Continuous Ultra Filtration - Chronic
G294	Arteriovenous slow continuous ultrafiltration init and acute
G295	Continuous aterivenous hemofiltration initial and acute
G323	Dialysis - Hemodialysis - Acute, repeat (max 3)
G325	Dialysis - Hemodialysis - Medical component(incl in unit fee)
G326	Dialysis - Chronic, contin. haemodialysis or haemofiltration each
G330	Peritoneal dialysis - Acute (up to 48 hrs)
G331	Peritoneal dialysis - Repeat acute (up to 48 hrs) max. 3
G332	Peritoneal dialysis - Chronic (up to 48 hrs)
G333	Home/self-care dialysis
R849	Dialysis - Hemodialysis - Initial & acute

APPENDIX 2: MAPPING OF PATIENT-BASED FUNDING BUNDLES AGAINST MODALITIES

Table 4.

Modality	Patient-Based Funding Bundle
PD	Bundle B APD – Home Automated Peritoneal Dialysis (APD) Patient
PD	Bundle B CAPD – Home Continuous Ambulatory Peritoneal Dialysis (CAPD) Patient
Home HD	Bundle C – Home HD Daily / Nocturnal Patient
Home HD	Bundle D – Home HD Conventional Patient
Facility-Based HD	Bundle E – Chronic In-Facility Or Satellite Hemodialysis Daily / Nocturnal
Facility-Based HD	Bundle F – Chronic In-Facility Or Satellite Hemodialysis Conventional

APPENDIX 3: LIST OF ACRONYMS

Table 5 provides descriptions for some of the acronyms used throughout the chapter.

Table 5.

Acronym	Description
AV	Arteriovenous
CCO	Cancer Care Ontario
CKD	Chronic Kidney Disease
ESRD	End Stage Renal Disease
HD	Hemodialysis
ID	Independent Dialysis
LHIN	Local Health Integration Network
MOHLTC	Ministry of Health and Long Term Care
OHIP	Ontario Health Insurance Plan
OHIP CHDB	Ontario Health Insurance Plan Claims History Database
ORN	Ontario Renal Network
ORP	Ontario Renal Plan
ORRS	Ontario Renal Reporting System
PD	Peritoneal Dialysis
RPDB	Registered Persons Database
SA	Strategic Analytics
WTIS	Wait Time Information System

Chapter 9
Non–Parametric Statistical Analysis of Rare Events in Healthcare:
Case of Histological Outcome of Kidney Transplantation

Soheila Nasiri
University of Ottawa, Canada

Bijan Raahemi
Unviersity of Ottawa, Canada

ABSTRACT

The assumption of Gaussian distribution of population does not always hold strongly in health studies. The sample size may not be large enough due to the limited nature of observations such as biopsies taken during kidney transplantation, the distribution of sample may not be Gaussian, or the observation may not even be possible for the far ends of a Gaussian distribution. In such cases, an alternative approach, called nonparametric tests can be applied. In this study, a non-parametric single center retrospective analysis of adult kidney transplant is performed to compare histological outcomes among three different groups of deceased kidney donors, based on the biopsies taken before and after kidney transplant at months 1, 3, and 12. A total of 107 transplants were observed in this study with 310 surveillance biopsy taken then classified based on the Banff 97 adequacy assessment. It is concluded that the recipient's internal condition after kidney transplant is as important as the donor's risk factors.

INTRODUCTION

Statistical analysis of sampled data has been extensively applied in many areas of health studies. The majority of the traditional statistical tests, such as ANOVA and the t-test, assume that the sampled data are from a population with a Gaussian (bell-shaped), or approximately Gaussian, distribution. However, the

DOI: 10.4018/978-1-5225-2515-8.ch009

assumption of a Gaussian population distribution does not always hold, especially in biology and health studies. The sample size may not be large enough, due to the limited nature of available observations, such as for kidney transplants performed in a particular state or country. Further, observation may not be possible for the far ends of a Gaussian distribution when examining biological tests. In such cases, an alternative approach, called *non-parametric* tests, can be applied, which do not assume that data follow a Gaussian distribution. In a non-parametric approach, instead of considering the actual values, they are ranked from low to high, and analysis is based on the distribution of ranks. This approach ensures that the test is not affected much by outliers, and does not require the assumption of any particular distribution.

In this study, we perform a non-parametric single-center retrospective analysis of consecutive deceased-donor adult kidney transplants. The goal is to compare histological and clinical outcomes among three different groups of deceased kidney donors, namely expanded criteria donor (ECD), standard criteria donor (SCD), and donation after cardiac death (DCD). We report on a study of 107 cadaveric kidney transplants with regard to histological changes, based on protocol biopsies taken before the transplant (month 0), and 1, 3 and 12 months after the transplant. The transplant recipients were selected based on a waiting list and histological compatibility, regardless of donor physiological characteristics. In some cases, the recipients' ages in the ECD, SCD, and DCD groups were the same. Consequently, we had the opportunity to compare the graft outcomes in the three groups of SCD, ECD and DCD, without considering age as a constraining factor.

It is observed that the relative increase in the Banff summation score, as an indicator of histological change, was similar among the SCD and ECD groups over the 12 months. However, in the DCD group, despite better organ condition at transplantation, its mean score was higher than that of the ECD group. It is further observed that the similar ages of recipients among the three groups highlights the influence of recipient's age on the outcome. We conclude that a recipient's internal condition after kidney transplant is as important as the donor's risk factors. In other words, it is not only the risk factors associated with donors that play a significant role in the outcome, but also the risk factors of recipients.

BACKGROUND

Non-Parametric Analysis

Many statistical methods, such as the t-test and ANOVA, are based on the assumption that the values are sampled from a Gaussian distribution. Because these tests are based on assumptions that can be defined by parameters, they are called parametric tests. Another family of methods makes no such assumption about the population distribution. These are called non-parametric methods, which most commonly work by ignoring the actual data, and instead, analyzing only their ranks. This approach insures that the test is not affected much by outliers, and does not require the assumption of any particular distribution.

The *Mann-Whitney* test is a non-parametric test used to compare two unpaired groups, to compute a *P*-value for the null hypothesis that the distribution of ranks is totally random. Under the null hypothesis, it would be equally likely for either of the two groups to have the larger mean ranks, and more likely to find the two mean ranks close together.

The *Wilcoxon* test compares two paired groups. It tests the null hypothesis that there is no difference in the populations, and so the differences between the matched pairs will be randomly positive or negative.

The *Spearman's rank correlation* is a non-parametric method for quantifying correlation. *Spearman's correlation* separately ranks the X and Y values, and then computes the correlation between the two sets of ranks. The *P*-value is then calculated, which tests the null hypothesis that there is no rank correlation in the overall population. The *Spearman* test quantifies the monotonic relationship between X and Y.

The non-parametric test analogous to one-way ANOVA is called the *Kruskal-Wallis* test, and the one analogous to repeated measure one-way ANOVA is called *Friedman's* test. These tests first rank the data from low to high, and then analyze the distribution of the ranks among groups.

The clear advantage of non-parametric tests is that they do not require the assumption of sampling from Gaussian population, and so can be used when the validity of that assumption is in doubt. When the assumption of Gaussian distribution does not hold, non-parametric tests have more power than parametric tests to detect differences.

Note that to be able to compute a *P*-value less than 0.05, the *Mann-Whitney* test requires more than 8 values, and *Wilcoxon's* matched-pair test requires more than 6 pairs.

Kidney Transplantation and Implications of Limited Donors

With improvement in life expectancy of the general population, increasingly accurate diagnosis of early-stage renal disease (ESRD), and a limited pool of kidney donors, the disparity between organ supply and demand is increasing. Proportionally, waiting lists for kidney transplants are getting longer. New approaches are needed to optimize the use of organs from potential donors. In the past, comparative studies on the recipients of expanded criteria donor (ECD) and standard criteria donor (SCD) transplants were biased toward the higher age of the recipients of the ECDs. The obvious statistical difference in clinical outcomes might have prevented us from discovering the impact of the recipients' ages on the graft function, regardless of the donors' ages.

ECD is defined as any brain-dead donor aged 60 years or over, or a donor aged 50 years or over with two of the following conditions: a history of hypertension (HTN), terminal serum creatinine level (sCr) > 1.5 mg/dL, or death resulting from a cerebrovascular accident (CVA) (Pascual, 2008). ECD and DCD were proposed in 1991 and 1999, respectively, to offer access to a larger number of donated organs. However, initial studies demonstrated higher risk of Delay Graft Function (DGF), and lower long-term survival in these two groups, while their Early Graph Survival rate was reported to be the same as that of the SCD group (Saidi, 2007).

Since the worldwide trend in kidney transplants is to place marginal kidneys in recipients older than 65 years or with a low life expectancy, the comparative studies between the recipients of ECD and SCD are biased toward the higher age of the recipients of the ECD and DCD donors. The European Senior Programme (ESP) is well-known for achieving acceptable outcomes using ECD kidneys from donors older than 65 years (Goplani, 2010). The obvious statistical difference in clinical outcomes between the recipients of the ECD and SCD donors might be due to the age or other confining factors in recipients, which might have prevented us from discovering the impact of the recipients' ages on the graft function regardless of the donors' ages. On the other hand, depriving young recipients of ECD kidneys could cause a longer waiting list for the young group of patients, who are potentially more suitable candidates for kidney transplants. Here are the important questions before us: Is the graft function tied to the donors' characteristics, the recipients', or both? Is the condition of the source of the kidney more important than the state of its destination? And what are the contributions of each in the outcomes of the transplantations?

Banff Score

The Banff Score is a standardized international classification of renal allograft biopsies, developed by a group of renal pathologists, nephrologists, and transplant surgeons, at a 1991 meeting in Banff, Canada. Before then, there was no standardized, international classification for renal allograft biopsies, which resulted in considerable heterogeneity among pathologists in characterization of renal allograft biopsies. The first Banff schema was published in 1993 (Solez, 1993) with the aim to standardize the histopathological diagnosis of renal allograft biopsies. The classification is expanded and updated every two years, at meetings organized by the Banff Foundation for Allograft Pathology (Racusen,1999), (Bhowmik, 2010). An evaluation of the Banff Classification, in March 2000, confirmed significant association between the revised Banff '97 classification and graft outcomes (Mueller, 2000).

The higher the Banff score, the higher the chance of kidney rejection. Accordingly, in this study we rely on Banff Score to evaluate and compare the graft outcomes of kidney transplants among ECD, SCD and DCD groups.

APPLYING NON-PARAMETRIC ANALYSIS TO STUDY HISTOLOGICAL OUTCOME OF KIDNEY TRANSPLANTATION

Method and Materials

In this study, we compare the histologic and clinical changes before and after kidney transplant in SCD, ECD, and DCD recipients. We report on the study of 107 cadaveric kidney transplants with regard to histological changes, based on protocol biopsies taken before the transplant (month 0), and 1, 3, and 12 months after the transplant.

Recipients were selected based on a waiting list and histological compatibility, regardless of the donors' characteristics. Cases were included where the recipients' ages in the ECD, SCD, and DCD groups were the same. Consequently, we had the opportunity to compare the graft outcome in the SCD, ECD and DCD groups without considering the age as a constraining factor.

Written informed consent was obtained from all patients in our kidney transplant program. Clinical and pre-clinical data were extracted from electronic databases and patient medical records.

We reviewed the deceased donors and kidney recipients between January 2008 and December 2011, meaning a period after the initiation routine ECD use in the clinical center. Consecutive deceased-donor kidney transplants were recorded in this retrospective cohort study. Simultaneous pancreas and kidney transplantation (SPK) was excluded, as well as one case of cardiac arrest in the operating room. The remaining population of 110 was divided into four groups, based on donor characteristics:

Group 1: Standard Criteria Donation (SCD)
Group 2: Donation after Cardiac Death (DCD)
Group 3: Expanded Criteria Donation (ECD)
Group 4: ECD+DCD

The ECD+DCD group was excluded from this study, as there were only three transplants in this group.

We examined the histologic findings in 310 surveillance biopsies from these 107 patients. Kidney biopsies were carried out just before transplantation (i.e. month 0), as well as in the first, third and twelfth months after implantation, and classified based on the Banff 97 (Racusen, 1999) adequacy assessment by a pathologist blinded to the patients' groups.

In the ECD group, all kidneys were from donors aged 60 years or older, or donors between the ages of 50 and 60 years who had two of three conditions of HTN, sCr >1.5 and CVA. The DCD group included donations after cardiac death, while DCD+ECD were donors who fulfilled both criteria. The SCD group included patients who did not meet any of the above criteria.

All patients but two received 20 mg of basiliximab at day 0 and 4, and Tacrolimus (Prograft;Fujisawa,Osaka,Japan) started at 0.075 mg/kg bd. Mycophenolate mofetil (MMF) (cellcept;Roche,Nutley,NJ) was started at 2 g per day, and prednisolone started at 20 mg a day, and decreased by 2.5 mg every two weeks for 3 months, when it was then kept at 10 mg. Recipients were stratified according to immunological risk, and immunosuppression therapy prescribed based on our local protocol.

The DGF(delayed graft function), patient and graft survival, cold ischemic time (CIT), the type and time of dialysis, GFR (Glomerular Filtration Rate) at twelve months, HLA (Human Leukocyte Antigens) mismatching data, the number of previous transplants, and sub-clinical and clinical rejection incidence at one year, were collected on all patients. The DGF is defined as the requirement of dialysis within one week post-transplant. Acute rejection was labelled when the serum creatinine were increased by 20% baseline, supported by histological findings of rejection according to Banff 97 criteria, and treated with methylprednisolone, 500 mg daily for three consecutive days, or anti-lymphocyte therapy for steroid resistance or vascular rejection.

Statistical Software Package

We performed the statistical analysis using the Predictive Analytics SoftWare (PASW) statistical package, version 19.0. (PASW is also known as SPSS statistical analysis software, which is now offered by IBM (IBM, 2017). We used a chi-square test for assessing the relationship of categorical variables with different type of patients (in the DCD, SCD, and EDC groups), and ANOVA analysis for comparison of numerical variables. For assessing the trend analysis between the observations at months 0, 1, 3 and 12, we used repeated-measure ANOVA. *P*-values less than 0.05 were considered statistically significant.

Results

A total of 107 transplants were observed in this study, of which 50 transplants (47%) were in the SCD group, 32 transplants (30%) in the ECD, and the remaining 25 transplants (23%) in the DCD group (see Table 1). Five patients died: three of them because of progression of underlying disease (wegner, breast cancer, and kidney cancer), and the other two because of severe sepsis.

Age, gender, type of dialysis, mean CIT and HLA mismatch were measured for each patient. There was no significant difference in the recipients' ages. Also, there was no significant difference in the type and time of dialysis (p=0.075), and there was no significant difference in gender and the number of previous transplants.

Table 2 compares the genders, ages, types and times of dialysis, and second or subsequent transplant, within the three groups of donors. The average age in the SCD group was recorded as 36.7 ± 14.5, in

Table 1. Recipients' demographic data

	SCD	ECD	DCD
Population, n	50	32	25
Male:female, n:n, (%:%)	27:23 (54:46)	20:12 (62.5:37.5)	16:9 (64:36)
Age (mean ± SD)	49.9 ± 12.7	53.1 ± 12.2	53.4 ±10.4
Cause of renal failure, n Diabetic nephropathy Hypertension GN Reflux PCKD FSGS IgA Other unknown	2 1 8 6 8 3 10 11 1	6 0 2 2 5 3 7 7 0	2 2 1 2 7 0 7 4 0
Type of dialysis, n (%) HD PD Pre-emptive	40 (80) 10 (20) 0	29 (91) 3 (9) 0	17 (68) 8 (36) 0
Time on dialysis (years) Mean (± SD)	6.4±3.0	5.5 ±3.2	6.0 ±3.0

SD: standard deviation; GN: glomerulonephritis; PCKD: polycystic kidney disease; FSGS: ; IGA: ; HD: hemodialysis; PD: peritoneal dialysis

Table 2. Donors and transplant details

	SCD	ECD	DCD	*P*-value
Number, n	50	32	25	
Donor sex Male, Female, n(%)	26:24 (52:48)	17:15 (53:47)	16:9 (64:36)	0.578
Donor age (mean ± SD)	36.7 ± 14.5	64.5 ± 6.8	43.0 ± 13.6	0.000
Mean CIT (minutes ± SD)	767 ± 258.5	853 ± 332	767 ± 180	0.726
Mean end sCr (umol/L ± SD)	93.3 ± 56.4	91.4 ± 59.2	93.6 ± 60.5	0.974
HLA MM (mean ± SD)	2.9 ± 1.8	2.8 ± 1.7	3.3 ± 1.9	0.856
DR MM (mean ± SD)	0.8 ± 0.8	0.8 ± 0.8	1.0 ± 0.9	0.818
Smoking, n(%)	10 (20%)	4 (2.5%)	5 (20%)	0.263
HTN, n(%)	1 (2%)	18 (56%)	1 (4.0%)	0.001
DM, n(%)	0 (0.0%)	1 (3.1%)	2 (8.0%)	0.106

DM: Diabetes Mellitus; HLA MM: HLA Mismatch; DR MM:DR Mismatch the ECD group as 64.5±6.8, and the DCD group as 43±13.6 with p=0.000. The ECD donors had the highest average age.

Donor hypertension had the highest frequency in the ECD group (18, 56%), and the lowest (1, 2%) in the SCD group, supported by a strong *P*-value (p<0.001). However, there was no statistically significant difference with regard to diabetes, smoking, gender, CIT, HLA Mismatch and DR Mismatch.

Clinical outcomes are presented in Table 3. The DGF value based on the requirement for dialysis within the first week, was maximum in the DCD group (60%), followed by the ECD (33.3%) and SCD (32.7%) groups (p<0.035). The DGF value based on the requirement for dialysis within the first 48 hours, or failure of creatinine to drop by more than 20%, was again maximum in the DCD group (68%), but nearly the same in the ECD (47%) and SCD (46%) groups (p<0.023). Other parameters including rejection, CNI toxicity (CNIT), graft survival, and patient survival showed no significant difference. The "any type of rejection" rate was maximum in the DCD group 16 (64%), followed by the ECD 18 (60.0%) and SCD 28(59.6%) groups, which were almost the same (p=0.381). No significant difference was observed in ATN (Acute Tubular Necrosis), CNIT and BKVAN (BK Viruses Associated Nephropathy) within the three groups, based on pathologic reports from biopsy samples taken within one year after transplantation.

ANALYSIS OF THE RESULTS

With the lack of similar studies in the literature, we faced the challenging task of comparing the histological changes in the three groups of ECD, DCD and SCD at the specific time intervals (1, 3, and 12 months). We decided to analyze the histological changes using three different statistical methods, as follows, and compare their results:

1.   We applied *Group Cross-tabulation* method on the 87 samples collected during the first phase of the study, and compared the frequency and percentage of the Banff Scores 0, 1, and 2, in different parts of tissues, including interstitium, tubules, vessels, and glomeruli, for the three groups of SCD, ECD, and DCD at months 0, 1, 3, and 12.

Table 3. Clinical outcomes

	SCD	**ECD**	**DCD**	**P-value**
Number, n	50	32	25	
DGF, n (%) (requirement for HD within 1 week)	16 (32.7%)	10 (33.3%)	15 (60%)	0.035
sCr at 12 months (mg/ dL, mean ± SD)	128.7 ± 69.8	146.3 ± 84.4	137.9 ± 84.8	0.381
ATN, n (%)	13 (26%)	10 (31%)	11 (44%)	0.269
CNIT, n (%)	3 (6%)	5 (15.62%)	2 (8%)	0.331
BKVAN, n (%)	3 (6%)	2 (6.25%)	1 (4%)	0.984
Any Rejection, n(%)	28 (59.6%)	18 (60.0%)	16 (64.0%)	0.382

ATN: Acute tubular necrosis; CNIT: CNI Toxicity; BKVAN: BK Viruses Associated Nephropathy;
DGF: Delay Graft Function;

Additionally, we classified the results into three categories: "no change," "increased score," and "decreased score." We observed no significant differences in the three groups of DCD, ECD, and SCD.

We applied *Kruskal-Wallis* non-parametric analysis to calculate the variances of histologic variables by groups at each month (months 0, 1, 3, 12), which showed no difference except for cases with chronic glomerular change at month 0, with *p*-value of 0.025.

2.   We also analyzed the results for the groups two-by-two, using the *Mann-Whitney* test of pathologic variables, which showed no significant difference in DCD vs. SCD, and ECD vs. DCD comparisons. However, in comparing SCD vs. ECD, there were differences in chronic glomerular change at month 0 (with *p*-value = 0.02), and hyalinosis at month 3 (with *p*-value=0.041).

     As we progressed through the study, we increased the sample size to include 107 transplantation samples. Similarly, we analyzed the Banff Scores of the three groups of SCD, ECD, and DCD at months 0, 1, 3, and 12 using cross-tabulation . Again, we observed no significant differences in the three groups.

3.   As the third statistical method, we applied Banff summation score to compare the histological changes in the three groups of SCD, ECD, and DCD at months 0, 1, 3 and 12. This analysis relies on the fact that a change in different parts of tissues — including the interstitium, tubules, vessels, and glomeruli — should cause an increase in Banff score (and hence, its summation score), which is an indication of more damages to the tissues.

The three statistical analyses resulted in similar conclusions. There was no significant difference across the three groups of SCD, ECD and DCD recipients.

We analyzed further details on the analysis of the results using the third method, the Banff summation score. We investigated the histologic changes within the first year of transplantation (at months 1, 3 and 12) compared to month 0 (the biopsy taken just before transplantation). We measured the sum of Banff scores at months 0, 1, 3 and 12 for the three groups, as shown in Figure 1. Also, since changes in CI (Chronic Interstitium) and CT (Chronic Tubule), also called chronicity index, are especially important, we measured and compared their mean Banff scores, as depicted in Figures 2 and 3.

As shown in Figure 1, the Banff summation score at month 0 in the SCD group is lower than those in the DCD and ECD groups. The mean sum score was 0.05 at month 0, reaching 0.37 within one year. In the DCD group, the mean sum score was 0.33 at month 0, reaching 0.86 in a year, which indicates a rapid move towards tissue damage. In the ECD group, however, the score increased gradually, from 0.38 at month 0, to 0.55 in one year.

The change in the scores in month 0 and 12 were the same for the ECD and SCD groups, but increased in the ECD and DCD groups, with a different slope (it increased more in the DCD group). We also observed an increase in the slope after month 3 in the ECD and DCD groups, while there was no such an increase in the slope in the SCD group.

With regard to the "Mean CI (Chronic Interstitium) Score," as shown in Figure 2, in the SCD group, a steady increasing trend and a plateau are seen between months 3 and 12 (0.05 – 0.42). In the ECD group, fluctuations with increasing slope are seen after month 3. In the DCD group, a sharp increase in slope is observed, which crosses the ECD graph at month 12.

In general, looking at the "Mean CT (Chronic Tubule) Scores," as shown in Figure 3, a decrease in score is observed in month 3 for the ECD group, and a sharp increase in slope is observed for the DCD and ECD groups, whereas a smooth increasing trend is observed in the SCD group.

Figure 1. The Average of Banff Summation Scores

GROUPS	TIME	Mean Sum Scores	95% Confidence Interval	
			Lower Bound	Upper Bound
SCD	0	0.05	-0.16	0.26
	1	0.16	-0.09	0.41
	3	0.26	-0.02	0.55
	12	0.37	0.04	0.70
DCD	0	0.33	0.02	0.64
	1	0.22	-0.15	0.59
	3	0.56	0.14	0.97
	12	0.89	0.41	1.37
ECD	0	0.36	0.08	0.64
	1	0.36	0.03	0.70
	3	0.18	-0.19	0.56
	12	0.55	0.11	0.98

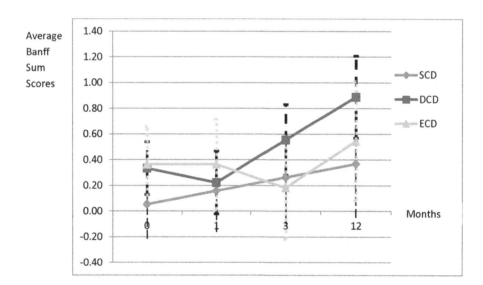

Discussion

With the scarcity of older donors, relying on the policy of "old kidney donors for old recipients" results in discarding a significant number of potential pools of kidney grafts. To alleviate the misbalance between the transplant necessities and the shortage of organs, transplant teams have expanded the criteria for accepting donors (Stratta, 2004). During the past years, several authors have studied the influence of donor factors on kidney transplant outcomes (Saidi, 2007, 2004; Andrés, 2009; Valcarce, 2009). The decreased number of donor organs versus the growth of waiting lists has led to a re-evaluation of these factors to include the ECD group (Singh, 2011).

Figure 2. Mean CI (Chronic Interstitium) scores

GROUPS	TIME	Mean CI Scores	95% Confidence Interval	
			Lower Bound	Upper Bound
SCD	0	0.37	-0.39	1.13
	1	0.84	0.18	1.51
	3	1.37	0.47	2.26
	12	1.84	0.69	2.99
DCD	0	1.63	0.46	2.79
	1	2.13	1.10	3.15
	3	2.63	1.25	4.00
	12	5.00	3.23	6.77
ECD	0	1.36	0.37	2.36
	1	1.73	0.85	2.60
	3	1.36	0.19	2.54
	12	3.09	1.58	4.60

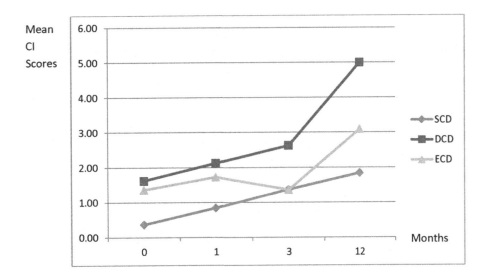

Conflicting results have been reported regarding the effects of donor age, recipient age and donor-recipient age difference on short- and long-term outcomes after kidney transplantation (Saidi, 2007, 2004; Marconi, 2011; Andrés, 2009; Ding, 2013; Jaffa, 2010; Callender, 2009). Kidneys are known to be affected by aging. Oxidative stress may be the most important cause of aging and aging-related disease, according to the "double-agent" aging theory (Ding, 2013). The contribution of oxidative stress to the development of aging has been perceived as a double jeopardy for outcomes after the kidney transplant. This is because older recipients of renal allografts have reduced antioxidative capacity, which may be associated with poorer outcomes.

Recently, in an experimental study, Rui Ding showed that the oxidative stress and gene expression profile were significantly different in the young donor and old recipient group, compared to the old donor

Figure 3. Mean CT (Chronic Tubule) scores

GROUPS	TIME	Mean CT Scores	95% Confidence Interval	
			Lower Bound	Upper Bound
SCD	0	0.05	-0.15	0.25
	1	0.26	-0.01	0.53
	3	0.42	0.14	0.70
	12	0.42	0.10	0.74
DCD	0	0.33	0.04	0.62
	1	0.33	-0.06	0.73
	3	0.67	0.26	1.08
	12	1.00	0.54	1.46
ECD	0	0.18	-0.08	0.44
	1	0.64	0.28	0.99
	3	0.36	-0.01	0.73
	12	1.00	0.58	1.42

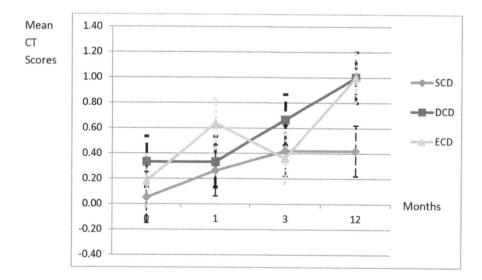

and young recipient group (Ding, 2013). The identified differences were mainly in the MAP (mitogen-activated protein) kinase and insulin signal pathways, making them potential targets for therapeutic intervention.

In other clinical studies, authors have evaluated the effects of donor factors on kidney transplant outcomes. Marconi et al. found that donor cause of death was not an independent risk factor for graft survival, or for the occurrence of chronic allograft nephropathy (Marconi, 2011). Zuckerman et al. showed that transplanting kidneys from deceased donors with terminal acute renal failure led to near-complete recovery after removal of the kidney from the donor environment, and transplanting it into the recipient (Zuckerman,, 2009).

We performed a single-center retrospective analysis of consecutive deceased donor adult kidney transplants, to compare histologic and clinical outcomes among the three different groups of SCD, ECD and DCD, at specific time intervals at month 0 and 1, 3, and 12. The Banff summation score was calculated as the sum of scores for the individual histological markers for all component and chronicity, as well as interstitial fibrosis, and tubular atrophy.

Despite older age and higher frequency of hypertension in the ECD donors (with p-value = 0.000 and 0.001, respectively), the DGF was the same in the ECD and SCD groups, but was more frequent in the DCD group (p-value<0.035). Moreover, we observed no significant differences in the three groups for other characteristics, including ATN, CNIT, BKVAN, and sCr within one year.

Relative increase in the Banff summation score, as an indicator of histological change, was similar among the SCD and ECD groups during 12 months. However, in the DCD group, despite better condition at transplantation, its score reached higher than that of the ECD.

Our study is notable for the similar age of recipients in the three different groups of SCD, ECD, and DCD, highlighting the effect of a recipient's age on the outcomes. We observed that it is not just the risk factors of donors (such as their age), but also, the risk factors of recipients that might play a significant role in the outcomes. We also note that the risk factors of donors and the risk factors of recipients could jointly affect the outcomes. This has been confirmed in genetic studies before. Consequently, we suggest revising the allocation system to better match the scores and the risk factors of the donors and recipients, regardless of whether the risk factors belong to the donors or recipients. We also suggest considering gene manipulation and therapeutic intervention to improve the outcomes.

CONCLUSION

Many statistical methods (such as the t-test and ANOVA) assume that the sampled data are from a population with a Gaussian distribution. However, such assumptions do not always hold strongly in health studies. The sample size may not be large enough, due to the limited nature of observations such as biopsies taken during kidney transplantation, that the distribution of sample may not be Gaussian, or that the observation may not even be possible for the far ends of a Gaussian distribution. In such cases, an alternative approach, called non-parametric tests, can be applied. The non-parametric methods work by ignoring the actual values, and instead, analyzing only their ranks. This approach ensures that the test is not affected much by outliers, and does not assume any particular distribution.

In this study, as a real case that calls for non-parametric tests, we performed a non-parametric single-center retrospective analysis of consecutive deceased donor adult kidney transplants, to compare histological and clinical outcomes among three different groups of deceased-kidney donors. With a limited pool of kidney donors and a long waiting list of recipients, we need new approaches to optimize the use of organs from potential donors. In the past, the comparative studies on the recipients of expanded criteria donor (ECD and standard criteria donor (SCD groups were biased toward the higher age of the recipients of the ECDs. The obvious statistical difference in clinical outcomes might have prevented us from discovering the impact of the recipients' age on the graft function, regardless of the donors' age.

Relative increase in the Banff summation score, as an indicator of histological change, was similar among the SCD and ECD groups during 12 months. However, in the DCD group, despite better condition at transplantation, its score reached higher than that of the ECD. We also observed the similar ages of recipients in the three groups, highlighting the influence of a recipient's age on the outcomes. We conclude that the recipient's internal condition after kidney transplant is as important as the donor's risk factors. In other words, it is not just the risk factors of donors, but also, the risk factors of recipients which play a significant role in the outcomes.

Factors associated with donors might be improved by transplantation into the physiological environment of a younger recipient. In other words, the recipient's internal condition after a kidney transplant can be as important as the donor's risk factors, or even more. The use of ECD and DCD would enable transplantation of kidneys from an expanded pool, with a low rate of DGF and rejection when factoring in recipient characteristics, genetic expressions and oxidative stress.

We will continue our studies, collecting and analyzing more data, and also, conducting long-term follow-ups with patients, to further investigate the promising observations of this research.

REFERENCES

Andrés, A., Polanco, N., Cebrian, M. P., Sol Vereda, M., Vazquez, S., Nuño, E., . . . Leiva, O. Aguirre, & F., Diaz, R. (2009). Kidneys From Elderly Deceased Donors Discarded for Transplantation. Proceedings of Transplantation, 41(6), 2379-2381.

Bhowmik, D. M., Dinda, A. K., Mahanta, P., & Agarwal, S. K. (2010). The evolution of the Banff classification schema for diagnosing renal allograft rejection and its implications for clinicians. *Indian Journal of Nephrology*, *20*(1), 2–8. doi:10.4103/0971-4065.62086 PMID:20535263

Callender, C. O., Cherikh, W. S., Traverso, P., Hernandez, A., Oyetunji, T., & Chang, D. (2009). Effect of Donor Ethnicity on Kidney Survival in Different Recipient Pairs: An Analysis of the OPTN/UNOS Database. Proceedings of Transplantation, 41(10), 4125-4130.

Ding, R., Chen, X., Wu, D., Wei, R., Hong, Q., Shi, S., & Xie, Y. et al. (2013). Effects of Aging on Kidney Graft Function, Oxidative Stress and Gene Expression after Kidney Transplantation. *Journal of Public Library of Science*, *8*(6), e65613. PMID:23824036

Goplani, K. R., Kute, V. B., Vanikar, A. V., Shah, P. R., Gumber, M. R., Patel, H. V., . . . Trivedi, H. L. (2010). Expanded Criteria Donor Kidneys for Younger Recipients: Acceptable Outcomes. In Proceedings of Transplantation, 42(10), 3931–3934.

IBM. (2017). *IBM SPSS Software*. Retrieved January 15, 2017, from http://www.ibm.com/analytics/us/en/technology/spss/

Jaffa, M. A., Woolson, R. F., Lipsitz, S. R., Baliga, P. K., Lopes-Virella, M., & Lackland, D. T. (2010). Analyses of renal outcome following transplantation Adjusting for informative right censoring and demographic factors: A longitudinal study. *Journal of Renal Failure*, *32*(6), 691–698. doi:10.3109/08860 22X.2010.486495 PMID:20540637

Marconi, L., Moreira, P., Parada, B., Bastos, C., Roseiro, A., & Mota, A. (2011). Donor Cause of Brain Death in Renal Transplantation: A Predictive Factor for Graft Function. Proceedings of Transplantation, 43(1), 74-76.

Mueller, A., Schnuelle, P., Waldherr, R., & van der Woude, F. J. (2000). Impact of the Banff 97 classification for histological diagnosis of rejection on clinical outcome and renal function parameters after kidney transplantation. *Transplantation, 69*(6), 1123–1127. doi:10.1097/00007890-200003270-00017 PMID:10762217

Pascual, J., Zamora, J., & Pirsch, J. D. (2008). A Systematic Review of Kidney Transplantation From Expanded Criteria Donors. *American Journal of Kidney Diseases, 52*(3), 553–586. doi:10.1053/j.ajkd.2008.06.005 PMID:18725015

Racusen, L. C., Solez, K., Colvin, R. B., Bonsib, S. M., Castro, M. C., Cavallo, T., & Yamaguchi, Y. et al. (1999). The Banff 97 working classification of renal allograft pathology. *Kidney International, 55*(2), 713–723. doi:10.1046/j.1523-1755.1999.00299.x PMID:9987096

Saidi, R. F., Elias, N., Kawai, T., Hertl, M., Farrell, M., Goes, N., & Ko, D. S. C. et al. (2007). Outcome of Kidney Transplantation using Expanded criteria Donors and Donation After Cardiac Death Kidneys: Realities and Costs. *American Journal of Transplantation, 7*(12), 2769–2774. doi:10.1111/j.1600-6143.2007.01993.x PMID:17927805

Singh, R. P., Farney, A. C., Rogers, J., Zuckerman, J., Reeves-Daniel, A., Hartmann, E., & Stratta, R. J. et al. (2011). Kidney Transplantation From donation after cardiac death donors: Lack of impact of delayed graft function on post-transplant outcomes. *Journal of Clinical Transplantation, 25*(2), 255–264. doi:10.1111/j.1399-0012.2010.01241.x PMID:20331689

Solez, K., Axelsen, R. A., Benediktsson, H., Burdick, J. F., Cohen, A. H., Colvin, R. B., & Yamaguchi, Y. et al. (1993). International standardization of criteria for the histologic diagnosis of renal allograft rejection: The Banff working classification of kidney transplant pathology. *Kidney International, 44*(2), 411–422. doi:10.1038/ki.1993.259 PMID:8377384

Stratta, R. J., Rohr, M. S., Sundberg, A. K., Armstrong, G., Hairston, G., Hartmann, E., & Adams, P. L. et al. (2004). Increased Kidney Transplantation Utilizing Expanded Criteria Deceased Organ Donors with Results Comparable to Standard Criteria Donor Transplant. *Annals of Surgery, 239*(5), 688–697. doi:10.1097/01.sla.0000124296.46712.67 PMID:15082973

Valcarce, E. G., Cerrato, A. O., Fuentes, F. L., Mondéjar, J. M., Fernández, G. M., Rubio, E. L., & Roldán, C. G. et al. (2009). Short Cold Ischemia Time Optimises Transplant results for kidneys from expanded criteria donors. *Journal of Nefrologia, 29*(5), 456–463. PMID:19820758

Zuckerman, J. M., Singh, R. P., Farney, A. C., Rogers, J., & Stratta, R. J. (2009). Single center experience Transplanting kidneys from deceased donors with terminal acute renal failure. *The Journal of Surgery, 146*(4), 686–695. PMID:19789028

KEY TERMS AND DEFINITIONS

Banff Score: A standardization of a renal allograft biopsy to establish an objective end-point for clinical trials. Banff 97 was developed by investigators using the Banff Schema and the Collaborative Clinical Trials in Transplantation (CCTT) modification, for diagnosis of renal allograft pathology.

Biopsy (Protocol Biopsy): A routine sampling of kidney tissue (with the use of biopsy needles and bioptic devices to obtain tissue cores, using ultrasound guidance for the biopsy procedure), particularly within the first few months of post-transplantation, to investigate potential rejection of a transplanted kidney. Multiple tissue samples are recommended for adequate sampling.

Donation After Cardiac Death (DCD): Defined as coming from a donor who has suffered irreversible brain injury and who may be near death, but who does not meet formal brain death criteria. In these cases, when the patient's heart stops beating, and with the permission of the family, the organs are then recovered in the operating room to be used for transplantation.

Expanded Criteria Donor (ECD): Defined as any brain-dead donor aged 60 years or more, or a donor aged 50 years or more with two of the following conditions: a history of hypertension, terminal serum creatinine level > 1.5 mg/dL, or death resulting from a cerebrovascular accident.

Gaussian Distribution: The Gaussian distribution is also commonly called the "normal distribution," and is often described as a "bell-shaped curve." If the number of events is very large, then a Gaussian distribution may be used to describe physical events. The normal distribution is useful because of the central limit theorem, which states that averages of random variables independently drawn from independent distributions become normally distributed when the number of random variables is sufficiently large.

Kruskal-Wallis Test: This non-parametric test is analogous to one-way ANOVA. This test first ranks the data from low to high, and then characterizes the distribution of the ranks among groups.

Mann-Whitney Test: A non-parametric test used to compare two unpaired groups, to compute a *P*-value for the null hypothesis that the distribution of ranks is totally random. Under the null hypothesis, it would be equally likely for either of the two groups to have the larger mean ranks.

Non-Parametric Tests: A family of methods which makes no assumptions about the population distribution. Non-parametric methods most commonly work by ignoring the actual values, and, instead, analyzing only their ranks. This approach ensures that the test is not affected much by outliers, and does not assume any particular distribution. The clear advantage of non-parametric tests is that they do not require the assumption of sampling from a Gaussian population. When the assumption of Gaussian distribution does not hold, non-parametric tests have more power than parametric tests to detect differences.

Standard Criteria Donor (SCD): Defined as a donor who is under 50 years of age and suffered brain death from any cause, including traumatic injuries or medical problems such as a stroke.

Chapter 10

Regression–Based Methods of Phase–I Monitoring Surgical Performance Using Risk–Adjusted Charts:
An Overview

Negin Asadayyoobi
Sharif University of Technology, Iran

ABSTRACT

Monitoring medical processes gained importance and researchers attempted to reduce death rates by quick detection mortality rate of surgical outcomes in recent years. The patient time until death (survival time) depends on risk factor of each patient, which reflects the patients' health condition prior to surgery. Ignoring differences in risk factors among specific patients, risk adjusted control charts could be considered as a corrective tool to minimize false alarms related to inhomogeneity in patients' health condition. A number of risk adjusted charting procedures have been developed on both phase I & II monitoring of aforementioned outcomes. This chapter will review both models and focus on phase-I risk-adjustment models in medical setting with a particular emphasis on monitoring for surgical context and describe each method's unique properties.

INTRODUCTION

Continuous improvement of healthcare systems requires the measuring and understanding of process variation. It is important to eliminate extraneous process variation wherever possible, while moving well-defined metrics toward their target values. Within this context, statistical process control (SPC) charts are very useful tools for studying important process variables and identifying quality improvements or quality deterioration. The role of patients in the definition of service quality can be considered as key competitive criteria. As a result, service providers are trying to apply quality assessment tools that sig-

DOI: 10.4018/978-1-5225-2515-8.ch010

nificantly emphasis on customer orientation (Houshmand et al., 2016). A control chart is a chronological time series plot of measurements of important variables. The statistics plotted can be averages, proportions, rates, or other quantities of interest. In addition to these plotted values, upper and lower reference thresholds called control limits are plotted. These limits are calculated using process data and define the natural range of variation within which the plotted points almost always should fall. Any points falling outside of these control limits therefore may indicate that all data were not produced by the same process, either because of a lack of standardization or because a change in the process may have occurred. Such changes could represent either quality improvement or quality deterioration, depending on which control limit is crossed. Control charts are thus quite useful both for monitoring if processes get worse and for testing and verifying improvement ideas (Faltin, Kenett, & Ruggeri, 2012).

Statistical monitoring for effective detection of the deteriorated mortality rate of surgical outcomes has increasingly attracted researchers' attention. Such detection can be further used to assist root cause identification and decision-making for surgical operation improvement. In order to more effectively detect the performance anomalies that go beyond the natural variability of surgical operations, the risk factor of each patient, which reflects the patient's health condition prior to surgery, must be taken into account (Paynabar, Jionghua, & Yeh, 2012). Drawing comparisons between Regression-based methods of phase-I monitoring surgical performance using risk adjusted charts is the main purpose of this chapter which hasn't been done before. This analysis is implemented by reporting key features of each work in the given context that could be considered beneficial hints for future work. The remainder of the chapter is structured as follows. In research methodology, the main properties of referenced articles are given. Background includes literature review on risk-adjusted charts from which four phase-I models are chosen and surveyed in selected methods. Finally, comparing different methods & discussion contains comparison between selected models presented in previous section and expresses discussion about strengths and weaknesses of each work that leads to recommendations for future study at the CONCLUSION & FUTURE WORK sections.

BACKGROUND: RISK-ADJUSTED CHARTS

Unlike monitoring of processes in the manufacturing industry, the monitoring of surgical performances is different and presented a unique problem because the patients are not homogeneous and hence the necessity of risk-adjustment. The Parsonnet scoring system (Parsonnet, Dean, & Bernstein, 1989) is widely used for estimating the risk of death of a patient who undergoes a cardiac operation. A competing scoring system was developed by Roques et al. (1999). Based on a patient's gender, age, morbid obesity, blood pressure, etc. integer scores are given and the total score is called the Parsonnet score. A Parsonnet score is an integer that ranges from 0 to 100; hence it is a discrete random variable. A small Parsonnet score represents a small risk and a high score represents a high risk.

Although monitoring the time until an event clearly has important applications in many fields, recent studies on the subject of health care monitoring focus on controlling a surgical process using risk-adjusted charting procedures, where the control limits are calculated typically based on a historical set of data. The analysis of historical data is referred to as Phase-I, whereas the prospective monitoring of future data is referred to as Phase-II monitoring. The control limits of charting procedures in a Phase-II monitoring to be accurate must be derived based on data taken from a process that is in control. However, the objective of a Phase-I study is to first remove out-of-control points from a historical dataset. The 'cleaned' data-set can then be used to determine the control limits of a charting procedure to be used in Phase-II monitoring (Zhang, Gan, & Loke, 2012).

To account for heterogeneity of individuals, some risk-adjusted cumulative sum (CUSUM)schemes have been suggested in the literature (see Grigg, Farewell, and Spiegelhalter (2003) for an overview.) Biswas and Kalbfleisch (2008) seem to be the first who used survival analysis (SURVREG) models for monitoring. They considered mortality monitoring of transplant patients during their first year after transplant. Another work is due to Sego, Reynolds, and Woodall (2009) who employed accelerated failure time (AFT) models for the in-control state as well as a change in the scale parameter as an alternative. Some other researchers who proposed risk adjusted procedures to monitor surgical performances include Steiner, Cook, Farewell, and Treasure (2000), Grigg and Spiegelhalter (2007) and Steiner and Jones (2010). Moreover, alternative schemes such as the one in Steiner et al. (2000) were proposed in this case. Loke and Gan (2012) proposed a joint scheme to monitor both clinical failures and predisposed risks of patients. The design of this scheme was demonstrated in detail using a real data-set. Interested readers are referred to review papers by Woodall (2006), pp. 89–104 and Hart, Mullany, Cook, Pilcher, and Duke (2008) for more details.

Since investigations in which poor performance of cardiac surgery centers remained undetected for a long time, tremendous research interests in improving Phase II monitoring of surgical outcomes have emerged. The relevant research on this topic can be divided into two groups, depending on the types of surgical outcome data used in the monitoring. The first group of monitoring methods focused on each patient's binary survival status at a specified time period after surgery. The second group of monitoring methods used continuous measures of each patient's survival time, or a fixed right censored time if a patient survives beyond a specified time period after surgery.

In the first group of monitoring methods, various risk-adjusted control charts have been developed. Steiner et al. (2000) introduced a risk-adjusted cumulative sum (RA-CUSUM) chart to monitor the binary survival status of any given patient during a thirty-day period after surgery. They adjusted the patient's risk using a logistic regression model and utilized a CUSUM chart to monitor the log-likelihood score corresponding to each operation. Grigg et al. (2003) proposed a more general monitoring approach, known as the resetting sequential probability ratio test (RSPRT) chart. They showed that the RA-CUSUM chart is a special case of the risk-adjusted RSPRT chart. Instead of directly monitoring the binary survival status of patients, Grigg and Farewell (2004a) proposed a risk-adjustment method to monitor the number of operations between two unsuccessful operations (two deaths). To evaluate the efficacy of the existing monitoring methods, Grigg and Farewell (2004b) compared the performance of the existing RA control charts in detecting changes based on the binary outcomes. Grigg and Spiegelhalter (2007) developed a risk-adjusted exponentially weighted moving average (RA-EWMA) chart, which, in addition to monitoring, can be used to estimate the risk of unsuccessful surgery for each patient. In the second group of monitoring methods, the control charts are developed based on continuous measures of the exact survival time or right censored time after surgery. Biswas and Kalbfleisch (2008) proposed an RA-CUSUM chart to monitor continuous survival time based on the Cox model. Sego et al. (2009) used location-scale regression models to monitor survival time, in which the corresponding observations are considered as censored data if a patient survives beyond thirty days after surgery. They proposed a risk-adjusted survival time CUSUM chart (RAST-CUSUM) based on the loglikelihood score of each operation. Steiner and Jones (2010) proposed an updated EWMA chart for monitoring risk-adjusted survival time. Pagel et al. (2013) introduced a method for paediatric cardiac surgery units to monitor their own program outcomes. This method was benchmarked to recent national outcomes using a new model for risk adjustment, where the data is fed back to the multi-disciplinary team. They concluded that timely and routine monitoring of risk-adjusted mortality following paediatric cardiac surgery is feasible. Asadzadeh, Aghaie, and Niaki (2013) proposed AFT models to devise two regression-adjusted control schemes based on Cox-Snell residuals. In their work, two scenarios with censored and non-censored data were considered. The competing control charts were compared in terms of zero-state and steady-state average run length criteria using the Markov chain approach. The comparison study revealed that the CUSUM-based monitoring procedure was superior and more effective.

All of the afore-mentioned research focuses on Phase II (prospective) monitoring, where it is assumed that the parameters of the risk-adjustment model are known or can be accurately estimated from historical data collected from a stable process. The Phase I (retrospective) control, however, is crucially needed in practice for checking the quality of historical data, and for obtaining accurate estimates of the model parameters, based on which the patient's risk factor can be correctly adjusted for Phase II monitoring. Despite the importance of Phase I control, very little work has been done in the literature on risk-adjusted control charts for Phase I control. Furthermore, for constructing risk-adjusted control charts in Phase I, since each sample represents an individual operation for each patient, it would be impossible to fit a risk-adjustment model for each patient based on individual observations. Therefore, it is necessary to check whether individual observations can be grouped together, which can then be adjusted by the same risk-adjustment model.

While all the above works are developed to monitor health care systems in Phase-II, Zhang et al. (2012) introduced a risk-adjusted Shewhart chart for a phase I study because of its ability to detect extreme observations from out of control processes. Paynabar et al. (2012) proposed a general risk-adjusted control-charting scheme for Phase-I control of surgical performance. This scheme not only accounts for patients' health conditions described by the Parsonnet scores, but also incorporates other categorical operational covariates such as the surgeons' group factor. Moreover, Mohammadian, Niaki, and Amiri (2016) proposed a Phase-I risk-adjusted geometric control chart using a logistic regression for patients' risks. Then Asadayyoobi and Niaki (2016) provided a general Phase-I accelerated failure time based risk-adjusted control chart to monitor continuous surgical outcomes based on a likelihood-ratio test derived from a change-point modelWhen the process is not stable due to assignable causes, the chart limits of any monitoring procedure are not determined properly. This may lead to incorrect inferences about the process being monitored. Therefore, a Phase-I investigation and checking the historical data is necessary. In general, there is often not a clear distinction between the two phases in health-related control charting but most existing researches focus on phase II monitoring, and very little work has been done on phase I control of surgical outcomes. In the following sessions, Due to the importance of Phase-I monitoring, author focuses on recent regression based methods of phase-I Monitoring patient survival times in surgical systems using risk adjusted charts to describe each method's unique properties compered others.

RESEARCH METHODOLOGY

Preparing this chapter required 21 references that consist of 20 journal papers and one text book which is available at Google books. Remaining papers are extracted from some databases such as Taylor & Francis, ProQuest, Wiley online library, etc. using aforementioned keywords. However most of these references are published in the past decade, ranging from 1989 to 2016.

MAIN FOCUS OF THE CHAPTER: SELECTED METHODS

Model 1: Phase-I Study of Surgical Systems Using Risk-Adjusted Shewhart Control Charts

In a phase I study, the Shewhart chart is usually preferred because the main objective in this phase, is to obtain an in-control data set by removing out-of-control points with assignable causes and the Shewhart chart is excellent in detecting extreme points resulting from out-of-control processes. If these points are left undetected, the chart limits of any charting procedure used in phase II monitoring will be calculated incorrectly and this might lead to incorrect inferences about the process being monitored.

For this study, Let Y denotes the outcome of a patient who undergoes an operation: 1 if the patient dies within 30 days or 0 if the patient survives. The surgical outcome is determined by two mainfactors: the surgeon who performs the operation and the condition of the patient which is summarized by the Parsonnet score (X). Historical data must first be collected from N patients operated by the m surgeons. The data set consists of N pairs of Parsonnet scores and surgical outcomes $(x_1, y_1), ..., (x_n, y_n)$. Z is predicted probability of death of a future patient who undergoes an operation. Although (x, y) and (z, y) contain the same information, the use of the latter is more popular because is a predicted probability of death.

In order to monitor the performance of a surgeon in phase II monitoring, one must first decide to whom this surgeon is to be compared to. One approach is to compare the surgeon to all the surgeons' immediate past performances in a hospital. The other approach is to compare the surgeon with the surgeon's own past performances. This study is described for the first approach and it can be modified easily for the second approach. They formulated the monitoring of surgical performance problem as testing the hypothesis:

$$H_0 : \ Pr(Y = 1 | Z = \ z) \ = \ z$$

Versus

$$H_1 : \ Pr\left(Y = 1 | Z = \ z\right) \ \neq \ z$$

Where the null hypothesis specifies an in-control process characterized by the average performance of all the surgeons based on a historical data set (Zhang et al., 2012). This study is described for the case when researchers want to monitor the performance of a surgeon with respect to the past performances of all the surgeons in a hospital. If they want to monitor a surgeon's performance with respect to the past performances of the surgeon alone, then the historical data should only contain data from the surgeon. The logistic regression model fitted in this case will provide the predicted risk of death of a patient to be operated by the surgeon. The statistic used is shown to be a likelihood ratio test statistic. The distribution of this statistic is bimodal with positive and negative values representing failed and successful operations respectively. Thus, it is reasonable to consider setting up the lower and upper control limits separately. The implementation of this procedure for a phase I study is illustrated with a real data set.

Model 2: Phase-I Study of Surgical Systems Using Risk-Adjusted Geometric Control Charts

In this model, the number of patients survived at least 30 days after a surgery is monitored using a novel risk-adjusted geometric control chart. In the chart, the patient risk is modeled using a logistic regression. The new scheme is proposed to be used in Phase-I where a likelihood ratio test derived from a change point model is employed and upper control limit was estimated using Monte Carlo simulation. Tests of hypothesis of this work are combined and the exam is performed only after a patient death. In this case, the number of patients before a death occurs is considered a random variable. Therefore, the overall probability of Type-I error would be smaller than the one for the Bernoulli random variable. The Phase-I control chart is constructed via a likelihood ratio test derived from a change-point model (LRTCP) based on the risk-adjusted logistic regression Phase-I monitoring of this process is equivalent to the test of hypothesis on whether the coefficients have changed or not, i.e.:

$$H_0 : \beta_0 = \beta_1$$

Versus

$$H_1 : \beta_0 \neq \beta_1$$

Where β is a vector of risk factors' coefficients denoted by $\beta T = (\beta 0, \beta_1, \beta p)$; Although $\boldsymbol{\beta 0}$ and $\boldsymbol{\beta 1}$ represent the parameters of the risk-adjusted model before and after the change, respectively (Mohammadian et al., 2016).

Most of the previous research considered patient's risk factors as the only continuous covariates in risk-adjustment models. However, there are often other variables that may also significantly affect surgical outcomes. For example, in addition to the preexisting health condition of a patient, certain operational variables such as surgeons, surgical procedures, and the types of surgery operations may also influence surgical outcomes. Generally, the performance of experienced surgeons may be different from that of inexperienced surgeons. As a result, the parameters of the risk-adjustment model would be different for surgeons with different levels of experience or skills. Hence, ignoring such important variables in the risk-adjustment model may result in an inaccurate estimation of the risk-adjustment model. Generally, these operational variables are often recorded as categorical covariates. Therefore, a regression model which includes dummy variables for categorical covariates, is first employed in the two next sessions to represent a unified risk-adjustment model. Change-point models have been widely used in various Phase I control chart applications for continuous responses (See for example, Sullivan and Woodall 2000, Zamba and Hawkins 2006). These studies intend to extend such work for binary/continuous responses with the focus on the Phase I control of risk-adjustment models. Specifically, the Phase I control chart is constructed via a likelihood ratio test derived from a change-point model (LRTCP) based on the risk-adjustment regression.

These models were based on binary outcomes while subsequent models are developed to include categorical covariates in the risk-adjustment model that uses continuous variables.

Model 3: Phase-I Study of Surgical Systems Using Risk-Adjusted Control Charts by Considering Categorical Covariates

In this model a general phase I risk-adjusted control chart is proposed for monitoring binary surgical outcomes based on a likelihood-ratio test derived from a change-point model. As mentioned before, Different from the existing methods, this model further shows that the binary surgical outcomes depend on not only the patient conditions described by the Parsonnet scores but also on other categorical operational covariates such as different surgeons. The proposed phase I risk-adjusted control chart was developed based on a likelihood-ratio test derived from a change-point model. The risk-adjustment model is fitted by incorporating dummy variables to reflect different surgeon groups' performance. The results show that the inclusion of surgeon groups as a categorical covariate in the risk-adjustment model can effectively reflect the inherent data heterogeneity, thus improving the estimation of the risk-adjustment model parameters. In this model $\psi^{(sl)}$ Defined as the vector of the risk-adjustment model parameters for observations $s + 1$ to l, Therefore, in order to control the process in phase I, it suffices to evaluate the following hypotheses:

$$H_0 : \Psi^{(0\tau)} = \Psi^{(\tau m)}$$

Versus

$$H_1 : \Psi^{(0\tau)} \neq \Psi^{(\tau m)}$$

Where $\tau = u, u+1, \ldots m\text{-}u$ and u ($u >$ the number of coefficients) is the minimum required sample size for estimating the parameters of the risk-adjustment model for m patients. The value of u is chosen so that at least one outcome with value 0 and one outcome with value 1 exist among sampled data from 1 to u and also from $m - u + 1$ to m. Thus, a likelihood-ratio test can be used to test the hypotheses (Paynabar et al., 2012).

The discovered data clusters of the mortality rate indicate that the inclusion of the categorical surgeon covariate in the risk-adjustment model can effectively model the heterogeneity of the surgical outcome data. Monte Carlo simulations were further conducted to demonstrate that the phase I risk-adjusted chart provides better detection power by including the surgeon covariate. It is expected that the improved estimation of model parameters based on the proposed phase I control will lead to better phase II monitoring performance. It is worth noting that the proposed RA-LRTCP chart can be potentially used for other applications in which a binary response variable follows a logistic regression model involving either continuous or categorical covariates, or both.

Model 4: Phase-I Study of Surgical Systems Using a Risk-Adjusted AFT Regression Chart

Most of RA monitoring methods have been proposed to monitor binary outcomes (such as whether a patient survives until 30 days after the operation or not). However, a monitoring scheme based on patient survival time may be more sensitive to the alarm of detecting increases in mortality rate than a procedure that only uses binary outcomes. In this model a general Phase-I accelerated failure time-based risk-adjusted control chart is proposed to monitor continuous surgical outcomes.

Censoring in this research occurs when there is no knowledge on the time of death for the patients being operated. This is principally due to the fact that some individuals outlive the experiment, while others leave the experiment before they die. Although the last time they have been seen alive is known, but there is no way of knowing their age at death. In other words, these individuals contribute something to the knowledge of the survivor function, but nothing to knowledge on their ages at death. Another reason for censoring occurs when individuals are lost from the study: they may be killed in accidents, they may emigrate, or they may lose their identity tags. To get rid of mixed data (which is a mixture of times at death and censored data) a censoring indicator is usually defined. If a time really is the time to death, then the censoring indicator takes the value 1. However, if a time is just the last time an individual has been seen alive, then the censoring indicator is set to 0. Let censoring indicator becomes:

$$d_i = \begin{cases} 1 & if \ X_i \leq C \\ 0 & if \ X_i > C \end{cases}.$$

Hence, in this study the data is collected in pair of (T_i, d_i) to distinguish between these two types of numbers, where $T_i = \text{Min } (X_i, C)$, C, X_i and d_i are the censoring time, the real survival time, and the censoring indicator of *i-th* patient, respectively (Asadayyoobi & Niaki, 2016).

It is reminded that the Phase-I accelerated failure time (AFT)-based risk-adjusted control chart of this model is proposed for monitoring continuous surgical outcomes based on a likelihood-ratio test derived from a change-point model. AFT survival models should not be viewed as models that are designed to predict long-term survival, especially when age, arguably the most influential factor in human survival, is not included in the regression model. Rather, for this purposes, the AFT survival models should be viewed as models that reflect the proximal survival patterns that are most likely to be influenced by the quality of the surgery. In contrast, parametric techniques are typically used for questions like this: 'what proportion of patients will die in 2 years based on data from an experiment that ran for just 4 months?' Moreover, unlike proportional hazards models, AFT models are predominately fully parametric and that the regression parameter estimates from AFT models are robust to omitted covariates. They are also less affected by the choice of probability distribution, where their results are easily interpreted. This is the reason of why it is chosen in this work to model the surgical process at hand.

The null and alternative hypothesis of this approach is the same as previous model and continuous outcomes in this model depend on not only the patient conditions described by the Parsonnet score, but also on other categorical operational covariates, such as surgeons which can improve the estimation of the parameters of the risk-adjustment model and hence can enhance the detection power of the proposed risk-adjusted control chart. The detailed specification of data used in all afore-mentioned studies is presented in the next session.

BENCHMARKING DATASET FOR PHASE-I MONITORING SURVIVAL TIME

All of mentioned papers used cardiac-surgery dataset from a single surgical center in the UK as a motivating example to illustrate the potential drawbacks of model fitting and compare it with others. The data set describes 6,994 operations that were performed at a single surgical center in the United Kingdom over a seven-year period, 1992–1998. The data consists of information on each patient including operation date, surgeon, type of procedure, age, the Parsonnet score, and the number of days the patient lived after the operation (if death was observed during the seven year period). The first two years were selected as a training data set to estimate the in-control values of the chart parameters and all authors assumed that recorded deaths in the training data set were related to the cardiac surgery. They used the data of first two years to estimate the parameters of the risk-adjustment model in order to monitor the rest of the Phase II data from 1994 to 1998.

The data used in models considering surgeons as categorical covariates, contain a total of six surgeons each designated as either a trainee or an experienced surgeon. The cardiac surgery data corresponding to the three experienced surgeons are chosen. This is because trainee surgeons operated on only relatively simple cases. Furthermore, during an operation by a trainee surgeon, an experienced surgeon has always been present to take over the operation if serious difficulties occur. In this case, the operation performance may not consistently reflect the performance of individual trainee surgeons. There are 1,112 records in Phase I data related to the selected experienced surgeons. The numbers of patients operated by surgeons 1, 2, and 3 are 565, 286, and 261, respectively. The numbers of dead patients are 54, 27, and 18 (99 in total) corresponding to surgeons 1, 2, and 3, respectively. The Parsonnet score is used as the risk factor in the model since it has been shown that it can effectively reflect the patients' risks prior to operation such as hypertension, diabetic status, and renal function (Steiner et al., 2000). The Parsonnet scores of patients operated by the selected surgeons range from 0 to 69.

COMPARING DIFFERENT METHODS AND DISCUSSION

The first model's strength relates to Shewhart chart superiority in the case of large shifts, alike the third model. These risk-adjusted Bernoulli control charts are Shewhart p-charts that consider the risk of each patient into account. As this control chart is designed to conduct test of hypothesis for each point (each patient), the number of hypothesis tests increases and as a result the overall probability of Type-I error would be large. One way to overcome this problem is to increase the upper control limit in order to achieve a desired probability of Type-I error. This leads to increasing probability of Type-II error and consequently decreasing power of the control chart. The next part of this section which focuses on conclusion & future work, presents a suggestion to overcome this challenge as future study.

Comparing Mohammadian et al. (2016) to Paynabar et al. (2012) showed better performance of the proposed risk-adjusted geometric scheme under all shifts and different locations of changes considered. They discussed that this improvement is due to decreasing number of hypothesis tests in the proposed geometric control chart compared to the one used in the Bernoulli control chart. This performance improvement is expected to happen in Phase-II monitoring of health care processes that use the proposed risk-adjusted geometric chart as well. Furthermore, in addition to have step shifts in the mortality rate, the performance of the proposed scheme can also be evaluated under the presence of outliers. Evaluated the performance of the change point estimator in the proposed geometric control chart in comparison with the one in the Bernoulli control chart showed the worse performance of the change point estimator in the proposed geometric control chart was due to decreasing number of observations used in the geometric control chart compared to the one used in the Bernoulli control chart, while the change occurs in the Bernoulli observations.

Ignoring the important categorical operational covariates (e.g., different surgeons) in fitting a risk-adjustment model may affect the control chart performance in Phase I as well as in Phase II. This point is the most obvious strength of The Paynabar et al. (2012) and Asadayyoobi and Niaki (2016). Major reason is that this may lead to higher variances of parameter estimators, and result in a poorer performance in detecting possible changes. Therefore, it is vital to consider important categorical operational covariates in the risk-adjustment model for examining historical data in Phase I control. A naive approach to account for the effect of a categorical operational covariate is to fit a risk-adjustment model for each level of the categorical variable. However, as the number of levels in the categorical operational covariates increases, the number of models and control charts required for monitoring the process also quickly increases. This results in not only more computing efforts, but an increase in the overall Type I error rate associated with the control charts. To tackle this problem, authors proposed to incorporate the categorical variables into one model by using dummy variables; so categorical covariates often exist and play a very important role in detection performance by including the surgeon covariate and ignoring important categorical covariates may bring about misleading results.

Throughout simulation studies, it is shown that the proposed control charts using continuous random variable is more effective in terms of power than the chart with a binary random variable. Hence Mohammadian et al. (2016) and Asadayyoobi and Niaki (2016) derived greater benefit from this hypothesis to enhance the detection power of their proposed risk-adjusted control chart.

CONCLUSION

Comparing the four focused researches with each other and previous works shows that in a phase I study, the Shewhart chart is usually preferred as the main objective in this phase is to obtain an in-control data set by removing out-of-control points with assignable causes and the Shewhart chart is excellent in detecting extreme points resulting from out-of-control processes. If these points are left undetected, the chart limits of any charting procedure used in phase II monitoring will be calculated incorrectly and this might lead to incorrect inferences about the process being monitored. After a phase I study, the 'cleaned' data set can then be used to set up control limits for any procedures to be used in phase II monitoring. The CUSUM and EWMA charts are usually not used in a phase I study because they are not as effective as a Shewhart chart in detecting extreme points. The CUSUM and EWMA charts are more sensitive to small and moderate process shifts than the Shewhart chart and hence are used in phase II monitoring if small and moderate shifts are considered more important to be detected. On the other hand, the Shewhart chart is preferred if large shifts are of major concern. The summarized features of mentioned models are shown in Table 1.

It should be noted that β_0 and β_1 are parameters of the risk-adjusted model so that β_0 represents the logit/AFT mortality probability for a healthy patient with parsonnet score equal to zero and β_1 shows the effect of parsonnet score on mortality when the parsonnet score changes one unit. These estimates show similar results in rounded estimates in model 1 & 3.

Table 1. summarized comparison of selected methods in phase-I risk-adjusted control charts

	Main features	Strengths / Weaknesses
Model 1	• Binary survival time • Fitting logistic regression model to data • Chart based on a Bernoulli-distributed random variable • $(\beta_0, \beta_1)=(-3.68, 0.08)$	S: Superiority of Shewhart chart in the case of large shifts W: large probability of Type-I error
Model 2	• Binary survival time • Categorical covariates inclusion • Fitting logistic regression model to data • Chart based on a Geometric-distributed random variable • $(\beta_0, \beta_1)=(-3.38, 0.07)$	S: Lower variances of parameter estimators due to included Categorical covariates
Model 3	• Continuous survival time • Fitting logistic regression model to data • Chart based on a Bernoulli-distributed random variable • $(\beta_0, \beta_1)=(-3.68, 0.08)$	S1: Improved performance under all shifts & different locations of changes due to decreasing number of hypothesis tests S2: higher power of control charts due to Continuous survival time W: Worse performance of the change point estimator
Model 4	• Continuous survival time • Categorical covariates inclusion • Fitting AFT regression model to data • Chart based on a Weibull-distributed random variable • $(\beta_0, \beta_1)=(-3.71, 0.02)$	S1: Lower variances of parameter estimators due to included Categorical covariates S2: higher power of control charts due to Continuous survival time

FUTURE WORK

As a future study on Phase-I risk-adjusted Bernoulli control chart (Shewhart p-chart), developing a method that decreases the number of hypothesis tests could be promising. Designing a chart based on counting the number of unsuccessful surgeries before a successful one may help to achieve a desired probability of Type-I error. Another future work could form by adjusting the patient's risk using a probit model which uses an error variable distributed according to a standard normal distribution instead of a standard logistic distribution. Although logistic regression and probit models tend to produce very similar predictions, comparing result of these assumptions can be interest too. In the case of Charts based on a Geometric-distributed random variable, to improve the performance of these risk-adjusted charts, covariates may be considered in Phase-I and Phase-II monitoring of health care systems in the future.

REFERENCES

Asadayyoobi, N., & Niaki, S. T. A. (2016). Monitoring patient survival times in surgical systems using a risk-adjusted AFT regression chart. *Quality Technology & Quantitative Management*, 1–12.

Asadzadeh, S., Aghaie, A., & Niaki, S. T. A. (2013). AFT regression-adjusted monitoring of reliability data in cascade processes. *Quality & Quantity*, *47*(6), 3349–3362. doi:10.1007/s11135-012-9723-2

Biswas, P., & Kalbfleisch, J. D. (2008). A risk-adjusted CUSUM in continuous time based on the Cox model. *Statistics in Medicine*, 27(17), 3382–3406. doi:10.1002/sim.3216 PMID:18288785

Faltin, F., Kenett, R. S., & Ruggeri, F. (Eds.). (2012). *Statistical methods in healthcare*. John Wiley & Sons. doi:10.1002/9781119940012

Grigg, O., & Farewell, V. (2004). An overview of risk-adjusted charts. *Journal of the Royal Statistical Society. Series A, (Statistics in Society)*, 167(3), 523–539. doi:10.1111/j.1467-985X.2004.0apm2.x

Grigg, O. A., & Farewell, V. T. (2004). A risk-adjusted Sets method for monitoring adverse medical outcomes. *Statistics in Medicine*, 23(10), 1593–1602. doi:10.1002/sim.1763 PMID:15122739

Grigg, O. A., Farewell, V. T., & Spiegelhalter, D. J. (2003). Use of risk-adjusted CUSUM and RSPRT charts for monitoring in medical contexts. *Statistical Methods in Medical Research*, 12(2), 147–170. doi:10.1177/096228020301200205 PMID:12665208

Grigg, O. A., & Spiegelhalter, D. J. (2007). A simple risk-adjusted exponentially weighted moving average. *Journal of the American Statistical Association*, 102(477), 140–152. doi:10.1198/016214506000001121

Hart, G. K., Mullany, D., Cook, D. A., Pilcher, D., & Duke, G. (2008). Review of the application of risk-adjusted charts to analyse mortality outcomes in critical care. *Critical Care and Resuscitation*, 10, 239–251. PMID:18798724

Houshmand, E., Ebrahimipour, H., Doosti, H., Vafaei, N. A., Mahmoudian, P., & Hosseini, S. E. (2016). *Validity and reliability of the Persian version of quality assessment questionnaire (SERVUSE model)*. Academic Press.

Loke, C. K., & Gan, F. F. (2012). Joint monitoring scheme for clinical failures and predisposed risks. *Quality Technology & Quantitative Management*, 9(1), 3–21. doi:10.1080/16843703.2012.11673274

Mohammadian, F., Niaki, S. T. A., & Amiri, A. (2016, February). Phase-I risk-adjusted geometric control charts to monitor health-care systems. *Quality and Reliability Engineering International*, 32(1), 19–28. doi:10.1002/qre.1722

Pagel, C., Utley, M., Crowe, S., Witter, T., Anderson, D., Samson, R., & Brown, K. (2013). Real time monitoring of risk-adjusted paediatric cardiac surgery outcomes using variable life-adjusted display: Implementation in three UK centres. *Heart (British Cardiac Society)*, 99(19), 1445–1450. doi:10.1136/heartjnl-2013-303671 PMID:23564473

Parsonnet, V., Dean, D., & Bernstein, A. D. (1989). A method of uniform stratifcation of risk for evaluating the results of surgery in acquired adult heart disease. *Circulation*, 79(6 Pt 2), I3–I12. PMID:2720942

Paynabar, K., Jionghua, J., & Yeh, A. B. (2012). Phase I risk-adjusted control charts for monitoring surgical performance by considering categorical covariates. *Journal of Quality Technology*, 44, 39–53.

Roques, F., Nashef, S. A. M., Michel, P., Gaducheau, E., De Vincentiis, C., Baudet, E., & Gams, E. (1999). Risk factors and outcome in European cardiac surgery: Analysis of the EuroSCORE multinational database of 19030 patients. *European Journal of Cardio-Thoracic Surgery*, 15(6), 816–823. doi:10.1016/S1010-7940(99)00106-2 PMID:10431864

Sego, L. H., Reynolds, M. R. Jr, & Woodall, W. H. (2009). Risk-adjusted monitoring of survival times. *Statistics in Medicine*, *28*(9), 1386–1401. doi:10.1002/sim.3546 PMID:19247982

Steiner, S. H., Cook, R. J., Farewell, V. T., & Treasure, T. (2000). Monitoring surgical performance using risk-adjusted cumulative sum charts. *Biostatistics (Oxford, England)*, *1*(4), 441–452. doi:10.1093/biostatistics/1.4.441 PMID:12933566

Steiner, S. H., & Jones, M. (2010). Risk-adjusted survival time monitoring with an updating exponentially weighted moving average (EWMA) control chart. *Statistics in Medicine*, *29*(4), 444–454. doi:10.1002/sim.3788 PMID:19908262

Woodall, W. H. (2006). The use of control charts in health-care and public-health surveillance. *Journal of Quality Technology*, *38*, 89–104.

Zhang, L., Gan, F. F., & Loke, C. (2012). Phase I study of surgical performances with risk-adjusted Shewhart control charts. *Quality Technology & Quantitative Management*, *9*(4), 375–382. doi:10.1080/16843703.2012.11673299

KEY TERMS AND DEFINITIONS

Accelerated Failure Time (AFT) Model: A parametric model that assumes the effect of a covariate is to accelerate or decelerate the life course of a disease by some constant.

Dummy Variable: One that takes the value "0" or "1" to indicate the absence or presence of some categorical effect that may be expected to shift the outcome.

Logistic Regression Model: A regression model where the dependent variable is categorical and can take only two values, "0" and "1" (the case of a binary dependent variable).

Parsonnet Score: A competing integer score based on a patient's gender, age, morbid obesity, blood pressure, etc. that estimates his/her risk of death.

Phase-I Monitoring: Monitoring historical data to remove out-of-control points from it and produce 'cleaned' data-set.

Phase-II Monitoring: Monitoring: Monitoring future data based on control limits which derived from the data of in control process (cleaned data-set).

Risk-Adjusted Control Chart: A monitoring chart that used to level the playing field regarding the reporting of patient outcomes by adjusting for the differences in risk among specific patients.

Section 3
Machine Learning and Data Mining

Chapter 11

Machine Learning Applications in Cancer Therapy Assessment and Implications on Clinical Practice

Mehrdad J. Gangeh
Sunnybrook Health Sciences Centre, Canada & University of Toronto, Canada

Hadi Tadayyon
Sunnybrook Health Sciences Centre, Canada & University of Toronto, Canada

William T. Tran
Sunnybrook Health Sciences Centre, Canada & University of Toronto, Canada

Gregory Jan Czarnota
Sunnybrook Health Sciences Centre, Canada & University of Toronto, Canada

ABSTRACT

Precision medicine is an emerging medical model based on the customization of medical decisions and treatments to individuals. In personalized cancer therapy, tailored optimal therapies are selected depending on patient response to treatment rather than just using a one-size-fits-all approach. To this end, the field has witnessed significant advances in cancer response monitoring early after the start of therapy administration by using functional medical imaging modalities, particularly quantitative ultrasound (QUS) methods to monitor cell death at microscopic levels. This motivates the design of computer-assisted technologies for cancer therapy assessment, or computer-aided-theragnosis (CAT) systems. This chapter elaborates recent advances in the design and development of CAT systems based on QUS technologies in conjunction with advanced texture analysis and machine learning techniques with the aim of providing a framework for the early assessment of cancer responses that can potentially facilitate switching to more efficacious treatments in refractory patients.

DOI: 10.4018/978-1-5225-2515-8.ch011

INTRODUCTION

Neoadjuvant chemotherapy is typically administered to patients with large breast tumours (> 5cm) that are inoperable and at risk of metastasis. Patients with this type of cancer, called *locally advanced breast cancer* (LABC), have a relatively poor prognosis with five-year survival rates below 50% due to variable response to chemotherapy (Yalcin, 2013). Currently, clinical tumour response to chemotherapy is determined based on changes in tumour size, using guidelines from Response Evaluation Criteria in Solid Tumours (RECIST 1.1) (Eisenhauer et al., 2009). Low survival rate is due to the late assessment of response (typically at the end of the full course of treatment, which takes several months) resulting in a missed opportunity for treatment intervention for refractory patients. Thus, there is growing interest in personalized medicine – delivering patient-tailored treatment based on their predicted response early on in the course of treatment.

In this book chapter, a review of machine learning techniques for cancer response assessment is presented. Specifically, a review of computer-aided cancer therapy assessment, referred to in this text as computer-aided-theragnosis (CAT) system, is provided, demonstrating how it can be utilized to assist physicians in making appropriate treatment decisions and improve patients' quality of life. The review begins with a survey of various imaging techniques for early cancer therapy assessment such as diffusion-weighted magnetic resonance imaging (DW-MRI), positron emission tomography (PET), diffuse optical spectroscopy (DOS), and quantitative ultrasound (QUS) methods. QUS Methods are described in conjunction with machine learning techniques for cancer therapy assessment and the design of a CAT system is presented. Examples of works in QUS–based cancer therapy assessment and CAT system design concepts can be found in (Gangeh, Tadayyon, et al., 2016; Gangeh, Hashim, Giles, Sannachi, & Czarnota, 2016; Sannachi et al., 2015; Tadayyon et al., 2016), on which this book chapter elaborates. The authors delve into the components of this system, which include data acquisition, feature extraction, feature selection, dissimilarity measurement, learning from imbalanced data, and response classification. The chapter ends with a discussion commenting on the performance of different machine learning methodologies, clinical implications, and future work.

BACKGROUND

Cancer Response Imaging

This section provides a brief overview of clinically relevant cancer response imaging techniques that can provide early indications (i.e., after one cycle of chemotherapy) of tumour response. The modalities that are described include PET, DW-MRI, DOS, and QUS. As QUS for cancer response imaging is the area of the authors' research expertise, a separate section is dedicated for this topic following the current section.

PET Imaging permits the probing of tumour metabolic activity, which can change during treatment as a sign of response. For instance, fluoro-deoxyglucose PET (FDG-PET) involves injecting the patient with FDG - a radiotracer/contrast agent - prior to imaging. Due to the preferential uptake of glucose-based molecules by tumours, the tumour region in the PET image will be enhanced and its metabolism can be tracked over the treatment period. FDG-PET has exhibited a specificity and sensitivity of near 90% for detecting primary cancers in various cancer patients (Czernin & Phelps, 2002). It has also been demonstrated to have capabilities for differentiating responding patients from non-responding ones early following therapy (Schelling et al., 2000; Spaepen et al., 2001; Weber et al., 2003).

DW-MRI is a special sequence of MR imaging that measures the degree of diffusion of water molecules through tissue. During chemotherapy in a responding tumour tissue, the apparent diffusion coefficient (ADC) increases due to the breakdown of tumour tissue and increased porosity. A study demonstrated that when percentage change in ADC was combined with tumour volume and diameter, a sensitivity and specificity of 84% and 60% could be achieved in detecting response (Sharma, Danishad, Seenu, & Jagannathan, 2009).

Diffuse Optical Spectroscopy (DOS) is a tomographic technique that employs near-infrared light to measure absorption and scattering properties of tissue (Ntziachristos & Chance, 2001; Tromberg et al., 2000) through quantitative spectral signal processing. In a recent study, DOS was used to monitor the response of breast cancer patients undergoing neoadjuvant chemotherapy (Falou et al., 2012). Results have shown that optical parameters, such as oxyhemoglobin, deoxyhemoglobin, water and scattering power, can provide an indication of response within 4 weeks of treatment. Responders showed a significant reduction in these optical parameters, whereas non-responders demonstrated insignificant changes after 4 weeks of treatment initiation.

Although DOS studies indicate a favorable sensitivity in detecting breast tumour response early on during treatment, DOS has limited tissue penetration depth, thereby limiting its application to superficial tumours. DW-MRI requires substantial capital investment and PET requires the injection of radioactive tracer isotopes, limiting repeated usability and imparting potential long-term health complications. The next section describes the advantages of ultrasound imaging and the potential of QUS methods in cancer imaging.

Quantitative Ultrasound Imaging in Cancer Response Assessment

Ultrasound is a pervasive clinical imaging modality with applications in screening, diagnosis, and image-guided procedures, due to its relatively low cost, high spatial and temporal resolutions, and its radiation-free nature. In ultrasound, brightness mode (B-mode) imaging provides gray-scale intensity images generated by reflections from tissue interfaces where there is a change in density and compressibility. B-mode ultrasound imaging is the standard mode used by sonographers and radiologists. Due to their distinct density and compressibility relative to surrounding tissue, tumours larger than 8 mm are readily detected in B-mode images as hypoechoic regions, requiring no external contrast agents (Insana & Oelze, 2006). However, the frequency-dependent information from tissue echo signals is lost during conversion of the raw ultrasound backscatter radiofrequency (RF) signal to B-mode images. Quantitative ultrasound (QUS) tissue characterization encompasses any signal analysis technique that involves the estimation of quantitative parameters from ultrasound data in order to characterize a tissue in *vivo, ex vivo,* or *in vitro*. Particularly, QUS spectroscopy aims to extract tissue-specific parameters through analysis of the frequency-dependent backscatter of the ultrasound RF signal. One of the common applications of QUS methods in biomedical research domain is in discriminating tissue abnormalities such as those of the prostate, lymph nodes, eye, as well as the myocardium (Coleman et al., 1985; Feleppa et al., 1996; Mamou et al., 2010; M. Yang, Krueger, Miller, & Holland, 2007), and also in detecting cell death in a tissue (Banihashemi et al., 2008; Czarnota et al., 1999; Lee et al., 2012; Vlad, Brand, Giles, & others, 2009).

Performing a linear regression analysis of the tissue power spectrum within the usable ultrasound bandwidth permits the estimation of linear regression parameters such as spectral slope (SS), spectral intercept (SI), as well as mid-band fit (MBF) - the value of the fit at the center of the frequency bandwidth. Through theoretical modeling and experimental validation, Lizzi *et al.* (Lizzi, Ostromogilsky, Feleppa, & Others, 1986) demonstrated that SS is related to the ultrasound scatterer size and SI is related to the ultrasound scatterer concentration. The SS and SI, among other QUS parameters, can be used to probe tissue microstructure, which can change with disease processes. In this light, the parameters MBF, SS, and SI have been used successfully to detect pathology in various types of tissues including prostate, lymph nodes, ocular tumours, as well as the myocardium (Coleman et al., 1985; Feleppa et al., 1996; Mamou et al., 2010; M. Yang et al., 2007), and have also been used to characterize therapeutic effects such as tumour response to radiotherapy, antivascular, and hyperthermia treatments (Banihashemi et al., 2008; Czarnota et al., 1999; Lee et al., 2012; Vlad et al., 2009). Moreover, the potential effectiveness of these parameters to grade breast cancer subtypes has recently been demonstrated in (Tadayyon, Sadeghi-Naini, & Czarnota, 2014; Tadayyon, Sadeghi-Naini, Wirtzfeld, Wright, & Czarnota, 2014).

Alternatively, advanced QUS parameters such as effective scatterer size and acoustic concentration have been used previously to differentiate mouse models of tumours from rat models of spontaneously occurring benign masses (Oelze, O'Brien, Blue, & Zachary, 2004). Effective/average scatterer diameter (ASD) and effective/average acoustic concentration (AAC) can be estimated by fitting a theoretical backscatter model to the measured backscatter signal from the tissue of interest. Previous studies found similarities between ASDs and the mean size of cells (for carcinoma and sarcoma) and glandular acini (fibroadenoma), which allowed carcinoma tumours in mice to be differentiated from fibroadenomas in rats (Oelze et al., 2004). The tissue types were found to be better differentiated when the ASD and AAC parameters were combined.

Using high-frequency ultrasound (20-25 MHz) imaging, previous *in vivo* studies have demonstrated that MBF and SS increase as a result of cell death in mouse xenograft models, treated with photodynamic therapy (Banihashemi et al., 2008) and radiation therapy (Vlad et al., 2009). Such increases in spectral characteristics were found to be associated histologically with morphological changes in the dying cell, including nuclear condensation and fragmentation. As well, parallel ultrasound observations were made at a clinically relevant ultrasound frequency range (4.5-9 MHz) when xenograft breast cancer tumours were treated with chemotherapy (Sadeghi-Naini, Falou, Tadayyon, et al., 2013). This finding suggested the potential for a new application of QUS: predicting tumour response to anticancer therapy using QUS techniques through surrogate measures of tumour cell death. More recently, ultrasound imaging applications have been extended to include therapy response monitoring in the clinical environment, particularly in breast cancer imaging. In a pilot study by Sadeghi-Naini *et al.* (Sadeghi-Naini, Falou, Zubovits, et al., 2013), abreast ultrasound images and RF data were acquired longitudinally from 25 patients undergoing neoadjuvant chemotherapy. Subsequently, QUS spectral parameters including MBF, SS, and SI were extracted from the ultrasound RF data prior to treatment initiation, at week 1, 4, and 8 of the treatment, and at completion of treatment (many months later prior to surgery). The study concluded that the combination of MBF and SI parameters could predict response with 100% sensitivity and 83% specificity at 4 weeks into the treatment. Taking a step further, statistical texture analysis of the QUS images using the gray-level co-occurrence matrices (GLCM) indicated an improvement in the discrimination of responsive patients from non-responsive ones (Sadeghi-Naini et al., 2014). Results of that study indicated that GLCM-based analysis could characterize tumour heterogeneity features, and predict treatment response. In the most recent work, the same group undertook a machine learning approach to the same problem and developed a multi-parametric QUS model employing a *k*-nearest-neighbor (*k*-NN) classifier that was cross-validated in a leave-one-subject-out evaluation scheme (Tadayyon et al., 2016). The results indicated that the best response prediction was achieved with 80% sensitivity and 79% specificity at week 4. In order to illustrate how QUS images can be used to visualize a responding tumour and a non-responding one, representative images of such tumours are presented in Figures 1 and 2 before treatment initiation and at 4 weeks after treatment initiation (2 cycles of chemotherapy), respectively. For each tumour, B-mode images, MBF images, power spectra before and 4 weeks after the start of treatment, and magnified hematoxylin and eosin (H&E) stained histology sections of whole-mount breast specimens obtained post-surgery (mastectomy/lumpectomy) are shown. Full color versions of these figures can be found in Tadayyon et al., 2016. Whereas B-mode images showed no appreciable changes in the tumour 4 weeks into treatment, a marked increase in MBF could be observed in the responding tumour region as a result of 4 weeks of chemotherapy (1-2 cycles). The non-responding tumour, in contrast, demonstrated no change or decrease in MBF. The before/after superimposed power spectra demonstrated the same concept graphically, where MBF is marked by a circle in the middle of the regression line (Figures 1C and 2C (*left*)). The histology image of the responding tumour indicates a stroma-filled tissue with small isolated patches of glands, demonstrating therapeutic effects. On the other hand, the histology of the non-responding tumour shows a gland-dominated tumour with low stromal collagen density, indicating little to no therapeutic effect.

The aforementioned studies mainly focused on the applications of QUS methods in cell death detection using simple features such as mean of intensity or classical texture methods like gray-level co-occurrence matrices (GLCM). Additionally, limited analytic tools such as linear discriminant analysis (LDA) or statistical tests of significance were used to provide a proof of principle of the developed systems based on QUS methods. This is while advanced textural methods and sophisticated machine learning techniques have extensively been used in the design of computer-aided systems to perform diagnosis – namely called computer aided-diagnosis (CAD) systems – in breast cancer using ultrasound data. For example, textural features (Chang, Wu, Moon, Chou, & Chen, 2003; Donohue, Huang, Burks, Forsberg, & Piccoli, 2001; Gomez, Pereira, & Infantosi, 2012; Huang & Chen, 2005; Lefebvre, Meunier, Thibault, Laugier, & Berger, 2000), fractal parameters (Chen et al., 2005), and morphological features (Alam, Feleppa, Rondeau, Kalisz, & Garra, 2011; Joo, Yang, Moon, & Kim, 2004; Lefebvre et al., 2000) have been used along with a variety of supervised learning methods such as a linear or quadratic discriminant analysis (Donohue et al., 2001; Lefebvre et al., 2000), neural networks (Joo et al., 2004), or support vector machines (Chang et al., 2003; Huang & Chen, 2005; M.-C. Yang et al., 2013) in CAD systems designed for breast cancer detection and classification (Cheng, Shan, Ju, Guo, & Zhang, 2010). However, the use of these techniques in the design of a computer-aided cancer therapy assessment system, known as a computer-aided-theragnostic (CAT) system, has remained far behind. Nonetheless, Gangeh *et al.* recently designed and developed CAT systems using ultrasound data in clinical applications (Gangeh, Tadayyon, et al., 2016; Gangeh, Tadayyon, Sannachi, Sadeghi-Naini, & Czarnota, 2015; Gangeh, Fung, Tadayyon, Tran, & Czarnota, 2016) as well as for preclinical data (Gangeh, Sadeghi-Naini, et al., 2014; Gangeh, El Kaffas, Hashim, Giles, & Czarnota, 2015; Gangeh, Hashim, Giles, & Czarnota, 2014; Gangeh, Sadeghi-Naini, Kamel, & Czarnota, 2013) in order to assess and monitor the early therapeutic responses. The remaining of this chapter mainly elaborates the components of a CAT system and describes their functionalities towards the design of a complete and automatic computer-assisted system for monitoring the therapeutic cancer responses.

Figure 1. Representative B-mode images (A), MBF images (B), power spectra (C left) before and 4 weeks after the start of chemotherapy treatment and hematoxylin and eosin histology histology images (C right) of an example responding breast tumour. MBF is measured in dBr, which represents dB relative to a tissue-equivalent reference phantom. Data in the left column represent pre-treatment data, obtained prior to treatment initiation, and data in the right column represent week 4 data. US scale bar represents 1 cm, histology scale bar represents 100 μm. Adopted from (Tadayyon et al., 2016).

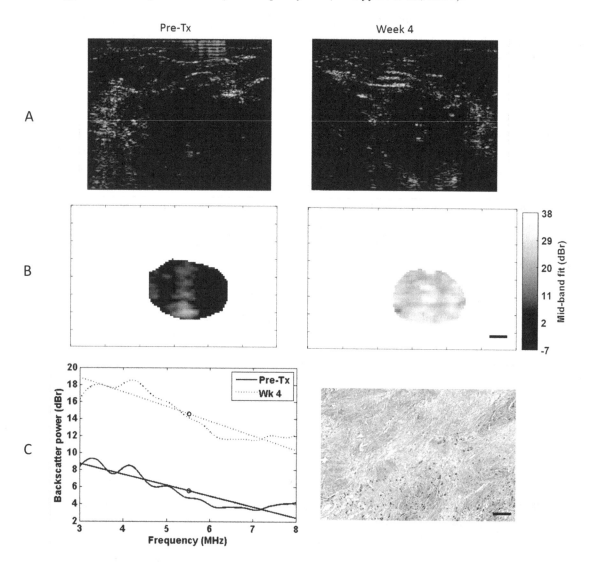

COMPUTER-AIDED THERAGNOSIS

Components of a Computer-Aided-Theragnosis System

A CAT system is a computer-assisted system that can reliably detect and classify cancer patients as responders or non-responders. The CAT system ideally performs the task non-invasively by employing images obtained from tumours using functional medical imaging modalities such as QUS methods as

Figure 2. Representative B-mode images (A), MBF images (B), power spectra (C left) before and 4 weeks after the start of chemotherapy treatment and hematoxylin and eosin histology histology images (C right) of an example non-responding breast tumour. MBF is measured in dBr, which represents dB relative to a tissue-equivalent reference phantom. Data in the left column represent pre-treatment data, obtained prior to treatment initiation, and data in the right column represent week 4 data. US scale bar represents 1 cm, histology scale bar represents 100 µm. Adopted from (Tadayyon et al., 2016).

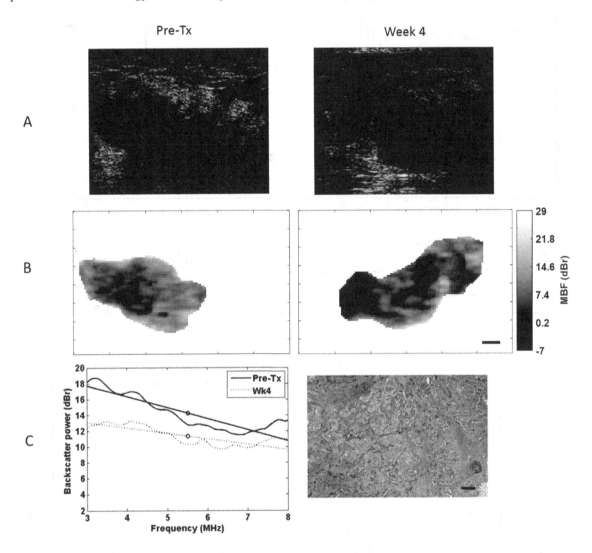

inputs. Further processing of input images are performed by the CAT system in order to extract discriminative features, measure the dissimilarities between the "pre" and "mid-treatment" scans as an indication of treatment effectiveness, and classify the patients as responders or non-responders. In addition, since the number of responders is usually much more than the number of non-responders, techniques for learning from imbalanced data should be employed before submission of the dissimilarity features to the classifier in order to prevent a poor classification performance on the minority (non-responder) class. Therefore, as shown in Figure 3, the main components of a CAT system are: feature extraction,

Figure 3. The schematic of a typical Computer-Aided-Theragnosis (CAT) system

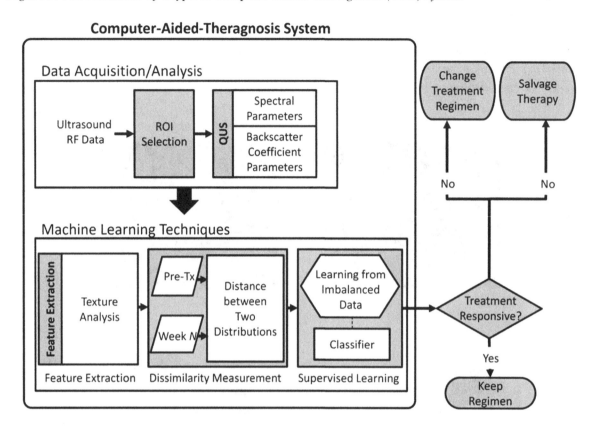

dissimilarity measure, learning from imbalanced data, and supervised learning based on a classification system. The main components of a CAT system are described in details in the next sections along with the motivations on choosing the specific methods in the design of the proposed CAT system. All algorithms and image analyses were developed and performed using MATLAB R2011 (Mathworks, Natick, MA).

Feature Extraction

QUS methods generate 2-D parametric maps, which are considered as inputs to the CAT system for further analysis to monitor and assess the responses to cancer treatment. The first step for the analysis is to extract discriminative features from these 2-D parametric maps in order to provide a more concise representation. Both parametric and non-parametric feature extraction methods might be considered for this purpose (Duda, Hart, & Stork, 2001). Parametric-based feature extraction methods assume a certain distribution for the data and rely on the estimation of the parameters of these underlying probability densities, which can be effective data descriptors for a large, multi-dimensional object, such as an image. However, it may not be well justified to assume a distribution on the data mainly because of the very high intrinsic dimensionality and unconstrained input environments of these domains. Alternatively, without making any assumptions on the underlying distribution of the data (whether it be Poisson, Gaussian, etc.), non-parametric density estimates of the features can be used to represent the data.

While the use of the mean of parametric maps does provide a means to interpret the status of the tumour cell over time, textural properties of parametric maps have shown a higher correlation to changes in the tumour tissue (Sadeghi-Naini, Falou, Tadayyon, et al., 2013). Specifically, texture properties derived from the grey level co-occurrence matrices (GLCM), for example, contrast and homogeneity, have been demonstrated to have a higher performance than the mean of intensity in response classification studies especially early on during a course of treatment (Sadeghi-Naini et al., 2014; Sadeghi-Naini, Falou, Tadayyon, et al., 2013). The reason for the improved classification performance when using more complex texture methods versus the simple mean method, may be due to the additional consideration of structures (manifested to pixel intensities) next to each other within a sufficiently sized neighbourhood. In addition, it has been demonstrated that the responses developed in tumours due to cancer therapy administration are often heterogeneous (Rice et al., 2010), which also motivates the use of texture methods in cancer response monitoring applications.

Texture Methods

There is a large body of work on texture analysis, as can be judged from its numerous applications in various fields (Materka & Strzelecki, 1998). Texture analysis has been applied to nine broad categories (Hadjidemetriou, Grossberg, & Nayar, 2004; Manjunath & Ma, 1996; Mirmehdi, Xie, & Suri, 2008; Muneeswaran, Ganesan, Arumugam, & Soundar, 2005; Petrou & Sevilla, 2006; Smeulders, Worring, Santini, Gupta, & Jain, 2000; Tuceryan & Jain, 1998):

1. *Texture classification* of stationary texture images that contain only one texture type per image.
2. Unsupervised t*exture segmentation* of non-stationary images that consist of more than one texture type per image.
3. *Texture synthesis*, which is important in computer graphics for rendering object surfaces to be as realistic looking as possible.
4. *3D shape from texture*, which investigates how a standard texel shape is distorted by 3D projections and relates it to the local surface orientation.
5. *Shape from texture*, in which texture is usually used in addition to other features such as shading, color, and so on to extract three-dimensional shape information.
6. *Color-texture analysis*, where joint color-texture descriptor improves discrimination over using color and texture features independently.
7. *Texture for appearance modeling*, which is fundamental in computer vision and graphics.
8. *Dynamic texture analysis* for dynamic shape and appearance modeling which is essential in video sequences with certain temporal regularity properties.
9. *Indexing* and image database retrieval usually based on similarity measure.
10. In cancer response monitoring, however, the focus is on texture classification among the texture analysis problems.

According to (Materka & Strzelecki, 1998) and (Tuceryan & Jain, 1998), texture analysis techniques are essentially classified into four types of approaches: statistical (Baraldi & Parmiggiani, 1995), structural/geometrical (Petrou & Sevilla, 2006), transform-/signal processing-based (Jain & Farrokhnia, 1991; Randen & Husøy, 1999), and model-based (Krishnamachari & Chellappa, 1997; Reed & du Buf, 1993). Furthermore, as a complicated phenomenon, there is no unique definition for textures that is agreed upon by the researchers (Ahonen & Pietikainen, 2009). As a consequence, there have been many different models proposed in the literature, each of which defined based on one or a few properties of textures (Mirmehdi et al., 2008). However, it has recently been demonstrated that small-sized local operators like local binary patterns (LBPs) (Ojala, Pietikäinen, & Mäenpää, 2002) and texton-based method based on patch representation of small local neighborhood (Varma & Zisserman, 2005, 2009) result in excellent texture classification performance on standard texture databases. As an explanation, it is worthwhile to mention here that small-sized local operators are desirable in situations where the region to be analyzed, often referred to as the region of interest (ROI), is relatively small. This is especially the case in medical applications, where pathology is often localized in small areas (Gangeh, Sørensen, Shaker, Kamel, de Bruijne, et al., 2010; Gangeh, Sørensen, Shaker, Kamel, & de Bruijne, 2010; Sørensen, Gangeh, Shaker, & de Bruijne, 2007). In these situations, convolving with large support filter banks suffers from boundary effects, and by using small-sized local operators, more patches can be extracted from an ROI that improves the reliability of estimating image statistics (Ojala et al., 2002).

A successful application of texture methods based on small-sized local operators has recently been demonstrated in clinical cancer response monitoring using QUS methods (Gangeh, Tadayyon, et al., 2016). In (Gangeh, Tadayyon, et al., 2016), the LBPs, which are *predefined* binary operators, were used as texture descriptors to represent 2-D QUS maps. On the other hand, texton-based approach, which is a *data-driven* texture method, can be employed as a textural feature descriptor. In the next paragraphs, these two state-of-the-art texture methods are described in the context of therapeutic cancer response assessment.

Local Binary Patterns

The LBPs (Ojala et al., 2002) can be considered an attractive tool for texture analysis. They are computationally efficient, theoretically simple, and achieve rather high performance in texture classification. The technique is based on the definition of local binary patterns, which are circularly symmetric operators with certain radius R, which defines the spatial resolution of the operator, and with P equally spaced pixels on this circle, which determines the quantization of angular space. These operators are defined in such a way that the operator is invariant to local gray-scale shifts.

Ojala *et al.* (Ojala et al., 2002) introduced rotation invariant *uniform* LBPs, denoted as $\text{LBP}_{P,R}^{riu}$, and demonstrated that they can be considered fundamental properties of image textures in the sense that computation of LBP responses on images mostly yields uniform ones (in some images more than 90%). Uniform LBPs have very few spatial transitions (less than three) and detect microstructures such as edges, lines, spots, and flat areas. Figure 4 depicts the nine *uniform* patterns with maximum two spatial transitions in $\text{LBP}_{8,1}^{ri}$. The frequency of the uniform patterns in the image is then computed, which has been shown to be a powerful texture descriptor. Hence, the LBP approach is considered as a combination of structural (because of defining microstructure operators) and statistical (due to using occurrence histogram of these operators in the image as a feature set) texture analysis technique. In the context of cancer response monitoring, the prevalence of primitive elements such as dots, corners, and edges in a parametric map indicates a more heterogeneous texture corresponding to more cell death, whereas availability of more flat areas indicates no cell death (corresponding to more homogeneous textures). This property of the LBPs was used in (Gangeh, Tadayyon, et al., 2016) to discriminate between responders and non-responder in LABC patients receiving neoadjuvant chemotherapy.

Figure 4. The nine uniform binary patterns with maximum two spatial transitions that appear in $\mathrm{LBP}_{8,1}^{ri}$.
Black and white dots correspond to 0 and 1, respectively. The corresponding binary number is shown under each operator. Each of the patterns correspond to one of the primitive textural features such as dots (pattern 0), edges (patterns 2-6), corners (patterns 1 and 7), and flat areas (pattern 8).

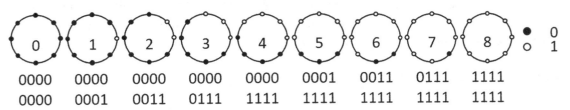

Multiresolution analysis can be achieved by using the LBPs at multiple spatial radii. The most common LBP operators in the literature are: $\mathrm{LBP}_{8,1}^{riu2}$, $\mathrm{LBP}_{16,2}^{riu2}$, and $\mathrm{LBP}_{24,3}^{riu2}$. The superscript in these operators stands for rotation invariant uniform 2 (uniform operator with maximum two spatial transition) and the first index in the subscript represents P and the second one is R.

The LBPs are, by design, invariant to gray-scale changes. However, in cancer response monitoring using QUS methods, the intensity levels of the 2-D parametric maps play an important role in detecting cell death levels. For example, it is well known from the previous studies on QUS methods that ultrasound backscatter increases with apoptosis (Czarnota & Kolios, 2010; Kolios & Czarnota, 2009), which consequently affects the levels of mid-band fit and 0-MHz intercept parametric maps. Therefore, to take into consideration the variations in intensity changes of QUS maps due to cell death, histogram of intensity can be combined with the histograms computed based on the LBPs to provide a richer feature descriptor (Gangeh, Tadayyon, et al., 2016).

Texton-Based Texture Analysis

Texton-based method, on the other hand, is considered a dictionary learning technique, where the dictionary atoms, namely called textons, are some primitive elements learned from texture images. One main advantage of using *data-driven* texture analysis over those based on *predefined* operators like the LBPs is the adaptability of the former approach to the type of the dataset.

The original concept of textons was originally introduced by Julesz (Julesz, 1981) to represent the elements of texture perception. However, it took about 20 years for the first proposal of a complete texture classification system based on Julesz's theory to be published (Leung & Malik, 2001). The approach was further optimized by several researchers including Cula *et al.* (Cula & Dana, 2004) and Varma and Zisserman (Varma & Zisserman, 2005, 2009), resulting in state-of-the-art results on benchmark texture datasets such as Columbia-Utrecht reflectance texture (CUReT) database (Dana, van Ginneken, Nayar, & Koenderink, 1999), and on medical images (Gangeh, Sørensen, Shaker, Kamel, de Bruijne, et al., 2010; Gangeh, Sørensen, Shaker, Kamel, & de Bruijne, 2010). There are three main representations associated with the texton-based approach including: raw-pixel representation (Varma & Zisserman, 2005, 2009), filter banks (Cula & Dana, 2004; Leung & Malik, 2001; Schmid, 2004), and the Markov random field (MRF) (Varma & Zisserman, 2005). In raw-pixel representation, the original pixels in patches extracted from a texture image are used without any further pre-processing, whereas in filter-bank representation, the patches are convolved with a filter as a pre-processing step. Finally in the MRF representation, the central pixel of a patch is modeled using the neighbouring pixels.

Irrespective of the type of representation used to describe local image (patch) information, there are mainly two steps in the texton-based approach: 1) learning a dictionary or codebook of textons, and 2) the construction of a model for each texture image using dictionary elements as illustrated in Figure 5. The two steps are elaborated in the next paragraphs as the core principles to texton dictionary learning approach in the context of cancer response monitoring.

Building the Codebook

In order to construct the codebook, patches of a specified size are extracted from each image in the dataset. These patches are converted to an appropriate representation such as raw-pixel representation, and vectorized. The vector elements representing the patches are subsequently submitted to a clustering algorithm, such as k-means, to cluster all the patch representations into a specified number of dictionary elements (the textons). In the application of cancer response monitoring, for each patient, sub-dictionaries are learned from the baseline ("pre-treatment") scans and "mid-treatment" scans separately, and composed into a single dictionary that is used for model learning for the patient's ROIs in the next step. The learning of dictionaries for each patient is separated due to the patient specific nature of ultrasound

Figure 5. The schematic of two stages of the texton-based approach: (A) codebook construction and (B) model learning. The ROIs from each Case include all "pre-treatment" scans and "mid-treatment" scans a t specific week (week 1, 4, or 8).

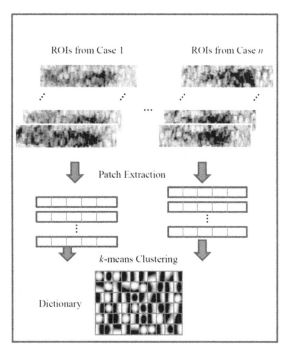

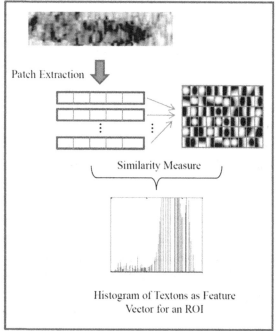

A   B

tumour data. The proposed CAT system represents a response classification system based upon differences between the "pre" and "mid-treatment" scan planes. In order to assign a representative measure that can quantify the difference between scans at a specific time during treatment versus the "pre-treatment" scans for a patient, the use of only a single patient's ROIs for dictionary learning provides a metric that better represents a dissimilarity feature that is independent from other individuals. If the dictionary was constructed using clustering of all features from all patients, the dissimilarity measure used to represent a patient would not have been the characteristic of solely the individual, potentially leading to a poorer classification performance.

Model Learning

After learning the codebook of textons for each patient, the models (feature sets) are built for the ROIs of each patient using the texton codebook constructed in the previous step for that particular patient. To this end, patches of the same size as the textons in the codebook are extracted by sliding a window pixel-by-pixel over each ROI of the patient. The patches are subsequently converted to the appropriate representation as used in the previous step and vectorized. Eventually, a histogram of textons is computed, as the model for each ROI, by comparing the extracted patches with the codebook textons constructed for each corresponding patient and finding the closest match using a similarity measure, such as Euclidean distance, to update the corresponding bin in the histogram of textons. Therefore, the model for an ROI is a histogram where the bin labels corresponded to textons, and the frequency of patches most similar to each of the textons determines the shape of the histogram. Figure 5 illustrates the codebook construction and model learning steps in the texton-based approach.

Remark on the Setup

This setup of codebook construction and model learning, which is based upon learning one dictionary per patient, also facilitates the implementation of a more efficient cross-validation step for evaluation of the classifier. In traditional machine learning experiments, cross-validation involves learning the dictionary for the training set, and using the dictionary on the test set. This requires many repetitions of the dictionary and model learning steps (as many as the number of folds in cross validation when evaluating the classifier), which makes the texton-based method computationally expensive. However, since in the implemented setup, one dictionary is learned per patient, and the texture models are learned exclusively using the patient dictionary, when the cross validation is performed at subject (patient) level, there is no need to build the dictionary again, as there is no risk of learning the dictionary on the test set. Consequently, the cross validation is performed in a much more efficient way.

As a final remark on comparing the LBPs and texton-based method as texture descriptors, it is worthwhile to highlight here that in texton-based approach based on raw-pixel representation, the intensity of extracted patches are taken into consideration in codebook and model learning. Therefore, texton-based method has an additional advantage over the LBPs as it includes the information on changes in intensity levels of QUS maps that occur due to cell death, whereas LBPs ignore this information as they are invariant to gray-scale variations. As mentioned before, the LBPs need to be, for example, combined with the histogram of intensities to include the information on variations in intensity levels of QUS parametric maps in the resulting feature descriptors.

Dissimilarity Measurement

Cancer response monitoring involves categorizing the patients into two categories: treatment responders and non-responders, thus classification is based upon measuring the dissimilarity of each time group after chemotherapy with the "pre-treatment" scans. This choice of categorization was the reason why the model histograms obtained from the previous feature extraction step (the histograms generated using the LBPs or texton-based method) are not arbitrarily submitted to train a classifier. Furthermore, a patient being categorized as a responder or non-responder depends on the changes since starting treatment. Thus, submitting the features of "pre-treatment" and "mid-treatment" ROIs separately will not prove useful in quantifying changes within these two populations that is crucial for characterizing treatment efficacy. Assigning a value for each patient that quantifies the differences between the scans taken "pre-" and "mid-treatment" is synonymous to identifying the treatment effectiveness, i.e., the larger the distance, the more success in treatment (Czarnota et al., 1999; Czarnota & Kolios, 2010). Finding the optimal dissimilarity measure that most accurately calculates the differences between the two populations is, therefore, important in the design of a CAT system.

One of the simplest and most straightforward formulations to measure the distance between the two distributions is to calculate the distance between the cluster means using:

$$d(p,q) = \| E(p) - E(q) \|_2^{1/2} \tag{1}$$

where E is the expectation function, p and q are the two distributions. The main drawback of the metric given in Equation (1), which is equivalent to Euclidean distance or $\ell 2$ norm, is that it only takes into account the first order statistics of the data samples taken from p and q. Therefore, if the two distributions have the same mean values, they cannot be discriminated using Equation (1) even if, e.g., their standard deviations (second order statistics) are different.

One approach to overcome this problem is to first, map the data to a higher dimensional feature space and then compute Equation (1) in the augmented feature space. By computing the expectation function in the augmented feature space, higher order statistics of the two distributions can be effectively taken into account resulting in potentially enhanced discrimination. This idea was effectively and efficiently implemented by (Gretton, Borgwardt, Rasch, Schölkopf, & Smola, 2012, 2006), leading to a nonparametric (i.e., making no assumption on the distributions p and q) kernel-based metric in reproducing kernel Hilbert spaces (RHKSs) called maximum mean discrepancy.

To provide a formal description, let $X = \{x_i\}_{i=1}^n$ and $Y = \{y_i\}_{i=1}^m$ be data samples drawn independently and identically distributed (i.i.d.) from p and q, respectively. A feature mapping function φ can be defined such that $X \sim p, X \xrightarrow{\varphi} \varphi(X)$, and likewise $Y \sim p, Y \xrightarrow{\varphi} \varphi(Y)$, which maps the data to a high dimensional feature space. By computing Equation (1) in this space, a metric is computed with the following formulation:

$$\mathrm{MMD}(\varphi, p, q) = \| E(\varphi(p)) - E(\varphi(q)) \|_2^{\frac{1}{2}}$$

$$= [E\{[\varphi(X) - \varphi(Y)]^T [\varphi(X) - \varphi(Y)]\}]^{\frac{1}{2}}$$

$$= [E\{\varphi(X)^T \varphi(X) - 2\varphi(X)^T \varphi(Y) + \varphi(Y)^T \varphi(Y)\}]^{\frac{1}{2}} \tag{2}$$

In practice, to compute Equation (2) using a finite number of data samples $X = \{x_i\}_{i=1}^n$ and $Y = \{y_i\}_{i=1}^m$ taken from the two distributions p and q, respectively, the following empirical formulation for MMD can be used:

$$\mathrm{MMD}(\varphi, X, Y) = [\frac{1}{n^2} \sum_{i,j} k(x_i, x_j) - \frac{2}{nm} \sum_{i,j} k(x_i, y_j) + \frac{1}{m^2} \sum_{i,j} k(y_i, y_j)]^{1/2} \tag{3}$$

where $k(x_i, x_j) = \langle \varphi(x_i), \varphi(x_j) \rangle$ and $\langle . \rangle$ is an inner product operator.

Intuitively, it is expected that empirical MMD will be small when $p = q$ and large when the two distributions are far apart. It can be computed in quadratic time, i.e., for $n + m$ data samples, the cost of computation is $O((n + m)^2)$ time, which is reasonably low for a real time computation. Moreover, an alternative approach has been proposed in (Gretton et al., 2012) with efficient linear time approximation, i.e., with a computational cost of $O(n + m)$ time. This is particularly important when larger volume of data is available. However, this is not the case in the application of cancer response monitoring as there are limited number of scan planes per subject.

The empirical MMD formulated in Equation (3) has been adapted here to compute the dissimilarity between the "pre" and "mid-treatment" samples of each patient at a specific time interval after the start of treatment. The MMD metric is expected to be useful in exploiting intra-group variance information available from multiple samples taken from each of the "pre" and "mid-treatment" populations. The computed MMD values are subsequently submitted to a classifier in a supervised learning paradigm to classify treatment response. MMD has already been proved to be useful to identify the changes between two populations in the application of scene change point detection (Diu, Gangeh, & Kamel, 2013), and on preclinical data (Gangeh, Hashim, et al., 2014) as well as in a clinical setting (Gangeh, Tadayyon, et al., 2016) in the application of cancer response monitoring.

Learning From Imbalanced Data

In machine learning, there are situations where the number of data samples is not equally distributed across different classes. For example, most clinical datasets naturally include many more data samples in the healthy class than the cancerous or abnormal class. Likewise, about 30% of LABC patients receiving neoadjuvant chemotherapy are non-responders, i.e., the ratio of responders to non-responders is approximately 3 to 1.

The fundamental problem in learning from imbalanced data is that without compensation for an uneven distribution of the data samples in two classes, the training of most classifiers is overwhelmed by the majority class, leading to a poor performance on the minority class. In clinical cancer response monitoring, the minority class is the patient non-responding population, meaning that misclassification will lead to the continued administration of an ineffective treatment regimen and worsening of the cancer. Similarly, in a computer-aided-diagnosis system with the goal of classifying cases to cancerous (usually minority class) and healthy (majority class), identifying a cancerous patient as non-cancerous can have dire consequences. Therefore, employing techniques for learning from imbalanced data is vitally important in these applications.

The techniques for learning from imbalanced data can broadly be categorized in three groups (He & Garcia, 2009): 1) Sampling, 2) cost-sensitive, and 3) kernel-based methods. Sampling methods employ some mechanisms to compensate for the uneven distribution of the data among the classes such that the final distribution is balanced. Cost-sensitive methods, on the other hand, provide different costs for the misclassification of the data samples, where the cost depends on the distribution of the data samples among different classes. Finally, kernel-based methods mainly centre on the most common kernel-based classifier, i.e., SVM by incorporating different weights into the computation of kernels depending on the distributions of the data samples in different classes. An extensive review of techniques for learning from imbalanced data has been provided in (Galar, Fernández, Barrenechea, Bustince, & Herrera, 2012; He & Garcia, 2009).

Among the approaches proposed for learning from imbalanced data as reviewed in (Galar et al., 2012; He & Garcia, 2009), sampling methods provide a simple yet effective mechanism, which strive to manipulate the size of the dataset submitted to the classifier (Estabrooks, Jo, & Japkowicz, 2004; Weiss & Provost, 2001). Sampling methods are broadly divided to random oversampling and random under-sampling. The former replicates the data samples from the minority class and append them to the training samples to balance the data, whereas the latter achieves this goal by sub-sampling the majority class. Gangeh *et al.* (Gangeh, Tadayyon, et al., 2016) have adapted random under-sampling in clinical cancer response monitoring. They have used the entire minority class and a random subsample of the majority class with the same size as the minority class for training the classifier. Under-sampling has been preferred over oversampling as the latter tends to lead to poorer classification on test data as a consequence of overfitting (Holte, Acker, & Porter, 1989; Mease, Wyner, & Buja, 2007; Rastgoo et al., 2016).

Supervised Learning

After extracting discriminative features using one of the described texture methods and the computation of the dissimilarities between the "pre-" and "mid-treatment" (week 1, 4, or 8) scans as an indication of cancer treatment effectiveness, the balanced data should be submitted to a classifier as indicated in Figure 3.

As for the choice of a classifier in the CAT system, while random forests classifier is considered as a strong methodological choice for supervised learning, it mainly relies on the bagging of features, which is especially useful in a high dimensional feature space (Criminisi & Shotton, 2013). An evidence is provided in (Uniyal et al., 2015) where a support vector machine (SVM) and a random forests classifier have been compared in the classification of breast lesions using low dimensional features resulting in a poorer performance of the random forests compared with the SVM. In cancer response monitoring, the features eventually submitted to the classifier are the dissimilarity measures between the "pre-" and "mid-treatment" scans, which is of very low dimensionality (can only be one, e.g., one MMD metric as the distance between the two population scans as being used in this study). In this application, the power of random forests cannot be fully employed and they are not considered as a good choice. According to Gangeh *et al.* (Gangeh, Tadayyon, et al., 2016, 2015; Gangeh, Fung, et al., 2016), among the classifiers tested, a naïve Bayes classifier achieves higher performance compared with an SVM with RBF kernel, and a *k* nearest neighbour (*k*-NN) classifier, and therefore has been adapted here in the application of clinical cancer response monitoring as the final stage in the design of the CAT system.

A naïve Bayes classifier is based upon the assumption that the features submitted for classification are independent from each other, and therefore simplifies the Bayes' theorem (Duda et al., 2001). The *k*-NN classifier is a non-parametric method that examines the labels of nearest neighbour training points in order to decide on the label of a test sample. This decision is based on the most common label among these nearest neighbours surrounding the test sample (Duda et al., 2001). An SVM is a classifier that finds the decision boundary such that the margin between the boundary points (support vectors) of the two classes is maximized. An SVM can perform a nonlinear classification by applying so called "kernel trick", where the input data is implicitly mapped to a (usually) high dimensional feature space (Duda et al., 2001).

Complete Computer-Aided-Theragnosis System

The proposed computer-aided-theragnosis system consisted of computing the spectral parametric maps for each selected ROI; extracting texture features using predefined LBPs and data-driven texton features based on raw-pixel representations on each parametric map; using the empirical estimate of the MMD given in Equation (3) to calculate the differences between "mid-treatment" (weeks 1, 4, or 8) and "pre-treatment" QUS features for each patient; compensation for the imbalanced data distribution between the two classes of responder and non-responder; and the submission of the balanced data to a classifier (Figure 3).

EXPERIMENTAL SETUP

The developed CAT system was evaluated on 56 patients with locally advanced breast cancer receiving neoadjuvant chemotherapy. The patients involved were in the age range of 29 to 67 years and tumour sizes ranged between 2 and 15 cm. Biopsy was performed on all patients to confirm a cancer diagnosis. Clinical and pathological data were used to determine tumour response, which was evaluated based on the guidelines from the RECIST (Eisenhauer et al., 2009). Based on this evaluation, 42 patients were identified as responders and 14 as non-responders.

Ultrasound B-mode and RF data were acquired from each patient using an L14-5/60 transducer with a transmission frequency of 10 MHz and centre frequency of 7 MHz, connected to a Sonix RP (Ultrasonix, Vancouver, Canada) ultrasound device. The RF sampling rate was set at 40 MHz and the depth of focus for each patient was kept constant throughout the study. Each patient was scanned before treatment and at three times during chemotherapy, i.e., at weeks 1, 4, and 8. The patients were also scanned within one week before lumpectomy surgery, which is typically performed 4 to 6 weeks after the completion of 2-4 months of chemotherapy administration. The "pre-treatment" scans were used as the baseline, with which the subsequent "mid-treatment" scans were compared for each patient. Scans were acquired to cover the entire tumour at approximately 1 cm spacing, resulting in 3-5 image planes from the tumour in each time interval.

QUS analysis was performed on the RF data across all scans with identifiable tumour regions. Spectral parametric maps including MBF, SI, and SS were extracted from each region of interest (ROI) using the techniques explained earlier in this chapter book (refer to Figures 1 and 2 for representative MBF parametric maps computed for typical responder and non-responder patients).

The performance of the developed CAT system was evaluated on four different feature extraction methods including the two state-of-the-art texture methods explained in previous sections (i.e., the LBP and texton-based methods), GLCM as a classical texture method and the mean of intensity as one of the simplest and earliest features used in the application of cancer response monitoring (Sadeghi-Naini, Falou, Zubovits, et al., 2013). Also, two different dissimilarity measures including the kernel-based metric MMD, and $\ell 2$ norm were used in association with the texture features. As for the mean of intensity, the difference of magnitude (denoted as DoF) was naturally employed as the dissimilarity measure between the "pre-" and "mid-treatment" scans.

Implementation Details and Software

Experiments were performed on spectral parametric maps. However, only the results on the MBF were reported as it yielded the best performance among the three parameters.

After the computation of the 2D parametric maps, features were extracted using the LBPs, texton method, GLCM, or the mean of intensity. As for the LBPs, rotation invariant uniform 2 local binary patterns $\text{LBP}_{P,R}^{\text{riu2}}$ were used at multiresolutions, i.e., at several (P,R) pair values including (8,1), (16,2), and (24,3) as suggested in (Ojala et al., 2002).

For the texton-based approach, the codebook construction was performed by making one dictionary per patient. Two subdictionaries were computed on "pre-" and "mid-treatment" scans of each patient by extracting 500 random patches from each scan and submitting to a k-means clustering algorithm. The two subdictionaries were subsequently composed into one dictionary for that particular patient. Raw-pixel representation was used for patch representation and five different k values from the set of {10, 20, ..., 50} were used for codebook construction, where k represents the number of clusters. To build the histogram of textons as the feature models per scan, patches were systematically extracted from each scan with one pixel sliding over the scan, and each patch was compared to the textons in the dictionary of the corresponding patient using a Euclidean metric to find the closest match. A histogram of textons was computed in this way for each scan.

As for the GLCM, the same settings as reported in (Sadeghi-Naini et al., 2014) were used. That is, the GLCMs were computed using 8 gray levels at 4 orientations (0°, 45°, 90°, and 135°), and 1 to 10 relative pixel distances. Four second order statistics were subsequently computed on each GLCM including homogeneity, energy, contract, and correlation. These statistics were then averaged over 40 different GLCMs (computed for 4 different orientation and 10 different relative pixel distances) to generate a vector of 4 features per scan.

Since the MMD dissimilarity measure is a kernel-based metric, a kernel should be selected to facilitate the computation of formulation provided in Equation (3). Gangeh *et al.* (Gangeh, Tadayyon, et al., 2016) proposed to choose a radial basis function (RBF) kernel in clinical cancer response monitoring. To avoid overfitting due to tuning using small data samples, a self-tuning approach can be used to set the kernel width for the RBF kernel. To this end, the median of all (Euclidean) distances among the "pre-" and "mid-treatment" samples are considered as the kernel width for each subject at a specific treatment interval.

All texture analysis and machine learning techniques described in this chapter were implemented using an in-house MATLAB software application (MATLAB R2011a, Mathworks, USA). The supervised learning algorithms such as Naïve Bayes, k-NN, and SVM algorithms were implemented using PRTools (van der Heijden, Duin, de Ridder, & Tax, 2004), a MATLAB-based pattern recognition toolbox mainly developed by the Pattern Recognition Lab at Delft University of Technology.

RESULTS AND DISCUSSION

The classification of patients' responses to treatment at each time interval during the course of treatment (weeks, 1, 4, and 8) was performed by the submission of computed dissimilarities to a naïve Bayes classifier. The classification was performed in a leave-one-subject-out (LOSO) scheme. All required tunings were performed on the training set in each fold of LOSO based on validation classification accuracy. Since the majority class was undersampled during training of the classifiers to compensate for the imbalanced distribution of the data samples in the two classes of responders and non-responders, the experiments were repeated 10 times using different subsampled sets of the majority class, and the results were averaged and reported.

Figure 6 provides the results of classification using different combinations of feature extraction-dissimilarity measures discussed in this book chapter on 56 LABC patients who received neoadjuvant chemotherapy assessed at weeks 1, 4, and 8 during the course of treatment administration. Mid-band fit (MBF) and spectral intercept (SI) parametric maps have been used here as representative QUS maps, which usually result in higher performance in cancer response monitoring applications as reported in many related studies compared with the spectral slope (SS) (Banihashemi et al., 2008; Gangeh, Tadayyon, et al., 2016; Sadeghi-Naini et al., 2014; Sadeghi-Naini, Falou, Tadayyon, et al., 2013; Sadeghi-Naini, Falou, Zubovits, et al., 2013; Sannachi et al., 2015; Tadayyon et al., 2016).

Four measures were used in order to evaluate the performance of the classifier: accuracy, area under curve (AUC) of the receiver operating characteristic (ROC), sensitivity, and specificity, as reported in Figure 6. The measure of focus is the sensitivity, which measures the true positive rate of the classifier corresponding to the correctly identified non-responders. Correctly identifying refractory patients and switching to more effective treatment regimens is necessary for preventing more serious cancer effects like metastasis. In contrast, if a responder is incorrectly identified as a non-responder, additional assessment for determining the patient's status will not prove harmful. As the treatment duration lengthens, predictions for the ultimate responsiveness of the treatment improve, at least for the well performing Texton-MMD approach. The LBP-MMD approach, which was the only other well performing method in this study, instead peaked in performance at week 4 for the MBF and week 1 for the SI parametric maps, respectively. Another rival method which obtained promising results was the mean of intensity feature, which was inferior to the other methods prior to week 8, but demonstrated the highest performance once that time was reached.

The proposed texton method using MMD as a kernel-based distance measure achieved the best results for 3 out of 4 of the measures, including a very high sensitivity value of 87% in week 1 on the MBF parametric map. In general, for the MBF parametric map, almost all of the best overall results were obtained by texton-based approach using both $\ell 2$ norm and MMD, with the Texton-MMD approach clearly achieving the highest AUC. As for the SI parametric map, LBP-MMD achieved higher

Figure 6. The classifier accuracy, area under (the receiver operating characteristic) curve (AUC), sensitivity (related to the percentage of non-responders correctly identified), and specificity (related to the percentage of responders correctly identified) for binary classification between responders/non-responders over three different time periods during neoadjuvant chemotherapy administration for (A) mid-band fit (MBF) and (B) spectral intercept (SI) as two representative spectral parametric maps. Leave-one-out at subject level has been used; results shown are averaged over ten runs over different random under-sampled sets of the majority class (responders). Error bars represent the standard deviations over ten runs.

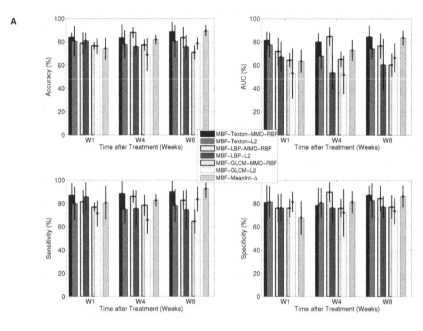

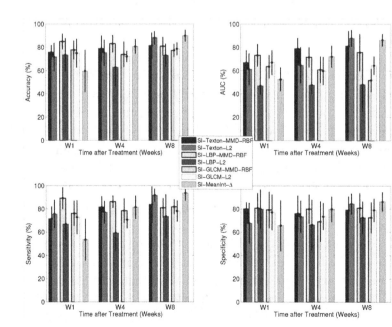

performance at week 1, whereas Texton-MMD approach outperformed at weeks 4 (at least based on the AUC measure) and 8.

Figure 6 indicates that a dissimilarity measure using a kernel-based metric such as the MMD combined with textons outperformed the mean of intensity method, i.e., representing the entire ROI with a single scalar value. Compared to using a simple Euclidean distance measure, MMD achieves much better results, except for GLCM at week 8.

FUTURE RESEARCH DIRECTIONS

Clinical imaging systems are conventionally operated by hand-held transducers, providing by default, a series of arbitrarily oriented 2-D images. 3-D reconstruction from hand-held ultrasound scanners is difficult due to the irregular spacing and orientation of the image planes. Reconstruction algorithms have been proposed with limited success. An alternative solution is the use of 3-D ultrasound imaging systems, such as ultrasound computed tomography and automated breast ultrasound (ABUS) technology (Gangeh, Raheem, et al., 2016; Zhuang et al., 2012), which have recently emerged in the market. These systems are equipped with RF data acquisition, permitting one to view ultrasound parametric images in a 3-D Cartesian volume. This can provide a better visualization of response/cell death in tumours (Figure 7). These technologies provide an operator-independent volume of the uncompressed breast (as opposed to free-hand transducers which cause breast compression during imaging), facilitating registration with other image modalities such as dynamic contrast enhanced magnetic resonance image (DCE-MRI) volume of the breast. The research on using 3-D QUS methods based on ABUS technology is an interesting avenue of research and currently underway by the authors of this book chapter.

CONCLUSION

In this book chapter, the application of a computer-aided-theragnostic system was demonstrated to predict, non-invasively, the early responses in patients with locally advanced breast cancer who received neoadjuvant chemotherapy. The CAT system was based on QUS methods as imaging system, state-of-the-art texture descriptors such as the LBPs and texton-based technique, and advanced machine learning techniques such as a kernel-based dissimilarity metric, learning from imbalanced data, and supervised learning paradigm.

Overall, the combination of a data-driven texture method and a kernel-based dissimilarly measure, i.e., Texton-MMD method, resulted in the strongest performance amongst other feature-distance combinations, particularly at week 1 using MBF spectral parametric map. The improvement was specifically important compared to the LBP-MMD approach at week 1, and the GLCM-MMD method on all weeks, which indicates the advantage of using a *data-driven* texture method over classical texture methods such as GLCM, and the texture methods relying on *predefined* operators such as the LBPs. Moreover, the performance was improved compared with the $\ell 2$ norm, which demonstrated the importance of using kernel-based dissimilarity measures in calculating the distances between the "pre-" and "mid-treatment" scans. The performance achieved by the proposed CAT system on weeks 1 and 4 validated its potential

Figure 7. Using a patented 360 degree rotating concave ultrasound transducer (Sonix Embrace Research) captures realistic, uncompressed images of a breast, while the patient lies in a comfortable prone position. The system captures 3-D ultrasound images, which is ideal for cancer detection research and treatment monitoring. A) Imaging system consisting of a bed with concave transducer in the center and a portable personal computer (PC), which handles the data acquisitions. B) LR-SI view of the reconstructed breast, C) AP-LR view, and D) AP-SI view. Photo credits: Analogic Ultrasound (Ultrasonix, Vancouver, BC).

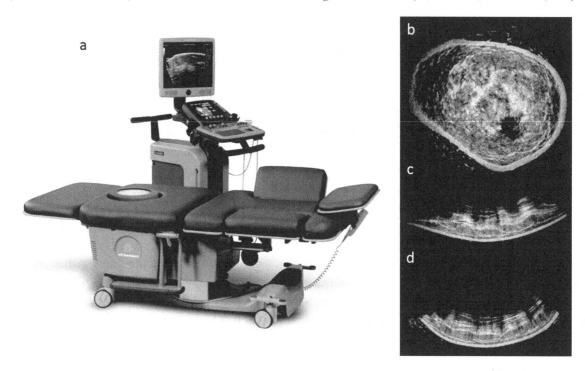

for assessing the effectiveness of treatment regimens in the early stages of neoadjuvant chemotherapy in LABC patients. Therefore, the QUS-based CAT system plays an integral role in association with other imaging modalities such as MRI and PET (Brindle, 2008) as treatment becomes more personalized and moves to molecular level.

The design of a high performance QUS-based CAT system demonstrates that cheap and accessible conventional frequency ultrasounds can effectively quantify tumour response to cancer treatment for human data. Other imaging modalities for detecting tumour response, including MRI and PET, require injecting contrast agents, prove to be less accessible, time-consuming, with the latter exposing the patients to unnecessary levels of radiation. The developed theragnostic system has been conducted using actual patient data and shown potential to be established as a clinical cancer monitoring protocol.

REFERENCES

Ahonen, T., & Pietikainen, M. (2009). Image description using joint distribution of filter bank responses. *Pattern Recognition Letters*, *30*(4), 368–376. doi:10.1016/j.patrec.2008.10.012

Alam, S. K., Feleppa, E. J., Rondeau, M., Kalisz, A., & Garra, B. S. (2011). Ultrasonic multi-feature analysis procedure for computer-aided diagnosis of solid breast lesions. *Ultrasonic Imaging, 33*(1), 17–38. doi:10.1177/016173461103300102 PMID:21608446

Banihashemi, B., Vlad, R., Debeljevic, B., Giles, A., Kolios, M. C., & Czarnota, G. J. (2008). Ultrasound imaging of apoptosis in tumor response: Novel preclinical monitoring of photodynamic therapy effects. *Cancer Research, 68*(20), 8590–8596. doi:10.1158/0008-5472.CAN-08-0006 PMID:18922935

Baraldi, A., & Parmiggiani, F. (1995). An investigation of texture characteristics associated with gray level co-occurrence matrix structural parameters. *IEEE Transactions on Geoscience and Remote Sensing, 33*(2), 293–304. doi:10.1109/36.377929

Brindle, K. (2008). New approaches for imaging tumour responses to treatment. *Nature Reviews. Cancer, 8*(2), 94–107. doi:10.1038/nrc2289 PMID:18202697

Chang, R.-F., Wu, W.-J., Moon, W.-K., Chou, Y.-H., & Chen, D.-R. (2003). Improvement in breast tumour discrimination by support vector machines and speckle-emphasis texture analysis. *Ultrasound in Medicine & Biology, 29*(5), 679–686. doi:10.1016/S0301-5629(02)00788-3 PMID:12754067

Chen, D.-R., Chang, R.-F., Chen, C.-J., Ho, M.-F., Kuo, S.-J., Chen, S.-T., & Moon, W.-K. et al. (2005). Classification of breast ultrasound images using fractal feature. *Clinical Imaging, 29*(4), 235–245. doi:10.1016/j.clinimag.2004.11.024 PMID:15967313

Cheng, H. D., Shan, J., Ju, W., Guo, Y., & Zhang, L. (2010). Automated breast cancer detection and classification using ultrasound images: A survey. *Pattern Recognition, 43*(1), 299–317. doi:10.1016/j.patcog.2009.05.012

Coleman, D. J., Lizzi, F. L., Silverman, R. H., Helson, L., Torpey, J. H., & Rondeau, M. J. (1985). A model for acoustic characterization of intraocular tumors. *Investigative Ophthalmology & Visual Science, 26*(4), 545–550. PMID:3884539

Criminisi, A., & Shotton, J. (2013). *Decision forests for computer vision and medical image analysis.* London: Springer. doi:10.1007/978-1-4471-4929-3

Cula, O. G., & Dana, K. J. (2004). 3D texture recognition using bidirectional feature histograms. *International Journal of Computer Vision, 59*(1), 33–60. doi:10.1023/B:VISI.0000020670.05764.55

Czarnota, G. J., & Kolios, M. C. (2010). Ultrasound detection of cell death. *Imaging in Medicine, 2*(1), 17–28. doi:10.2217/iim.09.34

Czarnota, G. J., Kolios, M. C., Abraham, J., Portnoy, M., Ottensmeyer, F. P., Hunt, J. W., & Sherar, M. D. (1999). Ultrasound imaging of apoptosis: High-resolution non-invasive monitoring of programmed cell death in vitro, in situ and in vivo. *British Journal of Cancer, 81*(3), 520–527. doi:10.1038/sj.bjc.6690724 PMID:10507779

Czernin, J., & Phelps, M. E. (2002). Positron emission tomography scanning: Current and future applications. *Annual Review of Medicine, 53*(1), 89–112. doi:10.1146/annurev.med.53.082901.104028 PMID:11818465

Dana, K. J., van Ginneken, B., Nayar, S. K., & Koenderink, J. J. (1999). Reflectance and texture of real-world surfaces. *ACM Transactions on Graphics*, *18*(1), 1–34. doi:10.1145/300776.300778

Diu, M., Gangeh, M. J., & Kamel, M. S. (2013). Unsupervised visual changepoint detection using maximum mean discrepancy. In *Proceedings of the 10th International Conference on Image Analysis and Recognition* (pp. 336–345). Berlin: Springer-Verlag. doi:10.1007/978-3-642-39094-4_38

Donohue, K. D., Huang, L., Burks, T., Forsberg, F., & Piccoli, C. W. (2001). Tissue classification with generalized spectrum parameters. *Ultrasound in Medicine & Biology*, *27*(11), 1505–1514. doi:10.1016/S0301-5629(01)00468-9 PMID:11750750

Duda, R. O., Hart, P. E., & Stork, D. G. (2001). *Pattern Classification (2nd ed.)*. New York: John Wiley & Sons.

Eisenhauer, E. A., Therasse, P., Bogaerts, J., Schwartz, L. H., Sargent, D., Ford, R., & Verweij, J. et al. (2009). New response evaluation criteria in solid tumours: Revised {RECIST} guideline (version 1.1). *European Journal of Cancer*, *45*(2), 228–247. doi:10.1016/j.ejca.2008.10.026 PMID:19097774

Estabrooks, A., Jo, T., & Japkowicz, N. (2004). A multiple resampling method for learning from imbalanced data sets. *Computational Intelligence*, *20*(1), 18–36. doi:10.1111/j.0824-7935.2004.t01-1-00228.x

Falou, O., Soliman, H., Sadeghi-Naini, A., Iradji, S., Lemon-wong, S., Zubovits, J., & Czarnota, G. J. et al. (2012). Diffuse optical spectroscopy evaluation of treatment response in women with locally advanced breast cancer receiving. *Translational Oncology*, *5*(4), 238–246. doi:10.1593/tlo.11346 PMID:22937175

Feleppa, E. J., Kalisz, A., Sokil-Melgar, J. B., Lizzi, F. L., Liu, T., Rosado, A. L., & Heston, W. D. W. et al. (1996). Typing of prostate tissue by ultrasonic spectrum analysis. *IEEE Transactions on Ultrasonics, Ferroelectrics, and Frequency Control*, *43*(4), 609–619. doi:10.1109/58.503779

Galar, M., Fernández, A., Barrenechea, E., Bustince, H., & Herrera, F. (2012). A review on ensembles for the class Imbalance problem: Bagging-, boosting-, and hybrid-based approaches. *IEEE Trans. on Systems, Man, and Cybernetics, Part C: Applications and Reviews*, *42*(4), 463–484. doi:10.1109/TSMCC.2011.2161285

Gangeh, M. J., El Kaffas, A., Hashim, A., Giles, A., & Czarnota, G. J. (2015). Advanced machine learning and textural methods in monitoring cell death using quantitative ultrasound spectroscopy. *Proceedings of the International Symposium on Biomedical Imaging: From Nano to Macro (ISBI)*, 646–650. doi:10.1109/ISBI.2015.7163956

Gangeh, M. J., Fung, B., Tadayyon, H., Tran, W. T., & Czarnota, G. J. (2016). Response monitoring using quantitative ultrasound methods and supervised dictionary learning in locally advanced breast cancer. *Proceedings of SPIE Medical Imaging*, 978406.

Gangeh, M. J., Hashim, A., Giles, A., & Czarnota, G. J. (2014). Cancer therapy prognosis using quantitative ultrasound spectroscopy and a kernel-based metric. *Proceedings of SPIE Medical Imaging*, 903406.

Gangeh, M. J., Hashim, A., Giles, A., Sannachi, L., & Czarnota, G. J. (2016). Computer aided prognosis for cell death categorization and prediction in vivo using quantitative ultrasound and machine learning techniques. *Medical Physics*, *43*(12), 6439–6454. doi:10.1118/1.4967265 PMID:27908167

Gangeh, M. J., Raheem, A., Tadayyon, H., Liu, S., Hadizad, F., & Czarnota, G. J. (2016). Breast tumour visualization using 3-D quantitative ultrasound methods. SPIE Medical Imaging, 979006.

Gangeh, M. J., Sadeghi-Naini, A., Diu, M., Tadayyon, H., Kamel, M. S., & Czarnota, G. J. (2014). Categorizing extent of tumour cell death response to cancer therapy using quantitative ultrasound spectroscopy and maximum mean discrepancy. *IEEE Transactions on Medical Imaging*, *33*(6), 1390–1400. doi:10.1109/TMI.2014.2312254 PMID:24893261

Gangeh, M. J., Sadeghi-Naini, A., Kamel, M. S., & Czarnota, G. J. (2013). Assessment of cancer therapy effects using texton-based characterization of quantitative ultrasound parametric images. *Proc. of the International Symposium on Biomedical Imaging: From Nano to Macro (ISBI)*, 1372–1375. doi:10.1109/ISBI.2013.6556788

Gangeh, M. J., Sørensen, L., Shaker, S. B., Kamel, M. S., & de Bruijne, M. (2010). Multiple classifier systems in texton-based approach for the classification of CT images of lung. In *Proceedings of the Medical Computer Vision: Recognition Techniques and Applications in Medical Imaging (MCV)* (pp. 153–163). Berlin: Springer-Verlag.

Gangeh, M. J., Sørensen, L., Shaker, S. B., Kamel, M. S., de Bruijne, M., & Loog, M. (2010). A texton-based approach for the classification of lung parenchyma in CT images. In *Proceedings of the International Conference on Medical Image Computing and Computer Assisted Intervention (MICCAI)* (pp. 595–602). Berlin: Springer-Verlag. doi:10.1007/978-3-642-15711-0_74

Gangeh, M. J., Tadayyon, H., Sannachi, L., Sadeghi-Naini, A., & Czarnota, G. J. (2015). Quantitative ultrasound spectroscopy and a kernel-based metric in clinical cancer response monitoring. *Proceedings of the International Symposium on Biomedical Imaging: From Nano to Macro (ISBI)*, 255–259. doi:10.1109/ISBI.2015.7163862

Gangeh, M. J., Tadayyon, H., Sannachi, L., Sadeghi-Naini, A., Tran, W. T., & Czarnota, G. J. (2016). Computer aided theragnosis using quantitative ultrasound spectroscopy and maximum mean discrepancy in locally advanced breast cancer. *IEEE Transactions on Medical Imaging*, *35*(3), 778–790. doi:10.1109/TMI.2015.2495246 PMID:26529750

Gomez, W., Pereira, W. C. A., & Infantosi, A. F. C. (2012). Analysis of co-occurrence texture statistics as a function of gray-level quantization for classifying breast ultrasound. *IEEE Transactions on Medical Imaging*, *31*(10), 1889–1899. doi:10.1109/TMI.2012.2206398 PMID:22759441

Gretton, A., Borgwardt, K., Rasch, M., Schölkopf, B., & Smola, A. (2006). A kernel method for the two-sample-problem. *Advances in Neural Information Processing Systems*, *19*, 513–520.

Gretton, A., Borgwardt, K. M., Rasch, M. J., Schölkopf, B., & Smola, A. (2012). A kernel two-sample test. *Journal of Machine Learning Research*, *13*, 723–773.

Hadjidemetriou, E., Grossberg, M. D., & Nayar, S. K. (2004). Multiresolution histograms and their use for recognition. *IEEE Transactions on Pattern Analysis and Machine Intelligence*, *26*(7), 831–847. doi:10.1109/TPAMI.2004.32 PMID:18579943

He, H., & Garcia, E. A. (2009). Learning from imbalanced data. *IEEE Transactions on Knowledge and Data Engineering, 21*(9), 1263–1284. doi:10.1109/TKDE.2008.239

Holte, R. C., Acker, L. E., & Porter, B. W. (1989). Concept learning and the problem of small disjuncts. In *Proceedings of the 11th International Joint Conference on Artificial Intelligence* (pp. 813–818). Morgan Kaufmann.

Huang, Y.-L., & Chen, D.-R. (2005). Support vector machines in sonography: Application to decision making in the diagnosis of breast cancer. *Clinical Imaging, 29*(3), 179–184. doi:10.1016/j.clinimag.2004.08.002 PMID:15855062

Insana, M. F., & Oelze, M. (2006). *Advanced ultrasonic imaging techniques for breast cancer research* (J. Suri, R. Rangayyan, & S. Laxminarayan, Eds.). Valencia, CA: American Scientific Publishers.

Jain, A. K., & Farrokhnia, F. (1991). Unsupervised texture segmentation using gabor filters. *Pattern Recognition, 24*(12), 1167–1186. doi:10.1016/0031-3203(91)90143-S

Joo, S., Yang, Y. S., Moon, W. K., & Kim, H. C. (2004). Computer-aided diagnosis of solid breast nodules: Use of an artificial neural network based on multiple sonographic features. *IEEE Transactions on Medical Imaging, 23*(10), 1292–1300. doi:10.1109/TMI.2004.834617 PMID:15493696

Julesz, B. (1981). Textons, the elements of texture perception, and their interactions. *Nature, 290*(5802), 91–97. doi:10.1038/290091a0 PMID:7207603

Kolios, M. C., & Czarnota, G. J. (2009). Potential use of ultrasound for the detection of cell changes in cancer treatment. *Future Oncology (London, England), 5*(10), 1527–1532. doi:10.2217/fon.09.157 PMID:20001791

Krishnamachari, S., & Chellappa, R. (1997). Multiresolution Gauss-Markov random field models for texture segmentation. *IEEE Transactions on Image Processing, 6*(2), 251–267. doi:10.1109/83.551696 PMID:18282921

Lee, J., Karshafian, R., Papanicolau, N., Giles, A., Kolios, M. C., & Czarnota, G. J. (2012). Quantitative ultrasound for the monitoring of novel microbubble and ultrasound radiosensitization. *Ultrasound in Medicine & Biology, 38*(7), 1212–1221. doi:10.1016/j.ultrasmedbio.2012.01.028 PMID:22579547

Lefebvre, F., Meunier, M., Thibault, F., Laugier, P., & Berger, G. (2000). Computerized ultrasound B-scan characterization of breast nodules. *Ultrasound in Medicine & Biology, 26*(9), 1421–1428. doi:10.1016/S0301-5629(00)00302-1 PMID:11179616

Leung, T., & Malik, J. (2001). Representing and recognizing the visual appearance of materials using three-dimensional textons. *International Journal of Computer Vision, 43*(1), 29–44. doi:10.1023/A:1011126920638

Lizzi, F. L., Ostromogilsky, M., Feleppa, E. J., & Others. (1986). Relationship of ultrasonic spectral parameters to features of tissue microstructure. *IEEE Trans. Ultrason. Ferroelect. Freq. Contr., UFFC-33*, 319–329.

Mamou, J., Coron, A., Hata, M., Machi, J., Yanagihara, E., Laugier, P., & Feleppa, E. J. (2010). Three-dimensional high-frequency characterization of cancerous lymph nodes. *Ultrasound in Medicine & Biology*, *36*(3), 361–375. doi:10.1016/j.ultrasmedbio.2009.10.007 PMID:20133046

Manjunath, B. S., & Ma, W. Y. (1996). Texture feature for browsing and retrieval of image data. *IEEE Transactions on Pattern Analysis and Machine Intelligence*, *18*(8), 837–842. doi:10.1109/34.531803

Materka, A., & Strzelecki, M. (1998). *Texture analysis methods - A review*. Academic Press.

Mease, D., Wyner, A. J., & Buja, A. (2007). Boosted classification trees and class probability/quantile estimation. *Journal of Machine Learning Research*, *8*, 409–439.

Mirmehdi, M., Xie, X., & Suri, J. E. (2008). *Handbook of Texture Analysis*. London: Imperial Collage Press. doi:10.1142/p547

Muneeswaran, K., Ganesan, L., Arumugam, S., & Soundar, K. R. (2005). Texture classification with combined rotation and scale invariant wavelet features. *Pattern Recognition*, *38*(10), 1495–1506. doi:10.1016/j.patcog.2005.03.021

Ntziachristos, V., & Chance, B. (2001). Breast imaging technology: Probing physiology and molecular function using optical imaging - applications to breast cancer. *Breast Cancer Research*, *3*(1), 41–46. doi:10.1186/bcr269 PMID:11250744

Oelze, M. L., OBrien, W. D., Blue, J. P., & Zachary, J. F. (2004). Differentiation and characterization of rat mammary fibroadenomas and 4T1 mouse carcinomas using quantitative ultrasound imaging. *IEEE Transactions on Medical Imaging*, *23*(6), 764–771. doi:10.1109/TMI.2004.826953 PMID:15191150

Ojala, T., Pietikäinen, M., & Mäenpää, T. (2002). Multiresolution gray-scale and rotation invariant texture classification with local binary patterns. *IEEE Transactions on Pattern Analysis and Machine Intelligence*, *24*(7), 971–987. doi:10.1109/TPAMI.2002.1017623

Petrou, M., & Sevilla, P. G. (2006). *Image Processing Dealing with Texture*. West Sussex, UK: John Wiley & Sons. doi:10.1002/047003534X

Randen, T., & Husøy, J. H. (1999). Filtering for texture classification: A comparative study. *IEEE Transactions on Pattern Analysis and Machine Intelligence*, *21*(4), 291–310. doi:10.1109/34.761261

Rastgoo, M., Lemaitre, G., Massich, J., Morel, O., Garcia, R., Meriaudeau, F., & Marzani, F. et al. (2016). Tackling the problem of data imbalancing for melanoma classification. *Bioimaging*.

Reed, T. R., & du Buf, J. M. H. (1993). A Review of recent texture segmentation and feature extraction techniques. *CVGIP. Image Understanding*, *57*(3), 359–372. doi:10.1006/ciun.1993.1024

Rice, S. D., Heinzman, J. M., Brower, S. L., Ervin, P. R., Song, N., Shen, K., & Wang, D. (2010). Analysis of chemotherapeutic response heterogeneity and drug clustering based on mechanism of action using an in vitro assay. *Anticancer Research*, *30*(7), 2805–2811. PMID:20683016

Sadeghi-Naini, A., Falou, O., Tadayyon, H., Al-Mahrouki, A., Tran, W., Papanicolau, N., & Czarnota, G. J. et al. (2013). Conventional frequency ultrasonic biomarkers of cancer treatment response in vivo. *Trasnlational Oncology*, *6*(3), 234–243. doi:10.1593/tlo.12385 PMID:23761215

Sadeghi-Naini, A., Falou, O., Zubovits, J., Dent, R., Verma, S., Trudeau, M. E., & Czarnota, G. J. et al. (2013). Quantitative ultrasound evaluation of tumour cell death response in locally advanced breast cancer patients receiving chemotherapy. *Clinical Cancer Research, 19*(8), 2163–2174. doi:10.1158/1078-0432. CCR-12-2965 PMID:23426278

Sadeghi-Naini, A., Sannachi, L., Pritchard, K., Trudeau, M., Gandhi, S., Wright, F. C., & Czarnota, G. J. et al. (2014). Early prediction of therapy responses and outcomes in breast cancer patients using quantitative ultrasound spectral texture. *Oncotarget, 5*(11), 3497–3511. doi:10.18632/oncotarget.1950 PMID:24939867

Sannachi, L., Tadayyon, H., Sadeghi-Naini, A., Tran, W. T., Gandhi, S., Wright, F., & Czarnota, G. J. et al. (2015). Non-invasive evaluation of breast cancer response to chemotherapy using quantitative ultrasonic backscatter parameters. *Medical Image Analysis, 20*(1), 224–236. doi:10.1016/j.media.2014.11.009 PMID:25534283

Schelling, M., Avril, N., Nährig, J., Kuhn, W., Römer, W., Sattler, D., & Schwaiger, M. et al. (2000). Positron emission tomography using [(18)F]Fluorodeoxyglucose for monitoring primary chemotherapy in breast cancer. *Journal of Clinical Oncology, 18*(8), 1689–1695. doi:10.1200/JCO.2000.18.8.1689 PMID:10764429

Schmid, C. (2004). Weakly supervised learning of visual models and its application to content-based retrieval. *International Journal of Computer Vision, 56*(1), 7–16. doi:10.1023/B:VISI.0000004829.38247.b0

Sharma, U., Danishad, K. K. A., Seenu, V., & Jagannathan, N. R. (2009). Longitudinal study of the assessment by MRI and diffusion-weighted imaging of tumor response in patients with locally advanced breast cancer undergoing neoadjuvant chemotherapy. *NMR in Biomedicine, 22*(1), 104–113. doi:10.1002/nbm.1245 PMID:18384182

Smeulders, A. W. M., Worring, M., Santini, S., Gupta, A., & Jain, R. (2000). Content-based image retrieval at the end of the early years. *IEEE Transactions on Pattern Analysis and Machine Intelligence, 22*(12), 1349–1380. doi:10.1109/34.895972

Sørensen, L., Gangeh, M. J., Shaker, S. B., & de Bruijne, M. (2007). Texture classification in pulmonary CT. In A. El-Baz & J. S. Sure (Eds.), *Lung Imaging and Computer Aided Diagnosis* (pp. 343–367). CRC Press.

Spaepen, K., Stroobants, S., Dupont, P., Van Steenweghen, S., Thomas, J., Vandenberghe, P., & Verhoef, G. et al. (2001). Prognostic value of positron emission tomography (PET) with fluorine-18 fluorodeoxyglucose ([18F]FDG) after first-line chemotherapy in non-Hodgkins lymphoma: Is [18F]FDG-PET a valid alternative to conventional diagnostic methods? *Journal of Clinical Oncology, 19*(2), 414–419. doi:10.1200/JCO.2001.19.2.414 PMID:11208833

Tadayyon, H., Sadeghi-Naini, A., & Czarnota, G. J. (2014). Noninvasive Characterization of Locally Advanced Breast Cancer Using Textural Analysis of Quantitative Ultrasound Parametric Images. *Translational Oncology, 7*(6), 759–767. doi:10.1016/j.tranon.2014.10.007 PMID:25500086

Tadayyon, H., Sadeghi-Naini, A., Wirtzfeld, L., Wright, F. C., & Czarnota, G. J. (2014). Quantitative ultrasound characterization of locally advanced breast cancer by estimation of its scatterer properties. *Medical Physics*, *41*(1), 12903. doi:10.1118/1.4852875 PMID:24387530

Tadayyon, H., Sannachi, L., Gangeh, M., Sadeghi-Naini, A., Tran, W. T., Trudeau, M. E., & Czarnota, G. J. et al. (2016). Quantitative ultrasound assessment of breast tumor response to chemotherapy using a multi-parameter approach. *Oncotarget*, *7*(29), 45094–45111. PMID:27105515

Tromberg, B. J., Shah, N., Lanning, R., Cerussi, A., Espinoza, J., Pham, T., & Butler, J. et al. (2000). Non-Invasive in vivo characterization of breast tumors using photon migration spectroscopy. *Neoplasia (New York, N.Y.)*, *2*(1–2), 26–40. doi:10.1038/sj.neo.7900082 PMID:10933066

Tuceryan, M., & Jain, A. K. (1998). Texture analysis. In C. H. Chen, L. F. Pau, & P. S. P. Wang (Eds.), *Handbook of Pattern Recognition and Computer Vision* (pp. 207–248). World Scientific Publishing Co.

Uniyal, N., Eskandari, H., Abolmaesumi, P., Sojoudi, S., Gordon, P., Warren, L., & Moradi, M. et al. (2015). Ultrasound RF time series for classification of breast lesions. *IEEE Transactions on Medical Imaging*, *34*(2), 652–661. doi:10.1109/TMI.2014.2365030 PMID:25350925

van der Heijden, F., Duin, R. P. W., de Ridder, D., & Tax, D. M. J. (2004). *Classification, Parameter Estimation and State Estimation*. John Wiley & Sons, Ltd. doi:10.1002/0470090154

Varma, M., & Zisserman, A. (2005). A Statistical approach to texture classification from single images. *International Journal of Computer Vision: Special Issue on Texture Analysis and Synthesis*, *62*(1–2), 61–81. doi:10.1007/s11263-005-4635-4

Varma, M., & Zisserman, A. (2009). A statistical approach to material classification using image patch exemplars. *IEEE Transactions on Pattern Analysis and Machine Intelligence*, *31*(11), 2032–2047. doi:10.1109/TPAMI.2008.182 PMID:19762929

Vlad, R. M., Brand, S., Giles, A., Kolios, M. C., & Czarnota, G. J. (2009). Quantitative ultrasound characterization of responses to radiotherapy in cancer mouse models. *Clinical Cancer Research*, *15*(6), 2067–2074. doi:10.1158/1078-0432.CCR-08-1970 PMID:19276277

Weber, W. A., Petersen, V., Schmidt, B., Tyndale-Hines, L., Link, T., Peschel, C., & Schwaiger, M. (2003). Positron emission tomography in non–small-cell lung cancer: Prediction of response to chemotherapy by quantitative assessment of glucose use. *Journal of Clinical Oncology*, *21*(14), 2651–2657. doi:10.1200/JCO.2003.12.004 PMID:12860940

Weiss, G., & Provost, F. (2001). *The effect of class distribution on classifier learning: An empirical study*. Academic Press.

Yalcin, B. (2013). Overview on locally advanced breast cancer: Defining, epidemiology, and overview on neoadjuvant therapy. *Experimental Oncology*, *35*(4), 250–252. PMID:24382433

Yang, M., Krueger, T. M., Miller, J. G., & Holland, M. R. (2007). Characterization of anisotropic myocardial backscatter using spectral slope, intercept and midband fit parameters. *Ultrasonic Imaging*, *29*(2), 122–134. doi:10.1177/016173460702900204 PMID:17679326

Yang, M.-C., Moon, W. K., Wang, Y.-C. F., Bae, M. S., Huang, C.-S., Chen, J.-H., & Chang, R.-F. (2013). Robust texture analysis using multi-resolution gray-scale invariant features for breast sonographic tumour diagnosis. *IEEE Transactions on Medical Imaging*, *32*(12), 2262–2273. doi:10.1109/TMI.2013.2279938 PMID:24001985

Zhuang, B., Chen, T., Leung, C., Chan, K., Dixon, J., Dickie, K., & Pelissier, L. (2012). Microcalcification enhancement in ultrasound images from a concave automatic breast ultrasound scanner. *Proceedings of IEEE International Ultrasonics Symposium*, 1662–1665. doi:10.1109/ULTSYM.2012.0417

KEY TERMS AND DEFINITIONS

Computer-Aided Theragnosis (CAT): A system based on machine learning algorithm(s) with the aim of predicting the response (typically cancer response) of a patient to a treatment regimen.

Gray-Level Co-Occurrence Matrix (GLCM): A statistical method of examining image texture that considers the spatial relationship of pixels, also known as the gray-level spatial dependence matrix.

Local Binary Pattern (LBP): A type of visual descriptor used for classification of images. It is a texture operator that labels the pixels of an image by thresholding the neighborhood of each pixel and considers the result as a binary number.

Maximum-Mean Discrepancy (MMD): A kernel-based approach aimed at measuring the distance between two probability distributions.

Quantitative Ultrasound Spectroscopy/ Quantitative Ultrasound (QUS): An ultrasound signal processing technique aimed at extracting frequency-dependent ultrasound parameters for the purpose of tissue characterization.

Response Evaluation Criteria in Solid Tumours (RECIST): A tumour response assessment guideline based on reduction of sum of diameters of tumour foci.

Ultrasound Imaging: In the medical field, a modality of imaging where the image is generated from the reflection of high-frequency (inaudible) sound waves from tissue(s).

Chapter 12
Application of Data Mining Techniques in Clinical Decision Making:
A Literature Review and Classification

Hakimeh Ameri
K. N. Toosi University of Technology, Iran

Somayeh Alizadeh
K. N. Toosi University of Technology, Iran

Elham Akhond Zadeh Noughabi
University of Calgary, Canada

ABSTRACT

Data mining techniques are increasingly used in clinical decision making and help the physicians to make more accurate and effective decisions. In this chapter, a classification of data mining applications in clinical decision making is presented through a systematic review. The applications of data mining techniques in clinical decision making are divided into two main categories: diagnosis and treatment. Early prediction of medical conditions, detecting multi-morbidity and complications of diseases, identifying and predicting the chronic diseases and medical imaging are the subcategories which are defined in the diagnosis part. The Treatment category is composed of treatment effectiveness and predicting the average length of stay in hospital. The majority of the reviewed articles are related to diagnosis and there is only one article which discusses the determination of drug dosage in successful treatment. The classification model is the most commonly practical model in the clinical decision making.

DOI: 10.4018/978-1-5225-2515-8.ch012

INTRODUCTION

Healthcare and medical researchers and practitioners have used different quantitative techniques in various areas of healthcare and medical decision-making. Among these techniques, statistical and artificial intelligence techniques methods have received considerable attention during the last few decades. Among these tools, data mining is becoming increasingly popular, if not increasingly essential. Different techniques of data mining are becoming of great interest and importance for healthcare practice and research. Data mining applications can greatly benefit all areas involved in the healthcare industry. For example, data mining can help healthcare insurers detect fraud, healthcare organizations make customer relationship management decisions, physicians identify effective treatments and best practices, and patients receive better and more affordable healthcare services (Koh & Tan, 2011; Berka, Rauch, & Zighed, 2009).

Based on the existing literature, we can categorize data mining applications in healthcare into three main categories: "clinical decision making", "public health" and "administration and policies". This chapter discusses data mining application in the first area. As the best of our knowledge, this is the first research which studies the applications of data mining in clinical decision making through a systematic literature review and presents a classification and framework for it. Actually, this study tries to do a systematic literature review on the application of data mining techniques in clinical decision making and presents a framework accordingly. In this regard, the exciting literature was studied. Accordingly, the applications of data mining in clinical decision making are categorized into two main categories: treatment and diagnosis. Each category has some sub-categories which are discussed in this chapter.

The organization of this chapter is as below:

At first the research methodology is explained. Next, the classification method is presented and then a classification and framework for applications of data mining in healthcare is discussed. Finally, the distribution of papers in this area is provided and the limitations and future works are discussed.

RESEARCH METHODOLOGY

The following online journal databases were searched to provide a bibliography of the clinical decision making and data mining.

- Science direct
- IEEE Transaction
- Hindawi Publishing
- Pub med
- Springer
- Weily online library
- Google scholar
- Online international conferences

Approximately 600 articles were read and reviewed. Those articles were not completely related to the subjects of applied data mining in clinical decision making were eliminated at the first step. Some conference papers with a low citations, text- books, masters and doctoral dissertations, and unpublished working papers were eliminated.

After this elimination we reached to about 200 papers for our research. Each article was reviewed again and two main categories and nine subcategories of clinical decision making were recognized. These categories and sub categories provide a comprehensive base for understanding of data mining research for clinical decision making.

CLASSIFICATION METHOD

As mentioned earlier, we categorized the applications of data mining techniques in clinical decision making into two main categories and nine sub-categories. These two categories include diagnosis and treatment that each one has some sub-categories. On the data mining side, six modeling types including classification, clustering, feature extraction, association analysis, regression and time series were recognized. We explain the categories and different types of modeling in the following in more details.

Classification Framework for Clinical Decision Making

The two main categories including diagnosis and treatment and the corresponding sub-categories are shown in Figure 1.

Figure 1. Categories and subcategories of clinical decision making

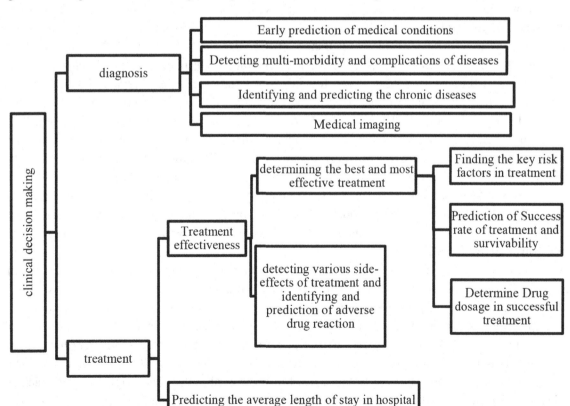

Diagnosis

Diagnosis is the act of the identification of a disease, illness, or a problem by the examination of something or someone's inspection. The diagnosis is based on information from some sources such as results of a physical examination, interview with the patient, family, or both, the medical history of the patient and family, and clinical findings that reported by laboratory tests and radiologic studies (diagnosis. In medical-dictionary online. Retrieved from http://medical-dictionary.thefreedictionary.com/diagnosis).

We have categorized the applications of data mining in diagnosis into four main categories which are: the early prediction of medical conditions, detecting multi-morbidity and complications of diseases, identifying and predicting the chronic diseases, and medical imaging.

The early prediction of medical condition involved with the prediction of disease probability and managing preventive measures in order to either prevent the disease altogether or significantly decrease its impact upon the patient. Individuals who are more susceptible to disease in the future can be offered lifestyle advice or medication with the aim of preventing the predicted illness (Abdar, Zomorodi-Moghadam, Das, & Ting, 2016; Abdi, Hosseini, & Rezghi, 2012a; Abdi, & Giveki, 2013; Aljumah, Ahamad, & Siddiqui, 2011a; Amin, Agarwal, & Beg, 2013; Aruna, Nandakishore, & Rajagopalan, 2012; Avci, 2009; Liu, Hu, Ma, Wang, & Chen, 2015; Babaoğlu, Fındık, & Bayrak, 2010a; Babaoğlu, Fındık, & Bayrak, 2010b; Balakrishnan, Narayanaswamy, Savarimuthu, & Samikannu, 2008 ; Banu, & Gomathy, 2013; Barker, et al., 2011; Bakar,Kefli, Abdullah, & Sahani, 2011; Barati, Saraee, Mohammadi, Adibi, & Ahmadzadeh, 2011; Cataloluk, & Kesler, 2012; Chang, & Chen, 2009; Chen, Xing, Xi, Chen, Yi, Zhao, & Wang, 2007; Escudero, Zajicek, & Ifeachor, 2011; Fei, 2010; Lee, Noh, & Ryu, 2007; Giri et al., 2013; Gürbüz, & Kılıç, 2014; Han, Rodriguez, & Beheshti, 2008; Harper, 2005; Harrison, & Kennedy, 2005; Heikes, Eddy, Arondekar, & Schlessinger, 2008; Hemant et al., 2012; Huang, Liao, & Chen, 2008; Karegowda, Jayaram, & Manjunath, 2012; Ilango, & Ramaraj, 2010; Ilayaraja, & Meyyappan, 2015; Inan, Uzer, & Yılmaz, 2013; Jayalakshmi, & Santhakumaran, 2010; Juan, Sen-lin, Hong-bo, Tie-mei, & Yi-wen, 2007; Karabatak, & Ince, 2009; Karimi, Amirfattahi, Sadri, & Marvasti, 2005; Karlik, & Harman, 2013; Kavitha, & Sarojamma, 2012; Kurt, Ture, & Kurum, 2008; Lekkas, & Mikhailov, 2010; Leroi, et al., 2007;Liu, et al., 2012; Luo, Wu, Guo, & Ye, 2008; Masethe, H. D., & Masethe, M. A., 2014; Meng, Huang, Rao, Zhang, & Liu, 2013; Moudani, Shahin, Chakik, & Rajab, 2011; Palaniappan, & Awang, 2008; Patil, & Kumaraswamy, 2009; Patil, Joshi, & Toshniwal, 2010b; Polat, 2012; Polat, Güneş, & Arslan, 2008; Santhanam, & Padmavathi, 2015; Soliman, Sewissy, & Abdel Latif, 2010; Soni, Ansari, Sharma, & Soni, 2011; Srinivas, Rani, & Govrdhan, 2010; Taneja, 2013; Temurtas, Yumusak, & Temurtas, 2009; Vijayarani, Dhayanand, & Phil, 2015; Wang, Richards, & Rea, 2005; Xie, Lei, Xie, Gao, Shi, & Liu, 2012; Yasodha, & Kannan, 2011; Zhao, & Ma, 2008; Zheng, Yoon, & Lam, 2014; Zuo, Wang, Liu, & Chen, 2013).

Comorbidity or more precisely multi-morbidity is a common condition, more frequent than the presence of a single disease. Complication means an unfavorable and severe evolution of a disease, a health condition or a therapy; the disease can become worse in its severity or show a higher number of signs and new signs, symptoms or new pathological changes (Ameri, & Alizadeh, 2015; Antonelli et al. 2013; Balakrishnan, Shakouri, & Hoodeh, 2013; Chan, Liu, & Luo, 2008; Chang, Wang, & Jiang, 2011; Cho, et al., 2008; Evirgen, & Çerkezi, 2014; Kasemthaweesab, & Kurutach, 2012; Lakshmi, & Kumar, 2014; Linares, et al., 2016; Marx, & Antal, 2015; McBride, et al., 2011; Nuwangi, Oruthotaarachchi, Tilakaratna, & Caldera, 2010a; Parthiban, & Srivatsa, 2012; Parthiban, Rajesh, & Srivatsa, 2011; Patel, et al., 2006; Radha, & Srinivasan, 2014; Sapna, & Tamilarasi, 2009; Skevofilakas, Zarkogianni, Karamanos, & Nikita, 2010; Tai, & Chiu, 2009; Tjandrasa, Arieshanti, & Anggoro, 2014).

The word chronic indicates a long term disease which may be controlled but not cured. Proper diagnosis, classification and prediction of the chronic diseases are essential due to the increase of disease prevalence and the augmentation of their controlling costs (Anbananthen, Sainarayanan, Chekima, & Teo, 2005; Anbarasi, Anupriya, & Iyengar, 2010; Badrinath, Gopinath, Ravichandran, & Soundhar, 2016; Chien, & Pottie, 2012; Chiu, Chen, Wang, Chang, & Chen, 2013; Dangare, & Apte, 2012; Das, Turkoglu, & Sengur, 2009; Dua, Du, SREE, & VI, 2012; Fong, et al., 2016; Huang, Chen, & Lee, 2007; Jen, Wang, Jiang, Chu, & Chen, 2012; Khanna, & Agarwal, 2013; Kolachalama, Bressloff, & Nair, 2007; Kurosaki, et al., 2010; Lahsasna, Ainon, Zainuddin, & Bulgiba, 2012; Neshat, Sargolzaei, Nadjaran Toosi, & Masoumi, 2012; Özçift, & Gülten, 2013; Polat, & Güneş, 2007; Purnami, Zain, & Embong, 2010; Sabariah, Hanifa, & Sa'adah, 2014; Sanakal, & Jayakumari, 2014; Saxena, & Sharma, 2016; Su, Yang, Hsu, & Chiu, 2006; Übeyli, & Doğdu, 2010; Xie, Lei, Xie, Shi, & Liu, 2013b; Yeh, Cheng, & Chen, 2011).

Medical imaging encompasses different imaging modalities and processes to visualize the human body for diagnostic and treatment purposes; therefore, it plays an important and initiative role in the improvement of public health (Cai, Chen, & Zhang, 2007; Celebi, Aslandogan, & Bergstresser, 2005; Chandra, Bhat, Singh, & Chauhan, 2009; Chang, & Teng, 2007; Chen, Zhang, Xu, Chen, & Zhang, 2012; El-Dahshan, Hosny, & Salem, 2010; Fu, & Zhang, 2010; Gao et al., 2010; Isa, Salamah, & Ngah, 2009; Jose, Sivakami, Maheswari, & Venkatesh, 2012; Kavitha, et al., 2016; Koley, & Majumder, 2011; Liu, Yuan, & Buckles, 2008; Ribeiro, Traina, Traina Jr, & Azevedo-Marques, 2008; Shen, Sandham, Granat, & Sterr, 2005; Smitha, Shaji, & Mini, 2011; Sulaiman, & Isa, 2010; Tabakove et al., 2006; Vimala, & Mohideen, 2013; Xu, Li, Chen, & Fan, 2013; Xuan, & Liao, 2007; Yun, & Mookiah, 2013; Zhang, et al., 2011; Zhou, Chan, Chong, & Krishnan, 2006)

Treatment

Treatment is defined as the management and medical care of a patient to combat disease or disorder (Treatment, In medical-dictionary online. Retrieved from http://medical-dictionary.thefreedictionary.com/treatment). We categorized the application of data mining in treatment into two main categories which are: treatment effectiveness and predicting the average length of stay (LOS) in hospital.

Treatment effectiveness involved with the prescription of an appropriate type of treatment, medication based on patient's demographic and clinical characteristics to improve the ability of the physicians to the rejection of nonessential measurements, time reductions and choose the best treatment type for the each group of patients. The treatment effectiveness includes two subcategories which are: determining the best and most effective treatment and detecting various side-effects of treatment and identifying and prediction of adverse drug reaction (ADR) (Arodz, Yuen, & Dudek, 2006; Bate, 2007; Chazard, Ficheur, Bernonville, Luyckx, & Beuscart, 2011; Chee, Berlin, & Schatz, 2011; Ibrahim, Saad, Abdo, & Eldin, 2016; Ji, et al., 2010a; 2011b; 2011c; 2013d; Liu, et al., 2012; Xu, & Wang, 2015). Determining the best and most effective treatment subcategory itself divided into three subcategories as finding the key risk factors in treatment which are: prediction of success rate of treatment, survivability, and determine drug dosage in successful treatment. The knowledge of the risk factors associated with disease helps health care professionals to identify patients at the high risk of disease. Data mining can present a good analysis by comparing causes, symptoms, and different patients' characteristics(Barakat, Bradley, & Barakat,

2010; Blagojević, Radović, Radović, & Filipović, 2015; Chen, Li, & Wei, 2007; Curiac, Vasile, Banias, Volosencu, & Albu, 2009; De Cos Juez, Suárez-Suárez, Lasheras, & Murcia-Mazón, 2011; Huang, Mc-Cullagh, Black, & Harper, 2007; Jilani, Yasin, Yasin, & Ardil, 2009; Kajabadi, Saraee, & Asgari, 2009; Karaolis, Moutiris, Hadjipanayi, & Pattichis, 2010; Liu, & Lu, 2009; Milewski, Malinowski, Milewska, Ziniewicz, & Wołczyński, 2010; Moon, Kang, Jitpitaklert, & Kim, 2012; Nahar, Imam, Tickle, & Chen, 2013; Noma, & Ghani, 2012; Nuwangi, Oruthotaarachchi, Tilakaratna, & Caldera, 2010b; Ordóñez, Matías, de Cos Juez, & García, 2009; Patil, Joshi, & Toshniwal, 2010a; Rajesh, & Sangeetha, 2012; Sangasoongsong, & Chongwatpol, 2012; Soni, & Vyas, 2010; Wren, & Garner, 2005). The measurement of clinical outcomes in patients is important to determine how well the treatment strategy is working. The main challenge is to report high-quality and detailed clinical outcomes in the large numbers of patients without relying on specialized data collection which can be expensive and laborious (Aljumah, Ahamad, & Siddiqui, 2013b; Bennett, & Doub, 2011; Belciug, Salem, Gorunescu, & Gorunescu, 2010b; Bertsimas et al., 2008; Chanthaweethip, & Guha, 2012; Chaurasia, & Pal, 2013; Chen, Hsu, Cheng, & Li, 2009; Cooper, Wei, Fernandez, Minneci, & Deans, 2015; Delen, Walker, & Kadam, 2005; Durairaj, & NandhaKumar, 2013; Gennings, Ellis, & Ritter, 2012; Guh, Wu, & Weng, 2011; Houthooft et al., 2015; Khan, Choi, Shin, & Kim, 2008; Kourou, et al., 2016; Kusiak, Dixon, & Shah, 2005; Lee, et al., 2012; Lin, Ou, Chen, Liu, & Lin, 2010; Liu, Sokka, Maas, Olsen, & Aune, 2009; Morales, et al., 2008; Shouman, Turner, & Stocker, 2012; Toussi, Lamy, Le Toumelin, & Venot, 2009; Tu, Wu, Hung, & Chen, 2010). A drug dose is the specific amount of medication to be taken at a given time. Determining the best drug dosage for specific patients is an important point (Yıldırım, Karahoca, & Uçar, 2011). The result of patient groups treated with different drug regimens for the same disease or condition were compared to determine the best and most cost-effective treatments actions.

Predicting the length of stay (LOS) of patients in a hospital is important in order to provide a better services and higher satisfaction for them. Moreover, it helps the manager of hospital to plan and manage the resources of hospital as meticulously as possible. Accurate inpatient LOS prediction has strong implications for health service delivery. This subcategory relies on a kind of regularity assumption demanding that patient traces of the specific treatment process as similar medical behaviors as LOS has (Azari, Janeja, & Mohseni, 2012; Belciug, 2009a; Hachesu, Ahmadi, Alizadeh & Sadoughi, 2013; Huang, Juarez, Duan, & Li, 2013a, 2014b; Houthooft, et al., 2015; Khairudin, Mohd, & Hamid, 2012; Negassa, & Monrad, 2011; Rowan, Ryan, Hegarty, & O'Hare, 2007; Suresh, Harish, & Radhika, 2015; Wu, et al., 2006; Yang, Wei, Yuan, & Schoung, 2010).

Classification Framework for Data Mining

Classification

Classification is the process of finding a model (or function) that describes and distinguishes data classes or concepts, for the purpose of being able to use the model to predict the class of objects whose class label is unknown. Classification predicts categorical (discrete, unordered) labels. The derived model is based on the analysis of a set of training data (i.e., data objects whose class label is known). The derived model may be represented in various forms, such as classification (IF-THEN) rules, decision trees, mathematical formulae, or neural networks (Han & Kamber, 2006)

Clustering

Clustering is the process of grouping the data into classes or clusters, so that objects within a cluster have high similarity in comparison to one another but are very dissimilar to objects in other clusters. Dissimilarities are assessed based on the attribute values describing the objects. Often, distance measures are used. Unlike classification and prediction, which analyze class-labeled data objects, clustering analyzes data objects without consulting a known class label. Additional advantages of a clustering-based process are that it is adaptable to changes and helps single out useful features that distinguish different groups. (Han & Kamber, 2006)

Feature Extraction

Feature extraction involves reducing the amount of resources required to describe a large set of data. In data mining approaches, feature extraction starts from an initial set of measured data and builds derived features intended to be informative and non-redundant, facilitating the subsequent learning and generalization steps, and in some cases leading to better human interpretations. Generalization on multimedia data can be performed by recognition and extraction of the essential features and/or general patterns of such data (Alpaydin, 2014; Han & Kamber, 2006).

Association Analysis

Association analysis, is useful for discovering interesting relationships hidden in large data sets. The uncovered relationships can be represented in the form of association rules or sets of frequent items. Association rule learning is a rule-based machine learning method for discovering interesting relations between variables in large databases. It is intended to identify strong rules discovered in databases using some measures of interestingness (Piateski, & Frawley, 1991; Tan, Steinbach, & Kumar, 2006).

Regression

Regression analysis is a statistical methodology that is most often used for numeric prediction, hence the two terms are often used synonymously. Regression analysis can be used to model the relationship between one or more independent or predictor variables and a dependent or response variable (which is continuous-valued). Regression analysis is a good choice when all of the predictor variables are continuous- valued as well. SVMs for regression attempt to learn the input-output relationship between input training tuples, and their corresponding continuous-valued outputs (Han & Kamber, 2006; Tan, Steinbach, & Kumar, 2006).

Time Series

A time series is a series of data points indexed (or listed or graphed) in time order or is a sequence taken at successive equally spaced points in time. Time series analysis comprises methods for analyzing time series data in order to extract meaningful statistics and other characteristics of the data. Time series forecasting is the use of a model to predict future values based on previously observed values. While regression analysis is often employed in such a way as to test theories that the current values of one or more independent time series affect the current value of another time series, this type of analysis of time series is not called "time series analysis", which focuses on comparing values of a single time series or multiple dependent time series at different points in time.(Pyle, 1999)

CLASSIFICATION OF DATA MINING APPLICATIONS IN CLINICAL DECISION MAKING

As shown in Table 1, data mining techniques have widely used in the field of clinical decision making in both diagnosis and treatment. We discuss the applications in these two categories as below:

Applications of Data Mining in Diagnosis

Several data mining and machine learning methods have developed for the diagnosis and management of disease. The employment of Computer Aided Diagnostic systems (CAD) as a "second opinion" has led to improved diagnostic decisions. Data mining techniques have widely used to either predict disease earlier or increase the success rate and decrease the decision-making time (Abdar, Zomorodi-Moghadam, Das, & Ting, 2016; Abdi, Hosseini, & Rezghi, 2012a; Abdi, & Giveki, 2013; Aljumah, Ahamad, & Siddiqui, 2011a; Amin, Agarwal, & Beg, 2013; Aruna, Nandakishore, & Rajagopalan, 2012; Avci, 2009; Liu, Hu, Ma, Wang, & Chen, 2015; Babaoğlu, Fındık, & Bayrak, 2010a; Babaoğlu, Fındık, & Bayrak, 2010b; Balakrishnan, Narayanaswamy, Savarimuthu, & Samikannu, 2008 ; Banu, & Gomathy, 2013; Barker, et al., 2011; Bakar,Kefli, Abdullah, & Sahani, 2011; Barati, Saraee, Mohammadi, Adibi, & Ahmadzadeh, 2011; Cataloluk, & Kesler, 2012; Chang, & Chen, 2009; Chen, Xing, Xi, Chen, Yi, Zhao, & Wang, 2007; Escudero, Zajicek, & Ifeachor, 2011; Fei, 2010; Lee, Noh, & Ryu, 2007; Giri et al., 2013; Gürbüz, & Kılıç, 2014; Han, Rodriguez, & Beheshti, 2008; Harper, 2005; Harrison, & Kennedy, 2005; Heikes, Eddy, Arondekar, & Schlessinger, 2008; Hemant et al., 2012; Huang, Liao, & Chen, 2008; Karegowda, Jayaram, & Manjunath, 2012; Ilango, & Ramaraj, 2010; Ilayaraja, & Meyyappan, 2015; Inan, Uzer, & Yılmaz, 2013; Jayalakshmi, & Santhakumaran, 2010; Juan, Sen-lin, Hong-bo, Tie-mei, & Yi-wen, 2007; Karabatak, & Ince, 2009; Karimi, Amirfattahi, Sadri, & Marvasti, 2005; Karlik, & Harman, 2013; Kavitha, & Sarojamma, 2012; Kurt, Ture, & Kurum, 2008; Lekkas, & Mikhailov, 2010; Leroi, et al., 2007;Liu, et al., 2012; Luo, Wu, Guo, & Ye, 2008; Masethe, H. D., & Masethe, M. A., 2014; Meng, Huang, Rao, Zhang, & Liu, 2013; Moudani, Shahin, Chakik, & Rajab, 2011; Palaniappan, & Awang, 2008; Patil, & Kumaraswamy, 2009; Patil, Joshi, & Toshniwal, 2010b; Polat, 2012; Polat, Güneş, & Arslan, 2008; Santhanam, & Padmavathi, 2015; Soliman, Sewissy, & Abdel Latif, 2010; Soni, Ansari, Sharma, & Soni, 2011; Srinivas, Rani, & Govrdhan, 2010; Taneja, 2013; Temurtas, Yumusak, & Temurtas, 2009; Vijayarani, Dhayanand, & Phil, 2015; Wang, Richards, & Rea, 2005; Xie, Lei, Xie, Gao, Shi, & Liu, 2012; Yasodha, & Kannan, 2011; Zhao, & Ma, 2008; Zheng, Yoon, & Lam, 2014; Zuo, Wang, Liu, & Chen, 2013).

Using data mining techniques help researchers and physician to understand the relationship between different life style, demographical and laboratory factors of patients and discover the most important and influential clinical and life style characteristics to avoid the complications of diseases and predict the multi-morbidity (Ameri, & Alizadeh, 2015; Antonelli et al. 2013; Balakrishnan, Shakouri, & Hoodeh, 2013; Chan, Liu, & Luo, 2008; Chang, Wang, & Jiang, 2011; Cho, et al., 2008; Evirgen, & Çerkezi, 2014; Kasemthaweesab, & Kurutach, 2012; Lakshmi, & Kumar, 2014; Linares, et al., 2016; Marx, &

Antal, 2015; McBride, et al., 2011; Nuwangi, Oruthotaarachchi, Tilakaratna, & Caldera, 2010a; Parthiban, & Srivatsa, 2012; Parthiban, Rajesh, & Srivatsa, 2011; Patel, et al., 2006; Radha, & Srinivasan, 2014; Sapna, & Tamilarasi, 2009; Skevofilakas, Zarkogianni, Karamanos, & Nikita, 2010; Tai, & Chiu, 2009; Tjandrasa, Arieshanti, & Anggoro, 2014).

Appropriate knowledge discovery from the historical data for chronic diseases would be a valuable tool for clinical researchers. Applying data mining techniques in chronic diseases data can facilitate sys-

Table 1. Data mining applications in clinical decision making

Category	Sub-Categories & Use Cases	Function	Techniques	References
Diagnosis	Early prediction of medical conditions	Classification	ANN	Harrison, & Kennedy, 2005; Karlik, & Harman, 2013
			CART, ANN and regression	Harper, 2005
			GDA +LS-SVM	Polat, Güneş, & Arslan, 2008
			ANN, Decision tree, Bayesian classifier and SVM	Chen, Xing, Xi, Chen, Yi, Zhao, & Wang, 2007
			ANN+ Levenberg–Marquardt	Temurtas, Yumusak, & Temurtas, 2009; Jayalakshmi, & Santhakumaran, 2010
			Adaptive SVM	Gürbüz, & Kılıç, 2014
			SVM +GA	Santhanam, & Padmavathi, 2015
			C4.5 & EM algorithm	Juan, Sen-lin, Hong-bo, Tie-mei, & Yi-wen, 2007
			Weighted KNN	Cataloluk, & Kesler, 2012
			PSO-SVM	Fei, 2010
			FUZZY –NN	Lekkas, & Mikhailov, 2010
			Classifier with SVM	Luo, Wu, Guo, & Ye, 2008
			Rule based, Decision tree, Naïve Bayes and ANN	Srinivas, Rani, & Govrdhan, 2010
			Random forest	Moudani, Shahin, Chakik, & Rajab, 2011
			Fuzzy KNN	Liu, et al., 2012
			Decision tree and NN	Wang, Richards, & Rea, 2005
			C5.0 and neural network	Chang, & Chen, 2009
			ID3 Algorithm and the Decision Tree	Han, Rodriguez, & Beheshti, 2008
			Decision tree, ANN, logistic regression	Meng, Huang, Rao, Zhang, & Liu, 2013
			ANN+GA	Amin, Agarwal, & Beg, 2013
			J48, Bayes Net, and Naive Bayes, Simple Cart, and REPTREE algorithm	Masethe, H. D., & Masethe, M. A., 2014
			SVM and ANN	Vijayarani, Dhayanand, & Phil, 2015
			Decision Trees, Naïve Bayes and NN	Palaniappan, & Awang, 2008; Bakar, Kefli, Abdullah, & Sahani, 2011; Taneja, 2013
			C5.0; Boosting technique; CHAID algorithm	Abdar, Zomorodi-Moghadam, Das, & Ting, 2016

continued on following page

Table 1. Continued

Category	Sub-Categories & Use Cases	Function	Techniques	References
		Clustering	K-Means clustering	Leroi, et al., 2007; Patil, & Kumaraswamy, 2009; Escudero, Zajicek, & Ifeachor, 2011; Barati, Saraee, Mohammadi, Adibi, & Ahmadzadeh, 2011
			k-means, GA and feature selection and KNN	Karegowda, Jayaram, & Manjunath, 2012
			K-means and SVM	Zheng, Yoon, & Lam, 2014; Soliman, Sewissy, & Abdel Latif, 2010
			K-Means and C4.5	Patil, Joshi, & Toshniwal, 2010b; Hemant et al., 2012; Banu, & Gomathy, 2013
			K-means with Fuzzy classifires	Polat, 2012
			KNN, Neural Networks, Classification based on clustering	Soni, Ansari, Sharma, & Soni, 2011
		Feature selection	Feature extraction with ANN	Zhao, & Ma, 2008
			Feature selection with GA +SVM	Babaoğlu, Fındık, & Bayrak, 2010b
			Feature selection with SVM	Huang, Liao, & Chen, 2008; Balakrishnan, Narayanaswamy, Savarimuthu, & Samikannu, 2008 ; Xie, Lei, Xie, Gao, Shi, & Liu, 2012
			Genetic SVM	Avci, 2009; Liu, Hu, Ma, Wang, & Chen, 2015
			Feature selection with Naïve bayes	Aruna, Nandakishore, & Rajagopalan, 2012
			PSO-SVM	Abdi, Hosseini, & Rezghi, 2012a; Abdi, & Giveki, 2013b
			SVM and K-means clustering	Ilango, & Ramaraj, 2010
			PCA+ SVM	Babaoğlu, Fındık, & Bayrak, 2010a
			FKnn	Zuo, Wang, Liu, & Chen, 2013
		Association analysis	Association rules and NN	Karabatak, & Ince, 2009
			Association rules with classifiers	Barker, et al., 2011
			Apriori with PCA and ANN	Inan, Uzer, & Yılmaz, 2013
			J48 and Bayes Network with appriori	Yasodha, & Kannan, 2011
			Association Rule Mining	Ilayaraja, & Meyyappan, 2015
		Regression	Logistic regression with CART classifier	Heikes, Eddy, Arondekar, & Schlessinger, 2008
			Regression	Aljumah, Ahamad, & Siddiqui, 2011a
			Linear regression with CART	Kurt, Ture, & Kurum, 2008; Kavitha, & Sarojamma, 2012
		Time series	Wavelet and ANN	Karimi, Amirfattahi, Sadri, & Marvasti, 2005
			Fourier and Princare plots for feature extraction + classifiers	Lee, Noh, & Ryu, 2007
			Discrete Wavelet Transform+ Gaussian Mixture Model	Giri et al., 2013

continued on following page

Table 1. Continued

Category	Sub-Categories & Use Cases	Function	Techniques	References
	Detecting multi-morbidity and complications of diseases	classification	Neural network	McBride, et al., 2011
			C5.0 and Neural network	Chan, Liu, & Luo, 2008; Ameri, & Alizadeh, 2015
			Fuzzy neural network	Evirgen, & Çerkezi, 2014; Sapna, & Tamilarasi, 2009
			Naïve Bayesian	Parthiban, Rajesh, & Srivatsa, 2011
			SVM	Parthiban, & Srivatsa, 2012
			C 5.0 and CBR	Balakrishnan, Shakouri, & Hoodeh, 2013
		clustering	K-means with RBFS	Tjandrasa, Arieshanti, & Anggoro, 2014
			Density based clustering	Antonelli et al. 2013
			expectation maximization (EM)	Patel, et al., 2006
		Feature selection	Linear SVM classifiers combined with wrapper or embedded feature selection	Cho, et al., 2008
			Logistic regression, 5.0. CHAID, executive CHAID with Voting principles	Chang, Wang, & Jiang, 2011
			feature selection by PSO Improved Fuzzy C Means (IFCM)	Radha, & Srinivasan, 2014
		Association analysis	Association rules	Tai, & Chiu, 2009
			Association rule and decision tree	Nuwangi, Oruthotaarachchi, Tilakaratna, & Caldera, 2010a
			Association rules with Apriori algorithm	Kasemthaweesab, & Kurutach, 2012
			Apriori algorithm and natural language processing	Lakshmi, & Kumar, 2014
			Bayesian networks	Marx, & Antal, 2015
			CART and other classifiers	Skevofilakas, Zarkogianni, Karamanos, & Nikita, 2010
			ecological time-series study and fit Poisson regression	Linares, et al., 2016
	Identifying and predicting the chronic diseases	classification	ANN	Anbananthen, Sainarayanan, Chekima, & Teo, 2005,; Das, Turkoglu, & Sengur, 2009; Chiu, Chen, Wang, Chang, & Chen, 2013
			Bayesian network	Kolachalama, Bressloff, & Nair, 2007
			PCA with ANFIS	Polat, & Güneş, 2007
			NN, Regression Logistic, DT, rough set	Su, Yang, Hsu, & Chiu, 2006
			C4.5	Saxena, & Sharma, 2016
			Modified spline SSVM	Purnami, Zain, & Embong, 2010
			FUZZY neural network	Lahsasna, Ainon, Zainuddin, & Bulgiba, 2012
			ANN, Decision tree, Bayesian classifier	Yeh, Cheng, & Chen, 2011

continued on following page

Table 1. Continued

Category	Sub-Categories & Use Cases	Function	Techniques	References
			3 layer artificial neural network and J48	Dangare, & Apte, 2012
			K-NN and Linear Discriminate Analysis	Jen, Wang, Jiang, Chu, & Chen, 2012
			Nonlinear features + PCA and MLP	Dua, Du, SREE, & VI, 2012
		clustering	k-means clustering	Übeyli, & Doğdu, 2010; Khanna, & Agarwal, 2013
			Fuzzy K-means with SVM	Sanakal, & Jayakumari, 2014
		Feature selection	Genetic Algorithm wrapped Bayesian Network (BN) Feature Selection	Özçift, & Gülten, 2013
			Feature extraction and SVM classifier	Chien, & Pottie, 2012; Xie, Lei, Xie, Shi, & Liu, 2013b; Badrinath, Gopinath, Ravichandran, & Soundhar, 2016
			Feature selection with genetic algorithm	Anbarasi, Anupriya, & Iyengar, 2010
		Association analysis	Integrated the decision tree induction algorithm and the case association with CBR	Huang, Chen, & Lee, 2007
			fuzzy unordered rule induction algorithm	Fong, et al., 2016
			PSO and CBR	Neshat, Sargolzaei, Nadjaran Toosi, & Masoumi, 2012
		Regression	CART	Kurosaki, et al., 2010; Sabariah, Hanifa, & Sa'adah, 2014
	Medical imaging	Classification	C 4.5 decision rules	Gao et al., 2010
			SVM and K-NN	Xu, Li, Chen, & Fan, 2013
			hybrid genetic swarm fuzzy (GSF) classifier	Kavitha, et al., 2016
			One class SVM	Zhou, Chan, Chong, & Krishnan, 2006
			SVM with Gaussian RBF kernel	Chandra, Bhat, Singh, & Chauhan, 2009
			PCA + FP-ANN and KNN	El-Dahshan, Hosny, & Salem, 2010
			ANN, logistic regression	Chen, Zhang, Xu, Chen, & Zhang, 2012
		Clustering	DBscan clustering	Celebi, Aslandogan, & Bergstresser, 2005
			fuzzy c-means (FCM) clustering with NN	Shen, Sandham, Granat, & Sterr, 2005
			two stage SOM	Chang, & Teng, 2007
			Fuzzy clustering	Isa, Salamah, & Ngah, 2009; Tabakove et al.(2006); Sulaiman, & Isa, 2010
			Fuzzy c-means	Cai, Chen, & Zhang, 2007
			cohesion based self-merging algorithm k-means	Koley, & Majumder, 2011
			K-Means Clustering and Self-Organizing Map	Yun, & Mookiah, 2013
			k-means and SVM	Vimala, & Mohideen, 2013

continued on following page

Table 1. Continued

Category	Sub-Categories & Use Cases			Function	Techniques	References
				Feature selection	Feature selection with SVM	Liu, Yuan, & Buckles, 2008; Zhang, et al., 2011
					edge density histogram and SVM .	Fu, & Zhang, 2010
					Feature selection and Adaboos classifier	Xuan, & Liao, 2007
				Association analysis	association rule-mining	Ribeiro, Traina, Traina Jr, & Azevedo-Marques, 2008; Smitha, Shaji, & Mini, 2011
					Apriori with Bayesian classifier	Jose, Sivakami, Maheswari, & Venkatesh, 2012
Treatment	Treatment effectiveness	determining the best and most cost-effective treatment	Finding the key risk factors in treatment	classification	Naïve Bayes and C5.0 with feature selection	Huang, McCullagh, Black, & Harper, 2007
					Bayesian belief networks	Liu, & Lu, 2009
					Bayesian network-based analysis	Curiac, Vasile, Banias, Volosencu, & Albu, 2009
					SVM and regression	Ordóñez, Matías, de Cos Juez, & García, 2009
					Neural network	De Cos Juez, Suárez-Suárez, Lasheras, & Murcia-Mazón, 2011; Blagojević, Radović, Radović, & Filipović, 2015
					C5.0 and Fuzzy	Karaolis, Moutiris, Hadjipanayi, & Pattichis, 2010
					SQRex-SVM	Barakat, Bradley, & Barakat, 2010
					Feature selection and C4.5	Rajesh, & Sangeetha, 2012
					logistic regression, decision tree, and ANN	Sa-ngasoongsong, & Chongwatpol, 2012
				Association analysis	Association rule	Wren, & Garner, 2005
					Multi kernerl SVM	Chen, Li, & Wei, 2007
					Apriori algorithm	Patil, Joshi, & Toshniwal, 2010a
					Margin based feature selection	Milewski, Malinowski, Milewska, Ziniewicz, & Wołczyński, 2010
					FP-tree algorithm	Noma, & Ghani, 2012
					Apriori, Predictive Apriori and Tertius	Nahar, Imam, Tickle, & Chen, 2013
					Assosiaction rule and classification	Nuwangi, Oruthotaarachchi, Tilakaratna, & Caldera, 2010b
					integrates association rule mining and classification rule mining	Soni, & Vyas, 2010
				Regression	Binary regression	Jilani, Yasin, Yasin, & Ardil, 2009
					CART regression	Moon, Kang, Jitpitaklert, & Kim, 2012; Kajabadi, Saraee, & Asgari, 2009

continued on following page

Table 1. Continued

Category	Sub-Categories & Use Cases				Function	Techniques	References
				Prediction of Success rate of treatment and survivability	classification	C5.0 with boosting	Toussi, Lamy, Le Toumelin, & Venot, 2009
						Decision tree	Shouman, Turner, & Stocker, 2012
						SVM	Aljumah, Ahamad, & Siddiqui, 2013b; Houthooft et al., 2015
						ANN, decision trees, and logistic regression	Delen, Walker, & Kadam, 2005
						Rough set theory and decision tree	Kusiak, Dixon, & Shah, 2005
						Basiyan classifier	Morales, et al., 2008
						Decision tree and NN	Khan, Choi, Shin, & Kim, 2008
						Genetic algorithm and decision tree	Chen, Hsu, Cheng, & Li, 2009
						Genetic algorithm and PSO	Guh, Wu, & Weng, 2011
						Bayesian Network, Neural Network, Random Forests,J48 Decision	Bennett, & Doub, 2011
						ANN	Chanthaweethip, & Guha, 2012
						CART, ID3, Decision table	Chaurasia, & Pal, 2013
					clustering	Clustering and classification	Bertsimas et al., 2008
						Clustering with SVM and KNN	Liu, Sokka, Maas, Olsen, & Aune, 2009
						K-means and association rule	Tu, Wu, Hung, & Chen, 2010
						Cohenen with SOM	Belciug, Salem, Gorunescu, & Gorunescu, 2010b
					Feature selection	Reduction algorithm And ANN	Durairaj, & NandhaKumar, 2013
						Wrapper feature selection with ANN predictor	Kourou, et al., 2016
					Regression	Logistic regression and ANN	Lee, et al., 2012
						Logistic regression	Gennings, Ellis, & Ritter, 2012; Cooper, Wei, Fernandez, Minneci, & Deans, 2015
						logistic regression and ANN	Lin, Ou, Chen, Liu, & Lin, 2010
				Determine Drug dosage in successful treatment	classification	Neural network(ANFIS and Rough Set methods)	Yıldırım, Karahoca, & Uçar, 2011

continued on following page

Table 1. Continued

Category	Sub-Categories & Use Cases		Function	Techniques	References
		detecting various side-effects of treatment and identifying and prediction of adverse drug reaction	classification	Bayesian confidence propagation neural network (BCPNN)	Bate, 2007
				linear discriminant analysis (LDA) with boosting	Arodz, Yuen, & Dudek, 2006
				Naïve Bayes (NB) and Support Vector Machine (SVM) with a RBF kernel	Chee, Berlin, & Schatz, 2011
				text classification(SVM), relationship extraction, signaling filtering, and signal prioritization	Xu, & Wang, 2015
				logistic regression, naïve Bayes, K-nearest neighbor, random forest and SVM	Liu, et al., 2012
			Association analysis	decision trees and association rules	Chazard, Ficheur, Bernonville, Luyckx, & Beuscart, 2011
				Fuzzy recognition	Ji, et al., 2010a; 2011b; 2011c; 2013d
				Modified Apriori	Ibrahim, Saad, Abdo, & Eldin, 2016
	Predicting the average length of stay in hospital		classification	SVM	Yang, Wei, Yuan, & Schoung, 2010
				Decision tree	Negassa, & Monrad, 2011
				ANN	Rowan, Ryan, Hegarty, & O'Hare, 2007
				decision tree, SVM, and ANN	Hachesu, Ahmadi, Alizadeh & Sadoughi, 2013
				PSO and Back propagation NN	Suresh, Harish, & Radhika, 2015
			clustering	the agglomerative hierarchical clustering	Belciug, 2009a
				K-means clustering and classifiers	Azari, Janeja, & Mohseni, 2012
			Association analysis	CBR +KNN	Huang, Juarez, Duan, & Li, 2013a
				CBR	Huang, Juarez, Duan, & Li, 2014b
			Regression	Logistic regression	Wu, et al., 2006
				Logistic regression and decision tree	Khairudin, Mohd, & Hamid, 2012
				SVM	Houthooft, et al., 2015

tematic analysis (Anbananthen, Sainarayanan, Chekima, & Teo, 2005; Anbarasi, Anupriya, & Iyengar, 2010; Badrinath, Gopinath, Ravichandran, & Soundhar, 2016; Chien, & Pottie, 2012; Chiu, Chen, Wang, Chang, & Chen, 2013; Dangare, & Apte, 2012; Das, Turkoglu, & Sengur, 2009; Dua, Du, SREE, & VI, 2012; Fong, et al., 2016; Huang, Chen, & Lee, 2007; Jen, Wang, Jiang, Chu, & Chen, 2012; Khanna, & Agarwal, 2013; Kolachalama, Bressloff, & Nair, 2007; Kurosaki, et al., 2010; Lahsasna, Ainon, Zainuddin, & Bulgiba, 2012; Neshat, Sargolzaei, Nadjaran Toosi, & Masoumi, 2012; Özçift, & Gülten, 2013; Polat, & Güneş, 2007; Purnami, Zain, & Embong, 2010; Sabariah, Hanifa, & Sa'adah, 2014; Sanakal, & Jayakumari, 2014; Saxena, & Sharma, 2016; Su, Yang, Hsu, & Chiu, 2006; Übeyli, & Doğdu, 2010; Xie, Lei, Xie, Shi, & Liu, 2013b; Yeh, Cheng, & Chen, 2011).

Medical imaging subcategory is related to a computer-aided diagnosis (CAD) system to assist the physicians to detect various wounds in medical images. It is done by merging the elements of data mining, artificial intelligence, and digital image processing with radiological image processing (Cai, Chen, & Zhang, 2007; Celebi, Aslandogan, & Bergstresser, 2005; Chandra, Bhat, Singh, & Chauhan, 2009; Chang, & Teng, 2007; Chen, Zhang, Xu, Chen, & Zhang, 2012; El-Dahshan, Hosny, & Salem, 2010; Fu, & Zhang, 2010; Gao et al., 2010; Isa, Salamah, & Ngah, 2009; Jose, Sivakami, Maheswari, & Venkatesh, 2012; Kavitha, et al., 2016; Koley, & Majumder, 2011; Liu, Yuan, & Buckles, 2008; Ribeiro, Traina, Traina Jr, & Azevedo-Marques, 2008; Shen, Sandham, Granat, & Sterr, 2005; Smitha, Shaji, & Mini, 2011; Sulaiman, & Isa, 2010; Tabakove et al., 2006; Vimala, & Mohideen, 2013; Xu, Li, Chen, & Fan, 2013; Xuan, & Liao, 2007; Yun, & Mookiah, 2013; Zhang, et al., 2011; Zhou, Chan, Chong, & Krishnan, 2006)

Different modeling types of classification, clustering, feature extraction, association analysis, regression and time series are used in this area. Some example are disused below:

For example, classification algorithms are used to find common key risk factors among patients' demographic and medicine conditions. The important of each feature is also measured. The greater understanding of the factors affecting the better understanding of diseases and can lead to the design of clinical trials, better diagnosis of the disease and enhance health care quality. Different classification methods are compared to identify the best overall accuracies in the early prediction of medical condition algorithms. This lead to create a more reliable decision support structure for physicians in identifying more influential clinical and personal features (Abdar, Zomorodi-Moghadam, Das, & Ting, 2016; Ameri, & Alizadeh, 2015; Amin, Agarwal, & Beg, 2013; Bakar,Kefli, Abdullah, & Sahani, 2011; Cataloluk, & Kesler, 2012; Chan, Liu, & Luo, 2008; Chang, & Chen, 2009; Chandra, Bhat, Singh, & Chauhan, 2009; Chen, Zhang, Xu, Chen, & Zhang, 2012; Chen, Xing, Xi, Chen, Yi, Zhao, & Wang, 2007; Evirgen, & Çerkezi, 2014; El-Dahshan, Hosny, & Salem, 2010; Fei, 2010; Gürbüz, & Kılıç, 2014; Gao et al., 2010 Han, Rodriguez, & Beheshti, 2008; Harper, 2005; Harrison, & Kennedy, 2005; Karlik, & Harman, 2013; Jayalakshmi, & Santhakumaran, 2010; Juan, Sen-lin, Hong-bo, Tie-mei, & Yi-wen, 2007; Kavitha, et al., 2016; Lekkas, & Mikhailov, 2010; Liu, et al., 2012; Luo, Wu, Guo, & Ye, 2008; Masethe, H. D., & Masethe, M. A., 2014; McBride, et al., 2011; Meng, Huang, Rao, Zhang, & Liu, 2013; Moudani, Shahin, Chakik, & Rajab, 2011; Palaniappan, & Awang, 2008; Parthiban, Rajesh, & Srivatsa, 2011; Parthiban, & Srivatsa, 2012; Polat, Güneş, & Arslan, 2008; Santhanam, & Padmavathi, 2015; Sapna, & Tamilarasi, 2009; Srinivas, Rani, & Govrdhan, 2010; Taneja, 2013; Temurtas, Yumusak, & Temurtas, 2009; Vijayarani, Dhayanand, & Phil, 2015; Wang, Richards, & Rea, 2005 Xu, Li, Chen, & Fan, 2013; Zhou, Chan, Chong, & Krishnan, 2006).

Classification method considers the impacts of different laboratory and demographic features that are presented in dataset for the severity of the diseases. Due to the severity of chronic diseases, finding accurate rules with the use of classifiers is essential. By yielding this, the gained knowledge is comprehensive and can enhance the process of decision making (Anbananthen, Sainarayanan, Chekima, & Teo, 2005; Balakrishnan, Shakouri, & Hoodeh, 2013; Chiu, Chen, Wang, Chang, & Chen, 2013; Dangare, & Apte, 2012; Das, Turkoglu, & Sengur, 2009; Dua, Du, SREE, & VI, 2012; Jen, Wang, Jiang, Chu, & Chen, 2012; Kolachalama, Bressloff, & Nair, 2007; Lahsasna, Ainon, Zainuddin, & Bulgiba, 2012; Polat, & Güneş, 2007; Purnami, Zain, & Embong, 2010; Saxena, & Sharma, 2016; Su, Yang, Hsu, & Chiu, 2006; Yeh, Cheng, & Chen, 2011).

Clustering methods are used by researchers to segment the most similar characteristics of patients into multi morbidity and complications. This help physicians to demonstrate the effectiveness of the method in the identification of patients groups with a similar examination history and the decrease or avoid of severity in complications (Antonelli et al. 2013; Banu, & Gomathy, 2013; Barati, Saraee, Mohammadi, Adibi, & Ahmadzadeh, 2011; Chang, & Teng, 2007; Cai, Chen, & Zhang, 2007; Celebi, Aslandogan, & Bergstresser, 2005; Escudero, Zajicek, & Ifeachor, 2011; Hemant et al., 2012; Isa, Salamah, & Ngah, 2009; Karegowda, Jayaram, & Manjunath, 2012; Khanna, & Agarwal, 2013; Koley, & Majumder, 2011; Leroi, et al., 2007; Patel, et al., 2006; Patil, Joshi, & Toshniwal, 2010b; Patil, & Kumaraswamy, 2009; Polat, 2012; Sanakal, & Jayakumari, 2014; Shen, Sandham, Granat, & Sterr, 2005; Sulaiman, & Isa, 2010; Soliman, Sewissy, & Abdel Latif, 2010; Soni, Ansari, Sharma, & Soni, 2011; Tabakove et al. 2006; Tjandrasa, Arieshanti, & Anggoro, 2014; Übeyli, & Doğdu, 2010; Vimala, & Mohideen, 2013; Yun, & Mookiah, 2013; Zheng, Yoon, & Lam, 2014).

Association rule mining technique determines the relations among the values of different kind of patient's attributes. The extracted frequent item set of association techniques are very easy to interpret and understand. Finding the relationship among clinical, personal and demographical patients' characteristic help doctors to find frequent item set from patient data to predict the symptoms causing disease (Anbarasi, Anupriya, & Iyengar, 2010; Abdi, Hosseini, & Rezghi, 2012a; Abdi, & Giveki, 2013b; Aruna, Nandakishore, & Rajagopalan, 2012; Avci, 2009; Babaoğlu, Fındık, & Bayrak, 2010a, 2010b; Badrinath, Gopinath, Ravichandran, & Soundhar, 2016; Balakrishnan, Narayanaswamy, Savarimuthu, & Samikannu, 2008; Barker, et al., 2011; Chang, Wang, & Jiang, 2011; Chien, & Pottie, 2012; Cho, et al., 2008; Fong, et al., 2016; Fu, & Zhang, 2010; Huang, Chen, & Lee, 2007; Huang, Liao, & Chen, 2008; Ilango, & Ramaraj, 2010; Ilayaraja, & Meyyappan, 2015; Inan, Uzer, & Yılmaz, 2013; Jose, Sivakami, Maheswari, & Venkatesh, 2012; Karabatak, & Ince, 2009; Kasemthaweesab, & Kurutach, 2012; Kurosaki, et al., 2010; Lakshmi, & Kumar, 2014; Linares, et al., 2016; Liu, Hu, Ma, Wang, & Chen, 2015; Liu, Yuan, & Buckles, 2008; Marx, & Antal, 2015; Neshat, Sargolzaei, Nadjaran Toosi, & Masoumi, 2012; Nuwangi, Oruthotaarachchi, Tilakaratna, & Caldera, 2010a; Özçift, & Gülten, 2013; Radha, & Srinivasan, 2014; Ribeiro, Traina, Traina Jr, & Azevedo-Marques, 2008; Sabariah, Hanifa, & Sa'adah, 2014; Skevofilakas, Zarkogianni, Karamanos, & Nikita, 2010; Smitha, Shaji, & Mini, 2011; Tai, & Chiu, 2009; Xie, Lei, Xie, Gao, Shi, & Liu, 2012; Xie, Lei, Xie, Shi, & Liu, 2013b; Xuan, & Liao, 2007; Yasodha, & Kannan, 2011; Zhang, et al., 2011; Zhao, & Ma, 2008; Zuo, Wang, Liu, & Chen, 2013).

Prediction the risk of disease and relationship between class of and laboratory and profile of patients based on hybrid methods of association rules and classifiers is favorable in early prediction or predict the multi-morbidity and chronic diseases.

Hybrid methods are used to enable researchers to gain the benefits of different data mining techniques (Wang, W., Richards, G., & Rea, S., 2005; Harper, P. R., 2005; Temurtas, H., Yumusak, N., & Temurtas, F., 2009; Jayalakshmi, T., & Santhakumaran, A., 2010; Santhanam, T., & Padmavathi, M. S., 2015; Juan, G., Sen-lin, L., Hong-bo, J., Tie-mei, Z., & Yi-wen, H., 2007; Fei, S. W., 2010; Lekkas, S., & Mikhailov, L. 2010). Use of Clustering with Feature selection and clustering with classifications as hybrid techniques make more accurate algorithms to predict the diseases (Karegowda, A. G., Jayaram, M. A., & Manjunath, A. S., 2012; Zheng, B., Yoon, S. W., & Lam, S. S., 2014; Soliman, T. H. A., Sewissy, A. A., & AbdelLatif, H., 2010; Patil, B. M., Joshi, R. C., & Toshniwal, D., 2010; Hemant, P., & Pushpavathi, T., 2012). Hybrid feature selection algorithms made more suitable methods which help researchers to find the best and more effective features for the classification and clustering methods as their inputs to early predict of medical conditions (Zhao, Z., & Ma, C., 2008; Babaoglu, İ., Findik, O., & Ülker, E., 2010; Huang, C. L., Liao, H. C., & Chen, M. C., 2008; Balakrishnan, S., Narayanaswamy, R., Savarimuthu, N., & Samikannu, R., 2008; Avci.E, 2009; Abdi, M. J., Hosseini, S. M., & Rezghi, M., 2012; Abdi, M. J., & Giveki, D.,2013; Ilango, B. S., & Ramaraj, N., 2010; Babaoğlu, I., Fındık, O., & Bayrak, M.,2010; Zuo, W. L., Wang, Z. Y., Liu, T., & Chen, H. L., 2013).

Applications of Data Mining in Treatment

Data mining techniques have been widely used in different dimensions of treatment. Data mining applications enables patients, doctors and everybody in a health care industry to make better decisions for the treatment of the large number of diseases at their early stages. The planning can be done by the development of some strategic solutions based on data mining for the treatment of the disease. We categorized the application of data mining in treatment into two main categories which are: treatment effectiveness and predicting the average length of stay (LOS) in hospital (Azari, Janeja, & Mohseni, 2012; Belciug, 2009a; Hachesu, Ahmadi, Alizadeh & Sadoughi, 2013; Huang, Juarez, Duan, & Li, 2013a, 2014b; Houthooft, et al., 2015; Khairudin, Mohd, & Hamid, 2012; Negassa, & Monrad, 2011; Rowan, Ryan, Hegarty, & O'Hare, 2007; Suresh, Harish, & Radhika, 2015; Wu, et al., 2006; Yang, Wei, Yuan, & Schoung, 2010).The treatment effectiveness includes two subcategories which are: determining the best and most effective treatment and detecting various side-effects of treatment and identifying and prediction of adverse drug reaction (ADR).

Application of data mining in analyzing the medical data to the best and most effective treatment is a good method for considering the existing relationships between different variables such as demographic, clinical, regimes and life style. Data mining techniques are powerful tools to do this. Drug side-effects, or adverse drug reactions, have become a major public health concern. It is one of the main causes of failure in the process of drug development, and of drug withdrawal once they have reached the market. Various number of conditions related to laboratory results, diseases, drug administration, and demographics can influence a person response to drug therapy. Data mining is used to enhance the early detection of previously unknown possible drug-ADR relationships, by highlighting combination of data mining methods that stand out quantitatively for clinical review (Arodz, Yuen, & Dudek, 2006; Bate, 2007; Chazard, Ficheur, Bernonville, Luyckx, & Beuscart, 2011; Chee, Berlin, & Schatz, 2011; Ibrahim, Saad, Abdo, & Eldin, 2016; Ji, et al., 2010a; 2011b; 2011c; 2013d; Liu, et al., 2012; Xu, & Wang, 2015).

Determining the best and most effective treatment subcategory itself divided into three subcategories as finding the key risk factors in treatment which are: Prediction of success rate of treatment, survivability, and Determine drug dosage in successful treatment. The Knowledge of the risk factors associated with disease helps health care professionals to identify patients at the high risk of disease. Data mining can present a good analysis by comparing causes, symptoms, and different patients' characteristics (Barakat, Bradley, & Barakat, 2010; Blagojević, Radović, Radović, & Filipović, 2015; Chen, Li, & Wei, 2007; Curiac, Vasile, Banias, Volosencu, & Albu, 2009; De Cos Juez, Suárez-Suárez, Lasheras, & Murcia-Mazón, 2011; Huang, McCullagh, Black, & Harper, 2007; Jilani, Yasin, Yasin, & Ardil, 2009; Kajabadi, Saraee, & Asgari, 2009; Karaolis, Moutiris, Hadjipanayi, & Pattichis, 2010; Liu, & Lu, 2009; Milewski, Malinowski, Milewska, Ziniewicz, & Wołczyński, 2010; Moon, Kang, Jitpitaklert, & Kim, 2012; Nahar, Imam, Tickle, & Chen, 2013; Noma, & Ghani, 2012; Nuwangi, Oruthotaarachchi, Tilakaratna, & Caldera, 2010b; Ordóñez, Matías, de Cos Juez, & García, 2009; Patil, Joshi, & Toshniwal, 2010a; Rajesh, & Sangeetha, 2012; Sa-ngasoongsong, & Chongwatpol, 2012; Soni, & Vyas, 2010; Wren, & Garner, 2005).

The measurement of clinical outcomes in patients is important to determine how well the treatment strategy is working. The main challenge is to report high-quality and detailed clinical outcomes in the large numbers of patients without relying on specialized data collection which can be expensive and laborious (Aljumah, Ahamad, & Siddiqui, 2013b; Bennett, & Doub, 2011; Belciug, Salem, Gorunescu, & Gorunescu, 2010b; Bertsimas et al., 2008; Chanthaweethip, & Guha, 2012; Chaurasia, & Pal, 2013; Chen, Hsu, Cheng, & Li, 2009; Cooper, Wei, Fernandez, Minneci, & Deans, 2015; Delen, Walker, & Kadam, 2005; Durairaj, & NandhaKumar, 2013; Gennings, Ellis, & Ritter, 2012; Guh, Wu, & Weng, 2011; Houthooft et al., 2015; Khan, Choi, Shin, & Kim, 2008; Kourou, et al., 2016; Kusiak, Dixon, & Shah, 2005; Lee, et al., 2012; Lin, Ou, Chen, Liu, & Lin, 2010; Liu, Sokka, Maas, Olsen, & Aune, 2009; Morales, et al., 2008; Shouman, Turner, & Stocker, 2012; Toussi, Lamy, Le Toumelin, & Venot, 2009; Tu, Wu, Hung, & Chen, 2010). A drug dose is the specific amount of medication to be taken at a given time. Determining the best drug dosage for specific patients is an important point. The result of patient groups treated with different drug regimens for the same disease or condition were compared to determine the best and most cost-effective treatments actions. Data mining can give researchers and physicians a good insight about the best drug dosage for the each patient's group (Yıldırım, Karahoca, & Uçar, 2011).

Different modeling types of classification, clustering, feature extraction, association analysis, and time series are used in this area. Some example are disused below:

The aim of the supervised classification system is to improve the overall success rate of treatment. For example, the classification methods are used in the identification of the most significant factors (Barakat, Bradley, & Barakat, 2010; Blagojević, Radović, Radović, & Filipović, 2015; Curiac, Vasile, Banias, Volosencu, & Albu, 2009; De Cos Juez, Suárez-Suárez, Lasheras, & Murcia-Mazón, 2011; Karaolis, Moutiris, Hadjipanayi, & Pattichis, 2010; Liu, & Lu, 2009; Ordóñez, Matías, de Cos Juez, & García, 2009; Sa-ngasoongsong, & Chongwatpol, 2012) and the relationship between a disease and diet and patients' lifestyle habits that cause some important diseases and their correlations, as well as finding the common important factors among patients' demographic, clinical characteristics, type of insurance, and the length of stay in hospital (Hachesu, Ahmadi, Alizadeh & Sadoughi, 2013; Negassa, & Monrad, 2011; Rowan, Ryan, Hegarty, & O'Hare, 2007; Suresh, Harish, & Radhika, 2015; Yang, Wei, Yuan, & Schoung, 2010).

Different classifier algorithms such as CART, C5.0, KNN, ANN and SVM with different feature selection techniques are compared to classify clinical data and predict the likelihood of a patient whether being affected with a specific disease or not (Huang, McCullagh, Black, & Harper, 2007; Rajesh, & Sangeetha, 2012). The classification methods are used to predict the ability of multiple prediction models for the survivability of patients (Aljumah, Ahamad, & Siddiqui, 2013b; Bennett, & Doub, 2011; Chanthaweethip, & Guha, 2012; Chaurasia, & Pal, 2013; Chen, Hsu, Cheng, & Li, 2009; Delen, Walker, & Kadam, 2005; Guh, Wu, & Weng, 2011; Houthooft et al., 2015; Khan, Choi, Shin, & Kim, 2008; Kusiak, Dixon, & Shah, 2005; Morales, et al., 2008; Shouman, Turner, & Stocker, 2012; Toussi, Lamy, Le Toumelin, & Venot, 2009).

Regression algorithms are used to gain useful relationships among the risk factors in diseases and estimate the relative risk for survivability of various medical conditions. The factors that have higher prevalence of the risk of disease can be found by data mining approaches and regression (Jilani, Yasin, Yasin, & Ardil, 2009; Kajabadi, Saraee, & Asgari, 2009; Moon, Kang, Jitpitaklert, & Kim, 2012).

The supervised rule induction methods (decision trees and association rules) are used to discover ADR detection rules, with respect to time constraints. Data mining algorithms are used to evaluate the associations between a drug and all potential ADRs in a real-world electronic health database (Arodz, Yuen, & Dudek, 2006; Bate, 2007; Chazard, Ficheur, Bernonville, Luyckx, & Beuscart, 2011; Chee, Berlin, & Schatz, 2011; Ibrahim, Saad, Abdo, & Eldin, 2016; Ji, et al., 2010a; 2011b; 2011c; 2013d; Liu, et al., 2012; Xu, & Wang, 2015).

Hybrid methods of clustering with classifiers are used to find the most successful treatment method and rate the survivability of patients (Belciug, Salem, Gorunescu, & Gorunescu, 2010b; Bertsimas et al., 2008; Liu, Sokka, Maas, Olsen, & Aune, 2009; Tu, Wu, Hung, & Chen, 2010).

In addition, hierarchical clustering approach is used for grouping the patients according to their length of stay in the hospital to enhance the capability of hospital resource management (Azari, Janeja, & Mohseni, 2012; Belciug, 2009a).

DISTRIBUTION OF PAPERS

The distribution of articles classified by the proposed classification model is shown in Table 2. Articles in decision making and data mining models are classified into two important categories which are diagnosis as well as treatment. Among them, data mining is mainly used in diagnosis (134 out of 203 articles, 66%). In addition, there were 65 articles presented for the early prediction of medical conditions, 22 articles for detecting multi-morbidity and complications of diseases, 21 articles for Identifying and predicting the chronic diseases, as well as 26 articles for the medical imaging.

Among the 69 treatment articles (34% of the all articles), 82.6% (57 articles) of them are related to the treatment effectiveness and 17.4% (12 articles) are related to predicting the average length of stay in hospital. 46 of 57 articles (80.7%) are related to determining the best and most cost-effective treatment. Moreover, 19.3% (11 out of 57) are about detecting various side-effects of treatment, identification, and the prediction of adverse drug reaction. Finally, 17.4% (12 out of 69 articles) are about Predicting the average length of stay in hospital.

The distribution of the articles by their publication year is shown in Figure 2.

CONCLUSION, RESEARCH IMPLICATIONS, AND LIMITATIONS

The data mining techniques are increasingly used in clinical decision support systems in order to aid physicians in the procedure of decision making. By the consideration of the data mining techniques they will be able to make more accurate and effective decisions, minimize medical faults, improve patient safety, as well as reduce costs. This chapter identifies 203 articles which are related to the applications of data mining techniques in clinical decision making. In addition, they are published between 2005 and 2016. The aim of the chapter is to give a research summary on the applications of data mining in the domain of clinical decision making and the introduction of most often used techniques. Although this review cannot claim to be exhaustive and comprehensive; however it presents a general framework and classification of the researches in this field and provides good insights for the researchers in this area. The presented results in this paper have several important implications:

Figure 2. The distribution of the articles by their publication year

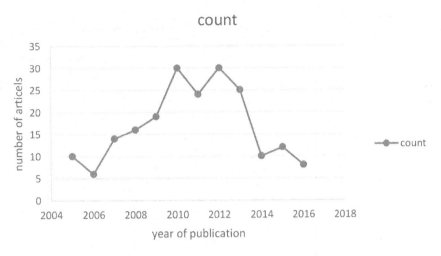

Table 2. Distribution of papers by clinical decision making and data mining categories

Dimension			Elements	Data Mining Model		Amount		
					65			
Diagnosis			Early prediction of medical conditions	Classification		28		
				Clustering		12		
				Feature selection		13		
				Association analysis		5		
				Regression		4		
				Time series		3		
					22			
			Detecting multi-morbidity and complications of diseases	Classification		8		
				Clustering		3		
				Feature selection		3		
				Association analysis		7		
					26			
			Identifying and predicting the chronic diseases	Classification		13		
				Clustering		3		
				Feature selection		5		
				Association analysis		3		
				Regression		2		
					22			
			Medical imaging	Classification		7		
				Clustering		8		
				Feature selection		4		
				Association analysis		3		

continued on following page

Table 2. Continued

Dimension			Elements	Data Mining Model	Amount			
								134
					22			
Treatment	Treatment effectiveness	determining the best and most cost-effective treatment	Finding the risk factors in treatment	Classification		10		
				Association analysis		8		
				Regression		4		
					23			
			Prediction the Success rate of treatment and survivability	Classification		13		
				Clustering		4		
				Feature selection		2		
				Regression		4		
					1			
			Determine Drug dosage in successful treatment	Classification		1		
							46	
					11			
		detecting various side-effects of treatment and identifying and prediction of adverse drug reaction		Classification		5		
				Association analysis		6		
							11	
								57
					12			
		Predicting the average length of stay in hospital		Classification		5		
				Clustering		2		
				Association analysis		2		
				Regression		3		
							12	12
							69	
					203	203	203	203

- The majority of the reviewed articles are related to diagnosis. By this taken into account, the 48.5% (65 articles) and 19.4% (26 articles) of them are related to early the prediction of medical conditions as well as the identification and prediction of the chronic diseases respectively. These articles could provide an insight to policy makers of organizations on the common data mining practices used in diagnosis of patients' medical conditions.

- Among the 46 articles related to the determination of the best and most cost-effective treatment category, only one of them discusses about the determination of drug dosage in successful treatment subcategory. The determination of drug dosage is very important in treatment stage and can be affected by many different factors. Furthermore, data mining techniques could be applied to discover unseen patterns of drug dosage from the determination of the best and most cost-effective treatment category database.

- Relatively fewer articles are discussing about the detection of the various side-effects of treatment as well as the identification and prediction of adverse drug reaction. The data mining techniques, such as neural networks and decision trees could be used to seek the most important risk factors of patients through the analysis of patient's laboratory results, diseases, drug administration, and demographics. Despite the fewer number of articles related to the detection of various side-effects of treatment, and the identification as well as prediction of adverse drug reaction, it does not mean that the application of data mining in this aspect is less mature than the others.
- The classification model is the most commonly practical model in the clinical decision making. This is not surprising that the classification models could be used to predict the effectiveness or profitableness of treatment and diagnosis through the clinical decision making strategy.
- Among the 203 articles, 43 papers have described the neural networks in the clinical decision making. Neural networks are used in classification, clustering, and prediction.
- In the case of popularity, after neural networks, decision trees and association rule mining techniques are placed in the next levels. Their logics are easier and more understandable by physicians and medical researchers than neural networks. Therefore, the two mentioned techniques could be a good choice for non-experts in data mining.

This study might have some limitations. Firstly, the surveyed articles are just published between 2005 and 2016, which were extracted based on some keywords such as "clinical decision making", "diagnosis", "treatment", "drugs", "survivability", "multi morbidity" and "data mining". Some other relevant articles which do not have that keywords could not be extracted. Secondly, in this research the articles just from the six online databases are used. There might be other academic journals which may be able to provide a more comprehensive picture of the articles related to the application of data mining in clinical decision making. Lastly, non-English publications were excluded in this study.

REFERENCES

Abdar, M., Zomorodi-Moghadam, M., Das, R., & Ting, I. H. (2016). (in press). Performance analysis of classification algorithms on early detection of Liver disease. *Expert Systems with Applications*.

Abdi, M. J., & Giveki, D. (2013b). Automatic detection of erythemato-squamous diseases using PSO–SVM based on association rules. *Engineering Applications of Artificial Intelligence*, 26(1), 603–608. doi:10.1016/j.engappai.2012.01.017

Abdi, M. J., Hosseini, S. M., & Rezghi, M. (2012a). A novel weighted support vector machine based on particle swarm optimization for gene selection and tumor classification. *Computational and Mathematical Methods in Medicine*.

Aljumah, A. A., Ahamad, M. G., & Siddiqui, M. K. (2011a). Predictive Analysis on Hypertension Treatment Using Data Mining Approach in Saudi Arabia. *Intelligent Information Management*, 3(6), 252–261. doi:10.4236/iim.2011.36031

Aljumah, A. A., Ahamad, M. G., & Siddiqui, M. K. (2013b). Application of data mining: Diabetes health care in young and old patients. *Journal of King Saud University-Computer and Information Sciences*, 25(2), 127–136. doi:10.1016/j.jksuci.2012.10.003

Alpaydin, E. (2014). *Introduction to machine learning*. MIT Press.

Ameri, H., & Alizadeh, S. (2015). Predicting complications of type 2 diabetes using decision tree algorithms. *Journal of Mitteilungen Saechsischer Entomologen, 114*, 1011–1028.

Amin, S. U., Agarwal, K., & Beg, R. (2013, April). Genetic neural network based data mining in prediction of heart disease using risk factors. In *Information & Communication Technologies (ICT), IEEE Conference on* (pp. 1227-1231). IEEE.

Anbananthen, S. K., Sainarayanan, G., Chekima, A., & Teo, J. (2005, November). Data mining using Artificial Neural network tree. In *Computers, Communications, & Signal Processing with Special Track on Biomedical Engineering, 2005. CCSP 2005. 1st International Conference on* (pp. 160-164). IEEE.

Anbarasi, M., Anupriya, E., & Iyengar, N. C. S. N. (2010). Enhanced prediction of heart disease with feature subset selection using genetic algorithm. *International Journal of Engineering Science and Technology, 2*(10), 5370–5376.

Antonelli, D., Baralis, E., Bruno, G., Cerquitelli, T., Chiusano, S., & Mahoto, N. (2013). Analysis of diabetic patients through their examination history. *Expert Systems with Applications, 40*(11), 4672–4678. doi:10.1016/j.eswa.2013.02.006

Arodz, T., Yuen, D. A., & Dudek, A. Z. (2006). Ensemble of linear models for predicting drug properties. *Journal of Chemical Information and Modeling, 46*(1), 416–423. doi:10.1021/ci050375+

Aruna, S., Nandakishore, L. V., & Rajagopalan, S. P. (2012). A hybrid feature selection method based on IGSBFS and naïve bayes for the diagnosis of erythemato-squamous diseases. *International Journal of Computers and Applications, 41*(7).

Avci, E. (2009). A new intelligent diagnosis system for the heart valve diseases by using genetic-SVM classifier. *Expert Systems with Applications, 36*(7), 10618–10626. doi:10.1016/j.eswa.2009.02.053

Azari, A., Janeja, V. P., & Mohseni, A. (2012, December). Predicting hospital length of stay (PHLOS): A multi-tiered data mining approach. In *2012 IEEE 12th International Conference on Data Mining Workshops* (pp. 17-24). IEEE.

Babaoğlu, I., Fındık, O., & Bayrak, M. (2010a). Effects of principle component analysis on assessment of coronary artery diseases using support vector machine. *Expert Systems with Applications, 37*(3), 2182–2185. doi:10.1016/j.eswa.2009.07.055

Babaoglu, İ., Findik, O., & Ülker, E. (2010b). A comparison of feature selection models utilizing binary particle swarm optimization and genetic algorithm in determining coronary artery disease using support vector machine. *Expert Systems with Applications, 37*(4), 3177–3183. doi:10.1016/j.eswa.2009.09.064

Badrinath, N., Gopinath, G., Ravichandran, K. S., & Soundhar, R. G. (2016). Estimation of automatic detection of erythemato-squamous diseases through adaboost and its hybrid classifiers. *Artificial Intelligence Review, 45*(4), 471–488. doi:10.1007/s10462-015-9436-8

Bakar, A. A., Kefli, Z., Abdullah, S., & Sahani, M. (2011, July). Predictive models for dengue outbreak using multiple rulebase classifiers. In *Electrical Engineering and Informatics (ICEEI), 2011 International Conference on* (pp. 1-6). IEEE. doi:10.1109/ICEEI.2011.6021830

Balakrishnan, S., Narayanaswamy, R., Savarimuthu, N., & Samikannu, R. (2008, October). SVM ranking with backward search for feature selection in type II diabetes databases. In *Systems, Man and Cybernetics, 2008. SMC 2008. IEEE International Conference on* (pp. 2628-2633). IEEE. doi:10.1109/ICSMC.2008.4811692

Balakrishnan, V., Shakouri, M. R., & Hoodeh, H. (2013). Developing a hybrid predictive system for retinopathy. *Journal of Intelligent & Fuzzy Systems*, *25*(1), 191–199.

Banu, M. N., & Gomathy, B. (2013). Disease Predicting System Using Data Mining Techniques. *International Journal of Technical Research and Applications*, *1*(5), 41–45.

Barakat, N., Bradley, A. P., & Barakat, M. N. H. (2010). Intelligible support vector machines for diagnosis of diabetes mellitus. *IEEE Transactions on Information Technology in Biomedicine*, *14*(4), 1114–1120. doi:10.1109/TITB.2009.2039485

Barati, E., Saraee, M., Mohammadi, A., Adibi, N., & Ahmadzadeh, M. R. (2011). A survey on utilization of data mining approaches for dermatological (skin) diseases prediction. *Journal of Selected Areas in Health Informatics*, *2*(3), 1–11.

Bate, A. (2007). Bayesian confidence propagation neural network. *Drug Safety*, *30*(7), 623–625. doi:10.2165/00002018-200730070-00011

Belciug, S. (2009a). Patient's length of stay grouping using the hierarchical clustering algorithm. *Annals of the University of Craiova-Mathematics and Computer Science Series*, *36*(2), 79–84.

Belciug, S., Salem, A. B., Gorunescu, F., & Gorunescu, M. (2010b, November). Clustering-based approach for detecting breast cancer recurrence. In *2010 10th International Conference on Intelligent Systems Design and Applications* (pp. 533-538). IEEE.

Bennett, C., & Doub, T. (2011). *Data mining and electronic health records: selecting optimal clinical treatments in practice.* arXiv preprint arXiv:1112.1668

Berka, P., Rauch, J., & Zighed, D. A. (2009). *Data Mining and Medical Knowledge Management: Cases and Applications*. IGI Global. doi:10.4018/978-1-60566-218-3

Bertsimas, D., Bjarnadóttir, M. V., Kane, M. A., Kryder, J. C., Pandey, R., Vempala, S., & Wang, G. (2008). Algorithmic prediction of health-care costs. *Operations Research*, *56*(6), 1382–1392. doi:10.1287/opre.1080.0619

Blagojević, M. D., Radović, M. D., Radović, M. M., & Filipović, N. D. (2015, November). Neural network based approach for predicting maximal wall shear stress in the artery. In *Bioinformatics and Bioengineering (BIBE), 2015 IEEE 15th International Conference on* (pp. 1-5). IEEE.

Cai, W., Chen, S., & Zhang, D. (2007). Fast and robust fuzzy c-means clustering algorithms incorporating local information for image segmentation. *Pattern Recognition*, *40*(3), 825–838. doi:10.1016/j.patcog.2006.07.011

Cataloluk, H., & Kesler, M. (2012, July). A diagnostic software tool for skin diseases with basic and weighted K-NN. In *Innovations in Intelligent Systems and Applications (INISTA), 2012 International Symposium on* (pp. 1-4). IEEE. doi:10.1109/INISTA.2012.6246999

Celebi, M. E., Aslandogan, Y. A., & Bergstresser, P. R. (2005, April). Mining biomedical images with density-based clustering. In *International Conference on Information Technology: Coding and Computing (ITCC'05): Vol. 2.* (Vol. 1, pp. 163-168). IEEE.

Chan, C. L., Liu, Y. C., & Luo, S. H. (2008, June). Investigation of diabetic microvascular complications using data mining techniques. In *2008 IEEE International Joint Conference on Neural Networks (IEEE World Congress on Computational Intelligence)* (pp. 830-834). IEEE. doi:10.1109/IJCNN.2008.4633893

Chandra, S., Bhat, R., Singh, H., & Chauhan, D. S. (2009). Detection of brain tumors from MRI using gaussian RBF kernel based support vector machine. *IJACT: International Journal of Advancements in Computing Technology, 1*(1), 46–51. doi:10.4156/ijact.vol1.issue1.7

Chang, C. D., Wang, C. C., & Jiang, B. C. (2011). Using data mining techniques for multi-diseases prediction modeling of hypertension and hyperlipidemia by common risk factors. *Expert Systems with Applications, 38*(5), 5507–5513. doi:10.1016/j.eswa.2010.10.086

Chang, C. L., & Chen, C. H. (2009). Applying decision tree and neural network to increase quality of dermatologic diagnosis. *Expert Systems with Applications, 36*(2), 4035–4041. doi:10.1016/j.eswa.2008.03.007

Chang, P. L., & Teng, W. G. (2007, June). Exploiting the self-organizing map for medical image segmentation. In *Twentieth IEEE International Symposium on Computer-Based Medical Systems (CBMS'07)* (pp. 281-288). IEEE. doi:10.1109/CBMS.2007.48

Chanthaweethip, W., & Guha, S. (2012). Temporal data mining and visualization for treatment outcome prediction in HIV patients. *Procedia Computer Science, 13*, 68–79. doi:10.1016/j.procs.2012.09.115

Chaurasia, V., & Pal, S. (2013). Early prediction of heart diseases using data mining techniques. *Carib. j. Sciences et Techniques (Paris), 1*, 208–217.

Chazard, E., Ficheur, G., Bernonville, S., Luyckx, M., & Beuscart, R. (2011). Data mining to generate adverse drug events detection rules. *IEEE Transactions on Information Technology in Biomedicine, 15*(6), 823–830. doi:10.1109/TITB.2011.2165727

Chee, B. W., Berlin, R., & Schatz, B. (2011, December). Predicting adverse drug events from personal health messages. *AMIA ... Annual Symposium Proceedings / AMIA Symposium. AMIA Symposium, 2011*, 217–226.

Chen, C. C., Hsu, C. C., Cheng, Y. C., & Li, S. T. (2009, June). Knowledge Discovery on In Vitro Fertilization Clinical Data Using Particle Swarm Optimization. In *Bioinformatics and BioEngineering, 2009. BIBE'09. Ninth IEEE International Conference on* (pp. 278-283). IEEE.

Chen, H., Zhang, J., Xu, Y., Chen, B., & Zhang, K. (2012). Performance comparison of artificial neural network and logistic regression model for differentiating lung nodules on CT scans. *Expert Systems with Applications, 39*(13), 11503–11509. doi:10.1016/j.eswa.2012.04.001

Chen, J., Xing, Y., Xi, G., Chen, J., Yi, J., Zhao, D., & Wang, J. (2007, June). A comparison of four data mining models: Bayes, neural network, SVM and decision trees in identifying syndromes in coronary heart disease. In *International Symposium on Neural Networks* (pp. 1274-1279). Springer Berlin Heidelberg. doi:10.1007/978-3-540-72383-7_148

Chen, Z., Li, J., & Wei, L. (2007). A multiple kernel support vector machine scheme for feature selection and rule extraction from gene expression data of cancer tissue. *Artificial Intelligence in Medicine*, *41*(2), 161–175. doi:10.1016/j.artmed.2007.07.008

Chien, C., & Pottie, G. J. (2012, August). A universal hybrid decision tree classifier design for human activity classification. In *2012 Annual International Conference of the IEEE Engineering in Medicine and Biology Society* (pp. 1065-1068). IEEE.

Chiu, R. K., Chen, R. Y., Wang, S. A., Chang, Y. C., & Chen, L. C. (2013). Intelligent systems developed for the early detection of chronic kidney disease. *Advances in Artificial Neural Systems*, *2013*, 1–7. doi:10.1155/2013/539570

Cho, B. H., Yu, H., Kim, K. W., Kim, T. H., Kim, I. Y., & Kim, S. I. (2008). Application of irregular and unbalanced data to predict diabetic nephropathy using visualization and feature selection methods. *Artificial Intelligence in Medicine*, *42*(1), 37–53. doi:10.1016/j.artmed.2007.09.005

Cooper, J. N., Wei, L., Fernandez, S. A., Minneci, P. C., & Deans, K. J. (2015). Pre-operative prediction of surgical morbidity in children: Comparison of five statistical models. *Computers in Biology and Medicine*, *57*, 54–65. doi:10.1016/j.compbiomed.2014.11.009

Curiac, D. I., Vasile, G., Banias, O., Volosencu, C., & Albu, A. (2009, June). Bayesian network model for diagnosis of psychiatric diseases. In *Information Technology Interfaces, 2009. ITI'09. Proceedings of the ITI 2009 31st International Conference on* (pp. 61-66). IEEE. doi:10.1109/ITI.2009.5196055

Dangare, C. S., & Apte, S. S. (2012). Improved study of heart disease prediction system using data mining classification techniques. *International Journal of Computers and Applications*, *47*(10), 44–48. doi:10.5120/7228-0076

Das, R., Turkoglu, I., & Sengur, A. (2009). Effective diagnosis of heart disease through neural networks ensembles. *Expert Systems with Applications*, *36*(4), 7675–7680. doi:10.1016/j.eswa.2008.09.013

De Cos Juez, F. J., Suárez-Suárez, M. A., Lasheras, F. S., & Murcia-Mazón, A. (2011). Application of neural networks to the study of the influence of diet and lifestyle on the value of bone mineral density in post-menopausal women. *Mathematical and Computer Modelling*, *54*(7), 1665–1670. doi:10.1016/j.mcm.2010.11.069

Delen, D., Walker, G., & Kadam, A. (2005). Predicting breast cancer survivability: A comparison of three data mining methods. *Artificial Intelligence in Medicine*, *34*(2), 113–127. doi:10.1016/j.artmed.2004.07.002

Dua, S., & Du, X., Sree, S. V., & Vi, T. A. (2012). Novel classification of coronary artery disease using heart rate variability analysis. *Journal of Mechanics in Medicine and Biology*, *12*(04), 1240017. doi:10.1142/S0219519412400179

Durairaj, M., & NandhaKumar, R. (2013). Data Mining Application on IVF Data for the Selection of Influential Parameters on Fertility. *Int J Eng Adv Technol*, *2*(6), 278–283.

El-Dahshan, E. S. A., Hosny, T., & Salem, A. B. M. (2010). Hybrid intelligent techniques for MRI brain images classification. *Digital Signal Processing*, *20*(2), 433–441. doi:10.1016/j.dsp.2009.07.002

Escudero, J., Zajicek, J. P., & Ifeachor, E. (2011, August). Early detection and characterization of Alzheimer's disease in clinical scenarios using Bioprofile concepts and K-means. In *2011 Annual International Conference of the IEEE Engineering in Medicine and Biology Society* (pp. 6470-6473). IEEE. doi:10.1109/IEMBS.2011.6091597

Evirgen, H., & Çerkezi, M. (2014). Prediction and Diagnosis of Diabetic Retinopathy using Data Mining Technique. *Turkish Online Journal of Science & Technology, 4*(3).

Fei, S. W. (2010). Diagnostic study on arrhythmia cordis based on particle swarm optimization-based support vector machine. *Expert Systems with Applications, 37*(10), 6748–6752. doi:10.1016/j.eswa.2010.02.126

Fong, S., Wang, D., Fiaidhi, J., Mohammed, S., Chen, L., & Ling, L. (2016). Clinical Pathways Inference from Decision Rules by Hybrid Stream Mining and Fuzzy Unordered Rule Induction Strategy. *Computerized Medical Imaging and Graphics*. doi:10.1016/j.compmedimag.2016.06.008

Fu, L. D., & Zhang, Y. F. (2010, November). Medical image retrieval and classification based on morphological shape feature. In *Intelligent Networks and Intelligent Systems (ICINIS), 2010 3rd International Conference on* (pp. 116-119). IEEE.

Gao, Z., Hong, W., Xu, Y., Zhang, T., Song, Z., & Liu, J. (2010, September). Osteoporosis Diagnosis Based on the Multifractal Spectrum Features of Micro-CT Images and C4. 5 Decision Tree. In *Pervasive Computing Signal Processing and Applications (PCSPA), 2010 First International Conference on* (pp. 1043-1047). IEEE.

Gennings, C., Ellis, R., & Ritter, J. K. (2012). Linking empirical estimates of body burden of environmental chemicals and wellness using NHANES data. *Environment International, 39*(1), 56–65. doi:10.1016/j.envint.2011.09.002

Giri, D., Acharya, U. R., Martis, R. J., Sree, S. V., Lim, T. C., Ahamed, T., & Suri, J. S. (2013). Automated diagnosis of coronary artery disease affected patients using LDA, PCA, ICA and discrete wavelet transform. *Knowledge-Based Systems, 37*, 274–282. doi:10.1016/j.knosys.2012.08.011

Guh, R. S., Wu, T. C. J., & Weng, S. P. (2011). Integrating genetic algorithm and decision tree learning for assistance in predicting in vitro fertilization outcomes. *Expert Systems with Applications, 38*(4), 4437–4449. doi:10.1016/j.eswa.2010.09.112

Gürbüz, E., & Kılıç, E. (2014). A new adaptive support vector machine for diagnosis of diseases. *Expert Systems: International Journal of Knowledge Engineering and Neural Networks, 31*(5), 389–397. doi:10.1111/exsy.12051

Hachesu, P. R., Ahmadi, M., Alizadeh, S., & Sadoughi, F. (2013). Use of data mining techniques to determine and predict length of stay of cardiac patients. *Healthcare Informatics Research, 19*(2), 121-129.

Han, J., & Kamber, M. (2006). *Data Mining: Concepts and Techniques* (2nd ed.). San Francisco: Morgan Kaufman Publisher.

Han, J., Rodriguez, J. C., & Beheshti, M. (2008, December). Diabetes data analysis and prediction model discovery using rapidminer. In *2008 Second International Conference on Future Generation Communication and Networking* (Vol. 3, pp. 96-99). IEEE. doi:10.1109/FGCN.2008.226

Harper, P. R. (2005). A review and comparison of classification algorithms for medical decision making. *Health Policy (Amsterdam)*, *71*(3), 315–331. doi:10.1016/j.healthpol.2004.05.002

Harrison, R. F., & Kennedy, R. L. (2005). Artificial neural network models for prediction of acute coronary syndromes using clinical data from the time of presentation. *Annals of Emergency Medicine*, *46*(5), 431–439. doi:10.1016/j.annemergmed.2004.09.012

Heikes, K. E., Eddy, D. M., Arondekar, B., & Schlessinger, L. (2008). Diabetes Risk Calculator A simple tool for detecting undiagnosed diabetes and pre-diabetes. *Diabetes Care*, *31*(5), 1040–1045. doi:10.2337/dc07-1150

Hemant, P., & Pushpavathi, T. (2012, July). A novel approach to predict diabetes by Cascading Clustering and Classification. In *Computing Communication & Networking Technologies (ICCCNT), 2012 Third International Conference on* (pp. 1-7). IEEE. doi:10.1109/ICCCNT.2012.6396069

Houthooft, R., Ruyssinck, J., van der Herten, J., Stijven, S., Couckuyt, I., Gadeyne, B., & De Turck, F. et al. (2015). Predictive modelling of survival and length of stay in critically ill patients using sequential organ failure scores. *Artificial Intelligence in Medicine*, *63*(3), 191–207. doi:10.1016/j.artmed.2014.12.009

Huang, C. L., Liao, H. C., & Chen, M. C. (2008). Prediction model building and feature selection with support vector machines in breast cancer diagnosis. *Expert Systems with Applications*, *34*(1), 578–587. doi:10.1016/j.eswa.2006.09.041

Huang, M. J., Chen, M. Y., & Lee, S. C. (2007). Integrating data mining with case-based reasoning for chronic diseases prognosis and diagnosis. *Expert Systems with Applications*, *32*(3), 856–867. doi:10.1016/j.eswa.2006.01.038

Huang, Y., McCullagh, P., Black, N., & Harper, R. (2007). Feature selection and classification model construction on type 2 diabetic patients data. *Artificial Intelligence in Medicine*, *41*(3), 251–262. doi:10.1016/j.artmed.2007.07.002

Huang, Z., Juarez, J. M., Duan, H., & Li, H. (2013a). Length of stay prediction for clinical treatment process using temporal similarity. *Expert Systems with Applications*, *40*(16), 6330–6339. doi:10.1016/j.eswa.2013.05.066

Huang, Z., Juarez, J. M., Duan, H., & Li, H. (2014b). Reprint of Length of stay prediction for clinical treatment process using temporal similarity. *Expert Systems with Applications*, *41*(2), 274–283. doi:10.1016/j.eswa.2013.08.036

Ibrahim, H., Saad, A., Abdo, A., & Eldin, A. S. (2016). Mining association patterns of drug-interactions using post marketing FDAs spontaneous reporting data. *Journal of Biomedical Informatics*, *60*, 294–308. doi:10.1016/j.jbi.2016.02.009

Ilango, B. S., & Ramaraj, N. (2010, September). A hybrid prediction model with F-score feature selection for type II Diabetes databases. In *Proceedings of the 1st Amrita ACM-W Celebration on Women in Computing in India* (p. 13). ACM. doi:10.1145/1858378.1858391

Ilayaraja, M., & Meyyappan, T. (2015). Efficient Data Mining Method to Predict the Risk of Heart Diseases Through Frequent Itemsets. *Procedia Computer Science*, *70*, 586–592. doi:10.1016/j.procs.2015.10.040

Inan, O., Uzer, M. S., & Yılmaz, N. (2013). A new hybrid feature selection method based on association rules and PCA for detection of breast cancer. *International Journal of Innovative Computing, Information, & Control, 9*(2), 727–729.

Isa, N. A. M., Salamah, S. A., & Ngah, U. K. (2009). Adaptive fuzzy moving K-means clustering algorithm for image segmentation. *IEEE Transactions on Consumer Electronics, 55*(4), 2145–2153. doi:10.1109/TCE.2009.5373781

Jayalakshmi, T., & Santhakumaran, A. (2010, February). A novel classification method for diagnosis of diabetes mellitus using artificial neural networks. In *Data Storage and Data Engineering (DSDE), 2010 International Conference on* (pp. 159-163). IEEE. doi:10.1109/DSDE.2010.58

Jen, C. H., Wang, C. C., Jiang, B. C., Chu, Y. H., & Chen, M. S. (2012). Application of classification techniques on development an early-warning system for chronic illnesses. *Expert Systems with Applications, 39*(10), 8852–8858. doi:10.1016/j.eswa.2012.02.004

Ji, Y., Ying, H., Dews, P., Farber, M. S., Mansour, A., Tran, J., . . . Massanari, R. M. (2010a, July). A fuzzy recognition-primed decision model-based causal association mining algorithm for detecting adverse drug reactions in postmarketing surveillance. In *Fuzzy Systems (FUZZ), 2010 IEEE International Conference on* (pp. 1-8). IEEE.

Ji, Y., Ying, H., Dews, P., Mansour, A., Tran, J., Miller, R. E., & Massanari, R. M. (2011b). A potential causal association mining algorithm for screening adverse drug reactions in postmarketing surveillance. *IEEE Transactions on Information Technology in Biomedicine, 15*(3), 428–437. doi:10.1109/TITB.2011.2131669

Ji, Y., Ying, H., Tran, J., Dews, P., Mansour, A., & Massanari, R. M. (2011c, December). Mining Infrequent Causal Associations in Electronic Health Databases. In *2011 IEEE 11th International Conference on Data Mining Workshops* (pp. 421-428). IEEE.

Ji, Y., Ying, H., Tran, J., Dews, P., Mansour, A., & Massanari, R. M. (2013d). A method for mining infrequent causal associations and its application in finding adverse drug reaction signal pairs. *IEEE Transactions on Knowledge and Data Engineering, 25*(4), 721–733. doi:10.1109/TKDE.2012.28

Jilani, T. A., Yasin, H., Yasin, M., & Ardil, C. (2009). Acute coronary syndrome prediction using data mining techniques-an application. *World Academy of Science. Engineering and Technology, 59*(4), 295–299.

Jose, J. S., Sivakami, R., Maheswari, N. U., & Venkatesh, R. (2012). An efficient diagnosis of kidney images using association rules. Int. J. Comput. Technol. Electron. *Eng, 12*(2), 14–20.

Juan, G., Sen-lin, L., Hong-bo, J., Tie-mei, Z., & Yi-wen, H. (2007, May). Type 2 diabetes data processing with EM and C4. 5 algorithm. In *Complex Medical Engineering, 2007. CME 2007. IEEE/ICME International Conference on* (pp. 371-377). IEEE.

Kajabadi, A., Saraee, M. H., & Asgari, S. (2009, October). Data mining cardiovascular risk factors. In *Application of Information and Communication Technologies, 2009. AICT 2009. International Conference on* (pp. 1-5). IEEE.

Karabatak, M., & Ince, M. C. (2009). An expert system for detection of breast cancer based on association rules and neural network. *Expert Systems with Applications*, *36*(2), 3465–3469. doi:10.1016/j.eswa.2008.02.064

Karaolis, M. A., Moutiris, J. A., Hadjipanayi, D., & Pattichis, C. S. (2010). Assessment of the risk factors of coronary heart events based on data mining with decision trees. *IEEE Transactions on Information Technology in Biomedicine*, *14*(3), 559–566. doi:10.1109/TITB.2009.2038906

Karegowda, A. G., Jayaram, M. A., & Manjunath, A. S. (2012). Cascading k-means clustering and k-nearest neighbor classifier for categorization of diabetic patients. *International Journal of Engineering and Advanced Technology*, *1*(3), 147–151.

Karimi, M., Amirfattahi, R., Sadri, S., & Marvasti, S. A. (2005, November). Noninvasive detection and classification of coronary artery occlusions using wavelet analysis of heart sounds with neural networks. In *Medical Applications of Signal Processing, 2005. The 3rd IEE International Seminar on (Ref. No. 2005-1119)* (pp. 117-120). IET.

Karlik, B., & Harman, G. (2013, April). Computer-aided software for early diagnosis of eerythemato-squamous diseases. In *Electronics and Nanotechnology (ELNANO), 2013 IEEE XXXIII International Scientific Conference* (pp. 276-279). IEEE. doi:10.1109/ELNANO.2013.6552035

Kasemthaweesab, P., & Kurutach, W. (2012, July). Association analysis of diabetes mellitus (DM) with complication states based on association rules. In *2012 7th IEEE Conference on Industrial Electronics and Applications (ICIEA)* (pp. 1453-1457). IEEE.

Kavitha, K., & Sarojamma, R. M. (2012). Monitoring of diabetes with data mining via CART Method. *International Journal of Emerging Technology and Advanced Engineering*, *2*(11), 157–162.

Kavitha, M. S., Ganesh Kumar, P., Park, S. Y., Huh, K. H., Heo, M. S., Kurita, T., & Chien, S. I. et al. (2016). Automatic detection of osteoporosis based on hybrid genetic swarm fuzzy classifier approaches. *Dento Maxillo Facial Radiology*, *45*(7), 20160076. doi:10.1259/dmfr.20160076

Khairudin, Z., Mohd, N., & Hamid, H. (2012, September). Predictive models of prolonged stay after Coronary Artery Bypass surgery. *In Statistics in Science, Business, and Engineering (ICSSBE), 2012 International Conference on* (pp. 1-5). IEEE.

Khan, M. U., Choi, J. P., Shin, H., & Kim, M. (2008, August). Predicting breast cancer survivability using fuzzy decision trees for personalized healthcare. In *2008 30th Annual International Conference of the IEEE Engineering in Medicine and Biology Society* (pp. 5148-5151). IEEE.

Khanna, S., & Agarwal, S. (2013, December). An Integrated Approach towards the prediction of Likelihood of Diabetes. In *Machine Intelligence and Research Advancement (ICMIRA), 2013 International Conference on* (pp. 294-298). IEEE. doi:10.1109/ICMIRA.2013.62

Koh, H. C., & Tan, G. (2011). Data mining applications in healthcare. *Journal of Healthcare Information Management*, *19*(2), 64–72.

Kolachalama, V. B., Bressloff, N. W., & Nair, P. B. (2007). Mining data from hemodynamic simulations via Bayesian emulation. *Biomedical Engineering Online*, *6*(1), 1. doi:10.1186/1475-925X-6-47

Koley, S., & Majumder, A. (2011, May). Brain MRI segmentation for tumor detection using cohesion based self-merging algorithm. In *Communication Software and Networks (ICCSN), 2011 IEEE 3rd International Conference on* (pp. 781-785). IEEE.

Kourou, K., Rigas, G., Exarchos, K. P., Goletsis, Y., Exarchos, T. P., Jacobs, S., & Fotiadis, D. I. et al. (2016). Prediction of time dependent survival in HF patients after VAD implantation using pre-and post-operative data. *Computers in Biology and Medicine*, *70*, 99–105. doi:10.1016/j.compbiomed.2016.01.005

Kurosaki, M., Matsunaga, K., Hirayama, I., Tanaka, T., Sato, M., Yasui, Y., & Nakanishi, H. et al. (2010). A predictive model of response to peginterferon ribavirin in chronic hepatitis C using classification and regression tree analysis. *Hepatology Research*, *40*(3), 251–260. doi:10.1111/j.1872-034X.2009.00607.x

Kurt, I., Ture, M., & Kurum, A. T. (2008). Comparing performances of logistic regression, classification and regression tree, and neural networks for predicting coronary artery disease. *Expert Systems with Applications*, *34*(1), 366–374. doi:10.1016/j.eswa.2006.09.004

Kusiak, A., Dixon, B., & Shah, S. (2005). Predicting survival time for kidney dialysis patients: A data mining approach. *Computers in Biology and Medicine*, *35*(4), 311–327. doi:10.1016/j.compbiomed.2004.02.004

Lahsasna, A., Ainon, R. N., Zainuddin, R., & Bulgiba, A. (2012). Design of a fuzzy-based decision support system for coronary heart disease diagnosis. *Journal of Medical Systems*, *36*(5), 3293–3306. doi:10.1007/s10916-012-9821-7

Lakshmi, K. S., & Kumar, G. S. (2014, February). Association rule extraction from medical transcripts of diabetic patients. In *Applications of Digital Information and Web Technologies (ICADIWT), 2014 Fifth International Conference on the* (pp. 201-206). IEEE.

Lee, H. G., Noh, K. Y., & Ryu, K. H. (2007, May). Mining biosignal data: coronary artery disease diagnosis using linear and nonlinear features of HRV. In *Pacific-Asia Conference on Knowledge Discovery and Data Mining* (pp. 218-228). Springer Berlin Heidelberg. doi:10.1007/978-3-540-77018-3_23

Lee, W. J., Chong, K., Chen, J. C., Ser, K. H., Lee, Y. C., Tsou, J. J., & Chen, S. C. (2012). Predictors of diabetes remission after bariatric surgery in Asia. *Asian Journal of Surgery*, *35*(2), 67–73. doi:10.1016/j.asjsur.2012.04.010

Lekkas, S., & Mikhailov, L. (2010). Evolving fuzzy medical diagnosis of Pima Indians diabetes and of dermatological diseases. *Artificial Intelligence in Medicine*, *50*(2), 117–126. doi:10.1016/j.artmed.2010.05.007

Leroi, I., Burns, A., Aarsland, D., Brønnick, K., Ehrt, U., De Deyn, P. P., & Cummings, J. et al. (2007). Neuropsychiatric symptoms in patients with Parkinsons disease and dementia: Frequency, profile and associated care giver stress. *Journal of Neurology, Neurosurgery, and Psychiatry*, *78*(1). doi:10.1136/jnnp.2006.101162

Lin, C. C., Ou, Y. K., Chen, S. H., Liu, Y. C., & Lin, J. (2010). Comparison of artificial neural network and logistic regression models for predicting mortality in elderly patients with hip fracture. *Injury*, *41*(8), 869–873. doi:10.1016/j.injury.2010.04.023

Linares, C., Martinez-Martin, P., Rodríguez-Blázquez, C., Forjaz, M. J., Carmona, R., & Díaz, J. (2016). Effect of heat waves on morbidity and mortality due to Parkinsons disease in Madrid: A time-series analysis. *Environment International*, *89*, 1–6. doi:10.1016/j.envint.2016.01.017

Liu, D. Y., Chen, H. L., Yang, B., Lv, X. E., Li, L. N., & Liu, J. (2012). Design of an enhanced fuzzy k-nearest neighbor classifier based computer aided diagnostic system for thyroid disease. *Journal of Medical Systems*, *36*(5), 3243–3254. doi:10.1007/s10916-011-9815-x

Liu, J., Yuan, X., & Buckles, B. P. (2008, August). Breast cancer diagnosis using level-set statistics and support vector machines. In *2008 30th Annual International Conference of the IEEE Engineering in Medicine and Biology Society* (pp. 3044-3047). IEEE.

Liu, K. F., & Lu, C. F. (2009, August). BBN-based decision support for health risk analysis. In *INC, IMS and IDC, 2009. NCM'09. Fifth International Joint Conference on* (pp. 696-702). IEEE.

Liu, M., Wu, Y., Chen, Y., Sun, J., Zhao, Z., Chen, X. W., & Xu, H. et al. (2012). Large-scale prediction of adverse drug reactions using chemical, biological, and phenotypic properties of drugs. *Journal of the American Medical Informatics Association*, *19*(e1), e28–e35. doi:10.1136/amiajnl-2011-000699

Liu, T., Hu, L., Ma, C., Wang, Z. Y., & Chen, H. L. (2015). A fast approach for detection of erythematosquamous diseases based on extreme learning machine with maximum relevance minimum redundancy feature selection. *International Journal of Systems Science*, *46*(5), 919–931. doi:10.1080/00207721.2013.801096

Liu, Z., Sokka, T., Maas, K., Olsen, N. J., & Aune, T. M. (2009). Prediction of disease severity in patients with early rheumatoid arthritis by gene expression profiling. *Human Genomics and Proteomics*, *1*(1).

Luo, Z., Wu, X., Guo, S., & Ye, B. (2008, June). Diagnosis of breast cancer tumor based on manifold learning and support vector machine. In *Information and Automation, 2008. ICIA 2008. International Conference on* (pp. 703-707). IEEE.

Marx, P., & Antal, P. (2015). Decomposition of Shared Latent Factors Using Bayesian Multi-morbidity Dependency Maps. In *First European Biomedical Engineering Conference for Young Investigators* (pp. 40-43). Springer Singapore. doi:10.1007/978-981-287-573-0_10

Masethe, H. D., & Masethe, M. A. (2014, October). Prediction of heart disease using classification algorithms. *Proceedings of the World Congress on Engineering and Computer Science*, *2*, 22-24.

McBride, J., Zhang, S., Wortley, M., Paquette, M., Klipple, G., Byrd, E., . . . Zhao, X. (2011, March). Neural network analysis of gait biomechanical data for classification of knee osteoarthritis. In Biomedical Sciences and Engineering Conference (BSEC), 2011 (pp. 1-4). IEEE. doi:10.1109/BSEC.2011.5872315

Meng, X. H., Huang, Y. X., Rao, D. P., Zhang, Q., & Liu, Q. (2013). Comparison of three data mining models for predicting diabetes or prediabetes by risk factors. *The Kaohsiung Journal of Medical Sciences*, *29*(2), 93–99. doi:10.1016/j.kjms.2012.08.016

Milewski, R., Malinowski, P., Milewska, A. J., Ziniewicz, P., & Wołczyński, S. (2010). The usage of margin-based feature selection algorithm in IVF ICSI/ET data analysis. Studies in Logic. *Grammar and Rhetoric*, *21*(34), 35–46.

Moon, S. S., Kang, S. Y., Jitpitaklert, W., & Kim, S. B. (2012). Decision tree models for characterizing smoking patterns of older adults. *Expert Systems with Applications*, *39*(1), 445–451. doi:10.1016/j.eswa.2011.07.035

Morales, D. A., Bengoetxea, E., Larrañaga, P., García, M., Franco, Y., Fresnada, M., & Merino, M. (2008). Bayesian classification for the selection of in vitro human embryos using morphological and clinical data. *Computer Methods and Programs in Biomedicine*, *90*(2), 104–116. doi:10.1016/j.cmpb.2007.11.018

Moudani, W., Shahin, A., Chakik, F., & Rajab, D. (2011). Intelligent predictive osteoporosis system. *International Journal of Computers and Applications*, *32*(5), 28–37.

Nahar, J., Imam, T., Tickle, K. S., & Chen, Y. P. P. (2013). Association rule mining to detect factors which contribute to heart disease in males and females. *Expert Systems with Applications*, *40*(4), 1086–1093. doi:10.1016/j.eswa.2012.08.028

Negassa, A., & Monrad, E. S. (2011). Prediction of length of stay following elective percutaneous coronary intervention. *ISRN Surgery*.

Neshat, M., Sargolzaei, M., Nadjaran Toosi, A., & Masoumi, A. (2012). Hepatitis disease diagnosis using hybrid case based reasoning and particle swarm optimization. *ISRN Artificial Intelligence*.

Noma, N. G., & Ghani, M. K. A. (2012, December). Discovering pattern in medical audiology data with FP-growth algorithm. In *Biomedical Engineering and Sciences (IECBES), 2012 IEEE EMBS Conference on* (pp. 17-22). IEEE.

Nuwangi, S. M., Oruthotaarachchi, C. R., Tilakaratna, J. M. P. P., & Caldera, H. A. (2010a, December). Utilization of Data Mining Techniques in Knowledge Extraction for Diminution of Diabetes. In *Information Technology for Real World Problems (VCON), 2010 Second Vaagdevi International Conference on* (pp. 3-8). IEEE.

Nuwangi, S. M., Oruthotaarachchi, C. R., Tilakaratna, J. M. P. P., & Caldera, H. A. (2010b, November). Usage of association rules and classification techniques in knowledge extraction of diabetes. In *Advanced Information Management and Service (IMS), 2010 6th International Conference on* (pp. 372-377). IEEE.

Ordóñez, C., Matías, J. M., de Cos Juez, J. F., & García, P. J. (2009). Machine learning techniques applied to the determination of osteoporosis incidence in post-menopausal women. *Mathematical and Computer Modelling*, *50*(5), 673–679. doi:10.1016/j.mcm.2008.12.024

Özçift, A., & Gülten, A. (2013). Genetic algorithm wrapped Bayesian network feature selection applied to differential diagnosis of erythemato-squamous diseases. *Digital Signal Processing*, *23*(1), 230–237. doi:10.1016/j.dsp.2012.07.008

Palaniappan, S., & Awang, R. (2008, March). Intelligent heart disease prediction system using data mining techniques. In *2008 IEEE/ACS International Conference on Computer Systems and Applications* (pp. 108-115). IEEE. doi:10.1109/AICCSA.2008.4493524

Parthiban, G., Rajesh, A., & Srivatsa, S. K. (2011). Diagnosis of heart disease for diabetic patients using naive bayes method. *International Journal of Computers and Applications*, *24*(3), 7–11. doi:10.5120/2933-3887

Parthiban, G., & Srivatsa, S. K. (2012). Applying machine learning methods in diagnosing heart disease for diabetic patients. *International Journal of Applied Information Systems*, *3*, 2249–0868.

Patel, S., Sherrill, D., Hughes, R., Hester, T., Huggins, N., Lie-Nemeth, T., & Bonato, P. et al. (2006, April). Analysis of the severity of dyskinesia in patients with Parkinson's disease via wearable sensors. In *International Workshop on Wearable and Implantable Body Sensor Networks (BSN'06)*. IEEE.

Patil, B. M., Joshi, R. C., & Toshniwal, D. (2010 a, February). Association rule for classification of type-2 diabetic patients. In *Machine Learning and Computing (ICMLC), 2010 Second International Conference on* (pp. 330-334). IEEE.

Patil, B. M., Joshi, R. C., & Toshniwal, D. (2010 b). Hybrid prediction model for Type-2 diabetic patients. *Expert Systems with Applications*, *37*(12), 8102–8108. doi:10.1016/j.eswa.2010.05.078

Patil, S. B., & Kumaraswamy, Y. S. (2009). Extraction of significant patterns from heart disease warehouses for heart attack prediction. *IJCSNS*, *9*(2), 228–235.

Piateski, G., & Frawley, W. (1991). *Knowledge discovery in databases*. MIT Press.

Polat, K. (2012). Application of attribute weighting method based on clustering centers to discrimination of linearly non-separable medical datasets. *Journal of Medical Systems*, *36*(4), 2657–2673. doi:10.1007/s10916-011-9741-y

Polat, K., & Güneş, S. (2007). An expert system approach based on principal component analysis and adaptive neuro-fuzzy inference system to diagnosis of diabetes disease. *Digital Signal Processing*, *17*(4), 702–710. doi:10.1016/j.dsp.2006.09.005

Polat, K., Güneş, S., & Arslan, A. (2008). A cascade learning system for classification of diabetes disease: Generalized discriminant analysis and least square support vector machine. *Expert Systems with Applications*, *34*(1), 482–487. doi:10.1016/j.eswa.2006.09.012

Purnami, S. W., Zain, J. M., & Embong, A. (2010, March). A new expert system for diabetes disease diagnosis using modified spline smooth support vector machine. In *International Conference on Computational Science and Its Applications* (pp. 83-92). Springer Berlin Heidelberg. doi:10.1007/978-3-642-12189-0_8

Pyle, D. (1999). *Data preparation for data mining* (Vol. 1). Morgan Kaufmann.

Radha, P., & Srinivasan, B. (2014, August). Feature Selection Using Particle Swarm Optimization for Predicting the Risk of Cardiovascular Disease in Type-II Diabetic Patients. *International Journal on Recent and Innovation Trends in Computing and Communication.*, *2*(8), 2503–2509.

Rajesh, K., & Sangeetha, V. (2012). Application of data mining methods and techniques for diabetes diagnosis. *International Journal of Engineering and Innovative Technology*, *2*(3).

Ribeiro, M. X., Traina, A. J., Traina, C. Jr, & Azevedo-Marques, P. M. (2008). An association rule-based method to support medical image diagnosis with efficiency. *IEEE Transactions on Multimedia*, *10*(2), 277–285. doi:10.1109/TMM.2007.911837

Rowan, M., Ryan, T., Hegarty, F., & OHare, N. (2007). The use of artificial neural networks to stratify the length of stay of cardiac patients based on preoperative and initial postoperative factors. *Artificial Intelligence in Medicine*, *40*(3), 211–221. doi:10.1016/j.artmed.2007.04.005

Sa-ngasoongsong, A., & Chongwatpol, J. (2012). An analysis of diabetes risk factors using data mining approach. Oklahoma State University.

Sabariah, M. M. K., Hanifa, S. A., & Sa'adah, M. S. (2014, August). Early detection of type II Diabetes Mellitus with random forest and classification and regression tree (CART). In *Advanced Informatics: Concept, Theory and Application (ICAICTA), 2014 International Conference of* (pp. 238-242). IEEE.

Sanakal, R., & Jayakumari, T. (2014). Prognosis of diabetes using data mining approach-fuzzy C means clustering and support vector machine. *International Journal of Computer Trends and Technology*, *11*(2), 94–98. doi:10.14445/22312803/IJCTT-V11P120

Santhanam, T., & Padmavathi, M. S. (2015). Application of K-means and genetic algorithms for dimension reduction by integrating SVM for diabetes diagnosis. *Procedia Computer Science*, *47*, 76–83. doi:10.1016/j.procs.2015.03.185

Sapna, S., & Tamilarasi, A. (2009, October). Fuzzy relational equation in preventing diabetic heart attack. In *Advances in Recent Technologies in Communication and Computing, 2009. ARTCom'09. International Conference on* (pp. 635-637). IEEE. doi:10.1109/ARTCom.2009.48

Saxena, K., & Sharma, R. (2016). Efficient Heart Disease Prediction System. *Procedia Computer Science*, *85*, 962–969. doi:10.1016/j.procs.2016.05.288

Shen, S., Sandham, W., Granat, M., & Sterr, A. (2005). MRI fuzzy segmentation of brain tissue using neighborhood attraction with neural-network optimization. *IEEE Transactions on Information Technology in Biomedicine*, *9*(3), 459–467. doi:10.1109/TITB.2005.847500

Shouman, M., Turner, T., & Stocker, R. (2012, March). Using data mining techniques in heart disease diagnosis and treatment. In *Electronics, Communications and Computers (JEC-ECC), 2012 Japan-Egypt Conference on* (pp. 173-177). IEEE.

Skevofilakas, M., Zarkogianni, K., Karamanos, B. G., & Nikita, K. S. (2010, August). A hybrid Decision Support System for the risk assessment of retinopathy development as a long term complication of Type 1 Diabetes Mellitus. In *2010 Annual International Conference of the IEEE Engineering in Medicine and Biology* (pp. 6713-6716). IEEE.

Smitha, P., Shaji, L., & Mini, M. G. (2011). A review of medical image classification techniques. *International Conference on VLSI, Communication & Instrumentation*, 34-38.

Soliman, T. H. A., Sewissy, A. A., & Abdel Latif, H. (2010, November). A gene selection approach for classifying diseases based on microarray datasets. In *Computer Technology and Development (ICCTD), 2010 2nd International Conference on* (pp. 626-631). IEEE. doi:10.1109/ICCTD.2010.5645975

Soni, J., Ansari, U., Sharma, D., & Soni, S. (2011). Predictive data mining for medical diagnosis: An overview of heart disease prediction. *International Journal of Computers and Applications*, *17*(8), 43–48. doi:10.5120/2237-2860

Soni, S., & Vyas, O. P. (2010). Using associative classifiers for predictive analysis in health care data mining. *International Journal of Computers and Applications*, *4*(5), 33–37. doi:10.5120/821-1163

Srinivas, K., Rani, B. K., & Govrdhan, A. (2010). Applications of data mining techniques in healthcare and prediction of heart attacks. *International Journal on Computer Science and Engineering*, *2*(02), 250–255.

Su, C. T., Yang, C. H., Hsu, K. H., & Chiu, W. K. (2006). Data mining for the diagnosis of type II diabetes from three-dimensional body surface anthropometrical scanning data. *Computers & Mathematics with Applications (Oxford, England)*, *51*(6), 1075–1092. doi:10.1016/j.camwa.2005.08.034

Sulaiman, S. N., & Isa, N. A. M. (2010). Adaptive fuzzy-K-means clustering algorithm for image segmentation. *IEEE Transactions on Consumer Electronics*, *56*(4), 2661–2668. doi:10.1109/TCE.2010.5681154

Suresh, A., Harish, K. V., & Radhika, N. (2015). Particle swarm optimization over back propagation neural network for length of stay prediction. *Procedia Computer Science*, *46*, 268–275. doi:10.1016/j.procs.2015.02.020

Tabakov, M. (2006, September). A fuzzy clustering technique for medical image segmentation. In *2006 International Symposium on Evolving Fuzzy Systems* (pp. 118-122). IEEE. doi:10.1109/ISEFS.2006.251140

Tai, Y. M., & Chiu, H. W. (2009). Comorbidity study of ADHD: Applying association rule mining (ARM) to National Health Insurance Database of Taiwan. *International Journal of Medical Informatics*, *78*(12), e75–e83. doi:10.1016/j.ijmedinf.2009.09.005

Tan, S. (2006). *Introduction to Data*. Pearson Addison Wesley.

Taneja, A. (2013). Heart disease prediction system using data mining techniques. *Orient. J. Comput. Sci. Technol.*

Temurtas, H., Yumusak, N., & Temurtas, F. (2009). A comparative study on diabetes disease diagnosis using neural networks. *Expert Systems with Applications*, *36*(4), 8610–8615. doi:10.1016/j.eswa.2008.10.032

Tjandrasa, H., Arieshanti, I., & Anggoro, R. (2014). Classification of non-proliferative diabetic retinopathy based on segmented exudates using K-Means clustering. *International Journal of Image. Graphics and Signal Processing*, *7*(1), 1–8. doi:10.5815/ijigsp.2015.01.01

Toussi, M., Lamy, J. B., Le Toumelin, P., & Venot, A. (2009). Using data mining techniques to explore physicians therapeutic decisions when clinical guidelines do not provide recommendations: Methods and example for type 2 diabetes. *BMC Medical Informatics and Decision Making*, *9*(1), 1. doi:10.1186/1472-6947-9-28

Tu, S. C., Wu, C. C., Hung, C. J., & Chen, J. S. (2010, August). A study for anaesthesia methods in total knee arthroplasties based on data mining. In *Electronics and Information Engineering (ICEIE), 2010 International Conference on* (Vol. *1*, pp. V1-61). IEEE. doi:10.1109/ICEIE.2010.5559838

Übeyli, E. D., & Doğdu, E. (2010). Automatic detection of erythemato-squamous diseases using k-means clustering. *Journal of Medical Systems*, *34*(2), 179–184. doi:10.1007/s10916-008-9229-6

Vijayarani, S., Dhayanand, M. S., & Phil, M. (2015). Kidney disease prediction using svm and ann algorithms. *International Journal of Computing and Business Research*, 2229-6166.

Vimala, G. A. G., & Mohideen, S. K. (2013, January). Automatic detection of optic disk and exudate from retinal images using clustering algorithm. In *Intelligent Systems and Control (ISCO), 2013 7th International Conference on* (pp. 280-284). IEEE.

Wang, W., Richards, G., & Rea, S. (2005, September). Hybrid data mining ensemble for predicting osteoporosis risk. *27th Int. Conf. on Engineering in Medicine and Biology*, 886-889. doi:10.1109/IEMBS.2005.1616557

Wren, J. D., & Garner, H. R. (2005). Data-mining analysis suggests an epigenetic pathogenesis for type 2 diabetes. *BioMed Research International, 2005*(2), 104-112.

Wu, C., Hannan, E. L., Walford, G., Ambrose, J. A., Holmes, D. R. Jr, King, S. B. III, & Jones, R. H. et al. (2006). A risk score to predict in-hospital mortality for percutaneous coronary interventions. *Journal of the American College of Cardiology*, *47*(3), 654–660. doi:10.1016/j.jacc.2005.09.071

Xie, J., Lei, J., Xie, W., Gao, X., Shi, Y., & Liu, X. (2012a, April). Novel hybrid feature selection algorithms for diagnosing erythemato-squamous diseases. In *International Conference on Health Information Science* (pp. 173-185). Springer Berlin Heidelberg. doi:10.1007/978-3-642-29361-0_21

Xie, J., Lei, J., Xie, W., Shi, Y., & Liu, X. (2013b). Two-stage hybrid feature selection algorithms for diagnosing erythemato-squamous diseases. *Health Information Science and Systems, 1*(1), 1.

Xu, R., & Wang, Q. (2015). Large-scale automatic extraction of side effects associated with targeted anticancer drugs from full-text oncological articles. *Journal of Biomedical Informatics*, *55*, 64–72. doi:10.1016/j.jbi.2015.03.009

Xu, Y., Li, D., Chen, Q., & Fan, Y. (2013). Full supervised learning for osteoporosis diagnosis using micro-CT images. *Microscopy Research and Technique*, *76*(4), 333–341. doi:10.1002/jemt.22171

Xuan, X., & Liao, Q. (2007, August). Statistical structure analysis in MRI brain tumor segmentation. In *Image and Graphics, 2007. ICIG 2007. Fourth International Conference on* (pp. 421-426). IEEE. doi:10.1109/ICIG.2007.181

Yang, C. S., Wei, C. P., Yuan, C. C., & Schoung, J. Y. (2010). Predicting the length of hospital stay of burn patients: Comparisons of prediction accuracy among different clinical stages. *Decision Support Systems*, *50*(1), 325–335. doi:10.1016/j.dss.2010.09.001

Yasodha, P., & Kannan, M. (2011). Analysis of a Population of Diabetic Patients Databases in Weka Tool. *International Journal of Scientific & Engineering Research*, *2*(5).

Yeh, D. Y., Cheng, C. H., & Chen, Y. W. (2011). A predictive model for cerebrovascular disease using data mining. *Expert Systems with Applications*, *38*(7), 8970–8977. doi:10.1016/j.eswa.2011.01.114

Yıldırım, E. G., Karahoca, A., & Uçar, T. (2011). Dosage planning for diabetes patients using data mining methods. *Procedia Computer Science*, *3*, 1374–1380. doi:10.1016/j.procs.2011.01.018

Yun, W. L., & Mookiah, M. R. K. (2013). Detection of diabetic retinopathy using k-means clustering and self-organizing map. *Journal of Medical Imaging and Health Informatics*, *3*(4), 575–581. doi:10.1166/jmihi.2013.1207

Zhang, D., Wang, Y., Zhou, L., Yuan, H., & Shen, D. (2011). Multimodal classification of Alzheimers disease and mild cognitive impairment. *NeuroImage*, *55*(3), 856–867. doi:10.1016/j.neuroimage.2011.01.008

Zhao, Z., & Ma, C. (2008, December). An intelligent system for noninvasive diagnosis of coronary artery disease with EMD-TEO and BP neural network. In *Education Technology and Training, 2008. and 2008 International Workshop on Geoscience and Remote Sensing. ETT and GRS 2008. International Workshop on* (Vol. 2, pp. 631-635). IEEE. doi:10.1109/ETTandGRS.2008.361

Zheng, B., Yoon, S. W., & Lam, S. S. (2014). Breast cancer diagnosis based on feature extraction using a hybrid of K-means and support vector machine algorithms. *Expert Systems with Applications*, *41*(4), 1476–1482. doi:10.1016/j.eswa.2013.08.044

Zhou, J., Chan, K. L., Chong, V. F. H., & Krishnan, S. M. (2006, January). Extraction of brain tumor from MR images using one-class support vector machine. In *2005 IEEE Engineering in Medicine and Biology 27th Annual Conference* (pp. 6411-6414). IEEE.

Zuo, W. L., Wang, Z. Y., Liu, T., & Chen, H. L. (2013). Effective detection of Parkinsons disease using an adaptive fuzzy k-nearest neighbor approach. *Biomedical Signal Processing and Control*, *8*(4), 364–373. doi:10.1016/j.bspc.2013.02.006

KEY TERMS AND DEFINITIONS

Data Mining: Data mining is the computing process of discovering patterns in large data sets involving methods at the intersection of artificial intelligence, machine learning, statistics, and database systems. The overall goal of the data mining process is to extract information from a data set and transform it into an understandable structure for further use.

Diagnosis: Diagnosis is the act of the identification of a disease, illness, or a problem by the examination of something or someone's inspection. The diagnosis is based on information from some sources such as results of a physical examination, interview with the patient, family, or both, the medical history of the patient and family, and clinical findings that reported by laboratory tests and radiologic studies.

Treatment: Treatment is defined as the management and medical care of a patient to combat disease or disorder.

Chapter 13

New Features Extracted From Renal Stone NCCT Images to Predict Retreatment After Shock Wave Lithotripsy (SWL)

Toktam Khatibi
Tarbiat Modares University (TMU), Iran

Mohammad Mehdi Sepehri
Tarbiat Modares University (TMU), Iran

Mohammad Javad Soleimani
Iran University of Medical Sciences (IUMS), Iran

Pejman Shadpour
Iran University of Medical Sciences (IUMS), Iran

ABSTRACT

Shock wave lithotripsy (SWL) is a noninvasive and safe treatment for small renal stones. In unsuccessful cases, retreatment procedures are needed after SWL. According to the previous studies, patient and stone descriptors are good predictors of SWL success. Some stone and kidney descriptors are measured from renal Non-Contrast Computed Tomography (NCCT) images. It is a tedious, time-consuming and error-prone process with large inter-user variability when performed manually. In this study, novel features are proposed automatically extracted from NCCT images to describe morphology and location of renal stones and kidneys to predict retreatments after SWL. The proposed features can distinguish between different kidney and stone morphologies and locations while being less sensitive to image segmentation errors. These features are added to other stone and patient features to predict retreatment within 3 months after SWL. The experimental results show that using the proposed stone features extracted from NCCT images can improve the accuracy of predicting retreatment.

DOI: 10.4018/978-1-5225-2515-8.ch013

INTRODUCTION

The general perspective of the chapter is two folded. The first is introducing new features that can be extracted from NCCT images of kidney stones automatically. The second one is investigating whether the proposed feature set can improve the performance of predicting SWL retreatment for patients or not. In this study, the research problem is to predict whether the patients after SWL would need retreatment procedures or not. For solving this problem, new features are proposed which will be extracted from NCCT images by using automatic methods. These features describe renal stone and kidney morphology and location descriptors. Object morphology is defined as its shape and size characteristics (Sparks & Madabhushi, 2013). The descriptors extracted from NCCT images and other stone and patient features are considered in this study for predicting retreatment within three months after SWL. For this, data mining methods are exploited.

The main contribution of this study is to introduce novel features which are automatically extracted from NCCT images of renal stones. These features are added to other stone and patient features to predict retreatment within three months after SWL. The experimental results show that using the proposed features extracted from NCCT images can improve the accuracy of predicting retreatment after SWL. In this study, for evaluating the significance of variables on the SWL success, data mining classifiers such as decision tree, k-nearest neighbor, support vector machines and Naïve Bayes are used.

BACKGROUND

Shock wave lithotripsy (SWL) is the treatment of choice for renal stones smaller than 2 cm in the renal pelvic and upper or middle pole calyces (Tiselius et al.,2001), whereas percutaneous nephrolithotomy (PCNL) is recommended for large or complex stones (Skolarikos, Alivizatos, & Delarosette, 2005). SWL has been introduced by Chaussy et al. (Chaussy, Brendel, & Schmiedt, 1980) as a noninvasive and safe therapy for small renal stones(Lee et al., 2015).

Goktas et al. have shown that SWL is very successful in pediatric patients for lower calyceal stones (Goktas et al., 2011). They have evaluated SWL for adults and children. For this purpose, stone free rate and the need for auxiliary procedures after the first SWL treatment have been considered. The results showed that the stone free rate after the first SWL for children was 66.6% and they have concluded that SWL is very successful for children.

In some cases, larger fragments remain after renal stone primary treatment and retreatment procedures are needed. Retreatment is a subsequent intervention for the disease condition. If SWL treats the stones successfully, there is no need for retreatment and the stone is completely fragmented. Therefore, retreatment rate and/or stone-free rate after the primary renal stone treatment show how the stone treatment is successful (G.V. et al., 2003; Pareek, Armenakas, Panagopoulos, Bruno, & Fracchia, 2005).

Retreatment rate can be estimated via Kidney, Ureter and Bladder X-ray (KUB radiography), and NCCT images. In this study, two class labels are considered as positive (if the patient has retreatment rate within three months after SWL) and negative (otherwise).

Some researchers have proposed different methods for predicting the success after stone treatment methods (Alger, Niederberger, & Turk, 2009; Chen, Liu, Hsieh, & Wang, 2016; Resorlu, Unsal, Gulec, & Oztuna, 2012; Zhu et al., 2011). Zhu et al. have used univariate and multivariate analysis (using logistic regression) of different variables for predicting stone free rate after PCNL. They have considered the variables such as patient age, sex, body mass index (BMI), stone side, size, number and position for this purpose. The results have shown that stone side, size, number and position are significant variables that affect the stone free rate after the initial treatment (Zhu et al., 2011). Resorlu et al. have investigated variables such as stone side, position, number, composition and patient age and sex, and kidney anatomic factors to predict stone free rate after stone treatment. Univariate analysis has shown that stone size, location, composition and kidney malformation can affect the stone free rate after the treatment. Multivariate analysis using logistic regression has shown that only stone location may has no effect on the stone free rate (Resorlu et al., 2012).

In an earlier pioneering research, the authors applied data mining to extract influential attributes for selecting between medical expulsive therapy, SWL, and transurethral lithotripsy, concluding that their model can bring 8 percent improvement in stone free rate outperforming the existing expert system developed in-house (Sepehri, Rahnama, Shadpour & Teimourpour, 2009).

The most common classifiers are used to predict the retreatment need after SWL based on the different feature sets. The reason of using classifiers in this study is because of their different abilities for different characteristics of dataset. For example, decision tree is a very good classifier for linearly separable datasets. Support vector machines is a very good classifier for nonlinearly separable datasets when trained by nonlinear kernels such as RBF. Naïve Bayes model classifies data based on estimating the prior and posterior probabilities from dataset. Finally, K-nearest neighbor uses the pair wise distance of the testing data with the training data to predict the class label of the testing data. They are common and popular classifiers (Han et al., 2012).

Selby et al. have used multivariate models for assessing whether total kidney stone volume was an independent predictor of stone events. For this purpose, features like the number of stones, largest stone diameter, and total kidney stone volume have been considered. They have shown that total stone volume can quantify stone burden for predicting stone events high accurately (Selby et al., 2015).

A previous study has compared the accuracy of predicting postoperative stone-free rate (SFR) for three different methods of estimating the stone burden including the cumulative stone diameter (M1), Ackermann's formula (M2), and the sphere formula (M3). The experimental results have shown that all of the three methods can predict SFR for stones smaller than 2 cm, and M2 and M3 can predict SFR for stones larger than 2 cm as well (Treigny et al., 2015).

Based on the above paragraphs, it can be concluded that SWL success rate depends on the patient properties including patient age, gender and BMI and stone features including stone size, side, position, number, composition(Budía, Lopez-Acon, Trassierra, & Boronat, 2015; Choi, Song, & Kim, 2012; El-Nahas, El-Assmy, Mansour, & Sheir, 2007; Goktas et al., 2011; Lee et al., 2015; Lin, Hsu, & Chen, 2008; Pareek et al., 2005; Wiesenthal, Ghiculete, Ray, Honey, & Pace, 2011) and renal anatomic factors (Lin et al.,2008)(Torricelli et al., 2015). Stone size can be described based on stone surface area(Nazim, Ather, & Khan, 2014) and stone volume(Saedi & Moulavi, 2012).Stone composition can be described based on Hounsfield Unit (HU) density (El-Nahas et al., 2007; Pareek et al., 2005). A well-known stone position descriptor is skin-to-stone distance (SSD)(Kim et al., 2013; Perks et al., 2008).

Some other descriptors can significantly affect the stone treatment success such as patient colic pain (Kang et al., 2015).

Therefore, in this study, patient features, stone descriptors and other features are considered for predicting stone retreatment after SWL.

Zhu et al. and Resorlue et al. have demonstrated that stone descriptors are important features for predicting stone treatment success (Zhu et al.,2011; Resorlu et al.,2012). Measuring stone features with high accuracy depends on the effective high-quality visualization of the stone. The more accurately the stone can be localized, the more likely it can be disintegrated (Bach & Buchholz, 2011).

Renal stone can be measured in ultrasound and NCCT images. The stone descriptors should be extracted from the ultrasound images or NCCT images. Dunmirea et al. have tried to estimate stone features such as stone size from ultrasound images (Dunmirea et al., 2016). Sternberg et al. have shown that extracting stone features such as stone size from ultrasound images is less accurate than NCCT images (Sternberg et al., 2016). Moreover, Geng et al. believe that NCCT images can be used for predicting SWL outcome because of the accurate stone measurement (Geng et al., 2015). Therefore, this study focuses on extracting stone descriptors from NCCT images.

Many stone and kidney descriptors can be computed from NCCT images of the renal stones. But, it is time-consuming and error-prone labor when measured manually.

RESEARCH METHODOLOGY

Figure 1 demonstrates the main steps of the research methodology which are data collection, preprocessing data, training the classifier and finally evaluating and validating the results.

As illustrated by Figure 1, the research methodology includes three main steps:

- Data collection
  - Collecting patient features and other stone descriptors from HIS and paper-based patient records
  - Selecting CT images containing the kidneys and finding the regions of interest (ROI)

Figure 1. The main steps of research methodology

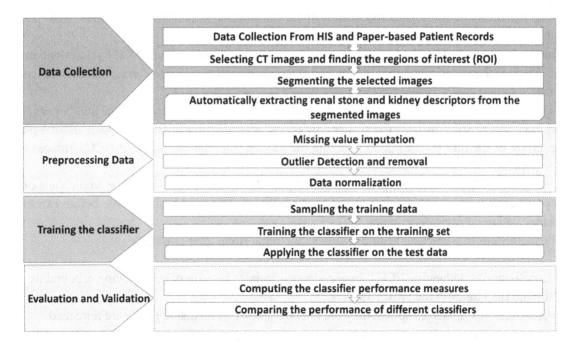

    ○   Segmenting the selected images and identifying the kidney stone in ROIs of the segmented images
    ○   Automatically extracting renal stone and kidney descriptors from the segmented images
- Preprocessing the collected data
    ○   Missing value imputation
    ○   Outlier detection and removal
    ○   Data normalization
- Training the classifier for predicting retreatment of three months after SWL
    ○   Sampling the training set from imbalanced data
    ○   Training the classifiers(Decision tree, SVM, k-NN and Naïve Bayes) on the training set
    ○   Applying the classifier on the test set
- Evaluation and validation
    ○   Computing the classifier performance measures including precision, recall, accuracy and F-measure
    ○   Comparing the performance of the classifiers trained on different subsets of the features including proposed stone descriptors (S_1), patient features (S_2), union of S_1 and S_2 (S_3), other stone descriptors (S_4), union of S_1 and S_4 (S_5), union of S_2 and S_4 (S_6), and union of S_1, S_2 and S_4 (S_7)

Each step is described in details, separately, in the following sections.

Data Collection

The data used in this research are collected from patients who have been treated with SWL at Hasheminejad Kidney Center (HKC) in 2015. From these patients, 150 ones having axial NCCT images of kidney stones are selected. The NCCT image slices have 512 * 512 pixel resolution with 33 dpi.

Some patient features are gathered from hospital information system (HIS) or paper-based patient records as illustrated by Table 1.

This study proposed a method to automatically extract other features from NCCT renal stone image slices. These features describe other kidney and stone characteristics, for instance, the shape, location and size.

CT scan produces cross-sectional image slices. The CT slice width determines the number of image slices. Each image slice displays the scanned tissue by assuming that it is sliced open along a plane. However, all of the image slices do not contain the kidney. Fig.2 shows different NCCT image slices for one patient.

Among the different image slices as shown in Figure 2, only image (c) shows the whole view of the kidneys. Therefore, it is required to find image slices that showing the kidney tissue before extracting the kidney and renal stone descriptors.

The main steps of extracting features from NCCT renal stone images include:

- Localizing the kidney in NCCT image slices manually by expert and drawing a bounding box around the kidney in the NCCT images.
- Cropping NCCT images so that only the bounding box and its inside pixels are remained.

Table 1. Description of features collected from HIS or paper-based patient records in HKC treated by SWL

Feature Set	Feature Code	Feature Name	values
S_2	$f_{2,1}$	Age	
S_2	$f_{2,2}$	SWL Date	
S_2	$f_{2,3}$	Stone treatment history	1: SWL 2: Open surgery 3: TUL 4: PCNL
S_2	$f_{2,4}$	Date of previous stone treatment	
S_2	$f_{2,5}$	Shockwave power	
S_2	$f_{2,6}$	Number of shockwaves	
S_2	$f_{2,7}$	Has pain	0: no 1: yes
S_2	$f_{2,8}$	Pain in left side	0: no 1: yes
S_2	$f_{2,9}$	Pain in right side	0: no 1: yes
S_2	$f_{2,10}$	Previous history of renal stone removal	1: occurred 2: not occurred
S_2	$f_{2,11}$	Drugs used: anticoagulant	0: no 1: yes
S_2	$f_{2,12}$	Diabetes	0: no 1: yes
S_2	$f_{2,13}$	Hypertension	0: no 1: yes
S_2	$f_{2,14}$	Ultrasound after SWL	0: not recommended 1: recommended
S_2	$f_{2,15}$	Isotope scan after SWL	0: not recommended 1: recommended
S_2	$f_{2,16}$	KUB after SWL	0: not recommended 1: recommended
S_2	$f_{2,17}$	CT-Scan after SWL	0: not recommended 1: recommended
S_2	$f_{2,18}$	Drugs prescribed after SWL: Drug Name	
S_2	$f_{2,19}$	Drugs prescribed after SWL: Drug Dosage	
S_2	$f_{2,20}$	Drugs prescribed after SWL: Drug usage pattern	
S_4	$f_{4,1}$	Stone Position	1: right kidney 2: left kidney 3: upper calyces 4: lower calyces 5: pelvis 6: right ureter 7: left ureter 8: upper ureter 9: lower ureter
S_4	$f_{4,2}$	Stone size	
S_4	$f_{4,3}$	Number of stones	
S_4	$f_{4,4}$	Stone type	
S_4	$f_{4,5}$	Stone localization method	1: Ultrasound 2: X-ray 3: both of them

Figure 2. Different NCCT image slices for one patient

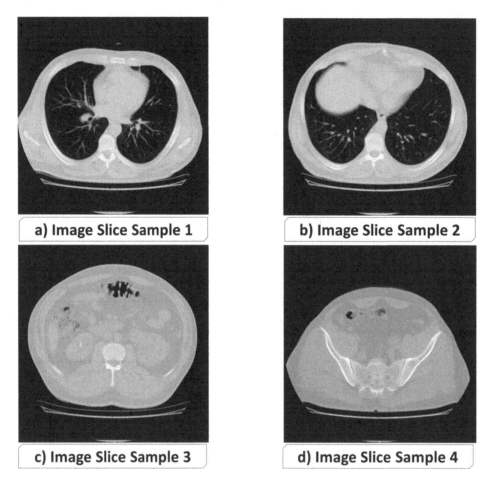

a) Image Slice Sample 1

b) Image Slice Sample 2

c) Image Slice Sample 3

d) Image Slice Sample 4

- Segmenting the NCCT image inside the bounding box and identifying the tissue and stone regions automatically.
- Computing the features from the segmented images.

Only some of the NCCT image slices for one patient show the kidney and renal stone. Therefore, at first, the expert verifies which NCCT image slices show the kidney and renal stone. Then, only the image slices containing kidney and renal stone are considered for further analysis.

The expert draws a bounding box around the kidney in each remaining NCCT image slices. Outside of the bounding box is removed from the image (as shown in Figure 3).

Then, the cropped image (region inside the red rectangle in Figure 3) must be segmented.

Image segmentation divides image pixels into some homogeneous regions. Many different methods have been proposed for medical image segmentation. CT scan images are gray-scale images. Color based segmentation methods and texture based methods are not applicable to CT images. Therefore, the segmentation methods which are appropriate for gray scale images, are considered. Sharma and Aggrawal have classified gray scale segmentation methods to three different classes based on the features used in the segmentation method. This classification includes methods based on histogram features, edge based

Figure 3. Marking the kidney in NCCT image slice by the expert

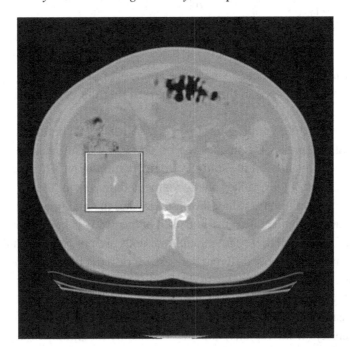

methods and region based methods (Sharma & Aggrawal, 2010). Segmentation based on thresholding the images is an example of the first class methods which is suitable for an image with regions of uniform brightness (Sharma & Aggrawal, 2010).

Since, NCCT images are gray-scale images with a few different intensities and the intensity of soft tissues like the kidney is known in advance, multi threshold segmentation method (Otsu, 1979) is appropriate for segmentation. Moreover, it is a simple and very fast method.

In this method, m different thresholds T_1, T_2, ..., T_m are calculated based on the different gray values of image pixels (considering the histogram of pixel intensities) and the image is converted to $(m+1)$ different level pixels.

Then, the intensity of each pixel in the segmented image is calculated based on Eq. 1:

$$intensity_{i.j}^{new} = \begin{cases} 0 & intensity_{i.j} \leq T_1 \\ 255 / m & T_1 \leq intensity_{i.j} \leq T_2 \\ ... & ... \\ 255 & intensity_{i.j} \geq T_m \end{cases} \quad (1)$$

where $intensity_{i.j}$ and $intensity^{new}_{i.j}$ are the intensities of the pixel in i^{th} row and j^{th} column of the image before and after the segmentation process, respectively.

In previous studies, a quality measure $Q(S)$ has been used for evaluating the quality of image segmentation methods. $Q(S)$ is defined in Eq. 2 (Borsotti, Campadelli, & Schettini, 1998):

$$Q(S) = \frac{1}{10000 * M * N} \sqrt{R \sum_{i=1}^{R} \left(\frac{e_i^2}{1 + logA_i} + \left(\frac{R(A_i)}{A_i} \right)^2 \right)} \qquad (2)$$

More details of the quality measure $Q(S)$ have been presented in (Borsotti et al., 1998).

The quality measure $Q(S)$ is used in this study for verifying the performance of the segmentation method.

In this study, after trying different m values ($m = 2,3,4,5,6,7$) the experimental results show that the best value of m for segmenting NCCT images (based on $Q(S)$ measure and experts' opinions) in the dataset is 4. Therefore, $m=4$ is used in the study for segmentation in NCCT images.

The summary of statistics of $Q(S)$ values on the segmented images for the dataset is listed in Table 2.

As shown in Table 2, the minimum value (the best one) and the maximum value (the worst case) are very low. It clarifies that the segmentation method used in this study is good enough for segmenting the images in the dataset. Therefore, other segmentation methods are not applied on the dataset.

But, each NCCT image may show different soft tissues or parts of them. Therefore, it is needed to determine which regions indicate the kidney. In this study, without loss of generality, it is assumed that the largest region among segmented regions of soft tissues (soft tissues are shown in medium gray color in NCCT images) indicates the kidney. Moreover, this study focuses on the calcium stones. These stones are shown in light intensity (white regions) and are bounded by the kidney tissue.

Therefore, it is known which segments show the soft tissues in NCCT images and which ones show renal stones (Figure 4).

Now, it is known which regions indicating the kidneys and renal stones. The next step is to extract the shape, size and location descriptors from these regions.

Let us assume that among all of the NCCT image slices from one patient, $I(=2J+1)$ consecutive image slices indicate the kidney. Therefore, among these I image slices, the image slice indicating the kidney with the largest area (in terms of pixels in the kidney segmented region) is considered as I_0. The jth previous image slice is considered as I_{-j} and the jth next image slice is considered as I_{+j}.

It is assumed that S_1 is the set of all features that it is proposed to be extracted from NCCT images. These features will be described in the following sections.

Stone Size Descriptors

Previous studies have shown that the renal stone volume, area and stone dimensions are important descriptors (Lin et al., 2008; Nazim et al., 2014; Saedi & Moulavi, 2012). But, most of them have been calculated manually by expert. In this study, the stone burden descriptors are extracted automatically from NCCT images with new proposed methods.

Table 2. Summary statistics of the quality measure on the segmented images of the dataset

Data	Min($Q(S)$)	Max($Q(S)$)	Mean($Q(S)$)
trainset	0.0114	0.0172	0.0138
testSet	0.0112	0.0169	0.0133

Figure 4. a) The original image, b) The kidney in the segmented image, c)The renal stone in the segmented image

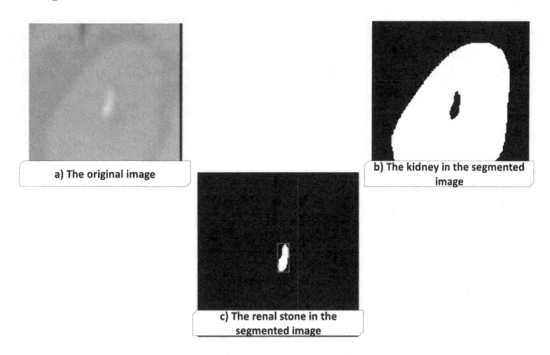

a) The original image

b) The kidney in the segmented image

c) The renal stone in the segmented image

One of the stone size descriptors is stone volume. Duan et al. have proposed a method for volume estimation of kidney stones from computerized tomography images. In their proposed method, the full width of stone has been estimated by applying a threshold equal to the average of the computerized tomography number of the object and the background. Then, their estimation has been corrected based on a model of a sphere and a 3-dimensional Gaussian point spread function(Duan et al., 2012). Since the Guassian function parameters can affect the estimation, therefore another method is used for stone volume estimation. In this method, the stone volume $(f_{1,1})$ is estimated as a summation of stone pixels in the K consecutive image slices multiplied by the slice width (Eq. 3):

$$f_{1,1} = Stone\, Volume = slice_{Width} \times \sum_{p=-J}^{J} A_{S\,p} \tag{3}$$

where $Slice_{Width}$ is the width of the consecutive image slices in NCCT images, and A_{S_p} is the area of the stone in the image I_p $(-J \leq p \leq J)$.

Stone area is described by two features including the maximal stone area $(f_{1,2})$ among the K consecutive image slices I_p(Eq.4) and the average of stone area $(f_{1,3})$ among these images (Eq.5).

$$f_{1,2} = max\left\{ A_{S_p} : -J \leq p \leq J \right\} \tag{4}$$

$$f_{1,3} = mean\left\{A_{S_p} : -J \le p \le J\right\} \tag{5}$$

For extracting the stone dimensions, large and small diameters of the oval bounded around the stone are calculated for each of K consecutive images. Then, the maximal and average values are considered as descriptors of stone dimensions. Maximal large (small) diameter is denoted by $f_{1,4}$ ($f_{1,5}$) and the average large (small) diameter is denoted by $f_{1,6}$ ($f_{1,7}$),

$$f_{1,4} = max\left\{LD_{S_p} : -J \le p \le J\right\} \tag{6}$$

$$f_{1,5} = max\left\{SD_{S_p} : -J \le p \le J\right\} \tag{7}$$

$$f_{1,6} = mean\left\{LD_{S_p} : -J \le p \le J\right\} \tag{8}$$

$$f_{1,7} = mean\left\{SD_{S_p} : -J \le p \le J\right\} \tag{9}$$

Where LDs_p and SDs_p are large diameter and small diameter of the oval bounded around the stone in image I_p, respectively.

Moreover, the ratio of the large diameter of oval bounded around the stone to the large diameter of oval bounded around the kidney ($f_{1,8}$), the ratio of maximal stone area to maximal kidney area ($f_{1,9}$) and the ratio of stone volume to the kidney volume ($f_{1,10}$) are calculated as follows:

$$f_{1,8} = f_{1,4} \,/\, Large\,Diameter\,of\,the\,oval\,bounding\,the\,kidney\,in\,I_0 \tag{10}$$

$$f_{1,9} = f_{1,2} \,/\, A_{K_0} \tag{11}$$

$$f_{1,10} = f_{1,1} \,/\, V_K \tag{12}$$

Where A_{K0} is the kidney area in I_0 and V_K is the kidney volume.

The ratio of small diameter to large diameter of stone ($f_{1,11}$), the ratio of large diameter of stone to stone area ($f_{1,12}$) and stone orientation (angle between the large diameter of stone and horizontal axis) ($f_{1,13}$) are calculated.

$$f_{1,11} = f_{1,5} \, / \, f_{1,4} \tag{13}$$

$$f_{1,12} = f_{1,4} \, / \, f_{1,2} \tag{14}$$

Stone Position Descriptors

The distance between stone center of gravity and kidney center of gravity is calculated ($f_{1,14}$).

The nearest distance ($f_{1,15}$) and the average distance ($f_{1,16}$) between the stone border and the kidney border are calculated.

Skin to stone distance ($f_{1,17}$) is calculated automatically from the NCCT images as well. For this purpose, the measures are used which have been proposed by Geng et al. (Geng et al., 2015).

Kidney Descriptors

Features including maximal kidney area ($f_{1,18}$) and the kidney volume ($f_{1,19}$) are calculated.

$$f_{1,18} = A_{K_0} \tag{15}$$

$$f_{1,19} = Kidney\,Volume = slice_{Width} \times \sum_{p=-J}^{J} A_{Kp} \tag{16}$$

Where A_{Kp} is the kidney area in I_p ($-J \leq p \leq J$).

Preprocessing the Collected Data

The second step is preprocessing and cleaning the collected data. This step includes missing value imputation, outlier detection and removal, and data normalization.

Features extracted from CT images have no missing values. Therefore, missing value imputation is performed on the features collected from HIS or paper-based patient records in HKC treated by SWL, as denoted as*S2* and *S4* features in Table 1.

Many algorithms have been proposed for missing value imputation in previous researches. In this study, KnnImpute method is used for missing value imputation (Troyanskaya et al., 2001). KnnImpute method is a weighted k-nearest neighbor method. The reason for using this method is that the previous studies showed that it has better performance in comparison with other imputation methods (Troyanskaya et al., 2001).

The next step is outlier detection and removal. For this purpose, distance-based outlier detection method is used which is an improved k-NN outlier detection method(Wang & Zheng, 2010). In this method, data is clustered at first. Then, all the clusters having no outlier are removed. The remaining clusters are considered for outlier detection. For each data in the remaining clusters, its K nearest neighbors are computed. If the distance between data and its k-nearest neighbors is more than a predefined threshold, then the data is considered as an outlier and consequently removed from the data set. Previous researches have shown that this method is fast enough and has reasonable accuracy in outlier detection (Wang & Zheng, 2010). In this study, after verifying different K values and different thresholds, the best results are obtained by using $K=3$ and threshold$=K*$ average of the pair wise distances belonging to the first, second and third quantile of the pair wise distance for different samples of the cluster.

Finally, the nominal attributes with m different levels are replaced with (m-1) binary variables. For more details, Han et al. book can be studied (Han et al., 2012).

The ordinal attributes and the numeric ones are normalized using min-max normalization method (Eq. 17):

$$F_i = (f_i - Min(f_i)) \ / \ (Max(f_i) - Min(f_i))$$
(17)

Where f_i and F_i are the ith attribute value before and after normalization, respectively. $Min(f_i)$ and $Max(f_i)$ are the minimum and maximum value among the f_i value for all patients, respectively.

Training Classifier for Predicting Retreatment After SWL

Afterwards, the classifiers must be trained on a training sample data. To this end, class-balanced random sampling (Han, Kamber, & Pei, 2012)is performed and some classifiers including Decision Tree, Support Vector Machines, k-Nearest Neighbors and Naïve Bayes(NB) are used(Han et al., 2012)to predict retreatment after SWL. The performance of each classifier is evaluated using 10-fold cross validation method.

Evaluation and Validation

The aim is to know which feature set can predict retreatment after SWL best. Therefore, different classifiers are trained on different feature sets and their performance measures are compared.

The performance measures used for comparing the classifiers and different feature sets include Precision (Eq.18), Recall (Eq. 19), Accuracy (Eq.20) and F-Measure (Eq.21)(Han et al., 2012).

$$\text{Precision} = \frac{TP}{TP + FP}$$
(18)

$$\text{Recall} = \frac{TP}{TP + FN}$$
(19)

$$\text{Accuracy} = \frac{TP + TN}{TP + FP + TN + FN}$$
(20)

$$F - Measure = 2.\frac{\text{Precision} \times \text{Recall}}{\text{Precision} + \text{Recall}} \qquad (21)$$

In the above equations, *TP*, *FP*, *TN* and *FN* denote true positive, false positive, true negative and false negative records, respectively.

Table 3 lists and compares the performance of the classifiers trained on different subsets of the features including proposed stone descriptors (*S1*), patient features (*S2*), union of *S1* and *S2* (*S3*), other stone descriptors (*S4*), union of *S1* and *S4* (*S5*), union of *S2* and *S4* (*S6*), and union of *S1*, *S2* and *S4* (*S7*).

Table 3. Comparing the performance of the classifiers trained on different feature sets

Feature Set	Classifier	Precision (%)	Recall (%)	Accuracy(%)	F-Measure(%)
S_1	Decision Tree	55	54	55	54
S_2	Decision Tree	53	52	53	52
$S_3 (S_1 + S_2)$	Decision Tree	75	75	75	75
S_4	Decision Tree	52	52	52	52
$S_5 (S_1 + S_4)$	Decision Tree	72	72	72	72
$S_6 (S_2 + S_4)$	Decision Tree	68	66	67	67
$S_7 (S_1 + S_2 + S_4)$	Decision Tree	82	79	81	80
S_1	K-NN	55	51	55	53
S_2	K-NN	52	51	52	51
$S_3 (S_1 + S_2)$	K-NN	73	75	74	74
S_4	K-NN	52	51	52	51
$S_5 (S_1 + S_4)$	K-NN	71	72	71	71
$S_6 (S_2 + S_4)$	K-NN	67	68	67	67
$S_7 (S_1 + S_2 + S_4)$	K-NN	80	76	78	78
S_1	SVM	60	64	61	62
S_2	SVM	57	57	57	57
$S_3 (S_1 + S_2)$	SVM	82	82	82	82
S_4	SVM	56	58	56	57
$S_5 (S_1 + S_4)$	SVM	76	75	76	75
$S_6 (S_2 + S_4)$	SVM	71	72	71	71
$S_7 (S_1 + S_2 + S_4)$	SVM	88	87	87	87
S_1	NB	60	60	60	60
S_2	NB	56	56	56	56
$S_3 (S_1 + S_2)$	NB	80	78	79	79
S_4	NB	55	58	55	56
$S_5 (S_1 + S_4)$	NB	75	76	75	75
$S_6 (S_2 + S_4)$	NB	70	72	70	71
$S_7 (S_1 + S_2 + S_4)$	NB	87	84	86	85

The proposed stone descriptors that are included in $S1$, are features describing stone volume ($f_{1,1}$), maximal stone area ($f_{1,2}$), average stone area ($f_{1,3}$), maximal large (small) diameter of stone $f_{1,4}$ ($f_{1,5}$) and the average large (small) diameter of stone $f_{1,6}$ ($f_{1,7}$), the ratio of the large diameter of oval bounded around the stone to the large diameter of oval bounded around the kidney ($f_{1,8}$), the ratio of stone area to kidney area ($f_{1,9}$) and the ratio of stone volume to the kidney volume ($f_{1,10}$), the ratio of the small diameter to the large diameter of stone ($f_{1,11}$), the ratio of large diameter of stone to the stone area ($f_{1,12}$) and stone orientation (angle between the large diameter of stone and the horizontal axis) ($f_{1,13}$), the distance between stone center of gravity and kidney center of gravity ($f_{1,14}$), the nearest distance ($f_{1,15}$) and the average distance ($f_{1,16}$) between the stone border and the kidney border, Skin to stone distance ($f_{1,17}$), maximal kidney area ($f_{1,18}$) and the kidney volume ($f_{1,19}$).

Patient features in $S2$ are age, SWL date, stone treatment history, date of previous stone treatment, Shockwave power, number of shockwaves, absence or presence of pain, absence or presence of pain in left side, absence or presence of pain in right side, previous history of renal stone removal,(anticoagulant, diabetes, hypertension) drugs used or not, ultrasound after SWL or not, isotope scan after SWL or not, KUB after SWL or not, CT-Scan after SWL or not, drugs prescribed after SWL, dosage of drugs prescribed after SWL and usage pattern of drugs prescribed after SWL.

Other stone descriptors in $S4$ include stone position, stone size, number of stones, stone type and stone localization method.

Figures 5-8 show the precision, recall, accuracy and F-measure of the different classifiers trained based on different feature sets.

Figure 5. The precision of different classifiers trained by different feature sets

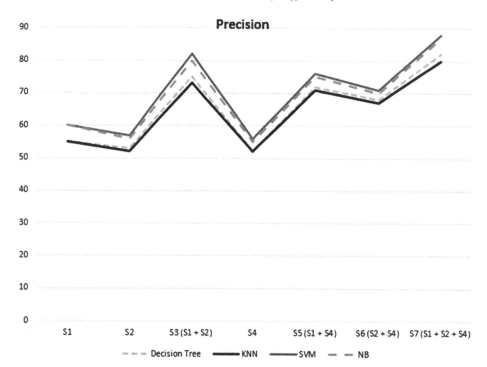

Figure 6. Recall of different classifiers trained by different feature sets

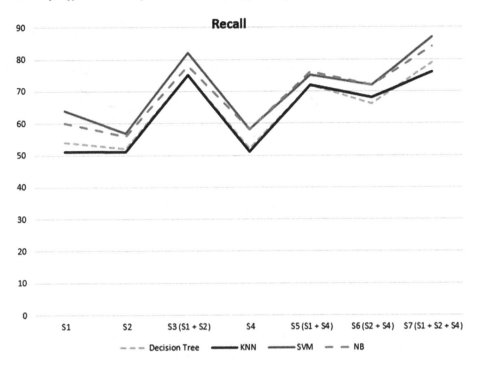

Figure 7. Accuracy of different classifiers trained on different feature sets

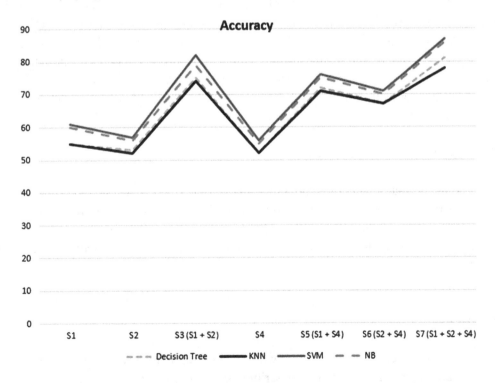

Figure 8. F-measure of the classifiers trained by different feature sets

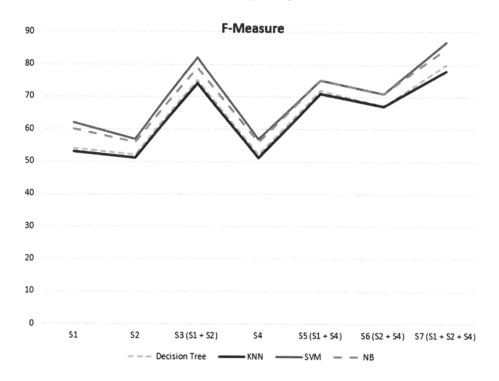

As illustrated by Table 3 and Figures 5-8, the experimental results show that S_3 is the best feature set for predicting retreatment after SWL among S_1, S_2 and S_3 and the second best one is S_1. Moreover, among S_4-S_7, the best feature set which can predict retreatment after SWL with the highest accuracy is S_7 and the second best one is S_5. This means that adding the proposed features to the other stone and patient features can improve prediction performance. On the other hand, the proposed features can be extracted fast and automatically. Therefore, there is no obstacle in using them for retreatment prediction.

FUTURE RESEARCH DIRECTIONS

In the future, the aim is to automatically identify the kidney in the NCCT image slices via image processing tools and remove the need for expert intervention to mark the kidney. Moreover, the automatic tracking of the kidney stone in the subsequent NCCT image slices is an interesting future research opportunity.

Other future research can propose more renal stone descriptors in order to predict SWL success rate more accurately.

CONCLUSION

In this study, some novel features are proposed which can be automatically extracted from renal NCCT images. These new features include features describing stone volume, stone area, large (small) diameter of stone, the ratio of the large diameter of oval bounded around the stone to the large diameter of oval bounded around the kidney, the ratio of stone area to kidney area and the ratio of stone volume to the kidney volume, the ratio of the small diameter to the large diameter of stone, the ratio of large diameter of stone to the stone area and stone orientation, the distance between stone center of gravity and kidney center of gravity, the distance between the stone border and the kidney border, Skin to stone distance, maximal kidney area and the kidney volume. This study proposes new algorithms for extracting the above mentioned features.

The experimental results showed that adding the proposed features to the patient and stone features which has been recorded in HIS and paper based records can improve the performance of retreatment prediction after SWL. The calculation modules for the proposed features can be added to NCCT image analysis software.

One of the limitations of this work is that the region of interest including the kidney from NCCT images must be specified by expert manually.

REFERENCES

Alger, P. W., Niederberger, C. S., & Turk, T. M. (2009). Neural Network to Predict Stone Free Rate Status After SWL, PCNL or Ureteroscopy. *The Journal of Urology*, *181*(4), 492. doi:10.1016/S0022-5347(09)61391-4 PMID:19110280

Bach, C., & Buchholz, N. (2011). Shock Wave Lithotripsy for Renal and Ureteric Stones. *European Urology Supplements*, *10*(5), 423–432. doi:10.1016/j.eursup.2011.07.004

Borsotti, M., Campadelli, P., & Schettini, R. (1998). Quantitative evaluation of color image segmentation results. *Pattern Recognition Letters*, *19*(8), 741–747. doi:10.1016/S0167-8655(98)00052-X

Budía, A., Lopez-Acon, J. D., Trassierra, M., & Boronat, F. (2015). Is an Increase in the Number of Shock Waves per Session Effective and Safe in Extracorporeal Lithotripsy? A Randomized, Prospective and Comparative Study. *European Urology Supplements*, *193*(4), 454–455.

Chaussy, C. H., Brendel, W., & Schmiedt, E. (1980). Extracorporeally induced destruction of kidney stones by shock waves. *Lancet*, *2*(8207), 1265–1268. doi:10.1016/S0140-6736(80)92335-1 PMID:6108446

Chen, P. C., Liu, Y. T., Hsieh, J. H., & Wang, C. C. (2016). *A practical formula to predict the stone-free rate of patients undergoing extracorporeal shock wave lithotripsy*. Urological Science. doi:10.1016/j.urols.2016.05.004

Choi, J. W., Song, P. H., & Kim, H. T. (2012). Predictive factors of the outcome of extracorporeal shockwave lithotripsy for ureteral stones. *Korean J Urol*, *53*(6), 424–430. doi:10.4111/kju.2012.53.6.424 PMID:22741053

Duan, X., Wang, J., Qu, M., Leng, S., Liu, Y., Krambeck, A., & McCollough, C. (2012). Kidney Stone Volume Estimation from Computerized Tomography Images Using a Model Based Method of Correcting for the Point Spread Function. *The Journal of Urology*, *188*(3), 989–995. doi:10.1016/j.juro.2012.04.098 PMID:22819107

Dunmirea, B., Harperb, J. D., Cunitza, B. W., Leeb, F. C., Hsib, R., Liud, Z., & Sorensen, M. D. et al. (2016). Use of the Acoustic Shadow Width to Determine Kidney Stone Size with Ultrasound. *The Journal of Urology*, *195*(1), 171–177. doi:10.1016/j.juro.2015.05.111 PMID:26301788

El-Nahas, A. R., El-Assmy, A. M., Mansour, O., & Sheir, K. Z. (2007). A Prospective Multivariate Analysis of Factors Predicting Stone Disintegration by Extracorporeal Shock Wave Lithotripsy: The Value of High-Resolution Noncontrast Computed Tomography. *European Urology*, *51*(6), 1688–1694. doi:10.1016/j.eururo.2006.11.048 PMID:17161522

Geng, J. H., Tu, H. P., Shih, P. M. C., Shen, J. T., Jang, M. Y., Wu, W. J., & Juan, Y. S. et al. (2015). Noncontrast computed tomography can predict the outcome of shockwave lithotripsy via accurate stone measurement and abdominal fat distribution determination. *The Kaohsiung Journal of Medical Sciences*, *31*(1), 34–41. doi:10.1016/j.kjms.2014.10.001 PMID:25600918

Goktas, C., Akca, O., Horuz, R., Gokhan, O., Albayrak, S., & Sarica, K. (2011). SWL in Lower Calyceal Calculi: Evaluation of the Treatment Results in Children and Adults. *Urology*, *78*(6), 1402–1406. doi:10.1016/j.urology.2011.08.005 PMID:21962877

Han, J., Kamber, M., & Pei, J. (2012). *Data Mining: Concepts and Techniques*. Morgan Kauffman. doi:10.1007/978-1-4419-1428-6_3752

Kang, D. H., Chung, D. Y., Cho, K. S., Lee, D. H., Han, J. H., Kang, H. W., & Lee, J. Y. et al. (2015). Impact of colic pain as a significant factor for predicting the stone free rate of one-session shock wave lithotripsy for treating ureter stones: A Bayesian logistic regression model analysis. *European Urology Supplements*, 14.

Kim, T. B., Lee, S. C., Kim, K. H., Jung, H., Yoon, S. J., & Oh, J. K. (2013). The feasibility of shockwave lithotripsy for treating solitary, lower calyceal stones over 1 cm in size. *Canadian Urological Association*, *7*(3), 156–160. doi:10.5489/cuaj.473 PMID:23589749

Lee, H. Y., Yang, Y. H., Lee, Y. L., Shen, J. T., Jang, M. Y., Shih, P. M. C., & Juan, Y. S. et al. (2015). Noncontrast computed tomography factors that predict the renal stone outcome after shock wave lithotripsy. *Clinical Imaging*, *39*(5), 845–850. doi:10.1016/j.clinimag.2015.04.010 PMID:25975631

Lin, C. C., Hsu, Y. S., & Chen, K. K. (2008). Predictive Factors of Lower Calyceal Stone Clearance After Extracorporeal Shockwave Lithotripsy (ESWL): The Impact of Radiological Anatomy. *Chinese Medical Associations*, *71*(10), 496-501.

Nazim, S. M., Ather, M. H., & Khan, N. (2014). Measurement of Ureteric Stone Diameter in Different Planes on Multidetector Computed Tomography e Impact on the Clinical Decision Making. *Urology*, *83*(2), 288–293. doi:10.1016/j.urology.2013.09.037 PMID:24275282

Otsu, N. (1979). A Threshold Selection Method from Gray-Level Histograms. *IEEE Transactions on Systems, Man, and Cybernetics*, *9*(1), 62–66. doi:10.1109/TSMC.1979.4310076

Pareek, G., Armenakas, N. A., Panagopoulos, G., Bruno, J. J., & Fracchia, J. A. (2005). Extracorporeal shock wave lithotripsy success based on body mass index and Hounsfield units. *Urology*, *65*, 33-36.

Perks, A. E., Schuler, T. D., Lee, J., Ghiculete, D., Chung, D. G., & Honey, R. J. (2008). Stone attenuation and skin-to-stone distance on computed tomography predicts for stone fragmentation by shock wave lithotripsy. *Urology*, *72*(4), 765–769. doi:10.1016/j.urology.2008.05.046 PMID:18674803

Raj, G., Auge, B. K., Weizer, A. Z., Denstedt, J. D., Watterson, J. D., Beiko, D. T., & Preminger, G. M. et al.G.V. (2003). Percutaneous Management of Calculi Within Horseshoe Kidneys. *The Journal of Urology*, *170*(1), 48–51. doi:10.1097/01.ju.0000067620.60404.2d PMID:12796642

Resorlu, B., Unsal, A., Gulec, H., & Oztuna, D. (2012). A New Scoring System for Predicting Stone-free Rate After Retrograde Intrarenal Surgery: The Resorlu-Unsal Stone Score. *Urology*, *80*(3), 512–518. doi:10.1016/j.urology.2012.02.072 PMID:22840867

Saedi, D., & Moulavi, M. (2012). Association between some CT characteristics of renal stones and extracorporeal shockwave lithotripsy success rate. *Tehran University Medical Journal*, *70*(3), 169–175.

Selby, M. G., Vrtiska, T. J., Krambeck, A. E., McCollough, C. H., Elsherbiny, H. E., Bergstralh, E. J., & Rule, A. D. et al. (2015). Quantification of Asymptomatic Kidney Stone Burden by Computed Tomography for Predicting Future Symptomatic Stone Events. *Urology*, *85*(1), 45–50. doi:10.1016/j.urology.2014.08.031 PMID:25440821

Sepehri, M. M., Rahnama, P., Shadpour, P., & Teimourpour, B. (2009). A data mining based model for selecting type of treatment for kidney stone patients. *Tehran University Medical Journal*, *67*(6), 421–427.

Sharma, N., & Aggrawal, L. (2010). Automated medical image segmentation techniques. *Journal of Medical Physics*, *35*(1), 3–14. doi:10.4103/0971-6203.58777 PMID:20177565

Skolarikos, A., Alivizatos, G., & Delarosette, J. (2005). Percutaneous Nephrolithotomy and its Legacy. *European Urology*, *47*(1), 22–28. doi:10.1016/j.eururo.2004.08.009 PMID:15582245

Sparks, R., & Madabhushi, A. (2013). Explicit shape descriptors: Novel morphologic features for histopathology classification. *Medical Image Analysis*, *17*(8), 997–1009. doi:10.1016/j.media.2013.06.002 PMID:23850744

Sternberg, K. M., Eisner, B., Larson, T., Hernandez, N., Han, J., & Pais, V. M. (2016). Ultrasonography Significantly Overestimates Stone Size When Compared to Low-dose, Noncontrast Computed Tomography. *Urology*, *95*, 67–71. doi:10.1016/j.urology.2016.06.002 PMID:27289025

Torricelli, F. C. M., Marchini, G. S., Yamauchi, F. I., Danilovic, A., Vicentini, F. C., Srougi, M., & Mazzucchi, E. et al. (2015). Impact of Renal Anatomy on Shock Wave Lithotripsy Outcomes for Lower Pole Kidney Stones: Results of a Prospective Multifactorial Analysis Controlled by Computerized Tomography. *The Journal of Urology*, *193*(6), 2002–2007. doi:10.1016/j.juro.2014.12.026 PMID:25524240

Treigny, O. M. D., Nasr, E. B., Almont, T., Tack, I., Rischmann, P., Souli, M., & Huyghe, E. (2015). The Cumulated Stone Diameter: A Limited Tool for Stone Burden Estimation. *Urology*, *86*(3), 477–481. doi:10.1016/j.urology.2015.06.018 PMID:26135811

Troyanskaya, O., Cantor, M., Sherlock, G., Brown, P., Hastie, T., Tibshirani, R., & Altman, R. B. et al. (2001). Missing value estimation methods for DNA microarrays. *Bioinformatics (Oxford, England)*, *17*(6), 520–525. doi:10.1093/bioinformatics/17.6.520 PMID:11395428

Wang, Q., & Zheng, M. (2010). An improved KNN based outlier detection algorithm for large datasets. *Advanced Data Mining and Applications, 6440*, 585–592. doi:10.1007/978-3-642-17316-5_56

Wiesenthal, J. D., Ghiculete, D., Ray, A., Honey, R. J. D., & Pace, K. T. (2011). A clinical nomogram to predict the successful shockwave lithotripsy of renal and ureteral calculi. *European Urology Supplements, 10*(2), 38. doi:10.1016/S1569-9056(11)60034-1

Zhu, Z., Wang, S., Xi, Q., Bai, J., Yu, X., & Liu, J. (2011). Logistic Regression Model for Predicting Stone-Free Rate After Minimally Invasive Percutaneous Nephrolithotomy. *Endourology and Stones, 78*(1), 32–36. PMID:21296398

KEY TERMS AND DEFINITIONS

Classification: Deciding which data record belongs to each class.

Data Preprocessing: Preparing and cleaning the data records.

Image Slices: 2D images captured by CT scan from a soft tissue.

Kidney Descriptors: Features describing the position, shape and size of the kidneys.

Non-Contrast CT Images: One type of imaging recommended for detecting and characterizing the renal stones.

Renal Stone Descriptors: Features describing the renal stone position, shape and size.

Shockwave Lithotripsy: A non-invasive treatment procedure for small renal stones.

Chapter 14
Applications of Image Processing in Laparoscopic Surgeries:
An Overview

Toktam Khatibi
Tarbiat Modares University (TMU), Iran

Mohammad Mehdi Sepehri
Tarbiat Modares University (TMU), Iran

Pejman Shadpour
Iran University of Medical Sciences (IUMS), Iran

Seyed Hessameddin Zegordi
Tarbiat Modares University (TMU), Iran

ABSTRACT

Laparoscopy is a minimally-invasive surgery using a few small incisions on the patient's body to insert the tools and telescope and conduct the surgical operation. Laparoscopic video processing can be used to extract valuable knowledge and help the surgeons. We discuss the present and possible future role of processing laparoscopic videos. The various applications are categorized for image processing algorithms in laparoscopic surgeries including preprocessing video frames by laparoscopic image enhancement, telescope related applications (telescope position estimation, telescope motion estimation and compensation), surgical instrument related applications (surgical instrument detection and tracking), soft tissue related applications (soft tissue segmentation and deformation tracking) and high level applications such as safe actions in laparoscopic videos, summarization of laparoscopic videos, surgical task recognition and extracting knowledge using fusion techniques. Some different methods have been proposed previously for each of the mentioned applications using image processing.

DOI: 10.4018/978-1-5225-2515-8.ch014

INTRODUCTION

The general perspective of the chapter is considering different applications of processing laparoscopic videos to extract the valuable knowledge. The main scope is considering the applications of image processing for laparoscopic videos. For this purpose, only the previous studies proposing methods for processing RGB videos of laparoscopic/endoscopic surgeries are considered. 3D videos like RGB-D images and videos augmented by supplementary data from the external sensors or other types of images such as MRI are not in the scope of this study.

The rest of the paper is organized as follows. Section 2 reviews the applications of image mining in laparoscopy. In section 3, the datasets being used in the previous studies are listed and the discussion is presented in section 4. Finally, section 5 summarizes and concludes the paper.

BACKGROUND

Laparoscopy lies in the category of endoscopic interventions. During the endoscopic interventions, a camera called endoscope is inserted into the patient body to display the internal organs. Endoscopes are divided into two categories including flexible endoscope used for inspecting the esophagus, stomach, small bowel, colon and airways; and rigid endoscope used for a variety of minimal invasive surgeries (i.e., laparoscopy, arthroscopy, endoscopic neurosurgery). The endoscopes have various sizes with a tiny video camera at the tip (Oh et al., 2007). The endoscope in the laparoscopic surgeries is called telescope.

Laparoscopy is a minimally-invasive procedure with a few small incisions on the patient's body. Therefore, the hospital stay and recovery time for the patients after the laparoscopic surgeries is shorter than the open surgeries for similar surgical operations.

The first laparoscopic surgery was performed about 100 years ago on dogs. The first laparoscopic surgery on human was about 30 years ago. Till now, many advancements in laparoscopy have been occurred by introducing robotics and new instruments. It leads to less invasive surgeries (Cwach & Kavoussi,2016).

The surgical tools and the telescope are inserted through the incisions to conduct an operation. The telescope displays the internal organs and can record the surgery as a laparoscopic video (Uecker, Wang, Lee, & Wang, 1995).

Laparoscopy is widely used for diagnosis and treatment of many diseases (Yu et al., 2015). It has many advantages such as reduced patient trauma, reduced pain, decreased rates of infection and sepsis, small scars, reduced hospitalization with improved prognosis, lower rate of returning to the operating room, reduced need for blood transfusion and a quicker recovery (Amodeo, L., J.V., E., & H.R., 2009; Grasso, Finin, Zhu, Joshi, & Yesha, 2009; S. L. Lee et al., 2010; Semerjian, Zettervall, Amdur, Jarrett, & Vaziri, 2015).

But, this procedure has some drawbacks such as a limited view because of two-dimensional imaging, challenging eye-hand coordination, absence of tactile feedback (Schols, Bouvy, Dam, & Stassen, 2013) and surface view of the organs (Ma°rvik et al., 2004).

Many types of surgical operations can be performed by laparoscopic procedure. For example, laparoscopic partial nephrectomy (LPN) is a standard therapy method for renal carcinomas (Baumhauer et al., 2008). Laparoscopic cholecystectomy is a surgical procedure to remove the gall bladder (Sánchez-González et al., 2011). Some other surgeries that can be performed via laparoscopic procedure in reduced hospital stays, faster recovery, reduced pain and improved results compared with open surgery include colorectal surgery (Braga et al., 2010; Choi, Lee, Park, & Lee, 2010), cholecystectomy (Navarra, Pozza, Occhionorelli, Carcoforo, & Donini, 1997), appendectomy (D'Alessio, Piro, Tadini, & Beretta, 2002), adrenalectomy (Castellucci et al., 2008), hernia repair (Podolsky, Mouhlas, Wu, Poor, & Curcillo, 2010) and etc.

The laparoscopic surgery consists of three main phases including before inserting the telescope in the patient body, when the telescope lies inside the patient body and after the telescope has brought out from the patient body. The laparoscopic videos can be taken during the second phase. In the first phase, the patient is prepared for the surgery and some activities such as positioning, anesthesia and making the incisions are performed for the patient. The telescope is inserted into the patient body via one of the incisions. At this time, the second phase is started. In the second phase, all of the surgical activities being performed inside the patient's body can be displayed on the monitor via the telescope and recorded simultaneously. This video taken by the telescope in the second phase of the laparoscopic surgery can be processed for further analysis purposes. When the telescope is taken out from the patient's body for the last time and turns off, the second phase terminated and the third phase is started. The third phase continues till the patient is transferred to the recovery room. We want to review the previous studies proposing methods for processing the videos recorded in the second phase of the laparoscopic surgery.

A technical improvement in laparoscopic procedures is the robotic surgery. Robotic technology can provide stable camera with 3D optics and more comfortable position for surgeons. Different surgical robotic systems have been proposed previously such as AESOP, telerobotic Zeus and da Vinci systems. Telerobotic Zeus and da Vinci systems can be used for remote surgery as well. The robotic instruments simulate the surgeon's motion (Ballantyne, 2002).

Some main disadvantages of the laparoscopic surgery are limited precision and poor ergonomics for surgeons in using the instruments (Amodeo et al., 2009) which can be reduced by robotic surgery.

Since, a video of the laparoscopic surgery can be captured and recorded by the telescope, processing this video can be helpful for extracting useful knowledge from the laparoscopic video to answer the surgeons' questions. For example, the surgeons may want to know which surgical tasks are performed in a laparoscopic video and in which style every task is performed, which surgical instruments are inserted into the patient's body and the motion pattern of each instrument. The prerequisite for answering these questions is applying the appropriate image processing algorithms on the laparoscopic video to enhance the video, segment regionally and/or temporally the video, extracting the color, texture and motion based features from the segmented regions in the laparoscopic video. And then, using the extracted features, the high level knowledge can be extracted from the laparoscopic videos. For example, which motion pattern each instrument has and which surgical activity is being performed in each temporal segment of the video by the instruments.

Image processing can be used to improve the performance of laparoscopic robotic surgery. One of the characteristics of robotic laparoscopic surgery is using the robots to hold and manipulate the endoscope to help the surgeon during the lengthy surgery (X. Zhang & Payandeh, 2002).

Visual tracking method is needed to achieve automated instrument localization and endoscope maneuvering in robot-assisted laparoscopic surgery (X. Zhang & Payandeh, 2002).

Depth perception in minimally invasive surgery is reduced because of two-dimensional and limited field of view in laparoscopic videos. Augmented reality uses patient's medical images (US, CT or MRI) to increase the surgeon's vision via 3D visualization of anatomical or pathological structures and the registration of this visualization on the real patient (S. Nicolau, Soler, Mutter, & Marescaux, 2011).

APPLICATIONS OF IMAGE PROCESSING IN LAPAROSCOPY

As mentioned in the previous sections, laparoscopic technique in surgery allows to record surgical videos captured by the telescope.

Laparoscopic video shows the tissues and surgical tasks performed on the tissues by the surgical instruments if the telescope is inside the patient's body. Therefore, many applications can be solved by image processing on laparoscopic videos.

Sometimes, the telescope is outpatient for some reasons. Camera position classification (whether the telescope is inpatient or outpatient), camera motion estimation and compensation, surgical instrument detection and tracking, tissue segmentation and navigation are some elementary problems can be solved by processing the laparoscopic images.

The mentioned applications can obtain the desired information to help solve some more complicated problems such as laparoscopic video summarization, safe action detection, and laparoscopic activity recognition.

There are some complicated problems that cannot be solved only by analyzing the laparoscopic videos. They need more information that must be obtained from other imaging techniques such as MRI, CT, and etc.

3D models can be obtained by augmenting the laparoscopic video with other information such as other imaging techniques or data obtained by external sensors. These models can be used in virtual reality for enhancing the surgical skills of the novice surgeons and mining these datasets is not in the scope of our study.

As illustrated by Figure 1, factors having visible effects on the laparoscopic videos are telescope, surgical instruments and soft tissues. Their related image processing problems are shown in Figure 1 as well.

Figure 1. Factors having visible effects on the laparoscopic videos and their corresponding image processing problems

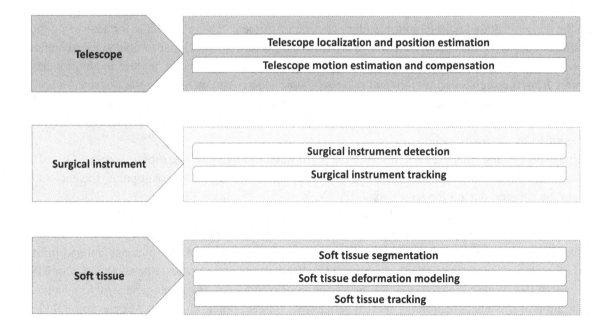

In this study, we will focus on applications that can be solved by processing the laparoscopic videos (as shown in Figure 2).

Figure 2 shows different image processing tasks that can be performed on the laparoscopic video. These tasks are classified into pre-processing task, low and mid-level tasks and high-level tasks. Pre-processing task includes image processing algorithms being exploited for enhancing the laparoscopic video frames by reducing noise, improving the contrast and etc.

Usually, before performing every image processing task on the laparoscopic video, it is required to pre-process the laparoscopic video frames. Therefore, the output of the laparoscopic image enhancement is the input of the tasks in the second category in Figure 2.

The second category illustrated in Figure 2 includes three different task types that try to extract features from the telescope, surgical instruments and soft tissues. The first task tries to estimate the position and motion of the telescope which is the camera of the video and tries to compensate the global motion pattern caused by the camera. The second task includes surgical instrument detection and tracking. The prerequisite task for surgical instrument tracking is the telescope motion estimation and compensation. It must be performed to improve the accuracy of estimation of the motion patterns of the surgical instruments. The last task in the second category is related to soft tissue segmentation and deformation tracking. The soft tissue deformation tracking has two prerequisites including the telescope motion estimation and compensation and surgical instrument tracking, because the global motion and the instrument motion can have influence on the neighboring soft tissues.

The tasks of the second category provide the necessary input for the third category tasks. The third category tasks are much more complicated tasks. They try to extract useful knowledge from the laparoscopic videos. These tasks include laparoscopic video summarization, detecting safe/unsafe actions,

Figure 2. The classification of laparoscopic video processing problems considered in this chapter

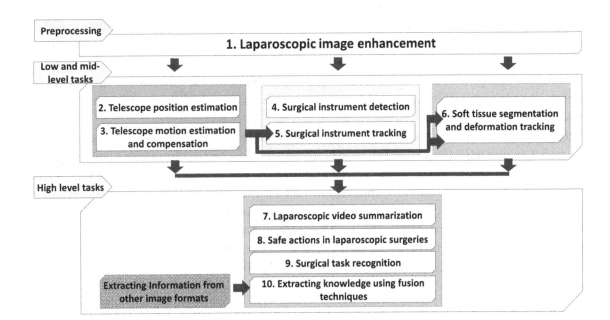

surgical task recognition and extracting knowledge using fusion techniques, in which the last item needs more inputs which can be collected from other external resources such as CT-scan or magnetic resonance images.

Laparoscopic Image Enhancement

Laparoscopic image enhancement is a preprocessing step that can improve the accuracy of extracting information from the video frames. Previous studies have proposed many different image enhancement methods (Giannarou, Visentini-Scarzanella, & Yang, 2012; Selka et al., 2015).

Enhancing images with the aim of improving the image quality is being performed and includes improving the image contrast, reducing unusual radiation, improving the image brightness, removing noise and etc.

Image enhancement must be performed using fast and simple algorithms for laparoscopic video frames because of their large number. Therefore, many of the previously proposed algorithms for enhancing images cannot be applicable on laparoscopic video frames because of their high computational complexity.

Generally image enhancement methods can be classified into simple pixel-level methods, filter-based methods and pseudo-color based methods. Simple pixel-level methods include intensity transformation and histogram equalization methods. Filter-based methods have used spatial or frequency domain filters to smooth or sharpen the images. Pseudo-color based methods have used false colors or pseudo color spaces.

Unfortunately, because of the limited number of published researches about laparoscopic image processing, the limited methods have been used for laparoscopic image enhancement.

Histogram equalization (HE) has been used to limit tracking failure (Wu, Chen, Liu, Chang, & Sun, 2004), adjust the image contrast and reduce the negative effects of the illumination changes on tracking the tissues (Giannarou et al., 2012). Selka et al. have shown that HE does not improve the tissue tracking performance (Selka et al., 2015).

In some researches, Gaussian smoothing filter has been performed to remove variations and noise, the brightness and contrast has been enhanced using classic brightness/contrast adjustment method and histogram thresholding has been used to remove specular reflections from laparoscopic video frames (Shu & Cheriet, 2005).

Both of the mentioned methods for enhancing the laparoscopic video frames are simple and fast. Therefore, they are applicable on the real laparoscopic video frames. But, they are sensitive to the parameter tuning.

Other than contrast enhancement, another challenging issue affecting laparoscopic image processing steps is specular reflection on the soft tissues. Therefore, a method for segmenting and recognizing specular reflection was proposed in the previous researches. For this purpose, dynamic thresholding technique is used to segment the video frames. Then the closed contours of the segmented regions are analyzed, and three different types of reflections are identified including non-reflection, small reflection with high brightness and reflections with small brightness. The contour shape is used to classify the regions into these three different classes (Marcinczak & Grigat, 2013).

This method is sensitive to parameter tuning as well. Moreover, for setting the dynamic thresholds, it needs the training data.

Telescope Position Estimation

Sometimes, it is important to know whether the telescope shows the inside of the patient's body or outpatient. If the telescope is outpatient, there is no need to process and archive the video frames. Surgical interruptions and problems occurred during the surgery may cause the telescope to exit the patient's body.

For example, when the telescope lens becomes foggy or dirty during the surgery, the surgeon's visibility is reduced and it is required to take out the telescope from the patient's body and clean it.

Sometimes, other problems occurring with the outpatient that may cause long interruptions leading to take out the telescope from the patient's body. For example, CO_2 capsule becomes empty and continuing the surgery before providing a new capsule is impossible. In these situations, the telescope is taken out from the patient's body.

The telescope position estimation can be seen as a classification problem in which the video frames are classified into outpatient and inpatient.

Stanek et al. have introduced novel color-based features to detect outpatient frames in endoscopic videos. The proposed features include Mean-red, mean-normalized-red, and accumulated mean-normalized-red. For classifying video frames, a threshold-based method has been used in (Stanek, Tavanapong, Wonga, Oh, & Groenc, 2012), and the results showed that the video frames could be classified based on the proposed features with high accuracy. But, the inpatient images of the laparoscopic surgery may have different color histogram pattern from the endoscopic video frames depending on the target tissue. Therefore, the proposed feature may not be sufficient to classify the laparoscopic video frames to inpatient and outpatient images.

Telescope Motion Estimation and Compensation

Camera motion estimation and compensation method is very important to process the laparoscopic videos. For example, for estimating local motions such as surgical instrument motion or tracking the instrument accurately, global motion can affect the local motion parameters and reduce the accuracy of local motion estimation and tracking. Therefore, camera motion estimation and compensation is a necessary pre-processing step in many applications of laparoscopic video processing.

Many previous studies have considered camera motion estimation and compensation. But, as the best of our knowledge, we have not seen any study considering camera motion estimation and compensation for laparoscopic videos specifically.

Camera motion estimation and compensation method has been studied in many researches generally (B. H. Chen et al., 2016). But, camera motion estimation and compensation in laparoscopic videos is different and more challenging task than camera motion estimation and compensation in indoor or outdoor scenes. Tissue respiratory motion can make camera motion estimation in laparoscopic videos a more challenging task. Moreover, very homogeneous tissue surfaces in very large magnified video frames, local motions of surgical instruments, their interaction with tissues and tissue deformation due to surgical instrument forces are other factors that can increase the complexity of camera motion estimation in laparoscopic videos.

Surgical Instrument Detection

If 3D pose of the surgical tools can be estimated, it will be valuable to extract data for the surgical training evaluation and using the knowledge of surgical instrument position to design new robotic systems. Since the laparoscopic video is recorded in two dimensions, surgical instrument shape and orientation can be useful to get its 3D position (Cano González, Vara Beceiro, Sánchez González, Pozo Guerrero, & Gómez Aguilera, 2008).

Surgical tools are solid objects. In the literature, detection and tracking of solid objects are easier than the soft tissues, because they have specified border and their shapes are less variant than the soft tissues. But, if the orientation of the solid object and its angle to the camera change, its shape may change as well. Therefore, the shape of surgical instrument in laparoscopic video frames depends on its orientation and relative position to the telescope. It makes instrument detection and tracking a challenging image processing task.

Another issue is the perceived color and texture of the surgical tool. Surgical tool tip is usually metallic and silver. Therefore, it is more sensitive to brightness and illumination variations. It may lead to inhomogeneous texture with a variety of colors and different brightness levels on the surface of the tool tip. Therefore, surgical tool segmentation and detection will be challenging.

The surgeon may need to adjust the camera magnification in different video frames. The camera magnification parameter can affect the perceived texture and color of the surgical tool tip.

According to the mentioned challenging issues, many researches have proposed methods for surgical instrument detection and tracking (Voros, Long, & Clinquin, 2007). In this section, some previous studies considering surgical instrument detection are reviewed. In the next section, some previous researches about tracking the surgical instruments are considered.

Segmenting the laparoscopic video frames into homogeneous segments is a necessary prerequisite step for surgical instrument detection. After segmenting the video frame, each segment is analyzed and the segments indicating the surgical instruments are detected. Therefore, detecting the surgical instrument consists of two main steps including image segmentation and then classifying the generated segments into surgical instrument and other regions.

Previously proposed methods for segmenting the video frames to detect the surgical instrument are classified into color-based segmentation methods, segmenting based on the combination of color and texture features, and edge-based segmentation methods.

Color-Based Segmentation Methods

Amini Khoyi et al. have proposed a segmentation algorithm based on combination of saturation and Value components of HSV color space to detect and track the tool tip (Amini Khoyi, Mirbagheri, & Farahmand, 2016).

Some researchers have proposed a fast color-based segmentation method to detect the gray regions in color images of laparoscopic videos. They have assumed that surgical tool's color is seen as gray in images which is not true all of the time. This method is based on recursive thresholds obtained from color histograms in HSI color space. Saturation component is enhanced and used in combination with hue component. Then a region growing approach is used for instrument segmentation. Some shape descriptors are extracted from the gray segmented regions including Fourier descriptors and moments. Then the gray regions are classified into instrument and non-instrument classes based on the extracted features (Doignon, Graebling, & Mathelin, 2005). The main advantage of this approach is its high speed. But, it is based on color features and region shape descriptors. Therefore, it is not robust to illumination variations and partially occlusion.

Some researchers have used artificial color markers on the surgical instruments to detect these markers in the images (Wei, Arbter, & Hirzinger, 1997; Zhao, 2014). It is a very fast approach and is more robust to the illumination variation and surgical tool partially occlusion. But, it may not be applicable in all the surgeries to use artificial markers on the instruments.

Segmenting Video Frames Based on the Combination of Color and Texture Features

Another approach has been proposed for surgical instrument detection in laparoscopic video frames based on color and texture features. At first, the images are segmented twice, one time based on color features and another time based on texture features. Then the segmented regions are merged if they have enough overlap. Finally, the regions having texture and color pattern similar to the surgical instruments are considered as surgical tool regions (Khatibi, Sepehri, & Shadpour, 2013). Using color and texture features simultaneously can reduce the error rate of surgical tool detection due to illumination variation and occlusion.

Edge-Based Segmentation Methods

Some researchers have tried to detect the surgical tools based on edge detection and applying the Hough transform on the detected edges in laparoscopic video frames. They have assumed that the surgical tool border is a combination of straight lines. Finally, motion information has been used to discriminate surgical tools from other structured elements in images (Climent & Mars, 2010). The Hough transform is robust under illumination variations, occlusion and distractions (Climent & Hexsel, 2012).

Finally, when the video frame is segmented, the segmented regions with similar color or motion pattern to the surgical instruments are considered as the surgical instrument regions.

Surgical Instrument Tracking

Instrument tracking can be used for autonomous control of a cameraman robot during the robotic laparoscopic surgery (Amini Khoyi et al., 2016). Prerequisite step for instrument tracking is the image segmentation for detecting the surgical instruments which is described in the previous section.

But in laparoscopic videos, a stable motion estimation is very complicated and challenging task and cannot be guaranteed generally (Öhsen, Marcinczak, Vélez, & Grigat, 2012).

Many different methods were proposed in the previous researches for tracking surgical instruments in the laparoscopic videos via image processing algorithms (Wolf, Duchateau, Cinquin, & Voros, 2011). The previously proposed methods for surgical instrument tracking can be divided into two main categories including tracking-based on image processing and tracking-based on the supplementary data.

Tracking the Surgical Instrument Only Based on Image Processing Methods

Some researchers have proposed an image processing method for tracking surgical instruments without artificial markers. The proposed method could estimate 2D/3D pose of visible instruments in real-time using Frangi filter for detecting edges and tool tips (Agustinos & Voros, 2016).

An adaptive mean-shift Kalman filter has been used to track the tool tip in another study. The filter can increase the accuracy of tracking when the tool tip is invisible in a few frames. This method is robust to the changes of size and shape of the instrument (Sa-Ing, Thongvigitmanee, Wilasrusmee, & Suthakorn, 2012).

In another study, a novel approach has been proposed for surgical instrument detection and tracking. The proposed image segmentation algorithm is based on training a decision tree on color features to classify the regions as surgical instrument or other regions. Then, the corner points of the surgical instruments are extracted and matched in two consecutive video frames. The instrument motion vector is estimated based on the replacement of the matching corner points in two consecutive frames (Khatibi, Sepehri, & Shadpour, 2014). This method is based on color and motion features and all the limitations of the color-based instrument segmentation and local motion estimation holds true, here.

Some researchers have used methods for segmenting and tracking the tools and organs to 3D reconstruct the surgical field (Sánchez-González et al., 2011).

Needle tracking is an assisting prerequisite of suturing which is a complex and difficult task in laparoscopy. Some researchers have used color and geometry-based segmentation to detect the needle (Speidel et al., 2015).

Other researchers have used texture and geometric features from edge-based descriptors as input to a spiking neural network for detecting the instrument. Tracking the instrument has been done using Kalman filter (C. J. Chen, Huang, & Song, 2013).

The mentioned methods have used color, texture, edge-based and/or motion features for surgical instrument tracking. Unfortunately, none of the color, texture and edge features can be extracted accurately in many real laparoscopic video frames, because of illumination variation, magnification changes and other challenging situations described before. Tracking objects based on motion vectors can be performed using filters such as Kalman filter with reasonable accuracy. Therefore, considering the combination of color, texture, edge and motion descriptors can improve the accuracy of instrument tracking. But, it may lead to more computational complexity of the tracking method.

Tracking the Surgical Instrument Based on the Supplementary Data

This category consists of methods using image processing techniques along with other supplementary data obtained by external sensors or other resources for tracking the surgical instruments.

Oropesa et al. have proposed an instrument tracking software based on tool edges, tool insertion point and focal point of camera to extract 3D position of the instruments (Oropesa et al., 2013). This method needs supplementary information and the tool tracking cannot be performed using only laparoscopic video frames. In robotic surgery, some researchers have proposed an approach for tracking surgical instruments to measure the distance between the instrument surface and a laser point illuminated on the tissue. For detecting the laser points, they have used high-pass filters, and then they have segmented the filtered image and used erosion morphologic operator (Krupa, Doignon, Gangloff, & Mathelin, 2002). This method needs laser point illumination which may not be available and safe in all situations.

Adding the supplementary data to the laparoscopic video may improve the accuracy of the surgical instrument tracking. But, it is not possible to use external devices and sensors to provide such supplementary data in many situations. Moreover, the synchronization of supplementary data with video data is another challenging issue that must be addressed.

Tissue Segmentation and Deformation Tracking

Sometimes, tissue deforms due to instrument forces and many other factors. Therefore, tissue deformation tracking is an important issue in laparoscopic video processing.

A preprocessing step for tissue tracking can be tissue segmentation. Tissue segmentation in laparoscopic videos can have many other advantages and is very helpful. For example, in gynecology, tissue segmentation can be performed to localize the uterus to facilitate and analyze the lesion on uterus and its surroundings. Therefore, a threshold-based segmentation has been proposed to segment the tissues, and then the regions are classified by SVM to uterus and other tissues (Yu et al., 2015). The threshold-based method for segmenting the soft tissues may divide a soft tissue into multiple regions because of illumination and contrast variations in different blocks of the image. Therefore, it is not an exact and accurate segmentation method.

Tissue navigation system which uses intraoperative imaging and real-time image processing can enhance the surgeon's perception and can guide surgeon's decisions and to provide some valuable information such as information about the tumor infiltrated tissue and risk structures (Baumhauer et al., 2008).

In the previous studies, some methods have been proposed for tissue deformation tracking (S. L. Lee et al., 2010; Stoyanov & Yang, 2011).

Collins et al. have introduced a method for 3D reconstruction of the tissue surface using the sliding windows approach (Collins, Compte, & Bartoli, 2011). Using fusion techniques and other imaging data such as MRI and/or CT images can improve the proposed method accuracy.

Stoyanov and Yang have proposed optical feature tracking method based on stereo-laparoscopic images. They have defined and used a constrained geometrical surface model that deforms with motion. Their proposed method is robust to occlusions and specular reflection, but it needs stereo camera (Stoyanov & Yang, 2011).

A previous study has proposed some context descriptors for tissue deformation tracking. They have considered tissue tracking as a classification problem and solved it using decision trees. They have argued that the proposed method is robust to drift, occlusion, orientation and scalingvariations (Mountney & Yang, 2012). Since the classifier trains in a supervised manner, the generalization ability for tissue deformation tracking may be reduced and for new deformations that are not seen in the training set, it may fail to recognize them.

Some researchers have proposed a technique to generate rough depth maps from laparoscopic video frames based on SURF features. This method can provide 3D visualization of 2D laparoscopic video (P. Y. Lee, Yan, Hu, & Marescaux, 2015). SURF features can be extracted from the interest points and matching the SURF features of the consecutive video frames can be used for estimating the motion of these points. SURF features are one of the highly accurate features that can be used for tracking the objects. But, it needs the number of the SURF features extracted from the tissue to be sufficient to estimate the tissue deformation with high accuracy.

Laparoscopic Video Summarization

One popular camera system for laparoscopic surgeries is the vision system of the daVinci-Si robotic surgical system (Intuitive Surgical, Sunnyvale, California) with high quality. Its generated video streams has approximately 360 MB of data per second (Ronaghi, Duffy, & Kwartowitz, 2015). This large volume of data shows the importance and necessity of laparoscopic video summarization.

On the other hand, all frames of a laparoscopic video do not contain valuable information. When the surgeons want to archive the laparoscopic videos for further analysis and training purposes, they are not interested in archiving all segments of a lengthy laparoscopic video. Therefore, summarizing a laparoscopic video by keeping only the valuable segments and removing the other segments can have high importance. It can reduce the review time of a summarized video and the required memory for archiving the video. But, the question is which segments of a laparoscopic video are valuable and which segments can be removed without information loss.

Simply, when the telescope is outside the patient's body or when there is no camera motion and/or surgical instrument movement, it can be concluded that no surgical activity is being performed inside the patient's body. Therefore, these video segments can be removed without loss of information.

The previously proposed methods for laparoscopic video summarization can be classified into two categories including key-frame selection and informative segment selection.

Key-Frame Selection

Key-frame selection tries to find the most desired video frames denoting the tissues and surgical activities with high quality. Therefore a video with N video frames may be summarized into K video frames ($K << N$) which every key-frame is selected from one temporal segment of the laparoscopic video. Therefore, the selected video frames are not immediately consecutive.

Some researchers have proposed algorithms for key-frame selection in laparoscopic/endoscopic videos (Öhsen et al., 2012; Wang et al., 2016). Ohsen et al. have scored all combination of frames in a sequence and they have tried to find the optimal solution. Finding the optimal solution have been described as a weighted directed graph problem and Dijkstras Algorithm has been used to find the best selection of frames (Öhsen et al., 2012).

Before extracting key-frames, video must be segmented temporally. Wang et al. have proposed a video segmentation method with an assumption that the semantic content of frames in a segment should change dramatically. Color and texture features are used for this purpose. Color features are the I component histogram in HSI color space, histogram of H and V components in HSV color space, RGB histogram, Normalized RGB histogram, RG histogram, Opponent histogram and HUE histogram. Local binary pattern (LBP) histogram is used for describing the texture. The reason of using histograms as the image features is their robustness against rotation and scaling variations. The similarity between two consecutive frames are calculated as their histogram intersection (Wang et al., 2016).

Another study has proposed a data reduction algorithm for extracting representative video frames (key-frames) from a Wireless Capsule Endoscopy (WCE) video. It can reduce significantly the reading time of WCE videos for experts without any loss of abnormalities. This method is used WCE video segments with fixed length, and features are extracted from video frames of each segment. Then the number of features are reduced using data reduction algorithms. The reduced feature set are clustered and the representative frames are selected from the clusters showing abnormalities in tissues (Iakovidis, Tsevas, & Polydorou, 2010).

In some researches, they have proposed methods for laparoscopic video summarization (Grasso et al., 2009). Grasso et al. have used support vector machines (SVM) for classifying the video frames to identify which frames are near to critical view and which frames are not. They have extracted feature vector of spectral and textural features such as energy, entropy, contrast, correlation and color descriptors. Then the feature selection have been performed using the Jeffrey Divergence with an experimentally derived threshold (Grasso et al., 2009).

In another study, similar video frames taken by a wireless capsule endoscope have been eliminated to minimize the redundancy in the images. For this purpose, enhanced intensity features, optical flow and Speed Up Robust Features (SURF) have been used to detect and reduce near-duplicate images (H. G. Lee, Choi, Shin, & Lee, 2013).

Some researchers have classified endoscopic video frames into informative and non-informative frames (Bashar, Kitasaka, Suenaga, Mekada, & Mori, 2010; Oh et al., 2007). For this purpose, Oh et al. have proposed two different approaches. In the first method, edge-based features are extracted by Canny edge detector and then the feature set are classified to informative, non-informative and ambiguous frames. In the second method, each frame is transformed using Discrete Fourier Transform (DFT) and the texture of the transformed image is analyzed. For this purpose, gray level co-occurrence matrix (GLCM) is extracted from the frequency spectrum image. Then seven texture features including Entropy, Contrast, Correlation, Homogeneity, Dissimilarity, Angular Second Moment and Energy are extracted from GLCM. The feature set is clustered using k-means algorithm into two clusters and each cluster is labeled as informative or non-informative cluster (Oh et al., 2007).

Informative Segment Selection

All of the above methods lay in the first category that tries to find key-frames. Now, the methods belonging to the second category tries to find the informative temporal segments which they will be reviewed.

The second class including informative segment selection tries to segment temporally the laparoscopic video and then classifies the temporal segments into informative and non-informative segments. Finally, only the informative segments are kept.

Temporal segmentation of laparoscopic video is an important prerequisite step for laparoscopic video summarization and identifying which temporal segments can be removed without the loss of information.

Khatibi et al. have proposed a novel approach for temporal segmentation of laparoscopic videos. They have extracted instrument motion parameters and defined temporal segmentation of video as an optimization problem. Then, they have solved this problem using multi-objective genetic algorithm in an unsupervised manner (Khatibi et al., 2014). The generated temporal segments can discriminate different surgical activities and each activity lies in a separate temporal segment. Because the surgical instruments have different motion patterns in different surgical activities. The temporal segments can be used for discriminating different surgical activities in surgical task recognition and finding the most desired activities. The laparoscopic video can be summarized by keeping only the segments corresponding to the most desired surgical activities. It is a more complicated type of the video summarization applications.

Other researches have proposed simpler methods for laparoscopic video summarization (Munzer et al.,2013; Stanek et al.,2012). They want to find inpatient segments and/or high quality segments. They do not distinguish different types of surgical activities.

Munzer et al. have defined three types of unrelated segments of laparoscopic videos including dark segments, segments which telescope is outside the patient's body and blurry segments. They have tried to discriminate these three different classes using features extracted from laparoscopic video. For this purpose, some preprocessing steps have been performed on the video frames including specular reflection removal, ignoring border pixels, low saturated pixels and dark segments. Then, HSV color features have been used. Their reason for choosing HSV color space has been its superiority to RGB color space. HSV color space is near to human perception (Münzer, Schoeffmann, & Böszörmenyi, 2013).

Stanek et al. have proposed an approach to automatically detect informative temporal segments of an endoscopic video and recorded only informative temporal segments. For this purpose, motion and color features have been used. Outpatient video frames have been detected and automatically discarded (Stanek et al., 2012). Their proposed method classifies the temporal segments into inpatient and outpatient segments and records only the inpatient segments using buffers.

In future, more deep researches can be performed for laparoscopic video summarization. For example, surgeons may be interested in keeping only special types of surgical tasks and remove other segments. It needs to recognize the laparoscopic surgical tasks from videos which will be discussed in section 3.4.

Safe Actions in Laparoscopic Surgeries

The surgeon wants to perform a safe surgical activity. For this purpose, the surgeon needs to know whether performing the surgical task by the instruments may hurt the tissues and/or arteries. For example, in cholecyctectomy, cystic artery must be avoided from the injury by the surgical instruments. Otherwise, injury to the cystic artery may lead to uncontrollable bleeding (Lahane et al., 2012).

Therefore, it is required to detect the blood vessels in laparoscopic video frames using image processing techniques. Lack of 3D view in laparoscopic videos makes it difficult to detect blood vessel positions accurately. Some researchers have used color and geometric features to detect blood vessels in laparoscopic video frames. But, this approach cannot recognize vessels occluded by fat or other tissues (Akbari & Kosugi, 2007).

Other researchers have used HSV color space information for detecting blood vessels among the enhanced laparoscopic video frames using multiple regression analysis (Hiroyasu, Tanaka, Hagiwara, & Ozamoto, 2015).

During the surgery, surgical instrument should not perform surgical activities near some critical tissues and vessels. For this purpose, surgical tool tip is detected in video frames using image processing techniques. Then, the fixed-size rectangular block around the surgical tool tip in laparoscopic video frames are drawn and analyzed to verify whether critical tissues or arteries exist there or not. If there is no critical tissue or artery in the block, it has been concluded that the block is safe. The regions around the tool tip are classified as safe or unsafe regions for surgical activities (Lahane et al., 2012).

Another study has proposed chromaticity moments of HSI color space as the features for bleeding and ulcer detection in WCE images and discriminating normal regions and abnormal regions. This classification problem has been solved using a neural network classifier (Li & Meng, 2009).

The mentioned above methods try to find blood vessels and/or discriminate normal/abnormal regions. In the laparoscopic surgery, these are two important applications of image processing for preventing unsafe actions. But, many other situations may exist that can cause the unsafe actions. In the future, the researchers can focus on finding and preventing other situations that may lead to unsafe surgical actions by image processing techniques.

Surgical Task Recognition in Laparoscopic Videos

An important and complex application of laparoscopic video processing is surgical task recognition for activities which are visible in the laparoscopic videos and performed in the patient's body.

Generally, several studies have been performed on human activity recognition in video clips (Moayedi, Azimifar, & Boostani, 2015; Yuan, Zheng, & Lu, 2016). Activity recognition problem is a complicated problem and there are many challenges yet. For example, same action can be performed in different styles and different speeds by different persons. Therefore, in literature, many different descriptors have been proposed for human activity recognition such as motion and shape descriptors (Dou & Li, 2014; Kviatkovsky, Rivlin, & Shimshoni, 2014).

There are some differences between human activity recognition and surgical activity recognition. Actors in the laparoscopic surgeries are surgical instrument. The surgical instrument can be hidden in the neighboring tissues for a few minutes during the surgery. They can cause soft tissue deformation. Therefore, the interaction between the actors and their neighboring tissues makes the surgical activity recognition problem different, more complicated and more challenging than the human activity recognition.

Recent approaches have demonstrated that video data can be used in surgical task recognition with high accuracy (Blum, Feuner, & Navab, 2010; Padoy et al., 2007).

The previously proposed methods for surgical activity recognition can be classified into two classes: the first class includes methods using only the information obtained from the laparoscopic videos and the second class includes the methods using other supplementary resources of data such as data obtained by external sensors being installed on the surgical instruments and capturing the instrument motion pattern or sensors detecting surgeon's eye motion.

Methods Using Only the Information Obtained From the Laparoscopic Videos

Some researchers have proposed an approach for recognition of surgical tasks in eye surgery videos. Short video subsequences have been classified into surgical tasks by fast nearest neighbor classifier. For this purpose, fixed-length feature vector including texture, color and motion features are extracted from each subsequence (Quellec et al., 2014). But, there are some differences between eye surgery videos and laparoscopic videos. Laparoscopic videos indicate different tissues and more variety of surgical activities. Moreover, the eye and its border are clear in eye surgery videos. Therefore, the video processing of laparoscopic surgery has more and different challenges.

Detection and segmentation of surgical motion can be used for evaluating surgical skill, obtaining surgical training feedback and archiving essential aspects of a procedure. Some researchers have used raw motion data to recognize surgical actions (H. C. Lin, Shafran, Yuh, & Hager, 2006). The motion data can be obtained by installing the appropriate sensors on the surgical instrument or by tracking the instruments in the video by image processing algorithms. Therefore, we lay this method in the first class.

Some researchers have proposed using Hidden Markov Models to recognize surgical tasks based on surgeon's motion analysis (Dosis et al., 2005). Some researchers have shown that surgical movement data can be used for laparoscopic surgical skill assessment with high accuracy (Z. Lin, Uemura, Zecca, & Sessa, 2012). But, extracting stable motion features is a challenging and complicated task.

Researchers have proposed generating surgical activity log from laparoscopic video as an information source. For this purpose, surgical instruments have marked and the markers have been tracked to produce a surgical activity log. Then, the workflow model has been extracted and the outliers have been detected using global pair-wise alignment (Bouarfa & Dankelman, 2012).

The Methods Using Other Supplementary Resources of Data

Many studies have used dynamic cues such as time to completion, speed, forces, torque or kinematic data such as robot trajectories and velocities to automatically recognize the surgical skills and gestures (Zappella, Béjar, Hager, & Vidal, 2013). They have assumed that the video has been segmented into video clips and each video clip has denoted a single gesture. Surgical gestures include grabbing the needle, passing the needle and etc. Three different models have been proposed for surgical gesture recognition based on video data and kinematic data. The first model has considered video clip as the output of a linear dynamical system (LDS) and has tried to classify the video clips. In the second one, spatio-temporal features are extracted from each video clip with bag-of-features representation for classification. The third one has used multiple kernel learning (MKL) to combine LDS and BOF approaches (Zappella et al., 2013).

After stating the methods of the two different categories of surgical action recognition, we must say which challenges and opportunities exist here. In laparoscopic videos, the actor is surgical instrument. Therefore, shape and motion descriptors can be extracted from the surgical instruments to recognize different types of surgical activities. Another information that can be used for surgical activity recognition is the interaction between the surgical tools and the soft tissues. Therefore, some extra descriptors must be extracted for describing different types of interaction between the instrument and the tissues.

Some researchers have shown that there is the statistical difference between expert surgeons and residents in terms of: (1) force/torque magnitude, (2) type of tool/tissue interactions and (3) time interval for each tool/tissue interaction and total completion time (Rosen, Solazzo, Hannaford, & Sinanan, 2002). Therefore, surgical activity recognition and recording the time intervals for each surgical task can improve the accuracy of surgical skill assessment methods. But, extracting the shape and motion of the surgical instruments and describing the interactions between the instruments and the soft tissue are very challenging and complex issue.

Extracting Knowledge From Laparoscopic Videos Using Fusion Techniques

Fusion techniques are not in the scope of this study. Therefore, this section is briefly described.

For robotic assisted minimally invasive surgery, knowing the 3D shape of tissues is important for guiding the robots and compensating the tissue respiratory motions (Stoyanov, Elson, & Yang, 2009).

Lack of 3D view in laparoscopic video frames makes it challenging to extract knowledge from laparoscopic videos in many applications. Therefore, it is required to use fusion techniques of surface information of laparoscope and supplementary information obtained from other image formats such as MRI, CT Scan and ultrasound images. For example, depth of blood arteries inside the target organs can be estimated by projecting the ultrasound image over a laparoscopic image (Zenbutsu, Igarashi, & Yamaguchi, 2013).

Many researches have used other images such as ultrasound images(Zenbutsu et al., 2013), MRI, CT scan images(Hayashi, Misawa, Hawkes, & Mori, 2016), multispectral imaging(Y. Zhang et al., 2016) and etc for extracting information from laparoscopic video frames more accurately.

Some papers have used stereoscopic video camera attached to a laparoscope to implement image-based 3D reconstruction of soft tissues (Kowalczuk et al., 2012).

In this chapter, we are interested in extracting knowledge using only laparoscopic video without fusion techniques.

Finally, the summary of many previous studies considered in this chapter is shown in Table 1.

Table 1. Summary of the previous studies considered in this chapter

Authors	Topic	Image Preprocessing	Features	Model
(Shu & Cheriet, 2005)	Laparoscopic image segmentation	Gaussian smoothing Enhancing brightness and contrast Histogram thresholding	intensity	Graph-based and region merging
(Marcinczak & Grigat, 2013)	Specular reflection segmentation	-	Intensity Region boundary shape descriptors	Dynamic thresholding technique Classifying the regions
(Lahane et al., 2012)	Unsafe action detection	Gaussian smoothing	HSV color features	Jeffrey divergence feature selection SVM classifier
(Akbari & Kosugi, 2007)	Blood vessel detection	-	RGB color features	LVQ neural network
(Hiroyasu et al., 2015)	Blood vessel detection	-	HSV color features	Multiple regression analysis
(Li & Meng, 2009)	Bleeding and ulcer detection	-	HSI color features	Neural network classifier
(Doignon et al., 2005)	Surgical instrument detection	-	HSI color features Region boundary shape features: Fourier descriptors and moments	Region growing algorithm
(Khatibi et al., 2013)	Surgical instrument detection	-	Color features Texture features	Novel region merging algorithm
(Climent & Mars, 2010)	Surgical instrument detection	-	Edge-based features Hough transform Motion features	-
(Wei et al., 1997)	Surgical instrument detection	-	Color features	-
(Zhao, 2014)	Surgical instrument detection	-	Color features	-
(Krupa et al., 2002)	Surgical instrument tracking	High-pass filtering Erosion morphologic operator	Color features Region boundary descriptors	-
(Speidel et al., 2015)	Surgical instrument detection	-	Color features Geometry features	-
(C. J. Chen et al., 2013)	Surgical instrument detection and tracking	-	Texture features Geometric features	Spiking neural network Kalman filter
(Amini Khoyi et al., 2016)	Surgical instrument detection	-	HSV Color features	-
(Sa-Ing et al., 2012)	Surgical instrument tracking	-	Color features	Mean-shift Kalman filter
(Oropesa et al., 2013)	Surgical instrument tracking	-	Edge features Tool insertion point	-
(Agustinos & Voros, 2016)	Surgical instrument tracking	-	Edge features Frangi filter	-
(Öhsen et al., 2012)	Video summarization: Key frame selection	-	Motion vectors	Dijikstra algorithm

continued on following page

Table 1. Continued

Authors	Topic	Image Preprocessing	Features	Model
(Wang et al., 2016)	Video summarization: Key frame selection	-	Color histograms: HIS-I histogram, HSV-HV histogram, RGB histogram, NormRGB histogram, RG histogram, Opponent histogram and HUE histogram. Texture features: LBP histogram	Similar-inhibition dictionary selection
(Iakovidis et al., 2010)	Video summarization: Extracting representative video frames	Subsampling video frames Dimensionality reduction of video segments	Non-negative matrix from intensity	Fuzzy clustering
(Grasso et al., 2009)	Video summarization	-	Color features Textural features: energy, entropy, contrast and correlation	Feature selection using Jeffrey Divergence SVM
(Münzer et al., 2013)	Irrelevant scene detection	Specular reflection detection Excluding border pixels dynamically Ignoring low saturated pixels	HSV color features	Fuzzy classification
(H. G. Lee et al., 2013)	Video summarization: eliminating similar frames	HE	Motion features: optical flow SURF Intensity	Egomotion classification
(Bashar et al., 2010)	Video summarization	-	Color features: local moments and HSV histogram Gauss Laguerre transformation (GLT) based multiresolution feature	SVM
(Oh et al., 2007)	Video summarization: informative frame detection	Identifying specular reflection using dynamic thresholding and outlier detection Discrete Fourier Transform	Edge-based features: using Canny Edge Detector Texture features: entropy, contrast, correlation, homogeneity, Angular second moment, energy	Clustering-based frame classification
(Stanek et al., 2012)	Video summarization: irrelevant scene detection	-	Color features Motion features	Novel proposed algorithms for identifying the start frames and end frames of a procedure
(Khatibi et al., 2014)	Video temporal segmentation Surgical instrument tracking	-	Color features Motion features	Decision tree for surgical instrument detection A novel proposed algorithm (based on Multi-objective GA) for temporal segmentation of video
(Yu et al., 2015)	Tissue segmentation	-	Color features	Threshold-based segmentation SVM region classifier
(Yip, Lowe, Salcudean, Rohling, & Nguan, 2012)	Tissue deformation tracking			
(Collins et al., 2011)				
(Stoyanov & Yang, 2011)				
(P. Y. Lee et al., 2015)				
(Dosis et al., 2005)	Surgical task recognition		Motion features	HMM
(Bouarfa & Dankelman, 2012)	Surgical task recognition	-	Motion features	Global pair-wise alignment
(Zappella et al., 2013)			Kinematic data Spatio-temporal features	Video clip classifiers

Datasets

Many researchers have stated that there is no publicly available dataset for laparoscopic image processing. Therefore, we present a list of datasets being used for validation of the previous studies in Table 2.

As listed in Table 1, many researches have used their datasets. One reason may be lack of any publicly available laparoscopic/endoscopic video dataset with ground-truth segmentation. This issue can introduce many limitations in implementing, improving and comparing the proposed works.

DISCUSSION

As mentioned in the previous sections, laparoscopic video processing is a challenging task due to moving background, respiratory motions of tissues, light reflection from the tissue surfaces, inhomogeneous and variable illumination in consequence video frames (Doignon et al., 2005), narrow field of view and lack of depth cue in conventional laparoscopy (Igarashi, Suzuki, & Naya, 2009).

Table 2. Datasets being used for validation of the previous studies for laparoscopic image processing applications

Authors	Research Problem	Dataset
(Marcinczak & Grigat, 2013)	Specular Reflection Segmentation	A dataset of 49 laparoscopic images taken from27 patients containing 269 true specular reflections. Ground truth segmentation of specular reflection has been performed manually.
(Lahane et al., 2012)	Unsafe action detection	900 image as train set 213 image as test set (positive and negative classes)
(Doignon et al., 2005)	segmentation of surgical instruments	Images from 3 video sequences of 500 color images
(Climent & Mars, 2010)	Instrument localization	128 images extracted from a real operation video
(Sa-Ing et al., 2012)	Instrument tracking	simulated videos for different situations
(Zhao, 2014)	3D visual tracking of laparoscopic instruments	a plastic phantom with a test-bench inside
(Collins et al., 2011)	deformable 3D surface reconstruction	Simulating a 3D kidney model comprising 1820 vertices
(Mountney & Yang, 2012)	tracking deforming tissue	simulated and in vivo MIS datasets of the liver, heart and abdomen
(Grasso et al., 2009)	Laparoscopic Video Summarization	378 images randomly selected from five laparoscopic cholecystectomy videos
(Iakovidis et al., 2010)	Endoscopic video summarization	annotated video frames with ground truth information labeled manually
(Oh et al., 2007)	Informative/ non-informative frame classification in endoscopic videos	70 frames were selected as a test set from three colonoscopy videos consisting of 35 informative frames and 35 non-informative frames
(Wang et al., 2016)	Laparoscopic video summarization and key-frame selection	a new gastroscopic video dataset has been proposed from 30 volunteers with more than 400k images
(Zappella et al., 2013)	Surgical gesture classification	Previously presented dataset

Many researches have tried to address some of the mentioned issues in their work. But, there is still need to propose more robust and stable methods for any of the mentioned applications in laparoscopic image processing.

CONCLUSION

In this study, an overview of the applications of image processing in laparoscopic surgeries are presented. The various applications include preprocessing video frames by laparoscopic image enhancement, telescope related applications (telescope position estimation, telescope motion estimation and compensation), surgical instrument related applications (surgical instrument detection and tracking), soft tissue related applications (soft tissue segmentation and deformation tracking) and high level applications such as safe actions in laparoscopic videos, summarization of laparoscopic videos, surgical task recognition and extracting knowledge using fusion techniques.

FUTURE PERSPECTIVES

A proposed direction in the future researches is tracking the surgical instruments and describing their interaction with soft tissues for surgical skill assessment.

Depth estimation is another important challenging issue in laparoscopic video processing (M. Nicolau, James, Benny, Darzi, & Yang, 2005). Another future research can be using depth information in laparoscopic videos. For this purpose, RGB-D cameras can be used as telescope in the laparoscopic surgeries.

Exploiting robotic technology in the laparoscopic surgeries with high popularity brings many advantages for single-port and multi-port laparoscopies such as 3D high-definition optics, better instrument performance and comforting the surgeon (Ramirez, Maurice, & Kaouk, 2016). It brings some new challenges and research opportunities by itself. For example, processing 3D images and using external sensors on the robots can be used. Moreover, detection and tracking the new instrumentation, describing the shape of surgical instruments and shape changes while performing different surgical activities are some other research opportunities that can be considered. Real-time image processing, finding the target region and magnifying it, adding more supplementary data for better describing the target region using the fusion techniques, and guiding the novice surgeons while performing the surgery are other future research directions.

REFERENCES

Agustinos, A., & Voros, S. (2016). 2D/3D Real-Time Tracking of Surgical Instruments Based on Endoscopic Image Processing. In X. Luo, T. Reichl, A. Reiter, & G. M. Mariottini (Eds.), *Computer-Assisted and Robotic Endoscopy* (pp. 90–100). Springer. doi:10.1007/978-3-319-29965-5_9

Akbari, H., & Kosugi, Y. (2007). Neural Network Blood Vessel Detection in Laparoscopy. *International Journal of Bioelectromagnetism, 9*(1), 37–38.

Amini Khoyi, K., Mirbagheri, A., & Farahmand, F. (2016). Automatic tracking of laparoscopic instruments for autonomous control of a cameraman robot. *Minimally Invasive Therapy & Allied Technologies, 25*(3), 121–128. doi:10.3109/13645706.2016.1141101 PMID:26872883

Amodeo, A., L., Q. A., J.V., J., E., B., & H.R., P. (2009). 2009, Robotic laparoscopic surgery: Cost and training. *The Italian journal of urology and Nephrology, 61*(2), 121-128.

Ballantyne, G. H. (2002). Robotic surgery, telerobotic surgery, telepresence, and telementoring. *Surgical Endoscopy and Other Interventional Techniques, 16*(10), 1389-1402.

Bashar, M. K., Kitasaka, T., Suenaga, Y., Mekada, Y., & Mori, K. (2010). Automatic detection of informative frames from wireless capsule endoscopy images. *Medical Image Analysis, 14*(3), 449–470. doi:10.1016/j.media.2009.12.001 PMID:20137998

Baumhauer, M., Simpfendörfer, T., Müller-Stich, B. P., Teber, D., Gutt, C. N., Rassweiler, J., & Wolf, I. et al. (2008). Soft tissue navigation for laparoscopic partial nephrectomy. *International Journal of Computer Assisted Radiology and Surgery, 3*(3-4), 307–314. doi:10.1007/s11548-008-0216-7

Blum, T., Feuner, H., & Navab, N. (2010). *Modeling and segmentation of surgical workflow from laparoscopic video.* Paper presented at the 13th international conference on Medical image computing and computer assisted intervention, Beijing, China. doi:10.1007/978-3-642-15711-0_50

Bouarfa, L., & Dankelman, J. (2012). Workflow mining and outlier detection from clinical activity logs. *Journal of Biomedical Informatics, 45*(6), 1185–1190. doi:10.1016/j.jbi.2012.08.003 PMID:22925724

Braga, M., Frasson, M., Zuliani, W., Vignali, A., Pecorelli, N., & Di Carlo, V. (2010). Randomized clinical trial of laparoscopic versus open left colonic resection. *Br J Surg, 97*(8), 1180-1186.

Cano González, A., Vara Beceiro, I., Sánchez González, P., Pozo Guerrero, F. D., & Gómez Aguilera, E. J. (2008). Laparoscopic image analysis for automatic tracking of surgical tools. *Computer Assisted Radiology and Surgery 22nd International Congress and Exhibition (CARS 2008).*

Castellucci, S. A., Curcillo, P. G., Ginsberg, P. C., Saba, S. C., Jaffe, J. S., & Harmon, J. D. (2008). Single port access adrenalectomy. *J Endourol, 22*(8), 1573-1576.

Chen, B. H., Kopylov, A., Huang, S. C., Seredin, O., Karpov, R., Kuo, S. Y., & Hung, P. C. et al. (2016). Improved global motion estimation via motion vector clustering for video stabilization. *Engineering Applications of Artificial Intelligence, 54*, 39–48. doi:10.1016/j.engappai.2016.05.004

Chen, C. J., Huang, W., & Song, K. T. (2013). *Image tracking of laparoscopic instrument using spiking neural networks.* Paper presented at the Control, Automation and Systems (ICCAS), Gwangju, China. doi:10.1109/ICCAS.2013.6704052

Choi, S. I., Lee, K. Y., Park, S. J., & Lee, S. H. (2010). Single port laparoscopic right hemicolectomy with D3 dissection for advanced colon cancer. *World J Gastroenterol, 16*(2), 275-278.

Climent, J., & Hexsel, R. A. (2012). Particle filtering in the Hough space for instrument tracking. *Computers in Biology and Medicine, 42*(5), 614–623. doi:10.1016/j.compbiomed.2012.02.007 PMID:22425691

Climent, J., & Mars, P. (2010). Automatic instrument localization in laparoscopic surgery. In H. Bunke, J. J. Villanueva, G. Sanchez, & X. Otazu (Eds.), *Progress in computer vision and image analysis* (Vol. 73). Singapore: World Scientific Publishing Co.

Collins, T., Compte, B., & Bartoli, A. (2011). *Deformable Shape-From-Motion in Laparoscopy using a Rigid Sliding Window*. Paper presented at the MIUA.

D'Alessio, A., Piro, E., Tadini, B., & Beretta, F. (2002). One-trocar transumbilical laparoscopic-assisted appendectomy in children: our experience. *Eur J Pediatr Surg, 12*(1), 24-27.

Doignon, C., Graebling, P., & Mathelin, M. D. (2005). Real-time segmentation of surgical instruments inside the abdominal cavity using a joint hue saturation color feature. *Real Time Imaging, 11*(5-6), 429–442. doi:10.1016/j.rti.2005.06.008

Dosis, A., Bello, F., Gillies, D., Undre, S., Aggarwal, R., & Darzi, A. (2005). Laparoscopic task recognition using Hidden Markov Models. *Studies in Health Technology and Informatics, 111*, 115–122. PMID:15718711

Dou, J., & Li, J. (2014). Robust human action recognition based on spatio-temporal descriptors and motion temporal templates. *Optik - International Journal for Light and Electron Optics, 125*(7), 1891-1896.

Giannarou, S., Visentini-Scarzanella, M., & Yang, G. Z. (2012). *Probabilistic tracking of affine-invariant anisotropic regions*. Paper presented at the IEEE Trans Pattern Anal Mach Intell.

Grasso, M. A., Finin, T., Zhu, X., Joshi, A., & Yesha, Y. (2009). *Video Summarization of Laparoscopic Cholecystectomies*. Paper presented at the the the AMIA 2009 Annual Symposium.

Hayashi, Y., Misawa, K., Hawkes, D. J., & Mori, K. (2016). Progressive internal landmark registration for surgical navigation in laparoscopic gastrectomy for gastric cancer. *International Journal of Computer Assisted Radiology and Surgery, 1*(5), 837–845. doi:10.1007/s11548-015-1346-3 PMID:26811079

Hiroyasu, T., Tanaka, N., Hagiwara, A., & Ozamoto, Y. (2015). *Emphasizing mesenteric blood vessels in laparoscopic colon cancer surgery video images*. Paper presented at the 37th Annual International Conference of the IEEE Engineering in Medicine and Biology Society (EMBC), Milan, Italy. doi:10.1109/EMBC.2015.7318780

Iakovidis, D. K., Tsevas, S., & Polydorou, A. (2010). Reduction of capsule endoscopy reading times by unsupervised image mining. *Computerized Medical Imaging and Graphics, 34*(6), 471–478. doi:10.1016/j.compmedimag.2009.11.005 PMID:19969440

Igarashi, T., Suzuki, H., & Naya, Y. (2009). Computer-based endoscopic image-processing technology for endourology and laparoscopic surgery. *International Journal of Urology, 16*(6), 533–543. doi:10.1111/j.1442-2042.2009.02258.x PMID:19226356

Khatibi, T., Sepehri, M. M., & Shadpour, P. (2013). SIDF: A Novel Framework for Accurate Surgical Instrument Detection in Laparoscopic Video Frames. *International Journal of Hospital Research, 2*(4), 163–170.

Khatibi, T., Sepehri, M. M., & Shadpour, P. (2014). A novel unsupervised approach for minimally-invasive video segmentation. *Medical Signals and Sensors, 4*(1), 53–71. PMID:24695410

Kowalczuk, J., Meyer, A., Carlson, J., Psota, E. T., Buettner, S., Pérez, L. C., & Oleynikov, D. et al. (2012). Real-time three-dimensional soft tissue reconstruction for laparoscopic surgery. *Surgical Endoscopy, 26*(12), 3413–3417. doi:10.1007/s00464-012-2355-8 PMID:22648119

Krupa, A., Doignon, C., Gangloff, J., & Mathelin, M. D. (2002). *Combined image-based and depth visual servoing applied to robotized laparoscopic surgery.* Paper presented at the IEEE/RSJ International Conference on Intelligent Robots and Systems, Lausanne, Switzerland. doi:10.1109/IRDS.2002.1041409

Kviatkovsky, I., Rivlin, E., & Shimshoni, I. (2014). Online action recognition using covariance of shape and motion. *Computer Vision and Image Understanding, 129,* 15–26. doi:10.1016/j.cviu.2014.08.001

Lahane, A., Yesha, Y., Grasso, M. A., Joshi, A., Park, A., & Lo, A. (2012). *Detection of unsafe action from laparoscopic cholecystectomy video.* Paper presented at the ACM SIGHIT International Health Informatics Symposium (ACM IHI). doi:10.1145/2110363.2110400

Lee, H. G., Choi, M. K., Shin, B. S., & Lee, S. C. (2013). Reducing redundancy in wireless capsule endoscopy videos. *Computers in Biology and Medicine, 43*(6), 670–682. doi:10.1016/j.compbiomed.2013.02.009 PMID:23668342

Lee, P. Y., Yan, S. L., Hu, M. H., & Marescaux, J. (2015). *A computed stereoscopic method for laparoscopic surgery by using feature tracking.* Paper presented at the IEEE international conference on Consumer Electronics, Taipai, Taiwan. doi:10.1109/ICCE-TW.2015.7217046

Lee, S. L., Lerotic, M., Vitiello, V., Giannarou, S., Kwok, K. W., Visentini-Scarzanella, M., & Yang, G. Z. (2010). From medical images to minimally invasive intervention: Computer assistance for robotic surgery. *Computerized Medical Imaging and Graphics, 34*(1), 33–45. doi:10.1016/j.compmedimag.2009.07.007 PMID:19699056

Li, B., & Meng, M. Q. H. (2009). Computer-based detection of bleeding and ulcer in wireless capsule endoscopy images by chromaticity moments. *Computers in Biology and Medicine, 39*(2), 141–147. doi:10.1016/j.compbiomed.2008.11.007 PMID:19147126

Lin, H. C., Shafran, I., Yuh, D., & Hager, G. D. (2006). Towards automatic skill evaluation: Detection and segmentation of robot-assisted surgical motions. *Computer Aided Surgery, 11*(5), 220-230.

Lin, Z., Uemura, M., Zecca, M., & Sessa, S. (2012). Objective Skill Evaluation for Laparoscopic Training Based on Motion Analysis. *IEEE Transactions on Bio-Medical Engineering, 60*(4), 977–985. PMID:23204271

Marcinczak, J. M., & Grigat, R. R. (2013). Closed Contour Specular Reflection Segmentation in Laparoscopic Images. *International Journal of Biomedical Imaging, 6.* PMID:23983675

Marvik, R., Langø, T., Tangen, G. A., Andersen, J. O., Kaspersen, J. H., Ystgaard, B., . . . Nagelhus Hernes, T. A. (2004). Laparoscopic navigation pointer for three-dimensional image-guided surgery. *Surg Endosc, 18,* 1242-1248.

Moayedi, F., Azimifar, R., & Boostani, R. (2015). Structured sparse representation for human action recognition. *Neurocomputing, 161,* 38–46. doi:10.1016/j.neucom.2014.10.089

Mountney, P., & Yang, G. Z. (2012). Context specific descriptors for tracking deforming tissue. *Medical Image Analysis*, *16*(3), 550–561. doi:10.1016/j.media.2011.02.010 PMID:21641270

Münzer, B., Schoeffmann, K., & Böszörmenyi, L. (2013). *Relevance Segmentation of Laparoscopic Videos*. Paper presented at the 2013 IEEE International Symposium on Multimedia (ISM), Anaheim, CA. doi:10.1109/ISM.2013.22

Navarra, G., Pozza, E., Occhionorelli, S., Carcoforo, P., & Donini, I. (1997). One-wound laparoscopic cholecystectomy. *British Journal of Surgery*, *84*(5), 695. doi:10.1002/bjs.1800840536 PMID:9171771

Nicolau, M., James, A., Benny, P. L., Darzi, A., & Yang, G. Z. (2005). *Invisible Shadow for Navigation and Planning in Minimal Invasive Surgery*. In Medical Image Computing and Computer-Assisted Intervention – MICCAI 2005 (Vol. 3750, pp. 25–32). Springer. doi:10.1007/11566489_4

Nicolau, S., Soler, L., Mutter, D., & Marescaux, J. (2011). Augmented reality in laparoscopic surgical oncology. *Surgical Oncology*, *20*(3), 189–201. doi:10.1016/j.suronc.2011.07.002 PMID:21802281

Oh, J. H., Hwang, S., Lee, J. K., Tavanapong, W., Wong, J., & Groen, P. C. D. (2007). Informative frame classification for endoscopy video. *Medical Image Analysis*, *11*(2), 110–127. doi:10.1016/j.media.2006.10.003 PMID:17329146

Öhsen, U. V., Marcinczak, J. M., Vélez, A. F. M., & Grigat, R. R. (2012). *Keyframe selection for robust pose estimation in laparoscopic videos*. Paper presented at the Medical Imaging 2012: Image-Guided Procedures, Robotic Interventions, and Modeling, San Diego, CA.

Oropesa, I., Sanchez-Gonzalez, P. J., Chmarra, M. K., Lamata, P., Fernandez, A. I., Sanchez-Margallo, J. A., & Gomez, E. J. et al. (2013). EVA: Laparoscopic Instrument Tracking Based on Endoscopic Video Analysis for Psychomotor Skills Assessment. *Surgical Endoscopy*, *27*(3), 1029–1039. doi:10.1007/s00464-012-2513-z PMID:23052495

Padoy, N., Blum, T., Essa, I., Feussner, H., Berger, M., & Navab, N. (2007). *A boosted segmentation method for surgical workflow analysis*. Paper presented at the Medical Image Computing and Computer Assisted Intervention. doi:10.1007/978-3-540-75757-3_13

Podolsky, E. R., Mouhlas, A., Wu, A. S., Poor, A. E., & Curcillo, P. G. (2010). Single Port Access (SPA) laparoscopic ventral hernia repair: initial report of 30 cases. *Surg Endosc, 24*(7), 1557-1561.

Quellec, G., Charrière, K., Lamard, M., Droueche, Z., Roux, C., Cochener, B., & Cazuguel, G. (2014). Real-time recognition of surgical tasks in eye surgery videos. *Medical Image Analysis*, *18*(3), 579–590. doi:10.1016/j.media.2014.02.007 PMID:24637155

Ramirez, D., Maurice, M. J., & Kaouk, J. H. (2016). Robotic Single-port Surgery: Paving the Way for the Future. *Urology*, *95*, 5–10. doi:10.1016/j.urology.2016.05.013 PMID:27211930

Ronaghi, Z., Duffy, E. B., & Kwartowitz, D. M. (2015). Toward real-time remote processing of laparoscopic video. *medical. Imaging*, *2*(4).

Rosen, J., Solazzo, M., Hannaford, B., & Sinanan, M. (2002). Task Decomposition of Laparoscopic Surgery for Objective Evaluation of Surgical Residents' Learning Curve Using Hidden Markov Model. *Computer Aided Surgery, 7*(1), 49-61.

Sa-Ing, V., Thongvigitmanee, S. S., Wilasrusmee, C., & Suthakorn, J. (2012). Adaptive Mean-Shift Kalman Tracking of Laparoscopic Instruments. *International Journal of Computer Theory and Engineering*, *4*(5), 685–689. doi:10.7763/IJCTE.2012.V4.557

Sánchez-González, P., Cano, A. M., Oropesa, I., Sánchez-Margallo, F. M., Del Pozo, F., Lamata, P., & Gómez, E. J. (2011). Laparoscopic video analysis for training and image-guided surgery. *Minimally Invasive Therapy & Allied Technologies*, *20*(6), 311–320. doi:10.3109/13645706.2010.541921 PMID:21247251

Schols, R. M., Bouvy, N. D., Dam, R. M. V., & Stassen, L. P. S. (2013). Advanced intraoperative imaging methods for laparoscopic anatomy navigation: An overview. *Surgical Endoscopy*, *27*(6), 1851–1859. doi:10.1007/s00464-012-2701-x PMID:23242493

Selka, F., Nicolau, S., Agnus, V., Bessaid, A., Marescaux, J., & Soler, L. (2015). Context-specific selection of algorithms for recursive feature tracking in endoscopic image using a new methodology. *Computerized Medical Imaging and Graphics, 40*, 49-61.

Semerjian, A., Zettervall, S. L., Amdur, R., Jarrett, T. W., & Vaziri, K. (2015). 30-Day morbidity and mortality outcomes of prolonged minimally invasive kidney procedures compared with shorter open procedures: National surgical quality improvement program analysis. *Journal of Endourology*, *29*(7), 830–837. doi:10.1089/end.2014.0795 PMID:25646859

Shu, Y., & Cheriet, F. (2005). *Segmentation of Laparoscopic Images: Integrating Graph-Based Segmentation and Multistage Region Merging*. Paper presented at the Computer and Robot Vision.

Speidel, S., Kroehnert, A., Bodenstedt, S., Kenngott, H., Müller-Stich, B., & Dillmann, R. (2015). *Image-based tracking of the suturing needle during laparoscopic interventions*. Paper presented at the Medical Imaging 2015: Image-based tracking of the suturing needle during laparoscopic interventions, Orlando, FL.

Stanek, S. R., Tavanapong, W., Wonga, J., Oh, J. H., & Groenc, P. C. D. (2012). Automatic real-time detection of endoscopic procedures using temporal features. *Computer Methods and Programs in Biomedicine, 108*, 524-535.

Stoyanov, D., Elson, D., & Yang, G. Z. (2009). *Illumination position estimation for 3D soft-tissue reconstruction in robotic minimally invasive surgery*. Paper presented at the 2009 IEEE/RSJ International Conference on Intelligent Robots and Systems, St. Louis, MO. doi:10.1109/IROS.2009.5354447

Stoyanov, D., & Yang, G. Z. (2011). *Soft tissue deformation tracking for robotic assisted minimally invasive surgery*. Paper presented at the 2009 Annual International Conference of the IEEE Engineering in Medicine and Biology Society, Minneapolis, MN.

Uecker, D. R., Wang, Y. F., Lee, C., & Wang, Y. (1995). Laboratory Investigation: Automated Instrument Tracking in Robotically Assisted Laparoscopic Surgery. *Journal of Image Guided Surgery*, *1*(6), 308–325. doi:10.1002/(SICI)1522-712X(1995)1:6<308::AID-IGS3>3.0.CO;2-E PMID:9080352

Voros, S., Long, J. A., & Clinquin, P. (2007). Automatic Detection of Instruments in Laparoscopic Images: A First Step Towards High-level Command of Robotic Endoscopic Holders. *The International Journal of Robotics Research*, *26*(11-12), 1173–1190. doi:10.1177/0278364907083395

Wang, S., Cong, Y., Cao, J., Yang, Y., Tang, Y., Zhao, H., & Yu, H. (2016). Scalable gastroscopic video summarization via similar-inhibition dictionary selection. *Artificial Intelligence in Medicine, 66*, 1–13. doi:10.1016/j.artmed.2015.08.006 PMID:26363682

Wei, G. Q., Arbter, K., & Hirzinger, G. (1997). Real-time visual servoing for laparoscopic surgery. Controlling robot motion with color image segmentation. *IEEE Engineering in Medicine and Biology Magazine, 16*(1), 40–45. doi:10.1109/51.566151 PMID:9058581

Wolf, R., Duchateau, J., Cinquin, P., & Voros, S. (2011). *3D Tracking of Laparoscopic Instruments Using Statistical and Geometric Modeling. In Medical Image Computing and Computer-Assisted Intervention-MICCAI 2011* (Vol. 6891, pp. 203–210). Springer. doi:10.1007/978-3-642-23623-5_26

Wu, C. H., Chen, Y. C., Liu, C. Y., Chang, C. C., & Sun, Y. N. (2004). *Automatic extraction and visualization of human inner structures from endoscopic image sequences.* Paper presented at the SPIE2004. doi:10.1117/12.535880

Yip, M. C., Lowe, D. G., Salcudean, S. E., Rohling, R. N., & Nguan, C. Y. (2012). Real-Time Methods for Long-Term Tissue Feature Tracking in Endoscopic Scenes. In P. Abolmaesumi, L. Joskowicz, N. Navab, & P. Jannin (Eds.), *Information Processing in Computer-Assisted Interventions* (pp. 33–43). Springer Berlin Heidelberg. doi:10.1007/978-3-642-30618-1_4

Yu, Z., Liu, J., Ding, H., Lu, M., Deng, M., Huang, Y., & Li, K. et al. (2015). An Image-Based Method of Uterus Segmentation in Gynecologic Laparoscopy. *Journal of Medical Imaging and Health Informatics, 5*(4), 819–825. doi:10.1166/jmihi.2015.1463

Yuan, Y., Zheng, X., & Lu, X. (2016). A discriminative representation for human action recognition. *Pattern Recognition, 59*, 88–97. doi:10.1016/j.patcog.2016.02.022

Zappella, L., Béjar, B., Hager, G., & Vidal, R. (2013). Surgical gesture classification from video and kinematic data. *Medical Image Analysis, 17*(7), 732–745. doi:10.1016/j.media.2013.04.007 PMID:23706754

Zenbutsu, S., Igarashi, T., & Yamaguchi, T. (2013). Development of Blood Vessel Depth Displaying Method for Laparoscopic Surgery Guidance. *Journal of Medical Imaging and Health Informatics, 3*(1), 101–106. doi:10.1166/jmihi.2013.1134

Zhang, X., & Payandeh, S. (2002). Application of Visual Tracking for Robot-Assisted Laparoscopic Surgery. *Journal of Robotic Systems, 19*(7), 315–328. doi:10.1002/rob.10043

Zhang, Y., Wirkert, S. J., Iszatt, J., Kenngott, H., Wagner, M., Mayer, B., . . . Maier-Hein, L. (2016). *Tissue classification for laparoscopic image understanding based on multispectral texture analysis.* Paper presented at the Medical Imaging: Image-Guided Procedures, Robotic Interventions, and Modeling.

Zhao, Z. (2014). Real-time 3D visual tracking of laparoscopic instruments for robotized endoscope holder. *Bio-Medical Materials and Engineering, 24*, 2665–2672. PMID:25226970

KEY TERMS AND DEFINITIONS

Global Motion Compensation: Trying to reverse the camera motion to improve the accuracy of the local motion estimation.

Image Enhancement: Trying to improve the image quality.

Image Segmentation: Dividing the image into several homogeneous regions.

Laparoscopy: A minimally-invasive surgical procedure using a camera to display the inside patient's body.

Soft Tissue Deformation Tracking: Trying to estimate the parameters of the soft tissue deformation model.

Surgical Activity Recognition: Trying to detect which surgical activity is being performed in the laparoscopic video.

Telescope: A camera inserted into the patient's body.

Section 4
Big Data

Chapter 15
Leveraging Applications of Data Mining in Healthcare Using Big Data Analytics:
An Overview

Mohammad Hossein Tekieh
University of Ottawa, Canada

Bijan Raahemi
University of Ottawa, Canada

Eric I. Benchimol
University of Ottawa, Canada

ABSTRACT

Big data analytics has been introduced as a set of scalable, distributed algorithms optimized for analysis of massive data in parallel. There are many prospective applications of data mining in healthcare. In this chapter, the authors investigate whether health data exhibits characteristics of big data, and accordingly, whether big data analytics can leverage the data mining applications in healthcare. To answer this interesting question, potential applications are divided into four categories, and each category into sub-categories in a tree structure. The available types of health data are specified, with a discussion of the applicable dimensions of big data for each sub-category. The authors conclude that big data analytics can provide more advantages for the quality of analysis in particular categories of applications of data mining in healthcare, while having less efficacy for other categories.

INTRODUCTION

While collecting, storing, and managing large amounts of digitized data are now technically feasible and affordable, only some useful information is still extracted from a small portion of the gathered data. To discover more information, strong analytical tools are needed for processing and analyzing the collected data, currently on the order of petabytes (Han, Kamber, & Pei, 2011). Data analysis algorithms have

DOI: 10.4018/978-1-5225-2515-8.ch015

also been developed to be able to handle big data collections. In addition, scalable and flexible software technologies have been introduced and are being improved to provide a suitable ecosystem to implement big data algorithms. The package comprising all these new components such as the technologies, algorithms, and methods is known as "big data analytics".

Data mining, as a strong analytical tool, has been applied to large amounts of digitized data collected in various fields – including healthcare – over the past decades. With the introduction of big data analytics, researchers are working to enhance data mining techniques to make the algorithms more scalable and faster. However, whether this enhancement resolves the existing limitations of data analysis studies in the field of healthcare remains unknown. It is necessary to first determine if all "health data" fit into the definition of "big data", before claiming big data analytics as the solution to overcome the limitations of health data analysis.

In this chapter, the authors investigate whether applications of data mining in healthcare can be leveraged by big data analytics by answering the following questions:

1. What are the applications of data mining in healthcare?
2. What are the different types of health data?
3. What are the characteristics of "big data"?
4. Is health data a form of "big data"?
5. Are all types of health data relevant in each application of data mining in healthcare?
6. To what extent do big data analytics enhance the quality of research in each application of data mining in healthcare?

In the introductory section, the application of data mining in healthcare is summarized, and the different types of health data and dimensions of big data are reviewed. Next, the methodology of achieving the above objective is presented and discussed in detail. Finally, the chapter will be concluded by summarizing the answers to the research questions.

BACKGROUND

Whether healthcare data can be considered "big data" is controversial. The phrase "health data" does not refer to a specific type or source of data. Some health data is gathered for specific research studies, but the majority is collected routinely without having pre-defined research questions in mind (Benchimol et al., 2015). There are many types of health data being collected routinely using various approaches, which will be presented later in this section. Often, the only characteristic they share is being related to the healthcare of patients. Each data type has its own characteristics and is collected for a specific reason, such as administration of a healthcare system. Since the majority of health data is not originally collected for research studies, they cannot necessarily be applicable for all types of data analysis studies. However, these health data instances can be valuable sources of information, and to which descriptive and predictive analytical tools such as data mining techniques can be applied to conduct novel analyses.

Data mining techniques have been applied to a large variety of data in many sectors and industries, such as healthcare, finance, retail, and telecommunication (Han et al., 2011). Although various applications of data mining in healthcare have been discussed in the literature, not all types of health data are suited to the requirements of each application. Due to the large and increasing volume of health data being collected on both ill and healthy subjects, a supportive infrastructure is required to process data with high scale, streaming, uncertain and multi-structural characteristics. However, the support for these limitations may not be necessary for all types of health data and research objectives, as not all limitations might be applicable. For instance, in studying a rare non-chronic health issue using administrative data collected annually, the rate of data acquisition may not limit the study, whereas mitigating the uncertainty in data could improve the quality of findings significantly.

In this background section, applications of data mining to healthcare are summarized and categorized based on past systematic reviews. Types of health data and big data dimensions are also reviewed.

Applications of Data Mining to Healthcare

The application of data mining to healthcare can be categorized into four groups; clinical decision making, population and public health, genetics and biomedicine, and health administration policies (Tekieh & Raahemi, 2015). Although "text mining" has important healthcare implications, it was excluded from this review as it is considered to be a separate and broader field of research with its own set of applications to healthcare. It focuses on natural-language processing techniques, and uses data mining as one of many components.

The categories and their descriptions are retrieved from past systematic reviews. Each is briefly introduced, along with an example.

Clinical Decision Making

Applying data mining techniques at a clinical level can help to predict high-risk patients, and provide additional information to clinicians. As an example, Healthways' data mining software discovers relationships to predict patient risk and suggests appropriate intervention and prevention plans based on the available evidence ("Healthways Heads Off Increased Costs with SAS," 2009).

Population and Public Health

Patterns, trends and causes of disease can be investigated using data mining, toward enhancing public health awareness and improving health status of the population. For instance, breast cancer patients have been classified and investigated epidemiologically using data mining techniques (Potter, 2007).

Genetics and Biomedicine

In contrast to studies done in the health of populations, biomedical data analysis research investigates diseases at the molecular level. Supporting data is retrieved from genomics, transcriptomics, and proteomics of humans and microbiota. Profiling gene expression in the diagnosis of leukemia is an example of applying data mining on human DNA microarray data (Haferlach et al., 2010).

Health Administration Policies

Health administration data systems are operated by healthcare providers, insurance companies and public sector institutions. Analyses are used to assess the accuracy and efficiency of their procedures and policies. A well-known study type in this category is insurance fraud detection using data mining ("First Things First—Highmark makes healthcare-fraud prevention top priority with SAS," 2006).

Types of Health Data

Health data has various types, and each has its own characteristics. The data collected for research purposes – via surveys, experiments, etc. – covers a small proportion of available health data. The majority is collected routinely as part of healthcare delivery. The health data being collected routinely, without having any pre-defined research question, can be divided into two categories based on their purpose for collection: administrative and clinical. In operating administration systems such as insurance claims, the administrative data is generated by system users, such as professional coders and hospitals. On the other hand, clinical data is created during the conduct of medical care by clinicians or through laboratory investigations. Health claims data, primary care databases, electronic health records and disease registries are examples of routinely collected health data. Health data may also be either routinely or non-routinely collected from other sources which introduce other types of health data, such as patient-generated data and machine-generated data (Benchimol et al., 2015; Deeny & Steventon, 2015).

Administrative Data

Health administrative data is collected as a result of operating modern administration of healthcare. The completeness of health administrative data depends on the requirements of associated health insurance plans, operating agencies, and regulators (Roos, Nickel, Romano, & Fergusson, 2014). Assessments of health outcomes and quality of care are typical secondary uses of administrative data. The sources of this type of health data include registries, life event records, insurance claims, and health service providers.

Clinically-Generated Data

This type of data is generated during clinical care, in providing diagnosis and treatment. Capture of information and input by clinicians results in deposition of data in the patient record, which can be retrieved on an ongoing basis or a per-project basis. Sources of this type of health data is electronic medical/health records (EMR/EHR) belonging to clinics, hospitals, laboratories and pharmacies. Depending on the regulatory nature of data collection, the data may be housed in the patient record, or deposited in a data warehouse for later use in research, administration, or clinical care.

Patient-Generated Data

This type of data is directly reported by the patient to a clinician or a healthcare system to monitor his/her health status. The data collection procedure can either be directed by a healthcare practitioner, or conducted individually by the patient. For example, the patient may decide to record this information by himself/herself for personal monitoring of symptoms, social networking or peer support. The sources of this type of health data include surveys, health web portals and social media.

Machine-Generated Data

A machine automatically generates this type of data, such as from computer processes and sensor signals, for passive monitoring of staff or patient behaviour and status. The sources of this type of data include remote sensors which collect or send data to a system and monitor for abnormalities. Examples include monitoring environmental exposures of a person, and remote holter ECG monitors.

Dimensions of Big Data

Enormous amounts of data of many different types and conditions are being collected on a regular basis. This includes streaming modes in various industries and sectors. In modern healthcare, due to the transition from paper-based systems to digitized systems using electronic means, large amounts of data are generated, often continuously. This recorded data is of different quantities, formats and conditions. Therefore, health data may qualify as being big data.

To evaluate this, the characteristics of big data need to be understood. Although an evolving concept, "big data" refers to data that is large in volume, varied in type, fast in generation velocity, and of uncertain veracity (accuracy) ("The Four V's of Big Data," 2013). Each of these dimensions can be defined briefly as following:

- **Volume:** Big data is large in scale (e.g. petabytes).
- **Velocity:** Big data is generated at a fast pace and often in real-time (e.g. streaming).
- **Variety:** Big data contains different forms of data – structured, semi-structured and unstructured.
- **Veracity:** Big data can lack high quality, and have uncertain accuracy.

Characterized by these four V's (and sometimes more), big data can be defined as a collection of data so large and complex that it becomes difficult to process using existing data analytics techniques. Analysis of big data relies on scalable distributed platforms, such as Hadoop and Spark, which support MapReduce structure optimized for analysis of massive data in parallel.

METHODOLOGY

The approach chosen for this chapter is to categorize and investigate the applications of data mining in healthcare using past systematic reviews. Therefore, each category represents an application of data mining to healthcare. One or more sub-categories are defined under each category. Each sub-category represents a set of studies with common characteristics from a data analysis perspective in that category. In other words, studies in each sub-category share similar technical concerns, limitations, and possible solutions in analyzing their data. For instance, two studies might not have much medical relationships with each other and still both fall into the same sub-category, while two other studies focusing on the same health condition have different data analysis characteristics. The available types of health data for particular applications are determined, as well as which dimensions of big data analytics (the four V's) are applicable to leverage analyses for each sub-category. Eventually, the possibility of enhancing the data analysis quality using big data analytics for each group of studies is assessed.

The collected information is presented and summarized in a hierarchical, tree-style format in Figure 1. The horizontal levels of the tree represent (1) the main categories of applications; (2) the sub-categories; (3) the associated health data types for the sub-category; and (4) the applicable dimensions of big data analytics for the same sub-category.

As an example, Population and Public Health is a category of data mining applications in healthcare, and studies with Responsive Conditions are grouped as a sub-category. For these particular studies, patient-generated data could be a source of information. Since the concerned conditions in this group are usually spread quickly among a population and/or require real-time analysis, the velocity of fetching data could be a limitation in running high quality analyses. This limitation can be mitigated using a big data analytics environment.

DISCUSSION

In this section, the authors discuss their investigations on each application of data mining in healthcare to introduce the known group of studies in each application, present the available health data and argue which big data dimensions are applicable.

Clinical Decision Making

Studies in this category are mainly at the clinical level. In practice, most of these studies are done either to develop treatment algorithms and clinical pathways, or to help recognize specific issues and patterns

Figure 1. Big data dimensions and accessible health data for applications of data mining in healthcare

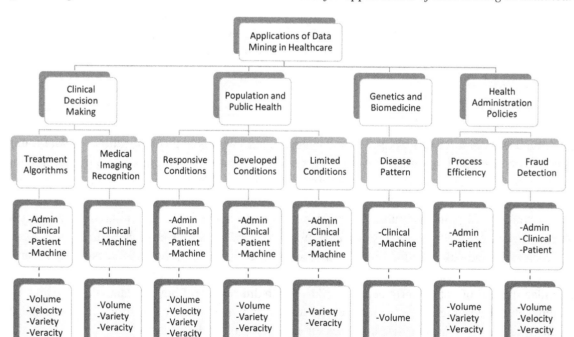

in medical imaging artifacts (Hardin & Chhieng, 2007). Suitable types of health data for these studies and applicable dimensions of big data are discussed for the two sub-categories.

Treatment Algorithms

In clinical care, developing a clinical pathway is typically a sensitive procedure, requiring attention to ethical considerations, as it deals with human lives. A clinical pathway or algorithm could be a stream of investigation, diagnosis, treatment, or some combination. Data mining techniques are employed to provide additional information in designing these algorithms based on experiences. In addition, clinicians would avoid under-estimating the effects of a symptom, and make treatment decisions with higher confidence by receiving supportive second opinions using analytical model. This could eventually reduce unnecessary costs for both care providers and insurance companies. Studies that attempt to predict high-risk outcomes for patients based on their symptoms and individual determinants fall in this category (Bandyopadhyay et al., 2015; Bates, Saria, Ohno-Machado, Shah, & Escobar, 2014; Easton, Stephens, & Angelova, 2014; Raju, Su, Patrician, Loan, & McCarthy, 2015). Data gathered by practitioners and stored in EMRs from examinations and lab tests, data reported by the patients themselves (either with directions from a clinician or not), and even data generated by health monitoring devices are potential sources of information to conduct these studies.

The number of EMR vendors is rapidly increasing, as is the choice of modules available within each system. Developing treatment algorithms to provide higher quality clinical service could be acute and time-sensitive, which would require analyzing streaming input data. Sources of information can involve both structured and unstructured text materials, including physician's notes and prescriptions. The collected data typically comes from different sources and individuals, which could introduce conflicts and inaccuracies within the data.

Since the available data for this set of studies contains all dimensions of big data – volume, velocity, variety and veracity – the possibility of enhancing the quality of analysis using big data analytics is "very high".

Medical Imaging Recognition

Examples of this set of studies include diagnosing melanoma by analyzing digitized images of skin lesions (Burroni et al., 2004), identifying minimal hepatic encephalopathy in patients with cirrhosis based on imaging of brain white matter (Chen, Chen, Yang, Teng, & Herskovits, 2015), discrimination of benign and malignant breast nodules using multiple ultra-sonographic features (Joo, Yang, Moon, & Kim, 2004), and differentiating neoplastic and non-neoplastic brain lesions based on magnetic resonance spectroscopy (Zellner, Rand, Prost, Krouwer, & Chetty, 2004). Data mining studies on anomaly detection in high-resolution high-dimensional medical imaging data which require extensive processing capacities also fall in this category.

The two main sources of information here are (1) the data gathered by clinicians as a result of examining patients prior to sending them for lab work (clinically-generated health data); and (2) the data generated by medical imaging machines in screening organs under study (machine-generated health data).

The quantity of screenings done using medical devices in health centers is usually high, supplementing clinical information gathered by clinicians. In addition, medical images are typically translated into high-dimensional data. The format of collected data includes images, videos and unstructured text, as well as other structured data. The collected data could include screening errors and vague images, increasing uncertainty of the data quality.

The possibility of enhancing the quality of analyses using big data analytics for this set of studies is "high" as the available data contains at least three dimensions of big data – volume, variety and veracity.

Population and Public Health

This type of research aims to determine the causes, trends and patterns of diseases (population health), and to analyze the practice of medicine associated with diseases (public health) at the population level. The goal is to improve the overall health of the public. Depending on what type of disease and under which condition is being analyzed, the requirements of a study might change. Therefore, they have been divided into three main groups, based on the commonality of their characteristics from a data analysis perspective: responsive conditions, developed conditions, and limited conditions. Note that this categorization is not classifying the diseases from medical point of view. The group naming is done based on sharing similar conditions and requirements to analyze data. Suitable types of health data for each of these studies and the applicable dimensions of big data are discussed following.

Responsive Conditions

Fast-spreading diseases usually infect a large proportion of the population in a short time, typically caused by viruses (e.g. H1N1, Ebola and influenza) or bacteria (e.g. *C. difficile* and *E. coli*). To control the spread, real-time analyses are conducted to anticipate the next at-risk regions. In overall, studies analyzing conditions that spread across or affect a proportion of population which require quick awareness and analysis fall in this group. Therefore, these studies are not just limited to controlling and monitoring fast-spreading diseases, and includes any high incidence conditions that need rapid response. Another example is predicting the number of asthma-related emergency department (ED) visits in a specific area in near-real-time using environmental and social media data to help public surveillance, ED preparedness, and targeted patient interventions (Ram, Zhang, Williams, & Pengetnze, 2015).

Data sources of this set of studies accumulate information from patient visits to healthcare centers (producing administrative data), examinations by clinicians and undergoing lab tests (creating clinically-generated data), sharing of their experiences and symptoms on social media to communicate with experts or other affected people (developing patient-generated data), and also environmental data collected by sensors as seen in the latest example (gathering machine-generated data).

When an outbreak occurs, such as the recent Zika virus in Brazil (Campos, Bandeira, & Sardi, 2015), large amounts of information and records are typically gathered. It is important for public health practitioners and the health system to react quickly and analyze data immediately, and as they change in real-time. The collected information could include both structured and unstructured materials such as experts' notes, affected people's video messages, and formal record capture. Usually the cause is unknown initially, and patient symptoms could overlap with those of other health issues; this can lead to capturing uncertain, irrelevant, and even incorrect information.

In this sub-category, the available data contains all dimensions of big data – volume, velocity, variety and veracity; hence, the possibility of enhancing the quality of analysis using big data analytics is "very high".

Developed Conditions

This group includes studies analyzing conditions that do not require real-time processing – as the critical stage of disease development has passed – or even cannot be processed instantly – due to the nature of disease which needs to develop to a certain point to provide further details. In addition, these conditions usually hit a large proportion of the population and typically have high prevalence. For instance, chronic diseases are not passed to other patients and do not have the same incidence rate as the fast-spreading diseases, but they often cause severe conditions and last longer in a population. The incidence of breast cancer, as an example, started to grow in most societies and now is still considered as a prevalent issue among a significant portion of global population which there were attempts in classifying and predicting the suffering patients (Potter, 2007). Another example is identifying the contributing factors of developing asthma in a population, from which more than 230 million people suffer worldwide, and is considered one of the most common chronic diseases among children (WHO, 2017).

Note that not all studies that focus on chronic diseases fall in this sub-category. As mentioned in the previous section, the study on anticipating the number of asthma-related emergency department visits (Ram et al., 2015) is considered a "responsive condition" as requires real-time analysis at population level. On the other hand, the study that predicts asthma attacks of the patient by analyzing sensor data (Bock, Scholz, Piller, & Böhm, 2016) is similar to Treatment Algorithms of Clinical Decision Making studies. Therefore, the category of every health data analysis study is determined based on its characteristics.

For analyzing this type of conditions, administrative health data can be used to track the development of the disease, in addition to clinical data provided by practitioners or patients themselves. Data generated by medical imaging devices for screening the involved organs can be considered as well.

Due to the high prevalence of the concerned condition in the focused population, the volume of data collected from both administrative and clinical perspective is large. However, in these cases the speed of generating and collecting data might not be high, comparing to the responsive conditions. The format of the collected data can be diverse, as well as the quality.

The available data for this set of studies contain at least three dimensions of big data – volume, variety and veracity –, therefore, the possibility of enhancing the quality of analysis using big data analytics is "high".

Limited Conditions

In this group, diseases have long duration and often unknown causes, hitting a smaller proportion of a population in contrast to the "developed conditions". Most immune-mediated diseases comply with this condition (e.g. inflammatory bowel disease and multiple sclerosis) in many societies; however, not all of them usually fall in this group (e.g. asthma). Note that a disease can be rear in one population, while quite common in another. No matter if the disease is considered rare in the focused population or not, as long as the amount of collected data to analyze the disease at a population level is no more than few millions of data cells of an ordinary structured data (e.g. hundreds of thousands of rows with tens of columns), the study is considered as "limited condition" in this categorization. There are generally attempts made in analyzing and investigating these diseases to narrow down the contributing risk factors. Although some genetic diseases may be rare, their root causes have usually been identified; therefore, the related analyses can focus on genetics data, which are introduced in the next category of applications. The sources of information for this group of studies can be the same as the previous group, as patients usually go through the same procedures: administrative data, clinically generated data, patient-generated data and machine-generated data.

In contrast to responsive conditions and developed conditions, studies dealing with limited conditions do not have the luxury of access to large amounts of data. Similar to the developed conditions, the input data is not collected at high rate. However, the format of the collected data can still be diverse, and the quality.

The possibility of enhancing the quality of analysis using big data analytics is "medium" for this sub-category as the available data contains at least two dimensions of big data – variety and veracity.

Genetics and Biomedicine

Research in this category focuses on disease caused at the molecular level, using data retrieved from genomics (DNA molecules), transcriptomics (RNA molecules), proteomics (proteins), and metabolomics (metabolites) of human hosts and their resident microbiota. These aspects can be used in determining an individual patient's unique biological profile toward applying the most effective therapy, also known as personalized medicine. The knowledge of gene and protein expression procedures has improved rapidly over recent years. Therefore, the amount of prepared microarray data has increased also. These developments allowed researchers to analyze health issues at the microscopic level, and to determine relationships among different aspects of the biology of humans and disease. Data mining is already being widely applied to microarray data, mainly for detecting patterns of diseases. Suitable types of health data for each of these studies and the applicable dimensions of big data are discussed below.

Disease Pattern

Examples of this form of research include profiling breast cancer subtypes based on pervasive differences in their gene expression patterns (Perou et al., 2000), and improving the prediction of colorectal cancer using gene expression signatures (Salazar et al., 2011). Initial data gathering is done in laboratories, by extracting genomic DNA samples (clinically-generated data). DNA segments are then sequenced by computer processes (machine-generated data), to provide microarray data after further procedures that demonstrate the expression level of genes.

Although the process of sequencing the human genome can now be done faster with much lower cost, the whole genome sequence consumes hundreds of gigabytes of storage space, and can require significant processing time and cost (Robison, 2014). When a disease with a known cause is being studied, only a specific part of the genome may need to be sequenced for analysis. However, for unknown diseases, the whole genome (or even the whole exome, including non-coding parts of the genome) may be required, and the amount of data produced becomes massive. On the bright side, typically whole genome sequencing is now done with high accuracy.

As the available data for this set of studies contain at least one dimension of big data – volume –, the possibility of enhancing the quality of analysis using big data analytics is "low".

Health Administration Policies

Studies that analyze healthcare administration policies at the system level fall under this category. Two main categories of research studies exist. First is evaluating and investigating the efficiency of processes, including policies, plans and procedures. Second is focusing on detection of fraud in the healthcare system. Suitable types of health data for each of these study areas, and the applicable dimensions of big data, are discussed below.

Process Efficiency

Any sort of systematic process within healthcare could potentially be assessed here, and improvements suggested through analysis of the associated data using data mining techniques. Examples of this form of research include evaluation of health insurance plans by identifying significant factors involved in improving health policies (Tekieh, Raahemi, & Izad Shenas, 2015), and identification of hospitals with potential quality problems (Geraci et al., 2000). Administrative data is considered to be the main source of information for evaluating healthcare systems. In addition, individually-directed patient-generated data could also contain useful "unofficial" information about the efficiency of various health systems, based on patients' experiences.

The collected data for this type of studies could potentially be large in scale, contain materials with different formats (e.g. unstructured text, video and structured data), and be highly uncertain in their accuracy. Optimally, health services research is conducted in a planned and orderly fashion, often repeated regularly, and hence real-time responses are probably not required.

The available data for this set of studies contains at least three dimensions of big data – volume, variety and veracity; hence, the possibility of enhancing the quality of analysis using big data analytics is "high".

Fraud Detection

Claiming reimbursement for unnecessary drugs or procedures by patients, doctors or even hospitals can cause a financial burden to insurance companies and governments. Data mining techniques have aided these organizations to detect cases of fraud ("First Things First—Highmark makes healthcare-fraud prevention top priority with SAS," 2006). Administrative data contain the details of what was claimed; however, the necessity and truthfulness of the claims can be verified based on conditions and patterns existing in clinically-generated data, as well as clinically-directed patient-generated data. An instance of such fraud is a patient who has claimed the use of a drug, but based on his health conditions and background, it would be unlikely that he would need that particular drug.

A large volume of administrative and/or clinical data may be necessary for the evaluation of fraud. Ideally, inspections would be better to be done in real-time as the claim is submitted, to avoid delayed prosecution. In addition to typical uncertainties that exist in health data, such as the linkage of various data sources, there will almost certainly be contradictions which require detection.

In this sub-category, the possibility of enhancing the quality of analysis using big data analytics is "high" as the available data contains at least three dimensions of big data – volume, velocity and veracity.

CONCLUSION

Data mining is a useful analytic tool, known for its ability to be used to analyze large datasets to discover latent patterns and trends. However, traditional algorithms of data mining have limitations in handling large collections of health data. Big data analytics have been introduced to exploit these algorithms.

Data mining has many different applications in healthcare, but the utility of using big data analytics for analyzing health data has not always been clear. It could be claimed that health data is a form of big data, and therefore using big data analytics is necessary when analyzing health data. However this assumption may not be correct in all situations or with all types of health data.

In this chapter, the applications of data mining in healthcare were divided into four categories (clinical decision making, population and public health, genetics and biomedicine, and health administration policies), and then into multiple sub-categories. Each sub-category represents a set of studies that are common in design and requirements. The accessible types of health data (from clinical, administrative, patient-generated, and machine-generated) and the applicable dimensions of big data (from volume, velocity, variety, and veracity) for each sub-category were presented and discussed.

In summary, not all datasets associated to every health data analysis study should be considered amenable to big data analytic techniques. Depending on the type of study and characteristics of the data, big data analytics can provide different degrees of enhancement of the quality of analysis. There cannot be one definitive statement about the efficacy of all data mining tools in healthcare because different types of health data may be used and different analytic techniques could be exploited. Accordingly, researchers, clinicians and health policy-makers should carefully examine the characteristics of the data and study conditions before making a decision on which (if any) big data analytic techniques can bring insights and add value in their study of the data.

REFERENCES

Bandyopadhyay, S., Wolfson, J., Vock, D. M., Vazquez-Benitez, G., Adomavicius, G., Elidrisi, M., … O'Connor, P. J. (2015). Data mining for censored time-to-event data: a Bayesian network model for predicting cardiovascular risk from electronic health record data. *Data Mining and Knowledge Discovery, 29*(4), 1033–1069. https://doi.org/10.1007/s10618-014-0386-6

Bates, D. W., Saria, S., Ohno-Machado, L., Shah, A., & Escobar, G. (2014). Big Data In Health Care: Using Analytics To Identify And Manage High-Risk And High-Cost Patients. *Health Affairs, 33*(7), 1123–1131. doi:10.1377/hlthaff.2014.0041 PMID:25006137

Benchimol, E. I., Smeeth, L., Guttmann, A., Harron, K., Moher, D., & Petersen, I. (2015). The REporting of studies Conducted using Observational Routinely-collected health Data (RECORD) Statement. *PLoS Med, 12*(10), e1001885. https://doi.org/10.1371/journal.pmed.1001885

Bock, N., Scholz, M., Piller, G., & Böhm, K. (2016). Capture and Analysis of Sensor Data for Asthma Patients (Research-in-Progress). In *ECIS 2016 Proceedings*. Istanbul, Turkey: Association for Information Systems.

Burroni, M., Corona, R., Dell'Eva, G., Sera, F., Bono, R., Puddu, P., … Rubegni, P. (2004). Melanoma Computer-Aided Diagnosis: Reliability and Feasibility Study. *American Association for Cancer Research, 10*(6), 1881–1886. https://doi.org/10.1158/1078-0432.CCR-03-0039

Campos, G. S., Bandeira, A. C., & Sardi, S. I. (2015). Zika Virus Outbreak, Bahia, Brazil. *Emerging Infectious Diseases, 21*(10), 1885–1886. doi:10.3201/eid2110.150847 PMID:26401719

Chen, H.-J., Chen, R., Yang, M., Teng, G.-J., & Herskovits, E. H. (2015). Identification of Minimal Hepatic Encephalopathy in Patients with Cirrhosis Based on White Matter Imaging and Bayesian Data Mining. *AJNR. American Journal of Neuroradiology*, *36*(3), 481–487. doi:10.3174/ajnr.A4146 PMID:25500314

Deeny, S. R., & Steventon, A. (2015). Making sense of the shadows: Priorities for creating a learning healthcare system based on routinely collected data. *BMJ Quality & Safety*, *24*(8), 505–515. doi:10.1136/bmjqs-2015-004278 PMID:26065466

Easton, J. F., Stephens, C. R., & Angelova, M. (2014). Risk factors and prediction of very short term versus short/intermediate term post-stroke mortality: A data mining approach. *Computers in Biology and Medicine*, *54*, 199–210. doi:10.1016/j.compbiomed.2014.09.003 PMID:25303114

First Things First—Highmark makes healthcare-fraud prevention top priority with SAS. (2006). SAS. Retrieved from http://www.sas.com/ success/pdf/highmarkfraud.pdf

Geraci, J. M., Johnson, M. L., Gordon, H. S., Peterson, N. J., Daley, J., Hur, K., & Wray, N. P. et al. (2000). Mortality after non-cardiac surgery: Prediction from administrative versus clinical data. *Journal of Investigative Medicine*, *48*(2).

Haferlach, T., Kohlmann, A., Wieczorek, L., Basso, G., Kronnie, G. T., Bene, M.-C., & Fo, R. et al. (2010). Clinical utility of microarray-based gene expression profiling in the diagnosis and subclassification of leukemia: Report from the international microarray innovations in leukemia study group. *Journal of Clinical Oncology*, *28*(15), 2529–2537. doi:10.1200/JCO.2009.23.4732 PMID:20406941

Han, J., Kamber, M., & Pei, J. (2011). *Data Mining: Concepts and Techniques*. Elsevier.

Hardin, J. M., & Chhieng, D. C. (2007). Data Mining and Clinical Decision Support Systems. In E. S. B. E. Fhimss Facmi (Ed.), *Clinical Decision Support Systems* (pp. 44–63). Springer New York. doi:10.1007/978-0-387-38319-4_3

Healthways Heads Off Increased Costs with SAS. (2009). SAS. Retrieved from http://www.sas.com/success/pdf/healthways.pdf

Joo, S., Yang, Y. S., Moon, W. K., & Kim, H. C. (2004). Computer-aided diagnosis of solid breast nodules: Use of an artificial neural network based on multiple sonographic features. *IEEE Transactions on Medical Imaging*, *23*(10), 1292–1300. doi:10.1109/TMI.2004.834617 PMID:15493696

Perou, C. M., Sørlie, T., Eisen, M. B., van de Rijn, M., Jeffrey, S. S., & Rees, C. A. … Botstein, D. (2000). Molecular portraits of human breast tumours. *Nature*, *406*(6797), 747–752. https://doi.org/10.1038/35021093

Potter, R. (2007). *Comparison of classification algorithms applied to breast cancer diagnosis and prognosis*. Presented at the 7th Industrial Conference on Data Mining, ICDM 2007, Leipzig, Germany.

Raju, D., Su, X., Patrician, P. A., Loan, L. A., & McCarthy, M. S. (2015). Exploring factors associated with pressure ulcers: A data mining approach. *International Journal of Nursing Studies*, *52*(1), 102–111. doi:10.1016/j.ijnurstu.2014.08.002 PMID:25192963

Ram, S., Zhang, W., Williams, M., & Pengetnze, Y. (2015). Predicting Asthma-Related Emergency Department Visits Using Big Data. *IEEE Journal of Biomedical and Health Informatics, 19*(4), 1216–1223. https://doi.org/10.1109/JBHI.2015.2404829

Robison, R. J. (2014, January 6). *How big is the human genome? In megabytes, not base pairs.* Retrieved September 14, 2016, from https://medium.com/precision-medicine/how-big-is-the-human-genome-e90caa3409b0

Roos, L. L., Nickel, N. C., Romano, P. S., & Fergusson, P. (2014). Administrative Databases. In *Wiley StatsRef: Statistics Reference Online.* John Wiley & Sons, Ltd. doi:10.1002/9781118445112.stat05227

Salazar, R., Roepman, P., Capella, G., Moreno, V., Simon, I., Dreezen, C., & Tollenaar, R. et al. (2011). Gene expression signature to improve prognosis prediction of stage ii and iii colorectal cancer. *Journal of Clinical Oncology, 29*(1), 17–24. doi:10.1200/JCO.2010.30.1077 PMID:21098318

Tekieh, M. H., & Raahemi, B. (2015). Importance of Data Mining in Healthcare: A Survey. In *Proceedings of the 2015 IEEE/ACM International Conference on Advances in Social Networks Analysis and Mining 2015* (pp. 1057–1062). New York: ACM. doi:10.1145/2808797.2809367

Tekieh, M. H., Raahemi, B., & Izad Shenas, S. A. (2015). Analysing healthcare coverage with data mining techniques. *International Journal of Society Systems Science, 7*(3), 198–221. doi:10.1504/IJSSS.2015.071315

The Four V's of Big Data. (2013). Retrieved May 31, 2016, from: http://www.ibmbigdatahub.com/infographic/four-vs-big-data

WHO. (2017). *Chronic respiratory diseases: Asthma.* Retrieved January 22, 2017, from: http://www.who.int/respiratory/asthma/en/

Zellner, B. B., Rand, S. D., Prost, R., Krouwer, H., & Chetty, V. K. (2004). A cost-minimizing diagnostic methodology for discrimination between neoplastic and non-neoplastic brain lesions: Utilizing a genetic algorithm scientific reports. *Academic Radiology, 11*(2), 169–177. doi:10.1016/S1076-6332(03)00654-8 PMID:14974592

KEY TERMS AND DEFINITIONS

Administrative Data: The data collected routinely due to operating a healthcare administration system, such as hospital's billing system and insurance claims. This data is generated automatically by the associated system.

Big Data: Big data is a collection of data sets so large and complex that it becomes difficult to process using traditional analytics algorithms. The challenges include capture, creation, storage, search, sharing, analysis, and visualization. The 4 V's of big data are Volume (large volumes of data), Velocity (speed of data generation), Variety (structured, unstructured), and Veracity (trust and integrity).

Big Data Analytics: The platform to process and analyze scalable, fast-streaming, and multi-formatted data using MapReduce techniques and related technologies such as Hadoop and Spark and their associated eco systems.

Clinical Data: The data collected routinely due to providing healthcare clinical services, usually gathered in Electronic Medical Records (EMR) systems. This data is generated by clinicians at bed-side, in addition to laboratory technicians as matter of conducting lab tests.

Data Mining: Data Mining is the process of extracting hidden, implicit, novel, and useful information from large volume of data. It has emerged as a unique combination of several fields of science and technology including statistics, database systems, computer programming, machine learning, and artificial intelligence. Data mining spans a wide range of applications in medicine and population health (study of drug implications, disease outbreak), bioinformatics (protein interactions, gene sequence analysis), engineering (intrusion detection and network security, flow classification, Web mining), business (fraud detection, decision support systems, risk analysis, forecasting market trend), and environmental studies (flood prediction).

Health Data: A data gathered as a matter of running a healthcare system, providing healthcare services, or conducting health research. Most health data are generated and collected routinely without a pre-defined research question, divided to administrative and clinical data.

Population Health: Investigating the cause, trends, and patterns of diseases in a population with the aim of improving the health of an entire human population.

Public Health: Analyzing the practice of medicine associated to diseases in a population leading to set of instructions to raise public awareness on different health issues.

Chapter 16
Overview of Big Data in Healthcare

Mohammad Hossein Fazel Zarandi
Amirkabir University of Technology (Tehran Polytechnic), Iran

Reyhaneh Gamasaee
Amirkabir University of Technology (Tehran Polytechnic), Iran

ABSTRACT

Big data is a new ubiquitous term for massive data sets having large, more varied and complex structure with the complexities and difficulties of storing, analyzing and visualizing for further processes or results. The use of Big Data in health is a new and exciting field. A wide range of use cases for Big Data and analytics in healthcare will benefit best practice development, outcomes analysis, prediction, and surveillance. Consequently, the aim of this chapter is to provide an overview of Big Data in Healthcare systems including two applications of Big Data analysis in healthcare. The first one is understanding disease outcomes through analyzing Big Data, and the second one is the application of Big Data in genetics, biological, and molecular fields. Moreover, characteristics and challenges of healthcare Big Data analysis as well as technologies and software used for Big Data analysis are reviewed.

INTRODUCTION

The last decade has experienced significant advances in the amount of data which is generally generated and stored in almost everyday activities, as well as the capability of utilizing technology to analyze and comprehend that data. The massive amount of data generated in healthcare systems is identified as Big Data and the ability to analyze that data is named Big Data analytics. Big Data supports businesses in various industries to become more productive and efficient. One of those industries in which Big Data is very useful is healthcare. Although health data is not always Big Data, there are some types of health data sets which are categorized as Big Data. Those data sets include massive data obtained from high-volume laboratory information system, electronic medical record (EMR), biomedical and biometrics data, test usage data, and gene expression data. In addition to profit boosting and decreasing squandered overhead, healthcare Big Data is being used to predict epidemics, cure disease, improve quality of life

DOI: 10.4018/978-1-5225-2515-8.ch016

and avoid preventable deaths. Both of the existing health data and the behavioral data could significantly increase opportunities to forecast long-term health conditions. Big Data also provides better diagnostics techniques, disease prevention, and enhance access and decrease healthcare costs.

The applications of Big Data are not limited to proposing more efficient healthcare systems. Big Data and analytics are applied in the healthcare industry showing very encouraging results. Integration and digitizing of Big Data as well as impressively using it, provide many advantages for physician offices, hospitals, and care organizations. Those advantages include disease diagnosis at its earlier stages providing the opportunity of easily treatment, controlling health conditions of individuals and groups, and detecting health care fraud promptly and effectively. Big Data and analytics support healthcare systems to achieve their goals. Two main categories for the "Big Data in Healthcare" have been reviewed in literature as follows.

The first category includes three important issues [IMIA]: (I) Big Data extracted from the health system such as health and medication history, lab reports, and pathology results, where these analyzes are aimed at improving physicians understanding of disease outcomes and their risk factors, decreasing health system costs, and enhancing its efficiency; (II) Massive data sets of biological and molecular fields are known as "Omics" data, genomics, proteomics, microbiomics, and metabolomics, where the goal of analyzing these data sets is to comprehend the mechanisms of diseases and expedite the medical treatments; (III) Data collected from social media along with the signs and behaviors of people who use Internet and software applications, for improving their health conditions (Hansen et al., 2014).

The second category includes five important issues according to [Big Data in healthcare]:

(I) Big Data which is used to manage healthcare delivery costs; (II) Big Data which is used for clinical decision making; (III) Big Data for extracting clinical information. (IV) Big Data for demographical analysis by investigating behavior and consumer category; (V) Big Data which is used as support information; this type of Big Data application is not categorized in one of the above categories (Groves et al., 2013; Hermon & Williams, 2014). Several researchers have studied those categories related to Big Data in healthcare.

As the first example, Archenaa and Anita (2015) reviewed the role of government in increasing quality of healthcare systems by reducing its costs which lies in the first category. This cost reduction is due to analyzing clinical Big Data of healthcare systems. For instance, diseases are detected at the earlier stages and the best medicine is prescribed by analyzing clinical Big Data and using genetic makeups. This leads to reduction of readmission rates, and as a result, it causes cost reduction for patients (Archenaa & Anita, 2015). Moreover, Hay et al. (2013) used statistical techniques such as Boosted Regression Tree method to predict the risk of disease outbreak in different geographical locations. That study is classified in the first category of Big Data analysis in healthcare.

In addition, Murphy et al. (2016) uses clinical Big Data to identify delays in follow-up of abnormal chest imaging results. That research is classified in the second category since its focus is on extracting clinical Big Data and clinical decision making. Another research which lies in the second category has been conducted by Bibault et al. (2016). In that study, machine learning techniques such as decision trees, naïve Bayes, support vector machines, neural networks, and deep learning which can be applied to aggregate clinical Big Data of radiation oncology were reviewed. Reviewing literature of both categories of Big Data analysis in healthcare shows that understanding disease outcomes, which lies in the first category, have significant impacts on diagnosis and curing people's diseases. Thus, in this chapter, we mainly concentrate on reviewing literature of understanding disease outcomes through analyzing Big Data. Since Big Data sets of genetics, biological, and molecular fields are very influential in understanding disease outcomes, we also review applications of Big Data in those fields. Furthermore, Big Data analysis in those fields encounters some challenges based on the characteristics of such data. Thus, at first, it is required to determine characteristics of healthcare Big Data and challenges that a researcher encounters during its analysis.

In summary, in this chapter, we will review the recent studies in the field of "Big data in healthcare. As examples, two applications of Big Data analytics in healthcare are discussed in this chapter. The rest of this chapter is organized as follows. Research methodology is presented in the next section. Then, characteristics and challenges of healthcare Big Data analysis are briefly reviewed. Afterwards, modern technologies and software for healthcare Big Data analysis is described. Thereafter, Big Data for understanding disease outcomes is presented. Big Data in genetics, biological, and molecular fields are illustrated in the last section.

RESEARCH METHODOLOGY

In this chapter, Big Data in healthcare has been overviewed by searching the "Google Scholar" databases which covers 16400 documents with the title of Big Data from 2004-2017 time scope. Choosing time scope from 2004 to 2017 is due to this fact that Big Data in healthcare is a new concept and older papers are not relevant to the subject. Documents extracted from Google Scholar include journal and conference papers as well as books from international, famous publishers. In order to choose the most appropriate and relevant documents, some criteria are introduced.

The first criterion is that only published peer-reviewed journal and conference papers were selected and unpublished works were omitted. Among those 16400 books and papers, 342 documents are about using Big Data in healthcare problems. Thus, we narrowed the selected papers to include ones about big healthcare data. Papers have been chosen based on both practical and conceptual studies. The other criterion for choosing manuscripts is their applicability. This criterion was verified by examining several phrases in title, keywords, abstract, and body of manuscripts. Finally, in order to filter the most relevant documents, several keywords were searched to as follows.

(1) Big healthcare data; (2) Big Data challenges; (3) big healthcare data applications; (4) big healthcare data technologies; (5) big healthcare data software; (6) big healthcare data infrastructure.

Reviewing the abovementioned references of Big Data analysis in healthcare shows that understanding disease outcomes have significant impacts on diagnosis and curing people's diseases. Thus, in this chapter, we mainly concentrate on reviewing literature of understanding disease outcomes through analyzing Big Data. Since Big Data sets of genetics, biological, and molecular fields are very influential in understanding disease outcomes, we also review applications of Big Data in those fields. Furthermore, Big Data analysis in those fields encounters some challenges based on the characteristics of such data. Thus, at first, it is required to determine characteristics of healthcare Big Data and challenges that a researcher encounters during its analysis.

CHARACTERISTICS AND CHALLENGES OF HEALTHCARE BIG DATA ANALYSIS

Big Data in healthcare problems include important characteristics such as incomplete and inexact data, as well as multi-spectral and heterogeneous observations. Those inexact, heterogeneous, and multi-spectral data sets collected from various sources are used in preventing disease outbreak, analyzing demographics, diagnosis, treatment, and mental impairments (Dinov, 2016). In addition to the abovementioned characteristics of Big Data sets, their two significant characteristics include energy and life-span (Dinov, 2016).

Energy encompasses information exists in the data indicating the joint distribution of healthcare process (Dinov, 2016). In other words, big healthcare data sets represent unidentified distribution of the clinical event using information extracted from observations not parametric models. Both characteristics of Big Data, energy and life span, has exponential model. The life span and value of data decays exponentially overtime named information devaluation (Dinov, 2016). For example, the most valuable predictors for forecasting Medicare spending are observed in years 2013-2017, and data collected in 2012 has less value.

The main characteristics of Big Data which shows how health data could be labeled as Big Data is summarized as follows.

The first characteristic of Big Data is its volume. Volume means the massive size of datasets. For instance, a 500-bed hospital includes more than 50 petabytes of data (Monteith et al., 2015). EMR generates 76 MB of imaging data for each patient in each year while genomic data need 50 times more storage than imaging data (Monteith et al., 2015). Big healthcare data will grow to 25,000 petabytes by 2020 due to the conversion of data from paper into electronical form as well as adding other types of data such as 3D images and genomics (Raghupathi, 2014). Big Data in healthcare is mainly collected from 1.2 billion ambulatory care visits, using electronic medical record (EMR) systems, smartphones with applications that record locations, and using sensors and RFID tags data (Monteith et al., 2015). High volume of Big Data leads to storage problem and complex data analysis. That high volume of data requires cloud-based platforms to be collected and stored.

The second characteristic of big healthcare data is its variety rising due to semistructured or unstructured data generated from new technologies including social media and the Internet (Alexandru, 2016). Variety refers to different types of Big Data in healthcare including structured data collected from a spreadsheet or relational database, unstructured data represented as text, video, image, and audio, and semi-structured data collected from XML documents (Monteith et al., 2015). The third characteristic of big healthcare data is its velocity which indicates the speed of data generation, retrieve, processing, and analyzing (Raghupathi, 2014). The other caharacteristic of Big Data is its veracity which means the preciseness and conformity of data to a specific format. Since Big Data sets are collected from different sources they are not in conformity to a specific formats (Alexandru, 2016). Another characteristic of Big Data is its variability which indicates the interpretability of that data. The sixth characteristic of big healthcare data is its visualization refering to accessibility of the data (Alexandru, 2016). The last characteristic of big healthcare data is its value indicating the possibility of extracting new knowledge from the existing data.

The abovementioned characteristics of Big Data leads to several challenges. Challenges of analyzing healthcare Big Data stems from its high dimensionality and large sample size which leads to three difficulties in Big Data problems. First, high dimensionality causes noise accumulation, incidental homogeneity, and correlations. Second, if the dataset has both characteristics of high dimensionality and large sample size, other difficulties such as algorithmic instability and heavy computational cost will rise.

Third, since Big Data samples are collected from various data bases some issues such as experimental variations, statistical biases, and heterogeneity will occur in data analysis (Fan et al., 2014).

Analyzing high dimensional Big Data requires dimension reduction techniques since correlations between response and covariates, endogeneity, and noise accumulation are pervasive in high dimensional datasets. In case of noise accumulation, the results of statistical analysis on datasets are not different from random guess (Fan et al., 2008; Fan et al., 2012; Pittelkow & Ghosh, 2008). Data heterogeneity refers to various characteristics of the pupolation which is under study (Patiño et al., 2013). Aggregation of heterogenous data itself leads to noise and error accumulation. Correlation between random variables grows in healthcare Big Data sets (Anderson et al., 2011). High dimensional Big Data deals with curse of dimensionality which adversely affects data analysis and statistical inferences (Spinello et al., 2010). In addition to above problems, endogeniety in healthcare Big Data analysis contradicts the primary assumption of regression analysis which emphasizes that exogenous variables and error terms need to be independence (Fan et al., 2014). The abovementioned challenges have significant impacts on healthcare Big Data analysis such as genomic and neuroscience datasets.

In genomic studies, Big Data is used to acquire biological sequences, investige biological functions, detect genetic disorders, and understand relations between gene sequences and diseases (Chen et al., 2012; Cohen et al, 2004; Fan et al., 2014; Han et al., 2010; Worthey et al., 2013). In addition to challenges that exist in Big Data in general such as heterogeneity (McAfee & Brynjolfsson, 2012), noise accumulation (Bollier & Firestone, 2010), correlations (Fan et al., 2014), and endogeneity (Fritsch et al., 2012), genomic Big Data encounter other issues which impose difficulties to data analysis. For example, because genomic data is usually qualitative and unstructured, data analysing is complex and computational extensive (Dinov, 2016).

In neuroscience, brain diseases such as Alzheimer are diagnosed by investigating brain networks. Functional magnetic resonance image (fMRI) data used to study brain networks is big, high dimensional, and noisy. Therefore, the problem of systematic biases arises due to experimental variations and aggregations of big datasets. The significant challenges of analysing neuroscience data are outlier rejection, removing biases, and voxels alignment (Fan et al., 2014; Mathur et al., 2014). Another problem of analyzing neuroscience Big Data is variable latency (Dinov, 2016; Wang & Yu, 2013). Big and heterogeneous data in healthcare industry encounters challenges for computational efficiency and reproducibility using classic statistical analysis methods. Due to the abovementioned challenges and special characteristics of healthcare Big Data, special data analytic methods are required.

Analytics has been defined as "the extensive use of data, statistical and quantitative analysis, explanatory and predictive models, and fact-based management to drive decisions and actions" (Hoyt and Yoshihashi, 2014). According to IBM, analytics refers to "the systematic use of data and business implemented through analytical methods such as statistical, contextual, quantitative, predictive, and cognitive techniques. Moreover, Adams and Klein (2011) have defined analytics in healthcare Big Data with three levels including: (I) Descriptive level which is explains current situations and problems; (II) Predictive level which includes simulation and modeling methods for determining trends in data; (III) Prescriptive level for optimizing clinical outcomes (Hoyt and Yoshihashi, 2014).

The main method which lies in those levels of data analytics is machine learning whose focus is to develop algorithms for learning from data. The other method is data mining, which is used to model massive amounts of data for extracting useful patterns. According to Kumar et al. (2013), the process of healthcare Big Data analytics have four main steps. The first step starts with input data sources including financial and clinical records, and genomics. The second step is feature extraction in which data is extracted using different techniques such as natural language processing (NLP). The third step is modeling by statistical methods such as machine learning to conclude from the data (Hoyt and Yoshihashi, 2014). Finally, the fourth step is predictions based on Big Data (Hoyt and Yoshihashi, 2014).

In order to apply those analytics for rectifying challenges and difficulties of Big Data analysis, advance techniques, technologies, and software are required to handle complex healthcare data. Thus, in the next section, we overview modern technologies and software for healthcare Big Data analysis.

MODERN TECHNOLOGIES AND SOFTWARE FOR HEALTHCARE BIG DATA ANALYSIS

Classic statistical data analysis techniques are no longer useful because of the challenges that exist in Big Data analysis which were explained in Section 2. Thus, modern technologies, software, and computing methods are used to overcome those challenges. Computing methods which have high processing performance include: (1) Graphical processing units (GPU); (2) Distributed systems (DSs); (3) Grid computing systems (GCS).

The first computing method is parallel data processing which is performed using GPU computing clusters (Owens, 2008; Satish et al., 2009). The second one is DSs consisting of a group of independent computers rectify the challenges of processing Big Data having high volume and variety of unstructured, structured, and semi-structured data (Coulouris et al., 2005). The third one is grid computing system (GCS) which boosts the computing performance by using resources such as CPUs and data storage of computers more efficiently. This feature of GCS provides ubiquitous and flexible accessibility to computing resources (Foster & Kesselman, 2003). However, DSs are different from GCSs.

The first distinction of GCSs from DSs is that GCSs facilitate computation amongst various administrative domains differing it from classic DSs. The second distinction is that DSs handle a lot of computer systems while the computing resources such as storage, CPU, and memory are restricted. Conversely, GCSs have the capabilities of managing utilization of heterogeneous systems with efficient workload management servers (Mohammed et al., 2014). Thus, parallel processing is a great method of dealing with Big Data which is done by MapReduce presented by Google (Dinov, 2016; Lämmel, 2008). MapReduce includes a mapper and a reducer which decompose processes to be implemented in parallel (Holmes, 2012).

MapReduce has the capability of facilitating Big Data processing by using computing clusters effectively. While MapReduce framework is resistant to hardware malfunctions, it is not appropriate for processing online transactions (Dean & Ghemawat, 2008; Jones, 1987; Mohammed, et al., 2014). The main merit of MapReduce programming software is its high performance in parallel computing incorporated with the simple programming framework as well as its various applications (Dean & Ghemawat, 2008; De Oliveira Branco, 2009; Mohammed, et al., 2014;]. In order to provide that capability for MapReduce software, workload among various computers should be divided, and according to the volume of input data, systems should work in parallel (Dean & Ghemawat, 2008). The input data sets (key1, value1) are processed using map function which converts those pairs to (key2, value2). Thereafter, the output pairs (key3, value3) are computed using reduce function. MapReduce parallelizes data processing using an open-source framework such as Hadoop (Holmes, 2012).

Hadoop framework includes distributed storage as well as computational infrastructures (Dean & Ghemawat, 2008). Hadoop was introduced primarily to rectify the scalability problem of an open source search engine and crawler named Nutch (Olson, 2010; Shvachko et al., 2010) using big-table (Olson, 2010) and MapReduce techniques. Hadoop is a distributed processing framework including the Hadoop Distributed File System (HDFS) for storage and the MapReduce infrastructure for computations (Dean & Ghemawat, 2008). The HDFS is responsible of storing data on the processing nodes which helps bandwidth to be more aggregated among the cluster (Dean & Ghemawat, 2008). The main characteristics of Hadoop are both division and parallel computation of Big Data sets. The computation and storage processes of Hadoop are improved by providing with the extra computing nodes for a Hadoop cluster (Dean & Ghemawat, 2008). The main advantage of Hadoop in comparison to other distributed systems approaches is its data processing framework. The former distributed systems iteratively transmit data between clients and servers which is an appropriate method for computationally intensive processes (De Oliveira Branco, 2009). However, when the data set is massive, moving between clients and server is not easily possible. Thus, Hadoop rectifies this problem by concentrating on transmitting code to data not data to code (Bryant, 2007; White, 2012). That transition of code to data is performed within the Hadoop cluster in which data is partitioned and distributed athwart the cluster (Dean & Ghemawat, 2008). Moreover, Hadoop programming framework and MapReduce are widely applied in healthcare issues.

For example, massive clinical data sets which are obtained and accumulated from test usage data, biomedical and biometrics data, high-volume laboratory information system data, electronic medical record (EMR), and gene expression data requires new data analysis frameworks. Analyzing those large data sets encounters significant difficulties applying former processing technologies. Big clinical data sets as well as queries are mapped into distinct elements using a MapReduce programming framework (Dean & Ghemawat, 2008). Two approaches are prevalent in processing of the mapped queries.

First, all of the mapped elements can be processes at the same time. Second, they are allowed to be reduced to expedite processing of the results (Dean & Ghemawat, 2008). MapReduce algorithms and Hadoop distributed systems have been prosperously implemented to analyze clinical, biometrics, and biomedical Big Data (Dean & Ghemawat, 2008). Moreover, both MapReduce and Hadoop frameworks have been applied in literature in bioinformatics (Dai et al., 2012; Taylor, 2010). According to Mohammed et al. (2014), MapReduce and Hadoop frameworks have been applied for analyzing clinical Big Data sets including five categories: (I) public datasets; (II) "Biometrics datasets" (Jonas et al., 2014); (III) "Bioinformatics datasets" (Wang et al., 2011); (IV) "Biomedical signal datasets" (Aphinyanaphongs et al., 2012); (V) "Biomedical image datasets".

An example of public data sets is adverse drug event (ADE) detection which is analyzed using a MapReduce algorithm proposed by Wang et al. (2011). That algorithm has been proposed to expedite biomedical data mining tasks such as pharmacovigilance cases (Dean & Ghemawat, 2008). It has been demonstrated that the MapReduce algorithm boosts the performance of signal detection algorithms for pharmacovigilance (Wang et al., 2011). Moreover, the MapReduce framework is used for dimension reduction through Markov feature selection techniques (Aphinyanaphongs et al., 2012; Yaramakala & Margaritis, 2005). This is done to diagnose unidentified cancer treatments.

The second application of MapReduce and Hadoop systems is in biometrics for fingerprint recognition and face matching (Kohlwey et al., 2011). A new biometrics system has been proposed in literature for investigating cloud-scale data and recognizing human images (Raghava, 2011). A biometric application for cell phones has been proposed for establishing availability of the cloud (Omri et al., 2012). A mobile user in the cloud is connected to the server via the Hadoop framework (Dean & Ghemawat, 2008).

The third application of MapReduce and Hadoop platforms is in bioinformatics including protein and genome data. For example, a new MapReduce algorithm has been developed for single-nucleotide polymorphism (SNP) selection (Chen et al., 2014; Dean & Ghemawat, 2008). In addition, a new algorithm for comparing genome sequences has been developed which uses both MapReduce and Hadoop for computation and data management respectively (Zhang et al., 2003). Another new bioinformatics technology which is named BioPig has been implemented using the Hadoop system as well as the Pig Latin language (Nordberg et al., 2013). Moreover, CloudBrush which is a new algorithm for compiling genomes has been developed using the MapReduce algorithm and string graphs (Chang et al., 2012). A new search engine has been proposed in literature for expediting computations of mass spectrometry based proteomics by the Hadoop frameworks (McKenna, et al., 2010; MacLean et al., 2006).

In addition to the abovementioned applications of Hadoop platforms in bioinformatics, a new parallel processing algorithm for aligning protein structures has been presented in literature (Lin, 2013; Thusoo et al., 2009). Another application of MapReduce algorithms was presented for DNA fragment assembly (Xu et al., 2012). A novel software named Cloudburst has been designed for genome mapping, single-nucleotide polymorphism detection, and genotyping (Schatz, 2009). As an example of a new platform proposed to increase MapReduce utilization in bioinformatics is Cloudgene (Schönherr et al., 2012). That platform is a graphical environment for implementing MapReduce programs (Lewis et al., 2012). Regression analysis and similarity learning of genes for big genetic data sets are facilitated by parallel processing of the random forest algorithm (Díaz-Uriarte & De Andres, 2006; Wang et al., 2013). That method has been used to investigate quantitative characteristic including neuroimaging phenotypes which demonstrate longitudinal alterations in individual's brain structure for analyzing Alzheimer disease.

Another application of MapReduce frameworks named Nephele which includes composition vector algorithm has been presented to show genome sequences (Colosimo et al., 2011; Gao & Qi, 2007). Moreover, a MapReduce algorithm has been proposed in literature to analyze high-volume gene networks by incorporating a parallel version of genetic algorithm and particle swarm optimization techniques (Juang, 2004; Lee et al., 2014).

The fourth application of MapReduce and Hadoop platforms is in biomedical signal processing. For example, a new parallel neural signal processing using ensemble empirical mode decomposition algorithm have been developed on the MapReduce and Hadoop frameworks in a novel cyber infrastructure (Wang et al., 2012; Wu & Huang, 2009). The results of implementing that algorithm demonstrate that the parallel ensemble empirical mode decomposition method drastically increases signal processing performance.

Finally, MapReduce and Hadoop programming frameworks are applied to process Big Data of biomedical images generated in hospitals (Wang et al., 2011). For example, in order to optimize parameters of use cases designed for image processing to classify lung texture, MapReduce algorithms have been applied in literature (Dean & Ghemawat, 2008; Markonis et al., 2012). Moreover, those algorithms have been proposed for wavelet processing for texture classification and medical image retrieval (Dean & Ghemawat, 2008; Markonis et al., 2012).

Some high level languages such as Hive (Xiaojing, 2010) and Pig Latin (Olston et al., 2008) which provide MapReduce frameworks are developed by Hadoop. MapR[1], Hortonworks[2], Cloudera[3], and DataStax[4] are other Hadoop based open source platforms for Big Data processing (Mohammed et al., 2014). Apache Spark is another infrastructure for Big Data process which is faster than MapReduce. Predictive Model Markup Language (PMML) is a data mining language for presenting predictive models using Big Data (Grossman, et al., 1999; Kliegr et al., 2011). In addition, cloud based services such as DataMining-as-a-Service (DMaaS) (Chen et al., 2012) and Decision Science-as-a-Service (DSaaS) (Granville, 2014) provide infrastructure for Big Data analysis.

The above mentioned technologies and software are applicable for analyzing many applications of Big Data in healthcare. However, reviewing literature of Big Data analysis in healthcare shows that understanding disease outcomes have significant impacts on diagnosis and curing people's diseases. Thus, in the next section, we mainly concentrate on reviewing literature of understanding disease outcomes through analyzing Big Data. Since Big Data sets of genetics, biological, and molecular fields are very influential in understanding disease outcomes, we also review applications of Big Data in those fields.

BIG DATA FOR UNDERSTANDING DISEASE OUTCOMES

Investigating diseases generates massive amount of data. Thus, we need to process those Big Data sets to find out the disease outcomes (Hughes, 2015). Big Data collected by controlling human's metabolism is significantly influential for diagnosis and curing people's diseases. Those Big Data sets help patient's reactions and side effects to medications to be more transparent. Hence, Big Data is widely used for diagnosis and treatment of various diseases. It is applicable in psychiatry for exploring and predicting of clinical and research problems. Mental illnesses such as depression require investigating Big Data of psychiatric disorders collected from people's communication as well as their physical movements and speech intents (Pentland et al., 2013). Following location of patients provides data about physical motions and places they went which is used to diagnose psychiatric disorders such as bipolar disorder, hyperactivity disorder, agoraphobia, and depression (Pentland et al., 2013).

The results of Big Data analysis in psychiatry have significant effects on clinical decision making. Those results are obtained from research and analytical tools which use Big Data as inputs (Monteith et al., 2015). Data mining models, which use Big Data as input of the models, are applied to find solutions for problems for which traditional clinical trials have no answers (Murdoch & Detsky, 2013). As an instance, data obtained from social media and event reporting tools is provided for drug surveillance (Harpaz et al., 2012; Monteith et al., 2015). Moreover, Big Data is useful for generalization of limited samples of clinical trials results to the greater population (Murdoch & Detsky, 2013). Hence, Big Data provides new, more generalizable hypotheses in clinical psychiatry research (Titiunik, 2015). In addition, Big Data supplies neuroimaging data studying brain processes in every stage of diseases (Van Horn & Toga, 2014). It also prepares adequate data to investigate specific samples like heroin addicts using integrative data analysis (Srinivasan et al., 2015). Big Data helps to find out the existence of heterogeneity in diagnosing psychiatric diseases like bipolar disorder and schizophrenia (Potash, 2015). Big Data improves analysing human behaviours. Such datasets including personality (Youyou et al., 2015), sexual orientation and ethnicity (Youyou et al., 2013), human motility (De Domenico et al., 2013), and friendships (Eagle et al., 2009) are collected from web, social media, monitoring applications, and smart phones (Monteith et al., 2015). Other applications of Big Data in psychiatry have reviewed by Monteith et al. (2015) in Table 1.

In addition, Big Data is applicable for investigating environment related diseases. That analysis would help to find correlations between people's exposure to air pollution and health status. The amount of air pollutants significantly alter in distinct distances and at different time horizons. Therefore, clinicians who study environmental health have recently concentrated on more accurate and dynamic patterns related to pollution exposure. They are able to collect those measures by monitoring location data provided by cell phones as well as environment air pollution at various locations (Hoge et al., 2008). Thus, Big Data analysis plays a key role in studying environment related diseases.

Moreover, Big Data could help to study diseases related to malnutrition (Pentland et al., 2013). Data accumulated from individuals' diet records is a great source for such a study. The imprecise data recorded from daily or weekly consumed food by people adversely influences on diagnosis and treatment of malnutrition related illnesses. Those imprecisions are now reduced by keeping track of individual's diet data collected form cell phones on which GPS applications are installed. GPS applications keep track of the places where consumers eat or provide food such as restaurants, farmer's markets, and snack-food shops (Pentland et al., 2013). Those comprehensive records provide three significant opportunities. First, it is a massive data source that contains people's diet records. Second, that Big Data helps health experts to study nutrition related diseases which rely on behavioral data. Third, nutrition based Big Data provides more food accessibility and security (Pentland et al., 2013).

Another health aspect that Big Data analysis helps it to improve is social health (Pentland et al., 2013). Big Data in social health is used to recognize social situations leading to behavioural changes and consequently health improvements. It is also used to define new health norms. Online social networks are useful for improving people's contributing in social activities like energy preservation. Moreover, Big Data sets recorded from cell phone calls help to find ethnic as well as poverty boundaries in society (Pentland et al., 2013). Another application of Big Data is analyzing of non-infectious diseases.

For example, Big Data of traumatic brain injury is analyzed to forecast its survival rates. In order to diagnose the difference among traumatic brain injury, anoxic brain injury, and stroke, clear description is required which is achievable by analyzing big healthcare data (Monteith et al., 2015). In addition, Big Data analysis is utilized for forecasting and curing Alzheimer's disease. Such an analysis helps to aggregate various levels of data including molecules and genes as well as cognitive performance and imaging (Husain, 2014).

Another example is Big Data of radiation oncology which is used to predict cancer (Bibault, et al., 2016). For analyzing Big Data of the above diseases some features are required to be considered. According to Lambin et al. (Lambin et al., 2013) the features for analyzing Big Data of radiation oncology include: (i) Clinical attributes such as grade and stage of the tumor, performance status of patient, patient questionnaires, results of blood test; (ii) Treatment attributes such as dose distribution and associated chemotherapy; (iii) Imaging attributes including metabolic uptake and tumor volume and size; (iv) molecular attributes as hypoxia (Le & Courter, 2008), tissue reactions (Okunieff et al., 2008), radiosensitivity (Bibault et al., 2013).

In addition to non-infectious disease analysis, Big Data analysis plays a significant role in diagnosis of infectious diseases (Lee et al., 2016). In order to control those kinds of diseases some spatial information is stored and a massive dataset is provided. The spatial Big Data is collected by investigating the population who are classified as higher risk for disease, the origins of the disease, and the geographical locations of future disease outbreaks. Big Data of infectious disease epidemiology enables researchers to access people upon time and space, personal behaviors, and disease outcomes (Lee et al., 2016).

Moreover, Big Data collected from the locations where the disease has been recorded, literature (Rogers et al., 2006), GenBank (Benson et al., 2012), and websites (Brownstein et al., 2008) helps to predict the risk of infectious disease (Hay et al., 2013). In order to forecast that risk, a disease map process is provided through extracting some environmental covariates such as temperature and rainfall related to epidemiological factors. Then, some statistical methods like Boosted Regression Tree are utilized to find the locations where the disease may be observed and its corresponding risk map (Salathe et al., 2012). The locations where diseases outbreak from are not static and should be dynamically updated when new disease occurrence data is recorded. That updating process is carried out using a feedback loop which

Table 1. Other applications of Big Data in psychiatry reviewed by Monteith et al. (2015)

Applications	Results	Number of Subjects
Big Data collected from patients is used for algorithms designed for predicting the risk of suicide due to the psychiatric disorder (Kessler, et al., 2015)	Among the hospitalized patients with the highest forecasted risks of suicide, 52.9% committed suicide	40,820 soldiers (Monteith et al., 2015)
Big Data collected from patients is used for investigating substance use disorders (SUD) outbreak among psychiatric patients (Wu et al., 2013)	Analyzing Big Data recorded from psychiatric patients shows that 24.9% of them had SUD which is associated with more inpatient and emergency care	40,999 psychiatric patients (Monteith et al., 2015)
Using Big Data of genetics and neuroimaging for investigating cognitive impairment (Weiner et al., 2012)	Neuroimaging phenotypes are drastically correlated with dementia	808 individuals identified as patients having Alzheimer's disease (Monteith et al., 2015)
Big Data collected from patients to analyze patients for whom psychotropic drugs was prescribed without psychiatric diagnosis (Wiechers, et al., 2013)	Among patients for whom a psychiatric medications were prescribed in 2009, 58% had no psychiatric diagnosis	5,132,789 patients (Monteith et al., 2015)
Big Data collected from patients is used for investigating prescription of psychotropic drugs (Mark et al., 2009)	"59% written by general practitioners, 23% by psychiatrists, 17% by other physicians and providers" (Monteith et al., 2015)	472 million prescriptions (Monteith et al., 2015)
Big Data collected from patients above 55 years old with traumatic (TBI) brain injury versus non-TBI trauma (NTT) is used to examine the risk of dementia (Gardner et al., 2014)	"TBI increased risk for dementia over NTT" (Monteith et al., 2015)	51,799 patients having trauma disease (Monteith et al., 2015)
Big Data collected from patients are used as inputs of machine learning techniques to forecast suicidal actions text in EMR (Ben-Ari & Hammond, 2015)	Specificity is significant in the model while sensitivity is low	250,000 soldiers (Monteith et al., 2015)
Big Data of patients are utilized to analyze the relations between parents age and risk of autism (Grether et al., 2009)	Increasing paternal and maternal ages leads to increasing the risk of autism	7,550,026 patients with autism (Monteith et al., 2015)
Big Data is used as an input of natural language processing (NLP) for classifying current mood state to diagnose depression (Perlis et al., 2012)	"NLP models better than those relying on billing data alone" (Monteith et al., 2015)	127,504 patients identified with major depression (Monteith et al., 2015)
Big Data of psychiatry is used to study the effect of medical authorization for irregular antipsychotics on propagation of schizophrenia in prisons (Goldman et al., 2014)	Former permissions correlated with the increasing rate of mental illness in prisoners	16,844 inmates (Monteith et al., 2015)
Analyzing Big Data of psychiatry to find severe psychiatric disorders as a consequent of head injury (Orlovska et al., 2014)	Head injuries increase risk of depression, bipolar disorder, organic mental disorders, and schizophrenia	113,906 patients with head injury (Monteith et al., 2015)
Big Data collected from prescription, EMR, and monitoring of depression are combined to rectify care in primary care (PC) (Valuck et al., 2012)]	Combination of those data sets leads to better diagnosis and treatment of depression in PC	61,464 patients (Monteith et al., 2015)

joins the risk map to the input data. Those evolving maps along with the massive digital data sets are categorized in the subject of Big Data (Brownstein et al., 2009; Hay et al., 2013; Salathe et al., 2012).

Because of high velocity, volume, and variety of those Big Data sets, the model on geographical locations and risks of disease outbreaks should be continuously revised (Hay et al., 2013). The noisy nature of Big Data sets requires machine learning techniques to be tuned for determining bias in statistical methods which are used to predict risk of infectious disease occurrence (Hay et al., 2013). In order to analyze infectious disease epidemiology, new technologies providing spatial Big Data are used. For example, climate forecasting through photos received from satellites as well as population data leads to figuring out spatial distributions of disease transmitting from mosquitos (Lee et al., 2016; Kraemer et al., 2015)

In order to find spatial distributions of some diseases like cholera through analyzing its spatial Big Data, an online prevalence aggregator named HealthMap is used (Tuite et al., 2011). Moreover, information collected from cell phone calls prepares data about dynamisms of people which have reported spatial dynamics and risk of malaria influx (Ruktanonchai et al., 2016). Another type of Big Data applied for testing spatial incongruity in intensity of influenza outbreak is collected from medical allegations (Gog et al., 2016; Lee et al., 2015; Lee et al., 2016). Social media data sets are also utilized for detecting spatial tendencies against vaccination (Salathé & Khandelwal, 2011). As mentioned earlier, since Big Data sets of genetics, biological, and molecular fields are very influential in understanding disease outcomes, we review applications of Big Data in those fields in the next section.

BIG DATA IN GENETICS, BIOLOGICAL, AND MOLECULAR FIELDS

Big Data of biological fields includes transcriptome, genome, epigenome, proteome, molecular pathways, molecular imaging, and metabolome data sets (Li & Chen, 2014). The biological data sets are massive require exabyte of memory space whose complexity is difficult to manage. The challenges in analyzing Big Data of biology are due to integrating the data from heterogeneous data bases and standard definitions (Li & Chen, 2014). The huge amount of biological data is extremely heterogeneous which shows correlation among some elements like proteins, pathways, and genes. Studies based on statistical hypothesis have significant impacts on massive biological data mining which decreases CPU time of data mining techniques (Li & Chen, 2014).

For example, using various data mining algorithms leads to different output even if the same gene expression data is used. Thus, one cannot be certain about the ability of a specific statistical method to solve the problem of heterogeneity of gene expression data (Li & Chen, 2014). In this case, according to Yuan et al. (2012), there is a biological assumption that ''If a number of genes that are conservatively co-expressed emerge as a dynamically-cooperative group across certain biological processes, these genes are most likely functionally closely related with physiological and pathological processes''(Yuan et al., 2012). Therefore, data mining methods are converted to find gene clusters which cooperate in cancer development stages (Li & Chen, 2014).

The Big Data which is used as the input of biological data mining methods includes: (I) hierarchy- various levels of data which varies from cells, tissues, and molecules to systems (Li & Chen, 2014); (II) heterogeneous – data created from imaging, physiology, genetics, and pathology by disparate techniques (Li & Chen, 2014); (III) complexity – data collected having the format of multi-level information (Li & Chen, 2014); (IV) dynamics – changes occur in biological states or processes over time. Two important issues in biology are dynamics and networks while previous studies have concentrated on static features of Big Data (Chen et al., 2009; Ma et al., 2014). In fact, failure of a single molecule does not lead to disease outbreak but malfunction of a specific network of molecules in the shape of biomarkers does (Li & Chen, 2014; Zeng et al., 2014).

Big Data of network of molecules are used for "preventive, predictive, participatory, and personalized medicine" (Li & Chen, 2014; Zeng et al., 2014). The network and dynamics specifications which were not observed previously are detectable using networks of biological elements instead of individual biological components (Li & Chen, 2014; Zeng et al., 2014). Not only does clinical aspect need biological networks data in the form of biomarkers, but also theoretical aspect does. Those biomarkers are progressing from single molecules to multiple molecules and associated molecules or from sole genes to gene sets and molecule network (Li & Chen, 2014). Big and high dimensional biological network data sets are classified as: "biomarkers (Zeng et al., 2014; Liu et al., 2014), network-based biomarkers (Ren et al., 2014; Wen et al., 2013; Zeng et al., 2014), network biomarkers (Yu et al., 2014; Zhang et al., 2014) and dynamical network biomarkers (DNBs) (Liu et al., 2014; Chen et al., 2012)"; (Li & Chen, 2014).

Big Data of biological networks are extracted to analyze EdgeMarkers. Investigating EdgeMarkers shows that non-differentially expressed genes are usually discarded using traditional methods. However, they are as useful as differentially expressed genes for categorizing various biological situations or phenotypes (Li & Chen, 2014; Zhang et al., 2014). Lately, new types of biomarkers known as DNBs are constructed using dynamic information of biological Big Data (Liu et al., 2014). While traditional biomarkers only have the capability of identifying disease states, DNBs are capable of detecting pre-disease state. Identifying pre-disease state helps to avoid disease happening or deteriorating (Li & Chen, 2014). That is, those newly developed types of biomarkers, DNBs, are able to detect ''pre-disease'' state using high-dimensional data including RNA-seq, imaging data, gene expression, and protein expression data (Li & Chen, 2014).

Another type of biological Big Data which is used to improve healthcare is pharmacogenomics data based on genomic information (Fan & Liu, 2013). Big Data of pharmacogenomics including genomes, transcriptomes, cells and tissues data as well as drug effects data along with other patient's information such as diseases, diet, environment, lifestyle, age, and state of health (Wu et al., 2013) are used to study the effect of genes on an individual's response to drugs. Analyzing Big Data of pharmacogenomics requires new statistical methods for handling the problem of determining correlation structures.

Those methods include approximating marginal and conditional correlations (Fan & Liu, 2013). Marginal correlation shows the correlation between two variables without the contribution of other variables whereas conditional correlation demonstrates the correlation between two variables by conditioning on the others (Fan & Liu, 2013). Other statistical techniques for managing Big Data of pharmacogenomics include: (I) thresholding approach for covariance estimation (Bickel & Levina, 2008), (II) Principal Orthogonal complEment Thresholding (POET) for covariance estimation (Fan et al., 2011; Fan et al., 2013), (III) inverse covariance calculation method known as "Constrained L1-Minimization for Inverse Matrix Estimation" (CLIME) (Cai et al., 2011). All those methods are used to statistically analyze Big Data in pharmacogenomics.

CONCLUSION

In this chapter, the recent studies in the field of Big Data in healthcare were reviewed. Analyzing health Big Data encounters significant challenges due to its high dimensionality and large sample size. High dimensionality causes noise accumulation, incidental homogeneity, algorithmic instability, heavy computational cost and correlations. Moreover, since Big Data samples are collected from various data bases some problems such as experimental variations, statistical biases, and heterogeneity will occur in data analysis (Fan et al., 2014). In addition to above problems, endogeniety in healthcare Big Data analysis contradicts the primary assumption of regression analysis which emphasizes that exogenous variables and error terms need to be independence (Fan et al., 2014). Due to the challenges exist in Big Data study, new technologies and methods are required for analyzing that kind of data. For example, parallel processing using MapReduce, Hadoop infrastructure, high level languages such as Hive and Pig Latin, MapR, Hortonworks, Cloudera, and DataStax are among tools for programming using Big Data. Other software and infrastructures include Apache Spark, Predictive Model Markup Language (PMML), DataMining-as-a-Service (DMaaS) (Chen et al., 2012) and Decision Science-as-a-Service (DSaaS) (Granville, 2014).

Big Data analysis has many applications in healthcare systems. Its first application is to forecast the disease outcomes. For instance, Big Data of psychiatry is used to explore and predict of clinical and research problems. Following location of patients provides data about physical motions and places they went which is used to diagnose psychiatric disorders such as bipolar disorder, hyperactivity disorder, agoraphobia, and depression (Pentland et al., 2013). In addition, Big Data is applicable for investigating environment related diseases. That analysis would help to find correlations between people's exposure to air pollution and health status. Big Data could also help to study diseases related to malnutrition (Pentland et al., 2013). Another health aspect that Big Data analysis helps it to improve is social health (Pentland et al., 2013). Other applications of Big Data are in genetics, biological, and molecular fields as well as analyzing non-infectious diseases.

The above information shows that analyzing Big Data has significant roles in improving healthcare issues. Thus, this chapter is a reference for researchers to become more familiar with applications of Big Data in healthcare systems as well as required technologies, infrastructures, and software for analyzing health Big Data.

REFERENCES

Adams, J., & Klein, J. (2011). Business Intelligence and Analytics in Health Care - A Primer. Washington, DC: The Advisory Board Company. Retrieved from http://www.advisory.com/Research/IT-Strategy-Council/Research-Notes/2011/Business-Intelligence-and-Analytics-in-Health-Care

Alexandru, A. et al.. (2016). Healthcare, Big Data and Cloud Computing. *WSEAS Transactions on Computer Research*, *4*, 123–131.

Anderson, D. R., Burnham, K. P., Gould, W. R., & Cherry, S. (2011). Concerns about finding effects that are actually spurious. *Wildlife Society Bulletin*, *29*, 311–316.

Aphinyanaphongs, Y., Fu, L. D., & Aliferis, C. F. (2012). Identifying unproven cancer treatments on the health web: Addressing accuracy, generalizability and scalability. *Studies in Health Technology and Informatics*, *192*, 667–671. PMID:23920640

Archenaa, J., & Mary Anita, E. A. (2015). A Survey of Big Data Analytics in Healthcare and Government. *Procedia Computer Science*, *50*, 408–413. doi:10.1016/j.procs.2015.04.021

Ben-Ari, A., & Hammond, K. (2015). Text mining the EMR for modeling and predicting suicidal behavior among US veterans of the 1991 Persian Gulf War. *2015 48th Hawaii International Conference on System Sciences*, 3168–75.

Benson, D. A., Karsch-Mizrachi, I., Clark, K., Lipman, D. J., Ostell, J., & Sayers, E. W. (2012, January 01). GenBank. *Nucleic Acids Research*, *40*(D1), D48–D53. doi:10.1093/nar/gkr1202 PMID:22144687

Brownstein, J. S., Freifeld, C. C., Reis, B. Y., & Mandl, K. D. (2008). Surveillance sans frontieres: Internet-based emerging infectious disease intelligence and the HealthMap project. *PLoS Medicine*, *5*(7), e151. doi:10.1371/journal.pmed.0050151 PMID:18613747

Bibault, J. E., Fumagalli, I., Ferté, C., Chargari, C., Soria, J. C., & Deutsch, E. (2013). Personalized radiation therapy and biomarker-driven treatment strategies: A systematic review. *Cancer and Metastasis Reviews*, *32*(3-4), 479–492. doi:10.1007/s10555-013-9419-7 PMID:23595306

Bibault, J.-E., Giraud, Ph., & Burgun, A. (2016). Big Data and machine learning in radiation oncology: State of the art and future prospects. *Cancer Letters*, 1–8. PMID:27241666

Bickel, P., & Levina, E. (2008). Covariance regularization by thresholding. *Annals of Statistics*, *36*(6), 2577–2604. doi:10.1214/08-AOS600

Bollier, D., & Firestone, C. M. (2010). *The promise and peril of big data, Communications and Society Program*. Washington, DC: Aspen Institute.

Brownstein, J. S., Freifeld, C. C., & Madoff, L. C. (2009). Digital disease detection - harnessing the Web for public health surveillance. *The New England Journal of Medicine*, *360*(21), 2153–2157. doi:10.1056/NEJMp0900702 PMID:19423867

Bryant, R. E. (2007). *Data-intensive supercomputing: The case for DISC*. Pittsburgh, PA: School of Computer Science, Carnegie Mellon University.

Cai, T., Liu, W., & Luo, X. (2011). A constrained l_1. *Journal of the American Statistical Association*, *106*(494), 594–607. doi:10.1198/jasa.2011.tm10155 PMID:22844169

Chang, Y. J., Chen, C. C., Ho, J. M., & Chen, C. L. (2012). De Novo Assembly of High-Throughput Sequencing Data with Cloud Computing and New Operations on String Graphs. Cloud Computing, 155–161. doi:10.1109/CLOUD.2012.123

Chen, L., Liu, R., Liu, Z. P., Li, M., & Aihara, K. (2012). Detecting early-warning signals for sudden deterioration of complex diseases by dynamical network biomarkers. *Scientific Reports*, *2*, 1–8. doi:10.1038/srep00342 PMID:22461973

Chen, T., Chen, J., & Zhou, B. (2012). A System for Parallel data mining service on cloud. *Second International Conference on Cloud and Green Computing*. doi:10.1109/CGC.2012.49

Chen, L., Wang, R., & Zhang, X. (Eds.). (2009). *Biomolecular networks: methods and applications in systems biology*. Hoboken, NJ: John Wiley & Sons. doi:10.1002/9780470488065

Chen, R., Mias, G., Li-Pook-Than, J., Jiang, L., Lam, H. Y. K., Chen, R., & Snyder, M. et al. (2012). Personal omics profiling reveals dynamic molecular and medical phenotypes. *Cell*, *148*(6), 1293–1307. doi:10.1016/j.cell.2012.02.009 PMID:22424236

Chen, W.-P., Hung, C.-L., Tsai, S.-J. J., & Lin, Y.-L. (2014). Novel and efficient tag SNPs selection algorithms. *Bio-Medical Materials and Engineering*, *24*(1), 1383–1389. PMID:24212035

Cohen, J., Kiss, R., & Pertsemlidis, A. (2004). Multiple rare alleles contribute to low plasma levels of HDL cholesterol. *Science, 305*(5685), 869–872. doi:10.1126/science.1099870 PMID:15297675

Colosimo, M. E., Peterson, M. W., Mardis, S. A., & Hirschman, L. (2011). Nephele: Genotyping via complete composition vectors and MapReduce. *Source Code for Biology and Medicine*, 6–13. PMID:21851626

Coulouris, G. F., Dollimore, J., & Kindberg, T. (2005). *Distributed Systems: Concepts and Design*. Pearson Education.

Dai, L., Gao, X., Guo, Y., Xiao, J., & Zhang, Z. (2012). Bioinformatics clouds for big data manipulation. *Biology Direct, 7*(1), 43. doi:10.1186/1745-6150-7-43 PMID:23190475

Dean, J., & Ghemawat, S. (2008). MapReduce: Simplified data processing on large clusters. *Communications of the ACM, 51*(1), 107–113. doi:10.1145/1327452.1327492

De Domenico, M., Lima, A., & Musolesi, M. (2013). Interdependence and predictability of human mobility and social interactions. *Pervasive and Mobile Computing, 9*(6), 798–807. doi:10.1016/j.pmcj.2013.07.008

De Oliveira Branco, M. (2009). *Distributed Data Management for Large Scale Applications*. Southampton, UK: University of Southampton.

Díaz-Uriarte, R., & De Andres, S. A. (2006). Gene selection and classification of microarray data using random forest. *BMC Bioinformatics, 7*(1), 3. doi:10.1186/1471-2105-7-3 PMID:16398926

Dinov, I. D. (2016). Methodological challenges and analytic opportunities for modeling and interpreting Big Healthcare Data. *GigaSci*, 5-12.

Dinov, I. D. (2016). Volume and Value of Big Healthcare Data. *J Med Stat Inform, 4*(1), 1–15. doi:10.7243/2053-7662-4-3 PMID:26998309

Eagle, N., Pentland, A. S., & Lazer, D. (2009). Inferring friendship network structure by using mobile phone data. *Proceedings of the National Academy of Sciences of the United States of America, 106*(36), 15274–15278. doi:10.1073/pnas.0900282106 PMID:19706491

Fan, J., & Fan, Y. (2008). High dimensional classification using features annealed independence rules. *Annals of Statistics, 36*(6), 2605–2637. doi:10.1214/07-AOS504 PMID:19169416

Fan, J., Guo, S., & Hao, N. (2012). Variance estimation using refitted cross-validation in ultrahigh dimensional regression. *Journal of the Royal Statistical Society. Series B. Methodological, 74*(1), 37–65. doi:10.1111/j.1467-9868.2011.01005.x PMID:22312234

Fan, J., Han, F., & Liu, H. (2014). Challenges of Big Data analysis. *National Science Review, 1*(2), 293–314. doi:10.1093/nsr/nwt032 PMID:25419469

Fan, J., Liao, Y., & Mincheva, M. (2011). High dimensional covariance matrix estimation in approximate factor models. *Annals of Statistics, 39*(6), 3320–3356. doi:10.1214/11-AOS944 PMID:22661790

Fan, J., Liao, Y., & Mincheva, M. (2013). Large covariance estimation by thresholding principal orthogonal complements (with discussion). *Journal of the Royal Statistical Society. Series B, Statistical Methodology, 75*(4), 603–680. doi:10.1111/rssb.12016 PMID:24348088

Fan, J., & Liu, H. (2013). *Statistical Analysis of Big Data on Pharmacogenomics. Advanced Drug Delivery Reviews.*

Foster, I., & Kesselman, C. (2003). *The Grid 2: Blueprint for a new Computing Infrastructure.* Houston, TX: Elsevier.

Fritsch, V., Varoquaux, G., Thyreau, B., Poline, J.-B., & Thirion, B. (2012). Detecting outliers in high dimensional neuroimaging datasets with robust covariance estimators. *Medical Image Analysis, 16*(7), 1359–1370. doi:10.1016/j.media.2012.05.002 PMID:22728304

Gardner, R. C., Burke, J. F., Nettiksimmons, J., Kaup, A., Barnes, D. E., & Yaffe, K. (2014). Dementia risk after traumatic brain injury vs nonbrain trauma: The role of age and severity. *JAMA Neurology, 71*(12), 1490–1497. doi:10.1001/jamaneurol.2014.2668 PMID:25347255

Goldman, D., Fastenau, J., Dirani, R., Helland, E., Joyce, G., & Conrad, R. et al.. (2014). Medicaid prior authorization policies and imprisonment among patients with schizophrenia. *The American Journal of Managed Care, 20*, 577–586. PMID:25295404

Granville, V. (2014). *Developing Analytic Talent: Becoming a Data Scientist.* John Wiley & Sons.

Grether, J. K., Anderson, M. C., Croen, L. A., Smith, D., & Windham, G. C. (2009). Risk of autism and increasing maternal and paternal age in a large North American population. *American Journal of Epidemiology, 170*(9), 1118–1126. doi:10.1093/aje/kwp247 PMID:19783586

Grossman, R., Bailey, S., Ramu, A., Malhi, B., Hallstrom, P., Pulleyn, I., & Qin, X. (1999). The management and mining of multiple predictive models using the predictive modeling markup language. *Information and Software Technology, 41*(9), 589–595. doi:10.1016/S0950-5849(99)00022-1

Groves, P., Kayyali, B., Knott, D., & Van Kuiken, S. (2013). *The 'big data' revolution in healthcare: Accelerating value and innovation. McKinsey & Company.*

Han, F., & Pan, W. (2010). A data-adaptive sum test for disease association with multiple common or rare variants. *Human Heredity, 70*(1), 42–54. doi:10.1159/000288704 PMID:20413981

Hansen, M. M., Miron-Shatz, T., Lau, A. Y. S., & Paton, C. (2014). Big Data in Science and Healthcare: A Review of Recent Literature and Perspectives Contribution of the IMIA Social Media Working Group. *IMIA Yearbook of Medical Informatics, 9*(1), 21–26. doi:10.15265/IY-2014-0004 PMID:25123717

Harpaz, R., DuMouchel, W., Shah, N. H., Madigan, D., Ryan, P., & Friedman, C. (2012). Novel data mining methodologies for adverse drug event discovery and analysis. *Clinical Pharmacology and Therapeutics, 91*(6), 1010–1021. doi:10.1038/clpt.2012.50 PMID:22549283

Hay, S. I., George, D. B., Moyes, C. L., & Brownstein, J. S. (2013). Big Data Opportunities for Global Infectious Disease Surveillance. *PLoS Medicine, 10*(4), e1001413. doi:10.1371/journal.pmed.1001413 PMID:23565065

Hermon, R., & Williams, P. A. H. (2014). Big data in healthcare: what is it used for?. *Proceedings of the 3rd Australian eHealth Informatics and Security Conference*, 40-49.

Hoge, C. W., McGurk, D., Thomas, J. L., Cox, A. L., Engel, C. C., & Castro, C. A. (2008). Mild traumatic brain injury in U.S. soldiers, returning from Iraq. *The New England Journal of Medicine, 358*(5), 15–27. doi:10.1056/NEJMoa072972 PMID:18234750

Holmes, A. (2012). *Hadoop in practice*. Manning Publications Co.

Hoyt, R.E., & Yoshihashi, A. (2014). *Healthcare Data Analytics. Health Informatics: Practical Guide for Healthcare and Information Technology Professionals*. Academic Press.

Hughes, G. (2015). *How big is 'big data' in healthcare?*. Retrieved 27 Sep, 2015, from http://blogs.sas.com/content/hls/2011/10/21/how-big-is-big-data-in-healthcare/

Husain, M., (2014). Big Data: could it ever cure Alzheimer's disease?. *Brain, a Journal of Neurology, 137*, 2623–2624.

Jones, S. L. P. (1987). *The Implementation of Functional Programming Languages*. Prentice-Hall International Series in Computer Science.

Jonas, M., Solangasenathirajan, S., & Hett, D. (2014). Patient Identification, A Review of the Use of Biometrics in the ICU. In Annual Update in Intensive Care and Emergency Medicine (pp. 679-688). New York: Springer.

Juang, C. F. (2004). A hybrid of genetic algorithm and particle swarm optimization for recurrent network design. *IEEE Transactions on Systems, Man, and Cybernetics. Part B, Cybernetics, 34*(2), 997–1006. doi:10.1109/TSMCB.2003.818557 PMID:15376846

Kessler, R. C., Warner, C. H., Ivany, C., Petukhova, M. V., Rose, S., Bromet, E. J., & Ursano, R. J. et al. (2015). Predicting suicides after psychiatric hospitalization in US Army soldiers: The army study to assess risk and resilience in service members (Army STARRS). *JAMA Psychiatry, 72*(1), 49–57. doi:10.1001/jamapsychiatry.2014.1754 PMID:25390793

Kliegr, T., Vojíř, S., & Rauch, J. (2011). Background knowledge and PMML: first considerations. *Proceedings of the 2011 workshop on Predictive markup language modeling*. doi:10.1145/2023598.2023606

Kohlwey, E., Sussman, A., Trost, J., & Maurer, A. (2011). Leveraging the cloud for big data biometrics: Meeting the performance requirements of the next generation biometric systems. *IEEE World Congress on Services (SERVICES)*, 597–601. doi:10.1109/SERVICES.2011.95

Kosinski, M., Stillwell, D., & Graepel, T. (2013). Private traits and attributes are predictable from digital records of human behaviour. *Proceedings of the National Academy of Sciences of the United States of America, 110*(15), 5802–5805. doi:10.1073/pnas.1218772110 PMID:23479631

Kraemer, M. U. G., Sinka, M. E., Duda, K. A., Mylne, A. Q. N., Shearer, F. M., Barker, C. M., & Hay, S. I. et al. (2015). The global distribution of the arbovirus vectors Aedes aegypti and Ae. Albopictus. *eLife, 4*, 1–18. doi:10.7554/eLife.08347 PMID:26126267

Kumar, A., & Niu, F., & Hazy, R. C. (2013). Making it easier to build and maintain big-data analytics. *Communications of the ACM, 56*(3), 40–49. doi:10.1145/2428556.2428570

Lambin, P., van Stiphout, R. G. P. M., Starmans, M. H. W., Rios-Velazquez, E., Nalbantov, G., Aerts, H. J. W. L., & Dekker, A. et al. (2013). Predicting outcomes in radiation oncology–multifactorial decision support systems. *Nat. Rev. Clin. Oncol*, *10*(1), 27–40. doi:10.1038/nrclinonc.2012.196 PMID:23165123

Lämmel, R. (2008). Googles MapReduce programming model—Revisited. *Science of Computer Programming*, *70*(1), 1–30. doi:10.1016/j.scico.2007.07.001

Le, Q. T., & Courter, D. (2008). Clinical biomarkers for hypoxia targeting. *Cancer and Metastasis Reviews*, *27*(3), 351–362. doi:10.1007/s10555-008-9144-9 PMID:18483785

Lee, E. C., Asher, J. M., Goldlust, S., Kraemer, J. D., Lawson, A. B., & Bansal, S. (2016). *Mind the scales: Harnessing spatial big data for infectious disease surveillance and inference*. Retrieved 2016, from https://arxiv.org/abs/1605.08740

Lee, W. P., Hsiao, Y. T., & Hwang, W. C. (2014). Designing a parallel evolutionary algorithm for inferring gene networks on the cloud computing environment. *BMC Systems Biology*, *8*(1), 5. doi:10.1186/1752-0509-8-5 PMID:24428926

Lee, E. C., Viboud, C., Simonsen, L., Khan, F., & Bansal, Sh. (2015). Detecting Signals of Seasonal Influenza Severity through Age Dynamics. *BMC Infectious Diseases*, *15*(587), 1–19. PMID:26715193

Lewis, S., Csordas, A., Killcoyne, S., Hermjakob, H., Hoopmann, M. R., Moritz, R. L., & Boyle, J. et al. (2012). Hydra: A scalable proteomic search engine which utilizes the Hadoop distributed computing framework. *BMC Bioinformatics*, *13*(1), 3–24. doi:10.1186/1471-2105-13-324 PMID:23216909

Li, Y., & Chen, L. (2014). Big Biological Data: Challenges and Opportunities. *Genomics, Proteomics & Bioinformatics*, *12*(5), 187–189. doi:10.1016/j.gpb.2014.10.001 PMID:25462151

Lin, Y. L. (2013). Implementation of a parallel protein structure alignment service on cloud. *Int J Genomics*, 1–8.

Liu, R., Wang, X., Aihara, K., & Chen, L. (2014). Early diagnosis of complex diseases by molecular biomarkers, network biomarkers, and dynamical network biomarkers. *Medicinal Research Reviews*, *34*(3), 4555–4578. doi:10.1002/med.21293 PMID:23775602

Liu, B., Yuan, Z., Aihara, K., & Chen, L. (2014). Reinitiation enhances reliable transcriptional responses in eukaryotes. *Journal of the Royal Society, Interface*, *11*(97), 1–11. doi:10.1016/j.jcis.2014.08.014 PMID:24850905

Liu, R., Yu, X., Liu, X., Xu, D., Aihara, K., & Chen, L. (2014). Identifying critical transitions of complex diseases based on a single sample. *Bioinformatics (Oxford, England)*, *30*(11), 1579–1586. doi:10.1093/bioinformatics/btu084 PMID:24519381

Ma, H., Zhou, T., Aihara, K., & Chen, L. (2014). Predicting time-series from short-term high dimensional data. *International Journal of Bifurcation and Chaos in Applied Sciences and Engineering*, *24*(12), 1–19. doi:10.1142/S021812741430033X

Mark, T. L., Levit, K. R., & Buck, J. A. (2009). Datapoints: Psychotropic drug prescriptions by medical specialty. *Psychiatric Services (Washington, D.C.)*, *60*(9), 1167. doi:10.1176/ps.2009.60.9.1167 PMID:19723729

Markonis, D., Schaer, R., Eggel, I., Müller, H., & Depeursinge, A. (2012). Using MapReduce for Large-Scale Medical Image Analysis. HISB.

Mathur, A. (2014). A new perspective to data processing: Big Data. *Computing for Sustainable Global Development (INDIACom), International IEEE Conference*.

McAfee, A., & Brynjolfsson, E. (2012). Big data: The management revolution. *Harvard Business Review*, *90*, 61–68. PMID:23074865

McKenna, A., Hanna, M., Banks, E., Sivachenko, A., Cibulskis, K., Kernytsky, A., & Daly, M. et al. (2010). The Genome Analysis Toolkit: A MapReduce framework for analyzing next-generation DNA sequencing data. *Genome Research*, *20*(9), 1297–1303. doi:10.1101/gr.107524.110 PMID:20644199

MacLean, B., Eng, J. K., Beavis, R. C., & McIntosh, M. (2006). General framework for developing and evaluating database scoring algorithms using the TANDEM search engine. *Bioinformatics (Oxford, England)*, *22*(22), 2830–2832. doi:10.1093/bioinformatics/btl379 PMID:16877754

Mohammed, E. A., Far, B. H., & Naugler, C. (2014). Applications of the MapReduce programming framework to clinical big data analysis: current landscape and future trends. *BioData Mining*, 7-22.

Monteith, S., Glenn, T., Geddes, J., & Bauer, M., (2015). Big data are coming to psychiatry: a general introduction. *Int J Bipolar Disord*, 3-21.

Murdoch, T. B., & Detsky, A. S. (2013). The inevitable application of big data to health care. *Journal of the American Medical Association*, *309*(13), 1351–1352. doi:10.1001/jama.2013.393 PMID:23549579

Murphy, D. R., Meyer, A. N. D., Bhise, V., Russo, E., Sittig, D. F., Wei, L., & Singh, H. et al. (2016). Computerized Triggers of Big Data to Detect Delays in Follow-up of Chest Imaging Results. *Chest*, *150*(3), 613–620. doi:10.1016/j.chest.2016.05.001 PMID:27178786

Nguyen, A. V., Wynden, R., & Sun, Y. (2011). HBase, MapReduce, and Integrated Data Visualization for Processing Clinical Signal Data. *AAAI Spring Symposium: Computational Physiology*.

Nordberg, H., Bhatia, K., Wang, K., & Wang, Z. (2013). BioPig: A Hadoop-based analytic toolkit for large-scale sequence data. *Bioinformatics (Oxford, England)*, *29*(23), 3014–3019. doi:10.1093/bioinformatics/btt528 PMID:24021384

Okunieff, P., Chen, Y., Maguire, D. J., & Huser, A. K. (2008). Molecular markers of radiation related normal tissue toxicity. *Cancer and Metastasis Reviews*, *27*(3), 363–374. doi:10.1007/s10555-008-9138-7 PMID:18506399

Olson, M. (2010). Hadoop: Scalable, flexible data storage and analysis. *IQT Quart*, *1*(3), 14–18.

Olston, C., Reed, B., Srivastava, U., Kumar, R., & Tomkins, A. (2008). Pig latin: a not-so-foreign language for data processing. *Proceedings of the 2008 ACM SIGMOD International Conference on Management of Data*, 1099–1110. doi:10.1145/1376616.1376726

Omri, F., Hamila, R., Foufou, S., & Jarraya, M. (2012). Cloud-Ready Biometric System for Mobile Security Access. In *Networked Digital Technologies* (pp. 192–200). New York: Springer. doi:10.1007/978-3-642-30567-2_16

Orlovska, S., Pedersen, M. S., Benros, M. E., Mortensen, P. B., Agerbo, E., & Nordentoft, M. (2014). Head injury as risk factor for psychiatric disorders: A nationwide register-based follow-up study of 113,906 persons with head injury. *The American Journal of Psychiatry*, *171*(4), 463–469. doi:10.1176/appi.ajp.2013.13020190 PMID:24322397

Patiño, J., Guilhaumon, F., Whittaker, R. J., Triantis, K. A., Gradstein, S. R., Hedenäs, L., & Vanderpoorten, A. et al. (2013). Accounting for data heterogeneity in patterns of biodiversity: An application of linear mixed effect models to the oceanic island biogeography of spore-producing plants. *Ecography*, *36*(8), 904–913. doi:10.1111/j.1600-0587.2012.00020.x

Pentland, A., Reid, T. G., & Heibeck, T. (2013). Revolutionizing medicine and Public Health. Report of the Big Data and Health Working Group, Doha.

Perlis, R. H., Iosifescu, D. V., Castro, V. M., Murphy, S. N., Gainer, V. S., & Minnier, J. (2012). Using electronic medical records to enable large-scale studies in psychiatry: Treatment resistant depression as a model. *Psychological Medicine*, *42*, 41–50.

Pittelkow, P. H., & Ghosh, M. (2008). Theoretical measures of relative performance of classifiers for high dimensional data with small sample sizes. *Journal of the Royal Statistical Society. Series B. Methodological*, *70*(1), 159–173. doi:10.1111/j.1467-9868.2007.00631.x

Potash, J. B. (2015). Electronic medical records: Fast track to big data in bipolar disorder. *The American Journal of Psychiatry*, *172*(4), 310–321. doi:10.1176/appi.ajp.2015.15010043 PMID:25827027

Raghava, N. (2011). Iris recognition on hadoop: A biometrics system implementation on cloud computing. *IEEE International Conference on Cloud Computing and Intelligence Systems*, 482–485.

Raghupathi, W., & Raghupathi, V. (2014). Big data analytics in healthcare: Promise and potential. *Health Information Science and Systems*, *7*(2-3), 1-10.

Ren, X., Wang, Y., Chen, L., Zhang, X. S., & Jin, Q. (2013). EllipsoidFN: A tool for identifying a heterogeneous set of cancer biomarkers based on gene expressions. *Nucleic Acids Research*, *41*(4), 1–8. doi:10.1093/nar/gks1288 PMID:23262226

Rogers, D. J., Wilson, A. J., Hay, S. I., & Graham, A. J. (2006). The global distribution of yellow fever and dengue. *Advances in Parasitology*, *62*, 181–220. doi:10.1016/S0065-308X(05)62006-4 PMID:16647971

Ruktanonchai, N. W., DeLeenheer, P., Tatem, A. J., Alegana, V. A., Trevor Caughlin, T., & Zu Erbach-Schoenberg, E. (2016). Identifying Malaria Transmission Foci for Elimination Using Human Mobility Data. *PLoS Computational Biology*, *12*(4), 1–19. doi:10.1371/journal.pcbi.1004846 PMID:27043913

Salathe, M., Bengtsson, L., Bodnar, T. J., Brewer, D. D., Brownstein, J. S., Buckee, C., & Vespignani, A. et al. (2012). Digital epidemiology. *PLoS Computational Biology*, *8*(7), e1002616. doi:10.1371/journal.pcbi.1002616 PMID:22844241

Salathé, M., & Khandelwal, Sh. (2011). Assessing vaccination sentiments with online social media: Implications for infectious disease dynamics and control. *PLoS Computational Biology*, *7*(10), 2011. doi:10.1371/journal.pcbi.1002199 PMID:22022249

Satish, N., Harris, M., & Garland, M. (2009). Designing efficient sorting algorithms for manycore GPUs. *IEEE International Symposium Parallel & Distributed Processing*, 1-10. doi:10.1109/IPDPS.2009.5161005

Schatz, M. C. (2009). CloudBurst: Highly sensitive read mapping with MapReduce. *Bioinformatics (Oxford, England)*, 25(11), 1363–1369. doi:10.1093/bioinformatics/btp236 PMID:19357099

Schönherr, S., Forer, L., Weißensteiner, H., Kronenberg, F., Specht, G., & Kloss-Brandstätter, A. (2012). Cloudgene: A graphical execution platform for MapReduce programs on private and public clouds. *BMC Bioinformatics*, 13(1), 200. doi:10.1186/1471-2105-13-200 PMID:22888776

Shvachko, K., Kuang, H., Radia, S., & Chansler, R. (2010). The hadoop distributed file system. In *IEEE 26th Symposium Mass Storage Systems and Technologies*, 1-10. doi:10.1109/MSST.2010.5496972

Spinello, L., Arras, K. O., Triebel, R., & Siegwart, R. (2010). A Layered Approach to People Detection in 3D Range Data. In *Twenty-Fourth AAAI Conference on Artificial Intelligence*. Atlanta, GA: AAAI Press.

Srinivasan, S., Moser, R. P., Willis, G., Riley, W., Alexander, M., Berrigan, D., & Kobrin, S. (2015). Small is essential: Importance of subpopulation research in cancer control. *American Journal of Public Health*, 105(S3), S371–S373. doi:10.2105/AJPH.2014.302267 PMID:25905825

Taylor, R. C. (2010). An overview of the Hadoop/MapReduce/HBase framework and its current applications in bioinformatics. *BMC Bioinformatics*, 11(Suppl 12), S1. doi:10.1186/1471-2105-11-S12-S1 PMID:21210976

Thusoo, A., Sarma, J. S., Jain, N., Shao, Z., Chakka, P., Anthony, S., & Murthy, R. et al. (2009). Hive: a warehousing solution over a map-reduce framework. *Proc VLDB Endowment*, 2(2), 1626–1629. doi:10.14778/1687553.1687609

Titiunik, R. (2015). Can big data solve the fundamental problem of causal inference? *PS Polit Sci Polit*, 48(01), 75–79. doi:10.1017/S1049096514001772

Tuite, A. R., Tien, J., Eisenberg, M., Earn, D. J. D., Ma, J., & Fisman, D. N. (2011). Cholera Epidemic in Haiti, 2010: Using a Transmission Model to Explain Spatial Spread of Disease and Identify Optimal Control Interventions. *Annals of Internal Medicine*, 154(9), 593–601. doi:10.7326/0003-4819-154-9-201105030-00334 PMID:21383314

Valuck, R. J., Anderson, H. O., Libby, A. M., Brandt, E., Bryan, C., Allen, R. R., & Pace, W. D. et al. (2012). Enhancing electronic health record measurement of depression severity and suicide ideation: A distributed ambulatory research in therapeutics network (DARTNet) study. *Journal of the American Board of Family Medicine*, 25(5), 582–593. doi:10.3122/jabfm.2012.05.110053 PMID:22956694

Van Horn, J. D., & Toga, A. W. (2014). Human neuroimaging as a Big Data science. *Brain Imaging and Behavior*, 8(2), 323–331. doi:10.1007/s11682-013-9255-y PMID:24113873

Wang, L., Chen, D., Ranjan, R., Khan, S. U., KolOdziej, J., & Wang, J. (2012). Parallel Processing of Massive EEG Data with MapReduce. ICPADS, 164–171.

Wang, Y., Goh, W., Wong, L., & Montana, G. (2013). Random forests on Hadoop for genome-wide association studies of multivariate neuroimaging phenotypes. *BMC Bioinformatics*, 14(16), 1–15. doi:10.1186/1471-2105-14-S4-S1 PMID:24564704

Wang, W., Haerian, K., Salmasian, H., Harpaz, R., Chase, H., & Friedman, C. (2011). A drug-adverse event extraction algorithm to support pharmacovigilance knowledge mining from PubMed citations. In *AMIA Annual Symposium Proceedings* (pp. 14-64). Bethesda, MD: American Medical Informatics Association.

Wang, F., Lee, R., Liu, Q., Aji, A., Zhang, X., & Saltz, J. (2011). Hadoop-gis: A high performance query system for analytical medical imaging with mapreduce. Emory University.

Wang, Y., & Yu, H. (2013). An ultralow-power memory-based big-data computing platform by non-volatile domain-wall nanowire devices. In *Proceedings of the International Symposium on Low Power Electronics and Design*. IEEE Press.

Weiner, M. W., Veitch, D. P., Aisen, P. S., Beckett, L. A., Cairns, N. J., Green, R. C., & Trojanowski, J. Q. et al. (2012). The Alzheimers disease neuroimaging initiative: A review of papers published since its inception. *Alzheimers & Dementia, 8*(1Suppl), S1–S68. doi:10.1016/j.jalz.2011.09.172 PMID:22047634

Wen, Z., Liu, Z. P., Liu, Z., Zhang, Y., & Chen, L. (2013). An integrated approach to identify causal network modules of complex diseases with application to colorectal cancer. *Journal of the American Medical Informatics Association, 20*(4), 659–667. doi:10.1136/amiajnl-2012-001168 PMID:22967703

White, T. (2012). *Hadoop: The Definitive Guide*. Sebastopol, CA: O'Reilly Media, Inc.

Wiechers, I. R., Leslie, D. L., & Rosenheck, R. A. (2013). Prescribing of psychotropic medications to patients without a psychiatric diagnosis. *Psychiatric Services (Washington, D.C.), 64*(12), 1243–1248. doi:10.1176/appi.ps.201200557 PMID:23999894

Worthey, E., Mayer, A., Syverson, G., Helbling, D., Bonacci, B. B., Decker, B., & Dimmock, D. P. et al. (2013). Making a definitive diagnosis: Successful clinical application of whole exome sequencing in a child with intractable inflammatory bowel disease. *Genetics in Medicine, 13*(3), 255–262. doi:10.1097/GIM.0b013e3182088158 PMID:21173700

Wu, L. T., Gersing, K. R., Swartz, M. S., Burchett, B., Li, T. K., & Blazer, D. G. (2013). Using electronic health records data to assess comorbidities of substance use and psychiatric diagnoses and treatment settings among adults. *Journal of Psychiatric Research, 47*(4), 555–563. doi:10.1016/j.jpsychires.2012.12.009 PMID:23337131

Wu, Z., & Huang, N. E. (2009). Ensemble empirical mode decomposition: A noise-assisted data analysis method. *Advances in Adaptive Data Analysis, 1*(1), 1–41. doi:10.1142/S1793536909000047

Wu, F. X., Wu, L., Wang, J., Liu, J., & Chen, L. (2014). Transittability of complex networks and its applications to regulatory biomolecular networks. *Scientific Reports, 4*, 1–10. PMID:24769565

Xiaojing, J. (2010). Google Cloud Computing Platform Technology Architecture and the Impact of Its Cost. *2010 Second WRI World Congress on Software Engineering*, 17–20. doi:10.1109/WCSE.2010.93

Xu, B., Gao, J., & Li, C. (2012). An efficient algorithm for DNA fragment assembly in MapReduce. *Biochemical and Biophysical Research Communications, 426*(3), 395–398. doi:10.1016/j.bbrc.2012.08.101 PMID:22960169

Yaramakala, S., & Margaritis, D. (2005). Speculative Markov blanket discovery for optimal feature selection. In *Fifth IEEE International Conference on Data Mining*. IEEE. doi:10.1109/ICDM.2005.134

Youyou, W., Kosinski, M., & Stillwell, D. (2015). Computer-based personality judgments are more accurate than those made by humans. *Proceedings of the National Academy of Sciences of the United States of America*, *112*(4), 1036–1040. doi:10.1073/pnas.1418680112 PMID:25583507

Yu, X., Li, G., & Chen, L. (2014). Prediction and early diagnosis of complex diseases by edge-network. *Bioinformatics (Oxford, England)*, *30*(6), 852–859. doi:10.1093/bioinformatics/btt620 PMID:24177717

Yuan, L., Ding, G., Chen, Y. E., Chen, Z., & Li, Y. (2012). A novel strategy for deciphering dynamic conservation of gene expression relationship. *Journal of Molecular Cell Biology*, *4*(3), 177–179. doi:10.1093/jmcb/mjs014 PMID:22498922

Zeng, T., Zhang, W., Yu, X., Liu, X., Li, M., Liu, R., & Chen, L. N. (2014). Edge biomarkers for classification and prediction of phenotypes. *Sci China Life Sci*, *57*(11), 1103–1114. doi:10.1007/s11427-014-4757-4 PMID:25326072

Zeng, T., Zhang, C. C., Zhang, W., Liu, R., Liu, J., & Chen, L. (2014). Deciphering early development of complex diseases by progressive module network. *Methods (San Diego, Calif.)*, *67*(3), 334–343. doi:10.1016/j.ymeth.2014.01.021 PMID:24561825

Zhang, K., Sun, F., Waterman, M. S., & Chen, T. (2003). Dynamic programming algorithms for haplotype block partitioning: applications to human chromosome 21 haplotype data. *Proceedings of the Seventh Annual International Conference on Research in Computational Molecular Biology*, 332–340. doi:10.1145/640075.640119

Zhang, W., Zeng, T., & Chen, L. (2014). EdgeMarker: Identifying differentially correlated molecule pairs as edge-biomarkers. *Journal of Theoretical Biology*, *362*, 35–43. doi:10.1016/j.jtbi.2014.05.041 PMID:24931676

Zhu, H., Rao, R. S., Zeng, T., & Chen, L. (2012). Reconstructing dynamic gene regulatory networks from sample-based transcriptional data. *Nucleic Acids Research*, *40*(21), 10657–10667. doi:10.1093/nar/gks860 PMID:23002138

KEY TERMS AND DEFINITIONS

Big Data: The massive amount of data which is identified by four characteristics including high volume, velocity, variety, and veracity.

Distributed Systems: Network of independent computers whose users utilize them as a single system connected with a middleware service.

Graphical Processing Units: Computing method which changes memory for rapidly creating images in a device used to show them.

Grid Computing Systems: A distributed computing method used for sharing resources collaboratively.

Healthcare Analysis: Analyzing healthcare data collected from different health resources including claims and cost data, clinical data, research and development data, and patient behavior data (Fan et al., 2014).

Healthcare Systems: The collection of people, resources, and organizations whose task is to deliver services related to health of patients to them.

MapReduce: A program which is used for processing Big Data by utilizing a distributed model on a cluster.

ENDNOTES

1   MAPR. Retrieved from [http://www.mapr.com/products/m3].
2   Hortonworks. Retrieved from [http://hortonworks.com/].
3   The Platform for Big Data and the Leading Solution for Apache Hadoop in the Enterprise - Cloudera. Retrieved from [http://www.cloudera.com/content/cloudera/en/home.html].
4   DataStax. Retrieved from [http://www.datastax.com/].

Section 5
Other Topics in Data Science

Chapter 17

Notifiable Disease Databases for Client Management and Surveillance

Ann M. Jolly
University of Ottawa, Canada

James J. Logan
University of Ottawa, Canada

ABSTRACT

The spread of certain infectious diseases, many of which are preventable, is widely acknowledged to have a detrimental effect on society. Reporting cases of these infections has been embodied in public health laws since the 1800s. Documenting client management and monitoring numbers of cases are the primary goals in collecting these data. A sample notifiable disease database is presented, including database structure, elements and rationales for collection, sources of data, and tabulated output. This chapter is a comprehensive guide to public health professionals on the content, structure, and processing of notifiable disease data for regional, provincial, and federal use.

INTRODUCTION

Under public health acts in all Canadian provinces, physicians, laboratories, nurses and other health professionals are required to report data on individuals with infections of public health importance to health departments. This chapter reviews legislation that requires the reporting of notifiable infections, the public health reasons behind reporting, and the design, use, and improvement of notifiable disease registries. There are few academic Canadian papers on legislation and implementation of notifiable disease programs. Therefore, this chapter references all of those and some from the United States, United Kingdom, and Europe so as to further elucidate the objectives, philosophy and processes behind disease reporting. The goal is to provide a thorough guide for developing and improving notifiable disease databases in order to accurately document public health surveillance and client management activities. This chapter is aimed at public health staff primarily in Canada, but also in other jurisdictions interested

DOI: 10.4018/978-1-5225-2515-8.ch017

in systematically collecting notifiable disease data, with attendant legal and public health rationales. Together with a flexible structure, these data will allow for proper management of cases and contacts, improves surveillance practices, and timely notification of outbreaks. The chapter includes data extraction standards for regular reports and outbreak detection.

The structure and content of notifiable disease registries varies substantially in Canada. As with many health databases, data are frequently collected and stored in a manner preventing easy access or analysis. To substantiate the data requirements, this chapter references various provincial public health acts. As many provincial acts contain the same provisions in similar language, the reader may refer to the relevant one in his/her own jurisdiction.

BACKGROUND

Public health laws stem from the industrial revolution. During that time, states were challenged with diseases emanating from undeveloped infrastructures for concentrated housing, migration to cities, and poor working conditions. Public health laws are an instrument of public health practice enacted through a democratic process which itemize measures to be taken by the government to preserve public health (Chorba, Berkelman, Safford, Gibbs, & Hull, 1989; Gostin, 2004; Sepulveda et al., 1992; Stephen B Thacker & Berkelman, 1988). This section describes the implementation of these laws, regulations, and policies as they affect data collection for the investigation and monitoring of notifiable infections.

Public Health Acts in Canada

In Canada, public health acts are enacted and administered by each province and their jurisdictions. Most start with a purpose clause, allowing the health minister or delegate (usually a medical officer of health) to prevent disease and promote the health of residents (Prince Edward Island Public Health Act, 2014; Quebec Public Health Act, 2016). They contain very broad powers for a minister of health or a delegated medical officer of health to do anything, including forbid or order an action to prevent a hazard (Ontario, 2015; Quebec Public Health Act, 2016).

As part of disease prevention, records of infected individuals are required to be reported to a medical officer or a delegate so that:

1. Sources are investigated (Ontario, 2015) and patients are treated appropriately (Chorba et al., 1989; Northwest Territories Public Health Act, 2011).
2. Incidence of infections are monitored regularly to distinguish unusual frequency, manifestations, demography, and locations with the goal of preventing disease (British Columbia, 2016; Quebec Public Health Act, 2016).
3. Mandated surveillance system is evaluated.
4. Patient management is audited.
5. The control program is evaluated.

The first two goals are most commonly cited in legislation and public health surveillance texts. Goals 3, 4, and 5 are also important for the purpose of quality public health professional practice, government financial accountability, and to clarify health department responsibilities for disease prevention efforts (Campbell, 2004; Gostin, 2000; Jajosky & Groseclose, 2004).

Medical Ethics, Privacy, and Data Security

The invasive nature of notifiable disease reporting seems contrary to privacy legislation and commonly held norms (Mallon & Kassinove, 1999). Privacy and individual rights challenges to public health laws have been resolved in favor of public health in all reported instances in Canada (Duggan, 2011; Vogel & Funk, 2008) and the U.S.

All clients and their contacts deserve to be treated with respect. Intrusions should be minimized whenever possible. If data have to be shared, only those elements relevant to the case should be transferred; source data should be kept confidential and secure. Published journal articles from France and Sweden provide legal requirements and technical standards for the storage of health data (Flahault et al., 2006; Rolfhamre, Janson, Arneborn, & Ekdahl, 2006). Some provincial public health acts state that access to communicable disease data is restricted to staff who need the data to fulfill their duties. Use of the data should be limited to the purpose for which they were collected. A Canadian method for maintaining security, allowing appropriate sharing, and providing prompt surveillance for notifiable disease data together with an encryption algorithm has been developed and tested (El Emam et al., 2011). Some of these principles may apply, although the method is designed specifically for transferring case counts from public health units to regional, provincial, and federal authorities, rather than for case management.

Data safety is also important. Therefore, careful consideration should be paid to implementing backup systems so that data, computers, and terminals are protected from physical damage due to floods or fires. In addition, backup systems must protect against electronic damage due to computer viruses, hacking, and ransom ware. Guidelines on the storage of medical records are available from provincial colleges of physicians and surgeons, institutions such as hospitals, and healthcare practice guidelines.

Notifiable Disease Reporting

Definitions of notifiable diseases or conditions differ depending on the jurisdiction for which the legislation was written. Most commonly, the definition of "communicable disease" is given, with the provision that it is reportable or notifiable under the list of infections included in the regulations. In Ontario (2015), "communicable disease" is specified in regulations made by the minister. Usually these infections meet one or more of the following criteria: common, severe, easily preventable, highly communicable, costly, instill fear in people, change in manifestation, population groups affected and/or geographic range. Interestingly, Australia uses a rating scheme developed by the Public Health Agency of Canada to determine which infections should be reported. It is based on the ability and responsibility of governments to intervene in order to protect the public, and monitoring the infection for effectiveness of prevention (Communicable Disease Network Australia, 2015b)(J.-A. Doherty, 2006).

In Canada, provinces voluntarily and by "mutual agreement" submit certain elements abstracted from notifiable disease reports which meet the federal case surveillance definitions, and send them electronically or on paper to the Public Health Agency; some jurisdictions forward only tabulated data (Totten, Maclean, Payne, & Severini, 2015).

In Australia, federal designation of notifiable infections depends on territorial and state requirements for notification. (Communicable Disease Network Australia, 2015a) This is formalized by all states and territories signing an agreement designated in the National Health Security Act of 2007. The Minister of Health must consult with the Chief Medical Officer and each territory and state on which infections should be notifiable. Under the act and the agreement, notifiable infections are reported to the Communicable Diseases Network Australia, which in turn disseminates aggregate counts widely through the National Notifiable Disease Surveillance System (Commonwealth of Australia, 2010; Department of Health Government of Australia, 2014; Kirby Institute for Infection and Immunity in Society 2015, 2015).

Definition of a Case

In most jurisdictions, case surveillance definitions issued by provincial health departments define the criteria for what constitutes a case of notifiable disease. The majority of these require a positive laboratory test as part of the case definition. A key distinction is the difference between a "case" of an infection (or disease) and an individual. An individual (denoted in records by a mandatory, unique, and personal identifier) can have multiple infections, or be tested and notified several times for the same infection. Each diagnosis constitutes a new, uniquely identified "case" and should be counted as such in surveillance reports. For example, definitions of new cases vs. continuing cases of bacterial STI are based on a standard period of time (28 days), (Public Health Ontario, 2104).

Historically, physician reports itemizing clinical and treatment information were matched with laboratory test reports at communicable disease control units. In some jurisdictions, nurses would call physicians who had ordered the laboratory tests and obtain information on the diagnosis. Recently, laboratory reports, which may include information on symptoms, form the backbone of most reporting systems. These reports are often supplemented by physician reports. In the absence of laboratory confirmation, a clinical diagnosis may be made and treatment administered. Clinical case definitions are helpful when specimens are transported long distances and are subject to differences in temperature and/or transit times.

Specific notifiable infections vary slightly from jurisdiction to jurisdiction. Most recognize the International Health Regulations in which a few serious infections, including SARS, are reportable within 48 hours (World Health Organization, 2005). In Canada, notifiable infections include the latter. Nationally notifiable infections are usually determined in collaboration with provincial public health authorities and include the majority of infections reported in the provinces (J. A. Doherty, 2000; Sockett, Garnett, & Scott, 1996).

Investigation and Management of Notifiable Disease

The obligation to investigate a source of infectious disease is inherent both in public health professions and legal literatures. The chain of investigation and control of infectious diseases begins with a notifiable disease report on a form specified in the public health act or regulations. The following minimum elements are usually required: patient name (Manitoba, 2016), patient address, patient demographics, laboratory, clinical, treatment, source, and physician data (Northwest Territories Public Health Act, 2011). Some jurisdictions include information on the contact information to whom the case was exposed (Manitoba, 2016). The investigation of possible sources of infection for an infected individual in a case report may include all possible exposures, including air-, food-, water-, vector-, and blood-borne, congenital, or sexually transmitted.

Food and water-borne exposure investigations are usually the least complicated. They are based on where the client was and what food he or she ingested approximately one incubation period before becoming ill, depending on the organism detected by the laboratory. No other general timelines for all enteric infections are available (Alberta Health, 2014; BC Enteric Policy Working Group Recommendations, 2007; Centers for Disease Control and Prevention, 2006; International Association of Food Protection, 2011; Manitoba, 2008, 2015b).

Vector-borne illnesses require more information about client's activities, location, and history of insect bites in the preceding days (Nova Scotia Department of Health and Wellness, n.d., 2013; State of New Jersey, 2013).

Air-borne exposures are more difficult to investigate, although exposure is usually determined by the pathogen isolated. Once air-borne transmission is suspected, information is required on locations of shared air space with someone who is already infected. Exposure to aerosolized water, hospitalization, travel, antibiotic treatment, and vaccine history are also important (Manitoba, 2011, 2015a).

Determining a source case is facilitated by the fact that a high proportion of sick individuals may have distinctive symptoms. These include coughing or spots (as is the case of many childhood infections), and/or local reports of others with the same symptoms. As vaccination is a mandated public health program in all jurisdictions in Canada, surveillance and investigation of vaccine-preventable diseases are the primary methods of evaluating outcomes (Government of Saskatchewan, 2014b; Public Health Ontario, 2015).

Contact Tracing

Investigating the source of tuberculosis (TB) or sexually transmitted and blood-borne infections (STB-BIs), is done by a formal process known as "contact tracing". In the case of STBBI, it is also known as "partner notification" (Brewer, 2005; Public Health Agency of Canada, 2014; Rothenberg, McElroy, Wilce, & Muth, 2003a). This is the formal process by which the case is interviewed and educated about his/her infections. Contacts are then elicited, located, and notified. The sex partner or contact is notified confidentially that he or she has been exposed, without divulging the name of the original patient (index case) and is encouraged to be tested and treated. The nature of contact is defined by the mode of transmission of the pathogen (for example, shared air space for TB, shared drug-use equipment for HIV or hepatitis C virus [HCV], or unprotected sex for chlamydia, gonorrhea, and syphilis). Contacts include those from whom the client may have contracted the infection (upstream or source contacts), and also those that the patient may have subsequently exposed (downstream or spread contacts). Contact tracing, or partner notification as it is known for STIs, is provided for in all the acts under the general title of "investigation." It is specifically mentioned in Manitoba's Public Health Act (Manitoba, 2016). If the contact is positive, then he/she becomes a case; is treated, and his/her diagnostic information is reported. The cycle of cases and contacts continues until all contacts test negative.

Investigating TB and STBBIs presents numerous challenges. In the case of TB, bacilli are transmitted by droplet nuclei. Particles of less than 5 microns in diameter can float in the air for up to 4 hours. Sharing air space with anyone infected with TB for at least four hours constitutes an exposure. Hence, investigations may result in large numbers of places and contacts outside of the home, including classrooms, bars, and homeless shelters (Cook, Shah, & Gardy, 2012). A comprehensive guide is given in the Canadian Tuberculosis Standards (Public Health Agency of Canada, 2014), presenting a unique opportunity to identify places as possible "sources" of infection, which is easier for people to recall than a large number of contacts (Brewer, 2002).

Recall of people with whom individuals have had sex is usually better than the same of have shared air space and injection drug use exposures (Brewer, Garrett, & Kulasingam, 1999). Yet sex partners may be anonymous, numerous, from diverse places, and exposures may have taken place over a long period of time. Overall, locations of exposure—bars, bathhouses, or shooting galleries—may be the most precise information obtainable.

Partner notification for STIs has the longest history (Rothenberg, McElroy, Wilce, & Muth, 2003a) and is the most complex of all contact investigations. We used it as the model for other investigations because STIs constitute a third to a half of all notifiable infections.

In-person partner notification for STIs can be performed by a healthcare provider, client, or by "contracting." In the first instance, the healthcare provider interviews the case, elicits names, and proceeds to locate and notify the contacts. Then, the provider coordinates testing and treatment. The second instance, also known as "self-referral" or "patient-based referral," does not require information to be recorded by public health staff because the patient assumes the responsibility for notifying his/her own contacts. In some jurisdictions, a public health nurse is required to review the case's capability and safety in partner notification. "Contracting" involves the nurse recording partner information and the patient notifies the partner. The nurse then arranges testing if the partner does not present during a specified period of time. The most common method of partner notification for chlamydia and gonorrhea are self-referrals, where notes or slips may be provided to patients to give to their partners. Registration of their return by the partner indicates that notification was completed. In many jurisdictions, partner notification is not performed for chlamydia and gonorrhea. Usually, notification is attempted for contacts exposed to HIV and syphilis.

Computerized applications for partner notification and nucleic acid detection methods of testing for STIs have engendered new possibilities for facilitating partner follow up. These applications allow the patients to send an electronic referral slip and testing information to their partners, which may streamline partner follow-up and record keeping.

Blood-borne infections contracted in healthcare settings are routinely investigated within the context of standard safety practices in using sharps, universal precautions, and workers' safety standards. (Centers for Disease Control and Prevention, 2001; Provincial Infectious Disease Advisory Committee on Communicable Disease, 2014). Investigation of the source of blood-borne infections (hepatitis B, C, and HIV) in the community includes sex or drug equipment partners (Government of Saskatchewan, 2014a), and history of: tattooing; coinfection with other blood-borne pathogens; STIs; sex with partners involving blood exposures; incarceration; and household contacts with whom razors or toothbrushes have been shared (Provincial Infectious Disease Advisory Committee on Communicable Disease, 2014).

The types of investigations, findings, contact tracing details, testing, treatment, and other prevention practices outlined above indicate the wide range of data and the structure of notifiable disease databases. Fortunately, much of the data collected for prevention is identical to that required for monitoring occurrence of infectious disease.

Surveillance

Surveillance is defined as the collection, compilation, analysis, and interpretation of health-related data, and dissemination of results to those who need to know in order to plan for or prevent illness (Thacker & Stroup, 1994). While goals of surveillance systems vary, they encompass four main areas:

1. Describe epidemiology, including: incidence, demography of people at risk, place, and timing (Chorba et al., 1989; Jajosky & Groseclose, 2004; Thacker & Berkelman, 1988).

2. Monitor the effectiveness of new or existing prevention programs, policies, and therapy, including collecting information for development of new prevention programs (Chorba et al., 1989; Jajosky & Groseclose, 2004; Thacker & Berkelman, 1988).

3. Detect outbreaks (World Health Organization, 1968).

4. Scan for incidence of re-emerging and anti-microbial resistant infections (Chorba et al., 1989), new manifestations of old pathogens, and changes in occurrence of agent and host factors; (registries should provide preliminary data for emerging natural history studies, generation of hypotheses [Thacker & Stroup, 1994], and allocation of resources [Jajosky & Groseclose, 2004]).

In summary, the reporting of notifiable diseases for surveillance involves setting objectives specifically to the monitor for that infection. (Foege, Hogan, & Newton, 1976; Thacker & Berkelman, 1988). The close association between information from surveillance reports and prevention activities emphasizes accountability of government agencies in disease control. Prevention and control includes direct intervention with patients, as well as investigations into causes of anomalies, supplementary analyses, enhanced surveillance (Foege, et al., 1976; Langmuir, 1963), and evaluations of the surveillance systems (Thacker & Berkelman, 1988). Maintenance of a good surveillance system with complete data can simplify or resolve outbreak investigations, resulting in significant savings in human resources, time, and expense. It can also prevent further cases.

DATABASE STRUCTURE

The structure of the data is directly linked to the nature of public health management and surveillance of individuals with notifiable infections. A data model captures the overall structure of data relevant to a problem, independent of its intended use (Cromley & McLafferty, 2012). It helps the database administrator identify potential data entities (for example, the contacts), attributes (such as addresses and health card numbers), and the relationship between multiple entities (e.g., a patient and their infections, a patient and all their named contacts, or a patient and their prescriptions). These data often involve multiple levels of relationships not easily expressed in individual tables of information. Given the complexity and comprehensive nature of the data collected through public health surveillance and client management activities, the exercise of constructing a data model is recommended for identifying local needs.

Data collected for surveillance systems is often entered from patient chart information into a single table (personal observation). They are sometimes entered in spreadsheets or may be kept on paper. Relational database management systems (RDBMS) allow for easier reporting and quick access to specific data queries. They manage the information as collections of tables. Data across multiple tables can share common attributes through which relationships can be drawn, linking connected information as needed (Cromley & McLafferty, 2012). Conceptualizing the information required by the public health surveillance system (see Figure 1) allows relationships among the data to be easily identified and expanded upon.

In Figure 1, a patient presents to a health practitioner. Ideally, the notifiable disease system is linked to the provincial patient insurance registry and/or a laboratory information system (LIS) containing a catalogue of possible patients. If the ideal linkages are infeasible, selecting an individual from the existing database of all those with notifiable infections minimizes but does not eliminate data entry errors, and duplication of records, both of which are common problems.

Figure 1. Tables of data connecting patient-specific information with case (infection episode) and contact information

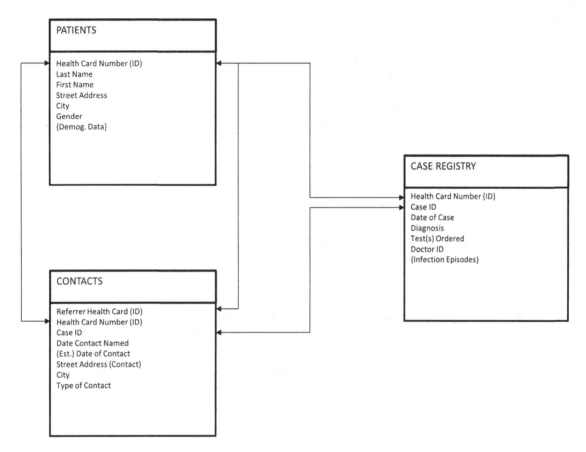

Diagnosis information can be populated from an algorithm based on test results, leaving only the treatment, contact, or source data to be entered. His or her health card number, if available, or a key identifier created by the system, connects all personal, demographic and locating information for that individual to the episode "case." It can be updated if there has been a change (for example, the patient has a new address). As the case episode results in a positive test, a contact record is created for each contact. It is then linked to the case patient through a unique identification number. Dates on these records (including the case, contact nomination, and estimated timing of contact) inform other data in the tables. The most recent dates of an infection episode for this individual would constitute a new case. The system would assign the next sequential episode number based on the patient's previous episodes. If the patient (John Doe) with health card number 111222333 presents for the third time and the case registry shows Doe has had gonorrhea on two prior occasions, a positive diagnosis of gonorrhea would populate the next number in sequence for the "gonorrhea episodes attribute."

The case record, in turn, is linked in a one-to-many relationship with tables for laboratory tests with results of: diagnoses, treatments (perhaps multiple for each diagnosis), sources, contacts, or places of exposure.

Below is a list of general attributes for the database, structure, appearance, and contents used to facilitate accurate record keeping and extraction. We have developed a prototype meeting these criteria and containing the variables itemized below in Epi Info 2000™, which we tested with 1,000 records.

1. Provide a data entry form showing "pages," "tabs," or other method indicating completion progress.
2. Keep data entry suitable for a variety of personnel, including clerical staff, public health nurses, inspectors, physicians, data entry experts, and epidemiologists.
3. Reduce missing data through mandatory fields (i.e., risks and sources).
    a. Client refusal to answer questions should be entered, as should those for which answers are unknown.
    b. Information commonly provided by healthcare providers (i.e., treatment or clinical data, like symptoms) should be entered as "not asked" or "unknown."
4. Enter dates using a calendar selection to minimize month/day errors.
    a. Restrict years so that patient birth dates must precede onset dates.
    b. A laboratory result must precede treatment dates.
    c. An investigation date must precede a case closed date.
5. Differentiate address fields into apartment number, building number, and street.
    a. Select cities, provinces, and countries with pick lists.
    b. Postcodes should be controlled entries of letters and numerals in six characters.
6. Separate risk factors and reasons for testing into multiple variables with check boxes.
    a. Add details in a separate field for the most important risk factor or reason.
7. Data entry algorithms should control pop up menus for test sites, symptoms and pregnancy based on sex (e.g. to avoid errors like 'pregnant men').
8. Systems should calculate and populate ages by using date of birth, onset, or report date.
    a. Range checks should be in place to alert user to unlikely entries.
9. Utilize pick lists and controlled entries as much as possible to avoid typographical errors.
10. Database users should be able to edit or add to fields or pick lists as new infections, treatments, risks, and modes of transmission arise.
    a. Logs of these changes should be kept in the system.
    b. Logs should also show the name of the person making the changes and the date.
11. Record creation and modification dates and the identity of the data entry person should be available.

SAMPLE DATABASE TABLES

To bridge theory and application, this chapter presents a list of definitions (see Table 2): standards, possible sources, and rationales for information essential to achieving the stated goals. Rationales for collecting variables include patient management, surveillance, and evaluation of both. This includes existing control programs. For ease of reference, the chapter replicates those in Table 1.

This sample database is intended for collecting STI data, which is more complicated and requires more information than water- or food-borne illnesses. Many of the variables or attributes in Table 2 are essential and identical to elements required for almost all other notifiable infections. These variables can be adapted, such as source instead of contact, and some can be omitted.

Table 1. Legal and public health practice rationales for notifiable disease data

Number	Rationale
1	Manage/treat patient, investigate source
2	Surveillance of infection to detect unusual frequencies in manifestation, demography, and location
3	Evaluate surveillance system
4	Audit patient care
5	Evaluate existing control programs

Table 2 includes information specific to an individual, whether a case or a contact. The demographic and locating information should be populated from the laboratory information system containing the positive result or provincial patient registry file. Privacy concerns about linking the databases are not valid. Technology is sufficiently developed to allow one-way access to the patient file by notifiable disease staff. At no time should staff handling physician or laboratory billings have access to notifiable disease information. Table 3 provides fields to update address information. Personal health insurance numbers are helpful in standardizing data entry and locating clients. They should not be essential for every client, as some may be unwilling to show identifying information in a sensitive situation or they may come from outside the province. Recent research has shown that people who recruit sex partners from places far away are more likely to have higher numbers of partners (Calzavara et al., 1998; Jolly & Wylie, 2013). Less prompt care and follow up between jurisdictions facilitates longer infectious periods and complicates partner notification (Wylie & Jolly, 2001).

Ethnic group, like marital status, has been omitted in some jurisdictions. However, it is useful because it may be tied to funding. First Nations people living on and off reserve, as well as the Inuit, bear a disproportionately high burden of infectious disease. This is often due to lack of public health infrastructures like sewage disposal and clean drinking water (Rosenberg et al., 1997). Documenting this is helpful in justifying adequate public health funding.

Aliases are useful in two instances: (1) street people and sex workers; and (2) internet dating. Including street people and sex worker aliases allows for use by outreach workers. Internet dating sites are useful in locating clients and partners for follow up. An alternate method of contact is provided for people who are on the streets. This field contains an answer to a question such as: "Is there anyone in your life with whom you check in periodically or who knows where you are?" These can be family members from another province, social workers, close friends, or foster parents. This can be very helpful in urgent cases (for example, a follow up for TB). Also worth mentioning is the variable to capture whether the index case or partner was aggressive or reported violence toward sex partners or healthcare workers.

The names of the people interviewing the client, or entering the data, and accompanying dates, are essential in the quality assurance process. An indicator field denoting whether the case was reported to the federal government is also helpful and can be generated from an algorithm of other entries to match federal case definitions.

Information on Each Infection Episode or Event "Case"

Table 3 details the information required for each event, linked by the unique case identification number (Figure 1). Although these elements are tailored to STIs, the variables can be used for water- or food-borne

Table 2. Basic demographic information of individuals with notifiable diseases

Variable	Special Information	Rationale for collection
Individual identification number	One unique key for each individual linking infection episode (case) tables related to that individual	1, 2, 4
Personal health insurance number	Select entry from provincial insurance registry file or populated from the LIS. This number can be linked with physician billing hospital discharge abstracts and other records for cohort studies.	1, 2, 4
Last name	Populated by LIS, provincial insurance or notifiable disease registry, select or auto fill	1, 2, 4
First name	Populated by LIS, provincial insurance or notifiable disease registry, select or auto fill	1, 2, 4
Middle name	Populated by LIS, provincial insurance or notifiable disease registry, select or auto fill	1, 2, 4
Sex	Populated by LIS, provincial insurance or notifiable disease registry, pick list or auto fill, must enter	1, 2, 4
Date of birth	Select or auto fill from LIS, provincial insurance or notifiable disease registry	1, 4, 5
Ethnic group	Pick list, align with population groups in Canada for which special funding is available	1, 2, 3, 4,5
Language note	Pick list, if client requires translation services	1, 4, 5
Alias surname	Select or auto fill from LIS, provincial insurance or notifiable disease registry; names on internet dating site	1, 4, 5
Alias given name	Select or auto fill from LIS, provincial insurance or notifiable disease registry; names on internet dating site	1, 2, 4
Apartment/Condo #	Select or auto fill from LIS, provincial insurance or notifiable disease registry	1
Street address	Populated by LIS, provincial insurance or notifiable disease registry, select or auto fill	1, 2
City	Populated by LIS, provincial insurance or notifiable disease registry, select or auto fill Lookup tables based on province	1, 2, 4, 5
E-mail		1
No fixed address	Move frequently, couch surf, use shelters, on the street	1, 3, 4, 5
Phone number		1
Postal code	Populated by LIS, provincial insurance or notifiable disease registry, select or auto fill Six digit postcodes map onto Statistics Canada's dissemination areas, small units of about 600 people or 200 households, for which detailed health and socioeconomic ecological data are available useful for planning interventions	2, 3, 4
Province	Populated by LIS, provincial insurance or notifiable disease registry, pick list, auto fill	1, 2, 5
Country	Pick list	1, 2
Health region	Pick list generated by city, town	1, 2, 5
Health unit	Pick list generated by city, town	1, 2, 5
Alternative locating information	Name and address of important person	1, 3, 4, 5
Interview date	Date of interview with public health nurse	1, 4, 5
Interviewer	Name of public health nurse who completed interview, pick list	1, 4, 5
Safety concerns	Does the case show signs of violence toward sex partners or public health workers?	1, 4, 5
Clerk who entered data	Pick list or auto fill based on login	1, 2, 3, 4, 5
Date record entered	Current date or auto fill based on login	1, 2, 3, 4, 5
Date record edited	Current date	1, 2, 3, 4, 5
User who edited record	Auto fill based on login	1, 2, 3, 4, 5
Case reported federally	May be an automatic feature based on the clinical case definition; Only those fields required for national disease surveillance may be reported	1, 2, 3, 4, 5

infections, such as salmonella. For example, variables on numbers of sex partners can be used to report how many ill people surrounded this case. Variables for sexual health recommendations can be adapted to detail hand washing and food safety education. Detailed symptom lists are helpful for distinguishing between enteric pathogens, as is duration of symptoms.

People may present to a healthcare provider and be tested for a variety of reasons. Therefore, conditions such as pregnancy are important to note so as to prioritize follow up for the client. Table 3 includes data relevant to each event. For this reason, other variables (i.e., patient's self-identified gender), which can change over time, are also included. To this end, the question "Do you have sex with men, women, or both?" focuses on the sexual interaction, rather than the sexual identity, of the client. In many jurisdictions, symptoms are recorded as being absent or present. For several reasons, it is crucial to be specific: (1) the patient may be unfamiliar with them; (in listing them, the healthcare provider is actually educating the patient); (2) symptoms may be the primary reason for testing; or (3) they are one of the few variables essential in evaluating patient care and prevention.

Table 3. Case table containing health provider visit, diagnosis, clinical, test, and treatment information

Variable	Special Information	Rationale for Collection
Episode number	Generated by the system based on the individual's unique key and dates of last episode.	1, 2, 4, 5
Case and contact indicator	Defines an individual as a confirmed case and/or whether he/she was named as a contact.	1, 2, 4, 5
Apartment/Condo #	Select or auto fill from LIS, provincial insurance or notifiable disease registry	1
Street address	Populated by LIS, provincial insurance or notifiable disease registry, select or auto fill	1, 2
City	Populated by LIS, provincial insurance or notifiable disease registry, look up tables based on province	1, 2, 4, 5
Physician billing code/Nursing practice license number or code	Select or auto fill from LIS	1, 2, 3, 4
Facility/clinic where patient visited physician, nurse practitioner, nurse	Select or auto fill from LIS	1, 2, 3, 4
Attending physician, nurse practitioner, nurse	Select or auto fill from LIS	1, 2, 3, 4
Pregnant	Must enter, only if sex is female (disable if sex is male)	1, 2, 3, 4
Marital status	Spouses of people with an STI may need to be informed	1, 4
Reasons for test	Checkboxes based on recommendations for screening and diagnostic testing	2, 4, 5
Gender	How does client identify?	1, 2, 4, 5
Sexual preferences	Sex with same sex and/or opposite sex	1, 2, 4, 5
Sexual health recommendations	Generated from guidelines, based on the entries in sex behavior risks	
Disease	Select or generate from LIS test result Auto fill from electronic physician report Include congenital infections	1, 2, 3, 4, 5

continued on following page

Table 3. Continued

Variable	Special Information	Rationale for Collection
Diagnosis date	Select or auto fill from LIS Auto fill from electronic physician report	1, 2, 3, 4, 5
Symptomatic	Auto fill if any symptoms below are checked off or populated from electronic physician report, include none and unknown	1, 2, 3, 4, 5
Symptom list	Pick list	1, 2, 3, 4, 5
Symptom onset date	Must enter, include unknown	1, 2, 3, 4, 5
Duration (days)	Calculated field based on symptom onset date and physician visit or lab specimen date	1, 2, 3, 4, 5
Test for specific infection(s)	Must enter Auto fill from LIS or pick list	1, 2, 3, 4, 5
Collection date	Must enter, code for missing Auto fill from LIS or pick list	1, 2, 3, 4, 5
Result(s)	Must enter, code for missing Auto fill from LIS or pick list	1, 2, 3, 4, 5
Result date(s)	Auto fill from LIS or pick list Must enter, code for missing	1, 2, 3, 4, 5
Specimen site/type(s)	Must enter, code for missing Auto fill from LIS or pick list	1, 2, 4, 5
Date infection formally reported	Auto fill from LIS laboratory report date, or date formally received at public health Must enter, code for missing	1, 2, 3, 4
Treatment(s)	Auto fill from electronic physician report Generated based on diagnosed infection, or pick list	1, 3, 4, 5
Administration(s)	Auto fill from electronic physician report or pick list	1, 3, 4, 5
Date(s) prescribed	Auto fill from electronic physician report or calendar	1, 3, 4, 5
Dosage(s)	Pick list generated from treatment Auto fill from electronic physician report, or	1, 3, 4, 5
Per day(s)	Pick list generated from treatment or auto fill from electronic physician report, or	1, 3, 4, 5
Duration(s)	Pick list generated from treatment Auto fill from electronic physician report,	1, 3, 4, 5
Other treatment	Free text field	1, 3, 4, 5
Contact investigation method selected	Options for contact tracing; self-referral, electronic notification, provider referral, contracting, none	1, 3, 4, 5
Date selected	Calendar	1, 3, 4, 5
Safer sex and STI education provided by;	Name of public health nurse and health unit who followed up with case, to select contact investigation options	1, 3, 4, 5
Syphilis specimen taken	Testing for syphilis is recommended in some places for all patients with gonorrhoea. Ever tested, date of last test, result	1, 4, 5
HIV specimen taken	Recommended depending on sexual history, Table 4. Ever tested, date of last test, result	1, 4, 5
Receiving HAART	Pick list	1, 4, 5
If receiving HAART, TB test history	Ever tested, date of last test, result	1, 4, 5

Information on Each Contact, Exposure, and Risk Interaction

Contact tracing for STBBI and TB are the most intensive and complicated. The health care provider referral method for partner notification requires the most information as in Table 4. The elements listed are useful in STI investigations and are easily transferrable to injection equipment using partners and contacts of TB cases. The variables can be adapted for cases of food- or water-borne illness such as: type of exposure (oral/fecal, water, food); symptoms; durations; administrative follow up data; tests; and treatment. Other variables may be omitted, including type of relationship to the index case.

Table 4. Contact management data

Variable	Special Information	Rationale for Collection
Contact ID	Selected from patient registry file, notifiable disease database or LIS	1, 4, 5
Mode of transmission	Congenital or sexual	1, 4, 5
Surname	Select or auto fill from LIS, provincial insurance or notifiable disease registry	1, 4, 5
Given name	Select or auto fill from LIS, provincial insurance or notifiable disease registry	1, 4, 5
Alias surname	Select or auto fill from LIS, provincial insurance or notifiable disease registry Include names on internet dating site	1, 4, 5
Alias given name	Select or auto fill from LIS, provincial insurance or notifiable disease registry Include names on internet dating site	1, 4, 5
Date of birth	Select or auto fill from LIS, provincial insurance or notifiable disease registry	1, 4, 5
Approximate age	As above	1, 4, 5
Sex	Pick list, must enter, (allow unknown as an option)	1, 4, 5
If female, pregnant?	If known	1, 4, 5
Ethnicity	Pick list	1, 4, 5
No fixed address	Yes, no or unknown entry	1, 4, 5
Apartment/Condo #	Select or auto fill from LIS, provincial insurance or notifiable disease registry	1, 4, 5
Street address	Select or auto fill from LIS, provincial insurance or notifiable disease registry	1, 4, 5
City	Select or auto fill from LIS, provincial insurance or notifiable disease registry Look up tables based on province	1, 4, 5
Province	Pick list	1, 4, 5
Country	Pick list	1, 4, 5
Postcode	Select or auto fill from LIS, provincial insurance or notifiable disease registry	1, 4, 5
*Phone number		1, 4, 5
*E-mail address		1, 4, 5

continued on following page

Table 4. Continued

Variable	Special Information	Rationale for Collection
Alternative locating information	Name and address of important person who knows where contact is	1, 4, 5
Condom used	Condom used at all sexual encounters; some jurisdictions don't follow these contacts	1, 4, 5
Public health unit to which the referral was sent	Pick list or generated from postcode or address of contact	1, 4, 5
Type of partner referral	Health provider by telephone, in person, self-referral, contracting, electronic partner referral service, expedited partner therapy	1, 4, 5
Name of public health nurse to which contact is assigned	Pick list	1, 4, 5
Date referral sent	Date referral sent to public health unit or electronic patient note sent to contact	1, 4, 5
Located	Enter if successfully located or not For electronic self-referral, note returned or acknowledged	1, 4, 5
Date located		1, 4, 5
Relationship with contact/sex partner	Client's self-designated relationship with partner (e.g., boy/girlfriend, spouse, client, pimp)	1, 4, 5
Type of sexual contact	Perform or receive oral, anal, or vaginal sex	1, 4, 5
Exposure dates	Dates of first and last sex	1, 4, 5
Symptomatic	Must enter, include unknown Auto fill if any symptoms below are checked off or from electronic physician report	1, 2, 3, 4, 5
Symptom list	Check boxes, must enter, include unknown	1, 2, 3, 4, 5
Symptom onset date	Must enter, include unknown	1, 2, 3, 4, 5
Duration (days)	Must enter, field calculation based on symptom onset date and date of interview	1, 2, 3, 4, 5
Tested	Provided by link to LIS	1, 4, 5
Date of test		1, 4, 5
Result		1, 4, 5
Result date		1, 4, 5
Treated	Generated by fields of drug prescribed under case, above.	1, 4, 5
Date treated	Generated by fields of drug prescribed under case, above	1, 4, 5
Educational points delivered	As per regional guidelines	1, 4, 5
Contact interviewed by	Name of public health nurse who interviewed the contact	1, 4, 5
Date of interview		1, 4, 5
Place of interview	Useful if outreach is completing the investigation	1, 4, 5
If no interview, reason	Pick list	1, 4, 5
Final disposition of contact/case closed	Located, notified, tested, treated, unknown	1, 4, 5
Date case closed	If lost to follow up, closed, or open	1, 4, 5
Referred out of jurisdiction	Enter if the location of the contacts' residence is out of health region, province, or Canada	1, 4, 5
Date referred		1, 4, 5

Risk behavior and sex practices of a person may differ depending on the partner (for example, between a man and his spouse vs. the same man and a sex worker). Accordingly, safe and risky behavior interaction variables are listed for each contact in Table 4: condom use; type of sex; and relationship with partner. Generalizing this to blood-borne infections allows us to specify more precisely which partners' injection drug equipment may be shared.

Summary Risk Behavior Information

Table 4 details the reasons for recording risk interactions with each contact or partner. However, where there are many sex partners, and in order to evaluate STI testing recommendations, it may be useful to collect more general indicators of engagement in risk practices (see Table 5). Unlike the contents of previous tables, these variables are relevant only for sexually transmitted or blood-borne infections.

Places of Exposure

The role of venues in the transmission of infectious disease extend to food-borne illnesses at community events or restaurants, tuberculosis in shelters and bars, and HIV in prisons and bath houses.(D'Angelo-Scott, Cutler, Friedman, Hendriks, & Jolly, 2015; De, Singh, Wong, Yacoub, & Jolly, 2004; Gardy et al., 2011; Klovdahl, 1985; Klovdahl et al., 2001; Logan, Jolly, & Blanford, 2016). Elements in Table 6 are required to adequately investigate source places (Table 1, rationales 1, 4, and 5).

COMPILATION AND DISSEMINATION OF SURVEILLANCE DATA

Surveillance is a balance between accuracy, completeness, and timeliness, in which a certain amount of completeness and accuracy are sacrificed in the interests of time. Fortunately, inaccuracies and incompleteness are often systemic and recurring, so that numbers of infections calculated over time are uniformly affected. For example, in a province or territory there may be laboratories which don't report cases. If this is ongoing, the surveillance data will obviously be incomplete; but it will be consistent. Thus, reasonable conclusions are still drawn about trends over time. Also, multiple laboratory reports on a single episode or event may occur despite our best attempts at deduplication. However, these usually recur at a constant rate, so that a similar proportion of duplicates reports each week do not necessarily disguise general trends. The most important indicator of unusual occurrence in infection incidence is *relative* change in weekly numbers, rather than absolute numbers.

The timing of compilation for reports is an important decision. Weekly reporting is a standard in the United States, where the most significant advances in surveillance have been made (Brammer et al., 2002). One week may be too short for cases to accumulate in many smaller areas. Yet monthly reporting is inadequate as whole outbreaks may occur without detection. A compromise may be reporting every two weeks, recognizing the possible insensitivity of the system and recognizing the challenge low numbers of events. It would certainly be worth conferring with a statistician to define methods if numbers are small over short periods of time. One of these methods is to smooth the weekly totals using a three week moving average. The outbreak threshold can be calculated by averaging the mean of the current week and the previous two weeks, then adding twice the standard deviation for all weeks on record. If no historical weekly data are available at the start of the surveillance system, six months lag

Table 5. STBBI risk behavior

Variable	Special Information	Rationale for Collection
Frequency of condom use	Use one or more standard measures of condom use, such as condom use at last sex	1, 4, 5
Reasons for condom use	Checklist and one free text field for "other" factors influencing the client to use condoms or ask that they be used	1, 4, 5
Number of partners	Number of partners over an average year, six months, month or week	1, 4, 5
Partners out of country	Number of partners from countries other than Canada	1, 4, 5
Client's self-rated risk of STI (non-HIV)	Standard scale from national health and social surveys	1, 4, 5
Syphilis specimen taken	Ever tested, date of last test, result	1, 4, 5
HIV specimen taken	Ever tested, date of last test, result	1, 4, 5
Receiving HAART	Pick list	1, 4, 5
If receiving HAART, TB test history	Ever tested, date of last test, result	1, 4, 5
Last STI history	Ever tested, date of last test, result	1, 4, 5
Survival sex	Ever accepted food, shelter, gifts, or other necessities for sex	1, 4, 5
Drugs for sex		1, 4, 5
Alcohol for sex		1, 4, 5
Ever injected drugs	Injection drug use (even in the distant past) may indicate risk of HCV, HIV	1, 4, 5
Recent injection drug use	Use standard measures for alcohol measures from Canadian Alcohol and Drug Use Monitoring Survey	1, 4, 5
Recent hard, non-injection drug use	As above	1, 4, 5
Recent non-injection drug use	As above	1, 4, 5
Casual or frequent use of marijuana	As above	1, 4, 5
Alcohol use patterns	As above	1, 4, 5
Alcohol during sex		1, 4, 5
Injection drugs just before sex		1, 4, 5
Non-injection hard drugs just before sex		1, 4, 5
Marijuana during sex		1, 4, 5
Syphilis test history	Ever tested, date of last test, result	1, 4, 5
HIV test history	Ever tested, date of last test, result	1, 4, 5
Receiving HAART	Pick list	1, 4, 5
If receiving HAART, TB test history	Ever tested, date of last test, result	1, 4, 5

time will allow sufficient data to accumulate so as to measure expected weekly totals against weekly observations. Another option is to combine regional data so that there are sufficient numbers. This is desirable not only for surveillance but control of many communicable infections, which, like their hosts, frequently cross administrative boundaries. Contact tracing and referral of cases and exposures across

Table 6. Locations

Variable	Special Information	Rationale for Collection
Location ID	Unique computer-generated identification number	1, 4, 5
Name	Auto look-up in registry for previous entries	1, 4, 5
Closest cross streets	One or more sets of cross streets	1, 4, 5
Location type	e.g. Bar, restaurant, bath house, prison, hospital	1, 4, 5
Apartment or unit number		1, 4, 5
Number of building on street		1, 4, 5
Street name		1, 4, 5
City	Pick list, depending on Province	1, 4, 5
Province	Pick list	1, 4, 5
Country	Pick list	1, 4, 5
Postcode		1, 4, 5
Phone number		1, 4, 5
E-mail address		1, 4, 5
Website	Copy and paste	1, 4, 5
Travel history	Places and dates	1, 4, 5
Additional information	Notes	1, 4, 5

jurisdictional boundaries may delay prompt treatment and source investigations, amply demonstrated in research findings. (D'Angelo-Scott et al., 2015; A. Jolly & Wylie, 2013; Wylie & Jolly, 2001) It should be noted that during outbreaks more frequent tabulations can be made.

A key concept in disseminating surveillance data, particularly during outbreaks, is that of reporting delay. Most communicable disease data are graphed by date of onset to most accurately depict events relative to exposure to the source. Of course there are delays in reporting diagnoses; seeking medical attention, specimen transit time to the lab, specimen processing and reporting results to the health authority. When reviewing the graphs or tables of cases or rates over time, it is absolutely crucial that interpretation of trends allow for this reporting delay. Figure 2, courtesy of Dena Schanzer, shows daily reports of influenza by date of onset which appear to decline. This is due to the fact that reports in the previous month have not yet been received (in grey), thereby producing a gross underestimate of the true numbers of cases. More accurate representation can be generated by graphing cases by report date, or by correcting current data for known reporting delays. This will prevent premature conclusions that outbreaks are over resulting in removal of prevention measures, and subsequent illness and loss of life. (Campbell, 2006)

It is also important to note the quality of the statistical tests performed. The repeated measurement of the mean and two standard deviations is subject to random error and will inevitably exceed the expected number of cases 5% of the time. However, the first step in outbreak investigation - to confirm that an outbreak exists - will resolve false positives. Preliminary checks are recommended to rule out data entry errors or unusually high numbers of duplicates. Indications of an outbreak include cases clustered in

Figure 2. Courtesy of Dena Schanzer, M.Sc., P. Stat

Reporting Delay Illustration

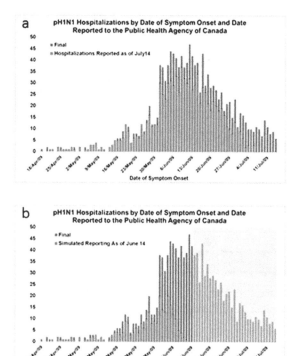

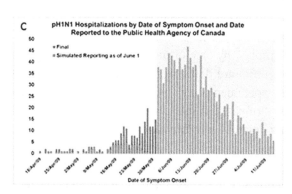

Hospitalizations with laboratory confirmed A(H1N1)pdm09 influenza plotted by date of symptom onset to illustrate the impact of reporting delays. The final epidemic curve for the spring wave from the first case on April 18, 2009 to July 14, 2009 is plotted against the number of cases reported to the Public Health Agency of Canada as of a) July 14th , b) June 14th and c) June 1st. a) July 14th corresponds to a period between the first and second wave, and the near real time epidemic curve shown in blue appears somewhat similar to the final curve shown in red. b) June 14th corresponds to approximately the peak the spring wave; a time when hospitals had considerable case load. Notice that the raw epidemic curve based on reported cases seems to suggest that the epidemic had peaked earlier in the month and was winding down with the approach of summer. c) June 1st corresponds to time when hospitals should have been preparing for a significant increase in case load. Instead the raw epidemic curve based on reported cases suggests that the spring was is winding down as summer approaches.

The most recent epidemic curves for hospitalizations, ICU admissions and deaths were posted by Public Health Agency of Canada throughout the pandemic period. The epidemic curves for June 14th and June 1st were simulated based on the reporting delay estimates.

one area of the jurisdiction, family names, ages, genders, exposures, risk factors or any combination of the above. If these findings are inconclusive, further investigation is indicated.

A weekly report of no more than three pages should be distributed to medical officers of health, infectious disease specialists, public health units and their staff, public health inspectors, statistical and data entry clerks, laboratory staff, and epidemiologists by secure e-mails, websites, or programmable fax machines. Two or three paragraphs may introduce the salient points of the report. The first might contain whether and which infections surpassed the mean and two standard deviations, the age ranges of cases, and general geographic area. The second could contain new information on strain types, unusual organisms identified, and their sources. A table should contain a list of notifiable infections, the number of cases reported in the current week, and the number expected (the outbreak threshold of the mean and two standard deviations). Unexpectedly high numbers of cases should be highlighted; comparisons to raw weekly or year-to-date totals are insufficient. If numbers are higher than expected, a preliminary description of the cases can be included with a graph showing the numbers of cases over time charted with the epidemic threshold.

An ideal situation was exemplified in Manitoba during laboratory based monitoring of infectious disease during the period 1996 to 1998. Data were extracted from the LIS every night in an automated download, imported into Epi Info v 6.04, frequencies compiled, and imported into MS Excel, where the final table was created. The reports were completed in the early afternoon of each Friday and disseminated. In one instance, positive results for giardia exceeded the threshold, affecting people in and around a small town following an unusually early thaw. The medical officer of health read the report, consulted with the epidemiologist and the director of the parasitology division, and issued a boil water order the next day (Saturday). There was a satellite cancer treatment center located in the town which immediately started providing bottled water to patients. The environmental health officer in the region confirmed that the particulates in the water were so high that an adequate volume of water could not be pumped through to test for *Giardia lamblia*. Further cases decreased over time subsequent to the boil water order.

In summary, we present a simple method of surveillance. With faster computing, evolving programming languages, and improved database software, more is certainly possible. However, given the erosion of public health resources, this basic minimum meets the obligations for surveillance under the public health acts in Canada.

EVALUATION OF SURVEILLANCE DATA AND PATIENT CARE

Consistent with the goal of providing appropriate care to patients with notifiable infections, regular programmed audits for inappropriate therapies, doses, routes and durations should be conducted. In the cases of TB and bacterial STI, routine assessments are all the more important in preventing and managing antimicrobial resistance. In at least two jurisdictions in Canada reminder letters to physicians who prescribed inappropriate therapies were routine through the 1980's and 90's. Ideally, the system could generate these letters from the individual's laboratory and treatment information, if it is linked to the registry of physicians authorized to receive payment under the provincial health insurance system. Reminder letters are particularly helpful in the treatment of bacterial STI and TB as they may elucidate possible misunderstandings of treatment guidelines or better define delays in implementation. They are also useful in educating physicians and health providers about management guidelines, which are rapidly changing.

Monitoring the disposition of clients and cases investigated is essential in documenting investigation status with respect to the source of infection, and quality of public health care received. With sexually transmitted, blood borne infections and tuberculosis, the number of contacts nominated, located, tested and treated are the measures of contact tracing effectiveness. (Iskrant & Khan, 1948; Rothenberg et al., 2003) Sources of food- water- and air-borne infections may never be conclusively defined, but the fact that a food questionnaire was sent; a well water sample was tested; or humidifier tests were completed provide concrete measures of public health activities and discharge of legal obligations. Delays in access to care and public health follow up can lead to long durations of infectiousness. At minimum, we recommend annual checks on (1) the delays between symptom onset and physician visit or specimen sampling date; (2) time elapsed between the date specimen taken and the date it was received at the lab; and (3) the time elapsed between the date a specimen is received at the lab and the date the results are reported to public health. Once public health authorities are notified of a case, delays between the receipt of the case report and referral to public health field staff to interview the person for contacts or sources, and the time between elicitation of contacts and their and notification and subsequent management should be monitored. Finally, primary data entry should be kept to a minimum. However, in jurisdictions where clerks are entering most of the data, monthly tabulations of error rates are recommended.

SECONDARY SURVEILLANCE AND CASE MANAGEMENT GOALS

Social Network Analysis

This technique has become more common in investigation of infections transmitted from person to person. A network is a group of people, items or locations connected by relationships or interactions. In the case of STI, each person is connected to his or her contacts by sexual intercourse. In contact tracing for TB, cases may be linked by time spent together in enclosed spaces and injection drug users, by sharing equipment. In addition, people may also be linked with places where risk activity took place, such as bars, shooting galleries, bath houses or homeless shelters. Social network analysis is most commonly used in STBBI and TB to define social interactions over time which may transmit infection between people, thus tracing all nominated source (upstream) and spread (downstream) cases and contacts. Disease investigation specialists from the CDC had already formulated the basic concept of drawing the likely transmission routes between interrelated cases. (Potterat et al., 1985) Social network analysis provided more rigorous interview methods, (Brewer D.D., 1999)(Brewer et al., 2005) together with measures denoting activity, such as number of people exposed by a particular case (degree centrality); importance defined by weighted path lengths between all in the network, (information centrality) (De et al., 2004) and parts of the network in which people are connected by more links than others (k-cores). (A S Klovdahl et al., 2001; Alden S Klovdahl, 1985) Its application has facilitated improved understanding of the context of transmission, crucial in improving prevention strategies. (Case et al., 2013; D'Angelo-Scott et al., 2015; De et al., 2004)

We have included all the data required to construct social networks in the tables above; specifically; single unique identifiers for cases, contacts and venues to minimize duplicate records; exposure and relationship types; timing of exposures; and clear links between records of cases and contacts, and between cases and venues. Construction of sexual or social networks for most social network software, such as Pajek, (Mrvar & Batagelj, n.d.) involves creating a single list of all cases, contacts and venues, with new, positive, consecutive numbers for use by the social network software. Obviously this list may contain contacts who became cases, and contacts who have been named multiple times; so standardization of names or record linkage is important. Individuals may be distinguished using their notification numbers or names, for ease of identification by public health staff. At minimum, case, contact, sex, and test status (positive, negative, untested or unknown) should accompany the identifying case data. Then a list of pairwise links is compiled using all the cases' named contacts and venues. The whole network or graph is then constructed in the social network software. This process can be automated such that drawings and reports of activity are updated and shared. We recommend routine construction of networks. Monthly reviews will suffice to identify contacts who have been named multiple times and are still presumably untreated. Cases with reinfections may also require testing more frequently in order to pre-empt long infectious periods. The proportions of reinfected cases and multiply named contacts is usually less than 10% of all individuals, facilitating enhanced interventions with a small group of people to great effect. (A. M. Jolly, Moffatt, Fast, & Brunham, 2005; A. M. Jolly & Wylie, 2001)

Detection of Infection Clusters in Space

Monitoring the occurrence of infection in geographic space is a natural extension of surveillance as cases are described by person, place, and time, in order to define common characteristics, which may indicate cause. Geography is intrinsic to epidemiologic investigation, amply demonstrated in the first infectious disease outbreak investigation of cholera by Dr. John Snow.(Snow, 1855) Places are important in almost all notifiable infections. Residences of cases are usually clustered around sources of contaminated water; food, air, and concentrations of infected vectors can also be narrowed down using residential information. Accordingly, we have listed all the location variables relevant to surveillance by place. The most obvious of these are patient and contact addresses; travel histories, social venues and other places of exposure including hospitals and prisons.

Software for identifying clusters of concentrated cases in space is available and free. SatScan requires the translation of street addresses into latitude and longitude, or "geocoding". (Kulldorff, 2015) Weekly or monthly tabulations of total cases and population statistics for defined geographic areas are used to build a model of proportionate numbers of cases expected if they were randomly distributed in space and/or time. Deviation from the expected, random, distribution reveals statistically significant clusters or concentrations of cases in space and or time which require investigation, but should not be considered as confirming the existence of an outbreak. Both cases and population counts can be stratified by age group and sex.

It is worth emphasizing here the importance of the full, six-character postcode; the smallest area in Canada for which census data are available. All postcodes are somewhat contiguous with Statistics Canada dissemination areas, except a small proportion mostly in rural areas (Statistics Canada, 2011). If postcodes of cases are complete and accurate, relatively fine-grained estimates of unusually high numbers of cases can be accurately detected. For example, clusters of people with unusually high rates of Lyme disease may be compared with areas of high concentrations of the vector.

Recent research has demonstrated the value of collecting geospatial information of people with sexually transmitted and blood borne infections. Social networks of street people selling sex and injecting drugs, among other things, were asked to list the places they lived; spent leisure time and engaged in risky activities; such as bars, shooting galleries and bath houses. Geographical analysis revealed that the mean distance between locations was 3.5 km, a relatively small space in which interventions could be focused. Additionally, people not directly nominated in each others' networks and who are likely to have anonymous sex, or pick up used drug equipment are included by virtue of colocation. Where specific venues are difficult to identify, the nearest cross streets may be used with success. (Logan, Jolly, & Blanford, 2016)

Virtual space has played a key role in recent outbreaks of syphilis, particularly in men who have sex with men. Both internet dating sites and physical places are important, as individuals may arrange online to meet up for sex at a specific location such as a bath house. (D'Angelo-Scott et al., 2015) For this reason websites, emails, phone numbers and online aliases have been included to assist in investigations.

Detection of Onset of Seasonal Infections

All the data required for calculating the start of the respiratory virus season is already included in the above tables; the most obvious being the dates of; onset, laboratory test result, or notification. Respiratory viruses are not usually notifiable, so any surveillance is usually done by using laboratory data only, with the exception of sentinel surveillance for physician visits of influenza like illness. Counts of laboratory test results for respiratory infections are used in calculating the mean and twice the standard deviation for all weeks over the years. When the upper threshold is exceeded, this indicates the start of the flu season. Such an indicator is helpful to physicians in diagnosing the flu within the mix of respiratory viruses at the start of the season. Note that monitoring positive laboratory tests of respiratory viruses especially influenza, are only part of what have become sophisticated influenza surveillance programs. Assessing the severity of one 'flu season over others should include only data from the winter months. Other infections with seasonal incidence patterns which could be monitored similarly include such pathogenic *E. coli*, and other food-borne bacteria, and water borne infections such as Shigella *spp* and giardia.

Antimicrobial Resistance Surveillance

Although there are some intricacies to monitoring antimicrobial resistance surveillance, it can be incorporated to some extent within a notifiable disease database. One of the differences is that resistant organisms are usually reported as a percentage of the total number of all isolated at the lab, rather than by population. If laboratory methods are standardized and the denominator is consistent over time it may be easier to incorporate it within the existing notifiable disease data than establishing a whole new system. Variables denoting standard panels of antimicrobials against which bacteria are tested at the lab(s), can easily be added to Table 3, along with minimum inhibitory concentrations. As above, recommended treatment algorithms can be programmed based on these indicators of reduced susceptibility. Other variables may be created for recording antimicrobial resistance detected by genetic sequencing of pathogens, and together with the denominator of all sequenced, can be used to develop a comprehensive overview of resistance trends over time.

Notifiable Diseases Requiring Immediate Attention

In smaller jurisdictions it may be unthinkable that illnesses which require prompt action or are reportable federally or internationally within short periods of time, are neglected. But in larger places with many different people working in communicable disease control it is advisable to build in alerts which appear once a record is saved. Examples of infections reportable to WHO include smallpox, wild type poliomyelitis, influenza in humans caused by a new subtype, SARS, cholera, pneumonic plaque, yellow fever, viral haemorrhagic fevers (Ebola, Lassa Marburg and West Nile), and others of concern in a WHO region, (dengue, Rift Valley fever, and meningococcal disease.) The inclusion of smallpox and haemorrhagic fevers is to address possible bioweapons attacks; these are thought to be the most likely pathogens in that event. (World Health Organisation, 2005). Due to their virulence and urgent need to administer immune globulin, alerts in the cases of animal bites, measles and tetanus, are also valuable.

Each jurisdiction may have different timelines for reporting different infections so incorporating this into the alert algorithm will be useful.

Special Surveillance Systems

Specialised surveillance of reinfections; strains, changes in risk behavior, modes of transmission, within the context of notifiable disease, is possible using variables provided in the tables, and a few additional ones.

Reinfections of bacterial STI are useful indicators of possible failures in the medical and or public health system, or of patients requiring intensive intervention. Repeated reinfections with chlamydia, for example, often indicate a patient whose partner(s) remain untreated. Delayed treatment of the partner can result in "ping pong" infections in which the index case is cured, and resumes sex with her partner, who is yet untreated. Once he is treated, he can contract infection from her a second time hence the name "ping pong" where the infection transmits back and forth. Inadequate treatment may be another reason for apparent reinfection. Recently, reinfection with syphilis in men who have sex with men, usually anonymously, in whom coinfection with HIV is common, indicates membership in a very high risk, active group with whom we have to engage constructively. A variable indicating reinfections within certain periods of time, usually 12 months, can be generated from entries in the episode table from test result dates, and added to the Table 2, after the episode number.

Strain surveillance, like antimicrobial resistance surveillance, can be accomplished by adding variables in Table 3 to designate strain types. A common example of this is the subtyping of salmonella, allowing us to count salmonella infections, but those associated with different subtypes. Obviously, the inclusion of subtypes in surveillance results is a far more accurate system to detect unusually high incidences. As each subtype is associated with birds, fish, or reptiles this can be immensely helpful in preliminary exposure questionnaires. Strain surveillance may be helpful in detecting evolutionary adaptation of organisms to evade antimicrobials, particularly in HIV and hepatitis C. Historically, certain strains have been associated with modes of transmission in certain subpopulations, and deviations in proportions of these may indicate changes in modes of transmission.

Variables to assess changes in risk behavior and modes of transmission are included in the tables above. The fact that they are associated with other data constitutes a valuable epidemiological tool. For example, proportions of syphilis infections in sex workers compared with those occurring in men who have sex with men, can calculated from the above variables. Changes in proportions over time may indicate shifts in trends, and explain changes in population incidence. Likewise, changes in modes of transmission for different infections can be assessed from percentages of cases transmitted in certain ways, Table 4 variable 2. Annual tables with summary data on the proportion of each risk behavior and mode of transmission contributing to total cases should be compiled.

Monitoring of vaccine coverage is best done through immunization record systems. However, it is valuable to add or link the vaccine history of people infected with vaccine preventable illness. These data can be found within vaccine registry systems; if the client is unvaccinated, vaccine administration should be included as part of follow up including thorough tracing of contacts. Variables on vaccine history can be added to Tables 2 and 3, with vaccines administered; lot numbers, health provider registration or billing numbers, and dates. Additionally it is good practice to include recommended vaccines within the management of people who have risk behaviours, or may contract co infections, such as verifying receipt of hepatitis B vaccine in those injecting drugs or those having unsafe sex, who have not already been vaccinated.

Hospital acquired infections may be monitored if they are notifiable in the jurisdiction. In some jurisdictions antimicrobial resistant organisms are notifiable, like vancomycin resistant enterococcus, and methicillin resistant *Staphloccocus aureus*. However, as with strain and antimicrobial resistance, denominator data of patient days or proportions of patients admitted are not available and so notifiable disease records can only supplement formal hospital based surveillance systems. (Canadian Hospital Epidemiology Committee, 2012) Results of investigations into exposure, contact and location included above, will facilitate monitoring. Health care acquired infections may become more important to track in the community due to ready exchange of genetic material between bacteria within and outside of hospitals, and continued use of antimicrobials as growth stimulants in feed animals. Similar to the above, compilations of weekly or monthly totals of people with specific strains and/or with susceptibility profiles of certain organisms can be totaled and compared with numbers from previous periods. This can be done in combination with source and exposure data to determine the relative proportion of community acquired and hospital acquired infection.

We have presented a comprehensive outline of a notifiable disease database which includes the modern realities of changing risk factors; assists active investigation, supports good public health practice, and facilitates sophisticated analyses. In addition, it is designed to be robust, flexible, fast, cheap, all of which are in essential in preventing infectious disease transmission. We have demonstrated how specialized surveillance systems can be operated within the notifiable disease collection process, and supplement other systems with routine counts of expected and unusually high numbers.

SUMMARY AND CONCLUSION

Reporting and monitoring infections of public health importance is as relevant today as it was in the days of smallpox. Pathogens develop resistance to antimicrobials and new infections emerge; we can meet the challenge. We have a legal mandate, duty of care and institutional processes to collect complete, accurate, relevant data to monitor and investigate infectious disease. We need sufficient, stable sources of funding and educated public health staff free to act objectively and scientifically in the interests of the public. In our favor, laboratory diagnostic techniques have vastly improved, as have electronic means of data collection and dissemination. Investing in the infrastructure for surveillance of notifiable diseases will serve us well against emerging and re-emerging infections, rather than spending resources on short term, ad hoc systems which only temporarily address public concerns.

REFERENCES

Alberta Health. (2013). *Public Health Notifiable Disease Management Guidelines; Measles*. Retrieved 21 January 2017 from http://www.health.alberta.ca/documents/Guidelines-Measles-2013.pdf

Alberta Health. (2014). *Public health notifiable disease management guidelines; salmonellosis*. Retrieved from http://www.health.alberta.ca/documents/Guidelines-Salmonellosis-2014.pdf

BC Enteric Policy Working Group. (2007). *Enteric diseases requiring follow-up in BC and standard follow-forms*. Retrieved from http://www.bccdc.ca/resource-gallery/Documents/Guidelines and Forms/ Guidelines and Manuals/Epid/CD Manual/Chapter 6 - SCD/BC enteric disease prioritisation_2007.pdf

Brammer, T., Murray, E., Fukuda, K., Hall, H., Klimov, A., & Cox, N. (2002). Surveillance for influenza; United States 1997/98, 1998/99, and 1999 to 2000 seasons. *Morbidity & Mortality Weekly Report, 51*(SS07), 1–10. Retrieved from https://www.cdc.gov/mmwr/preview/mmwrhtml/ss5107a1.htm PMID:12418623

Brewer, D. D. (2002). Supplementary Interviewing Techniques to Maximize Output in Free Listing Tasks. *Field Methods, 14*(1), 108–118. doi:10.1177/1525822X02014001007

Brewer, D. D. (2005). Case-finding effectiveness of partner notification and cluster investigation for sexually transmitted diseases/HIV. *Sexually Transmitted Diseases, 32*(2), 78–83. doi:10.1097/01.olq.0000153574.38764.0e PMID:15668612

Brewer, D. D., Garrett, S. B., & Kulasingam, S. (1999). Forgetting as a cause of incomplete reporting of sexual and drug injection partners. *Sexually Transmitted Diseases, 26*(3), 166–176. doi:10.1097/00007435-199903000-00008 PMID:10100775

Brewer, D. D., Potterat, J. J., Muth, S. Q., Malone, P. Z., Montoya, P., Green, D. L., … Cox, P. A. (2005). Randomized trial of supplementary interviewing techniques to enhance recall of sexual partners in contact interviews. *Sexually Transmitted Diseases, 32*(3), 189–193.

Brewer, D. D., & Webster, C. M. (1999). Forgetting of friends and its effect on measuring friendship networks. *Social Networks, 21*(4), 361–373. doi:10.1016/S0378-8733(99)00018-0

British Columbia. (2016). *Public Health Act.* Vancouver, Canada: British Columbia.

Calzavara, L. M., Burchell, A. N., Myers, T., Bullock, S. L., Escobar, M., & Cockerill, R. (1998). Condom use among Aboriginal people in Ontario, Canada. *International Journal of STD & AIDS, 9*(5), 272–279. doi:10.1258/0956462981922205 PMID:9639205

Campbell, A. (2004). The SARS Commission Interim Report: SARS and Public Health in Ontario' What went right. *Biosecurity and Bioterrorism: Biodefence Strategy, Practice and Science, 2*(2), 118–126.

Campbell, A. (2006). *The SARS Commission; the spring of fear.* Retrieved from http://www.archives.gov.on.ca/en/e_records/sars/report/v1-pdf/Volume1.pdf

Canadian Hospital Epidemiology Committee. (2012). *The Canadian Nosocomial Infection Surveillance Program.* Retrieved from http://www.phac-aspc.gc.ca/nois-sinp/survprog-eng.php

Case, C., Kandola, K., Chui, L., Li, V., Nix, N., & Johnson, R. (2013). Examining DNA fingerprinting as an epidemiology tool in the tuberculosis program in the Northwest Territories, Canada. *International Journal of Circumpolar Health, 72*(1), 1–8. doi:10.3402/ijch.v72i0.20067 PMID:23671837

Centers for Disease Control and Prevention. (2001). Updated U.S. Public Health Service Guidelines for the Management of Occupational Exposures to HBV, HCV, and HIV and Recommendations for Postexposure Prophylaxis. *Morbidity and Mortality Weekly Report, 50*(RR11), 1–42. PMID:11442229

Centers for Disease Control and Prevention. (2006). Guide to confirming an etiology in a foodborne disease outbreak. *Morbidity & Mortality Weekly Report, 49*(SS-1).

Chorba, T. L., Berkelman, R. L., Safford, S. K., Gibbs, N. P., & Hull, H. F. (1989). Mandatory reporting of infectious diseases by clinicians. *Journal of the American Medical Association, 262*(21), 3018–3026. doi:10.1001/jama.1989.03430210060031 PMID:2810646

Commonwealth of Australia. National Health Security Act 2007, Pub. L. No. 174. (2010). Retrieved from https://www.legislation.gov.au/Details/C2013C00147

Communicable Disease Network Australia. (2015a). *Protocol for making a change to the national notifiable disease list in Australia.* Retrieved January 4, 2017, from http://www.health.gov.au/internet/main/publishing.nsf/Content/ohp-protocol-NNDL-list.htm

Communicable Disease Network Australia. (2015b). *Protocol for making a change to the national notifiable diseases list (NNDL) in Australia.* Retrieved 21 Jnauary 2017 from http://www.health.gov.au/internet/main/publishing.nsf/Content/8DF6148BCAC589D6CA257EE5001D0DF7/$File/Protocol-change-NNDL.pdf

Cook, V. J., Shah, L., & Gardy, J. (2012). Modern contact investigation methods for enhancing tuberculosis control in aboriginal communities. *International Journal of Circumpolar Health, 71*(1), 18643. doi:10.3402/ijch.v71i0.18643

Cromley, E., & McLafferty, S. (2012). *GIS and Public Health* (2nd ed.). New York: The Guidford Press.

DAngelo-Scott, H., Cutler, J., Friedman, D., Hendriks, A., & Jolly, A. M. (2015). Social network investigation of a syphilis outbreak in ottawa, Ontario. *The Canadian Journal of Infectious Diseases & Medical Microbiology, 26*(5), 268–272. doi:10.1155/2015/705720 PMID:26600816

De, P., Singh, A. E., Wong, T., Yacoub, W., & Jolly, A. M. (2004). Sexual network analysis of a gonorrhoea outbreak. *Sexually Transmitted Infections, 80*(4), 280–285. doi:10.1136/sti.2003.007187 PMID:15295126

Department of Health Government of Australia. (2014). *National framework for communicable disease control.* Retrieved 21 January 2017 from http://www.health.gov.au/internet/main/publishing.nsf/Content/E5134F29919E9D74CA257CFB0082C7C5/$File/National-framework.pdf

Doherty, J. A. (2000). Establishing priorities for national communicable disease surveillance. *The Canadian Journal of Infectious Diseases, 11*(1), 21–4. Retrieved January 4 2017 from http://www.pubmedcentral.nih.gov/articlerender.fcgi?artid=2094737&tool=pmcentrez&rendertype=abstract

Doherty, J.-A. (2006). Final report snd recommendations from the national notifiable diseases working group. *Canada Communicable Disease Report, 32*(19), 211–225. PMID:17076030

Duggan, E. (2011, January). Dairy farmer to challenge raw milk rules. *Globe and Mail.* Retrieved 21 January 2017 from http://www.theglobeandmail.com/news/british-columbia/dairy-farmer-to-challenge-raw-milk-rules/article562804/

El Emam, K., Hu, J., Mercer, J., Peyton, L., Kantarcioglu, M., Malin, B., & Earle, C. et al. (2011). A secure protocol for protecting the identity of providers when disclosing data for disease surveillance. *Journal of the American Medical Informatics Association.* PMID:21486880

Flahault, A., Blanchon, T., Dorleans, Y., Toubiana, L., Vibert, J. F., & Valleron, A. J. (2006). Virtual surveillance of communicable diseases: A 20-year experience in France. *Statistical Methods in Medical Research*, *15*(5), 413–421. doi:10.1177/0962280206071639 PMID:17089946

Foege, W. H., Hogan, R. C., & Newton, L. H. (1976). Surveillance projects for selected diseases. *International Journal of Epidemiology*, *5*(1), 29–37. doi:10.1093/ije/5.1.29 PMID:944166

Gardy, J. L., Johnston, J. C., Ho Sui, S. J., Cook, V. J., Shah, L., Brodkin, E., & Tang, P. et al. (2011). Whole-genome sequencing and social-network analysis of a tuberculosis outbreak. *The New England Journal of Medicine*, *364*(8), 730–739. doi:10.1056/NEJMoa1003176 PMID:21345102

Gostin, L. O. (2000). Public health law in a new century: part I: law as a tool to advance the communitys health. *Journal of the American Medical Association*, *283*(21), 2837–2841. doi:10.1001/jama.283.21.2837 PMID:10838654

Gostin, L. O. (2004). Health of the people: The highest law?. *Journal of Law Medicine & Ethics, 32*(3), 509. http://doi.org/DOI 10.1111/j.1748-720X.2004.tb00164.x

Government of Saskatchewan. (2014a). *Communicable Disease Control Manual; Blood and body fluid pathogens; hepatitis C*. Retrieved 21 January 2017 from https://www.ehealthsask.ca/services/manuals/Documents/cdc-section-6.pdf#page=18

Government of Saskatchewan. (2014b). *Communicable Disease Control Manual; Respiratory and direct contact; measles*. Retrieved 21 January 2017 from http://www.ehealthsask.ca/services/manuals/Documents/cdc-section-2.pdf#page=87

International Association of Food Protection. (2011). *Procedures to investigate foodborne illness* (6th ed.). New York: Springer.

Iskrant, A., & Khan, H. (1948). Statistical indices used in the evaluation of syphilis contact investigation. *Journal of Venereal Disease Information*, *29*(1), 1–6. PMID:18917634

Jajosky, R. A., & Groseclose, S. L. (2004). Evaluation of reporting timeliness of public health surveillance systems for infectious diseases. *BMC Public Health*, *4*(1), 29. doi:10.1186/1471-2458-4-29 PMID:15274746

Jolly, A., & Wylie, J. L. (2013). Sexual networks and sexually transmitted infections; the strength of weak (long distance) ties. In S. O. Aral, K. A. Fenton, & J. Lipshutz (Eds.), *The New Public Health and STD/HIV Prevention: Personal, Public and Health Systems Approaches* (pp. 77–109). Springer-Verlag. doi:10.1007/978-1-4614-4526-5_5

Jolly, A. M., Moffatt, M. E. K., Fast, M. V., & Brunham, R. C. (2005). Sexually transmitted disease thresholds in Manitoba, Canada. *Annals of Epidemiology*, *15*(10), 781–788. doi:10.1016/j.annepidem.2005.05.001 PMID:16168671

Jolly, A. M., & Wylie, J. L. (2001). Sampling individuals with large sexual networks - An evaluation of four approaches. *Sexually Transmitted Diseases*, *28*(4), 200–207. doi:10.1097/00007435-200104000-00003 PMID:11318250

Kirby Institute for infection and immunity in society 2015. (2015). *HIV, viral hepatitis and sexually transmitted infections in Australia; annual surveillance report 2015*. Retrieved 21 January 2015 from http://kirby.unsw.edu.au/sites/default/files/hiv/resources/NBBVSTI%20Surveillance%20and%20Monitoring%20Report%202015_0.pdf

Klovdahl, A. S. (1985). Social networks and the spread of infectious diseases: The AIDS example. *Social Science & Medicine, 21*(11), 1203–1216. doi:10.1016/0277-9536(85)90269-2 PMID:3006260

Klovdahl, A. S., Graviss, E. A., Yaganehdoost, A., Ross, M. W., Wanger, A., Adams, G. J., & Musser, J. M. (2001). Networks and tuberculosis: An undetected community outbreak involving public places. *Social Science & Medicine, 52*(5), 681–694. doi:10.1016/S0277-9536(00)00170-2 PMID:11218173

Kulldorff, B. M. (2015). *SaTScan User Guide V9.4*. Retrieved 21 January 2017 from http://www.unc.edu/~emch/gisph/SaTScan.pdf

Langmuir, A. (1963). The surveillance of communicable diseases of public health importance. *The New England Journal of Medicine, 268*(4), 182–194. doi:10.1056/NEJM196301242680405 PMID:13928666

Logan, J. J., Jolly, A. M., & Blanford, J. I. (2016). The sociospatial network: Risk and the role of place in the transmission of infectious diseases. *PLoS ONE, 11*(2), 1–14. doi:10.1371/journal.pone.0146915 PMID:26840891

Mallon, W., & Kassinove, A. (1999). Mandatory Reporting Laws and the Emergency Department. In *Topics in Emergency Medicine*. Aspen Publishers, Inc. Retrieved from http://ovidsp.ovid.com/ovidweb.cgi?T=JS%7B&%7DPAGE=reference%7B&%7DD=ovftd%7B&%7DNEWS=N%7B&%7DAN=00007815-199909000-00009

Manitoba Health. (2008). *Enteric illness protocol*. Retrieved 21 January 2017 from http://www.gov.mb.ca/health/publichealth/cdc/protocol/enteric.pdf

Manitoba Health. (2011). *Communicable Disease Management Protocol; Invasive meningococcal disease*. Retrieved 21 January 2017 from http://www.gov.mb.ca/health/publichealth/cdc/protocol/mid.pdf

Manitoba Health. (2015a). *Communicable Disease Management Protocol; Legionellosis*. Retrieved 21 January 2017 from http://www.gov.mb.ca/health/publichealth/cdc/protocol/legion.pdf

Manitoba Health. (2015b). *Communicable disease management protocol;shigellosis*. Retrieved 21 January 2017 from http://www.gov.mb.ca/health/publichealth/cdc/protocol/shigellosis.pdf

Manitoba. Public Health Act. (2016). Retrieved 21 January 2017, from http://www.gov.mb.ca/health/publichealth/act.html

Mrvar, A., & Batagelj, V. (n.d.). *Pajek: Program for Analysis and Visualization of Large Networks (Reference Manual)* (A. M. V. Batagelj, Ed.). Retrieved from http://pajek.imfm.si/doku.php?id=pajek

Northwest Territories. Public Health Act. (2011). *Yellowknife: Territorial Assembly*. Retrieved 21 January 2017 from https://www.justice.gov.nt.ca/en/files/legislation/public-health/public-health.a.pdf

Nova Scotia Department of Health and Wellness. (2013). *Nova Scotia Communicable Diseases Manual; Lyme disease*. Retrieved from 21 January 2017 http://novascotia.ca/dhw/cdpc/cdc/documents/Lyme.pdf

Nova Scotia Department of Health and Wellness. (n.d.). *Nova Scotia Communicable Diseases Manual; West Nile Virus*. Retrieved 21 January 2017 http://novascotia.ca/dhw/cdpc/cdc/documents/West-Nile-Virus.pdf

Ontario. Health Protection and Promotion Act. (2015). Ontario Provincial Parliament. Retrieved 21 January 2017 from https://www.ontario.ca/laws/statute/90h07

Potterat, J. J., Rothenberg, R. B., Woodhouse, D. E., Muth, J. B., Pratts, C. I., & Fogle, J. S. (1985). Gonorrhea as a social disease. *Sexually Transmitted Diseases*, *12*(1), 25–32. doi:10.1097/00007435-198501000-00006 PMID:4002091

Prince Edward Island. Public Health Act. (2014). Retrieved 21 January 2017 from https://www.princeedwardisland.ca/en/legislation/public-health-act

Provincial Infectious Disease Advisory Committee on Communicable Disease. (2014). *Recommendations for the public health response to hepatitis C in Ontario*. Retrieved 21 January 2017 from http://www.publichealthontario.ca/en/eRepository/Recommendations_Public_Health_Response_Hepatitis_C.pdf

Public Health Agency of Canada. (2014). *Canadian tuberculosis standards* (VII). Ottawa, Ontario: Public Health Agency of Canada, Canadian Lung Association. Retrieved 21 January 2017 from http://www.respiratoryguidelines.ca/tb-standards-2013

Public Health Ontario. (2015). *How to complete the measles and rubella enhanced surveillance form*. Retrieved 21 January 2017 from http://www.publichealthontario.ca/en/eRepository/How_to_complete_MR_Surveillance_Form_2015.pdf

Public Health Ontario. (2014). *Provincial Case Definitions for Reportable Diseases; Chlamydia trachomatis infections*. Retrieved 21 January 2017 from http://www.health.gov.on.ca/en/pro/programs/publichealth/oph_standards/docs/mumps_cd.pdf

Quebec. Public Health Act. (2016). Quebec National Assembly. Retrieved 21 January 2017 from http://www.gov.pe.ca/law/statutes/pdf/p-30_1.pdf

Rolfhamre, R., Janson, A., Arneborn, M., & Ekdahl, K. (2006). SmiNet-2: Description of an internet-based surveillance system for communicable diseases in Sweden. *Eurosurveillance*, *11*(5). PMID:16757847

Rosenberg, T., Kendall, O., Blanchard, J., Martel, S., Wakelin, C., & Fast, M. (1997). Shigellosis on Indian Reserves in Manitoba, Canada : Its Relationship to Crowded Housing, Lack of Running Water, and Inadequate Sewage Disposal. *American Journal of Public Health*, *87*(9), 1547–1551. doi:10.2105/AJPH.87.9.1547 PMID:9314814

Rothenberg, R. B., McElroy, P. D., Wilce, M. A., & Muth, S. Q. (2003). Contact tracing: Comparing the approaches for sexually transmitted diseases and tuberculosis. *The International Journal of Tuberculosis and Lung Disease*, *7*(12Suppl 3), S342–S348. PMID:14677820

Sepulveda, J., Lopez-Cervantes, M., Frenk, J., Gomez de Leon, J., Lezana-Fernandez, M. A., & Santos-Burgoa, C., & (CDC), C. for D. C. (1992). Key issues in public health surveillance for the 1990s. *Morbidity and Mortality Weekly Report*, *41*(Suppl), 61–76. PMID:1344267

Snow, J. (1855). *On the mode of communication of cholera*. London: UCLA. Retrieved 21 January 2017 from http://www.ph.ucla.edu/epi/snow/snowbook.html

Sockett, P., Garnett, M., & Scott, C. (1996). Communicable disease surveillance; Notification of infectious diseases in Canada. *The Canadian Journal of Infectious Diseases & Medical Microbiology*, 7(5), 293–295. PMID:22514452

State of New Jersey. (2013). *Communicable disease outbreak manual - vectorborne diseases*. Retrieved from http://njlmn2.rutgers.edu/sites/default/files/Appendix_T3_Vectorborne_outbreak_investigations.pdf

Statistics Canada. (2011). *Postal code conversion file*. Retrieved January 4, 2017, from http://www.statcan.gc.ca/daily-quotidien/110720/dq110720f-eng.htm

Thacker, S. B., & Berkelman, R. L. (1988). Public health surveillance in the united states. *Epidemiologic Reviews*, 10. PMID:3066626

Thacker, S. B., & Stroup, D. F. (1994). Future Directions for Comprehensive Public Health Surveillance and Health Information Systems in the United States. *American Journal of Epidemiology*, 140(5), 383–397. doi:10.1093/oxfordjournals.aje.a117261 PMID:8067331

Totten, S., Maclean, R., Payne, E., & Severini, A. (2015). Chlamydia and lymphogranuloma venereum in Canada: 2003- 2013 summary report. *Canada Communicable Disease Report, 41*(2). Retrieved from http://www.phac-aspc.gc.ca/publicat/ccdr-rmtc/15vol41/dr-rm41-02/surv-1-eng.php

Vogel, C., & Funk, M. (2008). Measles Quarantine—The Individual and the Public. *Journal of Travel Medicine*, 15(2), 65–67. doi:10.1111/j.1708-8305.2008.00182.x PMID:18346237

World Health Organisation. (1968). *National and global surveillance of communicable disease*. Retrieved 21 January 2017 from http://apps.who.int/iris/bitstream/10665/143764/1/WHA21_TD-2_eng.pdf

World Health Organisation. (2005). *International Health Regulations*. Geneva: Author.

Wylie, J. L., & Jolly, A. (2001). Patterns of Chlamydia and Gonorrhea Infection in Sexual Networks in Manitoba, Canada. *Sexually Transmitted Diseases*, 28(1), 14–24. doi:10.1097/00007435-200101000-00005 PMID:11196040

KEY TERMS AND DEFINITIONS

Notifiable Disease: A communicable infection which is designated as such under the public health act and regulations of a jurisdiction. Usually these are; common, severe, easily prevented, highly communicable, costly, generate fear in people, and/or show changes in manifestation, population affected, or geographic range.

Chapter 18
Brain–Machine Interface:
Human–Computer Interaction

Manoj Kumar Mukul
BIT Mesra, India

Sumanta Bhattaharyya
BIT Mesra, India

ABSTRACT

The brain-machine interface (BMI) is a very recent development in the area of the human machine interaction (HCI) and emerged as the sister technology of BCI. A physiological signal related to these electrical potentials in response of the mental thoughts is known as Electroencephalogram (EEG) signals. The BMI is most commonly known as the BCI because there is a direct communication between the brain and the external machine via a computer, which analyses and interprets the incoming physiological signals, which contain the shadow of the mental activity and the different types of artefacts. A multi-channel recording of the electromagnetic waves emerging from the neural currents in the brain generate a large amounts of the EEG data. The neural activity of the human brain recorded non-invasively is sufficient to control the external machine, if advanced methods of signal analysis and feature extraction are used in combination with the machine learning techniques either supervised or unsupervised.

INTRODUCTION

Many patients become afflicted with neurological conditions or neurodegenerative diseases (Wolpaw et. al., 2000) hat disrupt the normal information flow from the brain to the spinal cord, and eventually, to the targets of that information,(i.e., the muscles) which affect the person's intent. Amyotrophic lateral sclerosis (ALS also called Lou Gehrig's disease),spinal cord injury, strokes, and many other conditions can impair either the neural pathways controlling muscle's, or impair the muscles themselves. Individuals that are most affected may lose all their abilities to control their muscles. Thus, they lose all options to communicate and become completely locked inside their bodies. In absence of ways to reverse the effects of these disorders, there are three principal options for restoring function. The first option is to substitute the damaged neural pathways or muscles with pathways or muscles that are still functional. While

DOI: 10.4018/978-1-5225-2515-8.ch018

this substitution is often limited, it can still be useful. For example, patients can use eye movements to communicate or hand movements to produce synthetic speech. The second option is to restore function by detecting nerve or muscle activity above the level of the injury. For example, freehand prosthesis is a method of restoring hand function to patients with spinal cord injuries. The third option for restoring function is to provide the brain with a new and non-muscular output channel, a brain–computer interface (BCI) (Wolpaw et.al., 2000), for conveying the user's intent to the external world.

The brain-machine interface (BMI) is a very recent development in the area of the human machine interaction (HCI) and emerged as the sister technology of BCI. However, there is not a clear cut difference between the BCI and the BMI. In fact, a computer is always between the brain and the machine for the interface. Different mental thoughts generate the electrical potentials over the surface of the scalp. These are recorded with sensors placed on the surface of the head. A form of physiological signals related to these electrical potentials of thoughts are known as Electro-encephalogram (EEG) (Carlson, 2007) signals. The BMI based on the EEG signals is called the EEG-based BMI (Carlson, 2007) system. The BMI pertains to the manipulation or operation of an external machine as per thoughts of a user, and such machine is called a though controlled machine. Thus, there is a direct communication between human and machine via a computer. The BMI is most commonly known as the BCI because there is a direct communication between the brain and the external machine via a computer, which analyses and interprets the incoming physiological signals (electroencephalograms), which contain the shadow of the mental activity and the different types of artifacts. A multi-channel recording of the electromagnetic waves emerging from the neural currents in the brain shows large amounts of EEG data. The neural activity of the human brain recorded non-invasively is sufficient to control the external machine, if advanced methods of signal analysis and feature extraction are used in combination with the machine learning techniques either supervised or unsupervised. A suitable feature extraction and classification methods are useful to generate a control command for controlling the external machine.

BCI provides a direct interface between the human brain and a computer. BCI is an emerging application of HCI. The first international BCI workshop was held in June 1999, in Rensselaerville, New York. More than twenty research groups from the different part of the world participated in that workshop. In it, a formal definition of the BCI was proposed (Wolpaw, 2000):

A brain-computer interface is a communication system that does not depend on the brain's normal output pathways of peripheral nerves and muscles.

BCI involves monitoring brain activity using brain pattern identification and analyzing the characteristics of the brain pattern using signal processing algorithms. In a BCI, system messages and commands generated to control any machine are nothing but the electrophysiological signals generated within the brain. The motivation that inspired to extend the research in the field of BCI is to develop an alternative way of the conventional communication system between the human and the computer. The BCI systems are bridging gap between the human and the machine used to interact with the world. BCI systems provide assistance to the human being with paralytic disability like Amyotrophic lateral sclerosis (ALS), Traumatic Brain Injury (TBI), Cerebral Palsy (CP), Spinal Cord Injury (SCI) etc.

The Brain and Its Functions

The weight of the average adult human brain is around 1.4 kg. The human brain is surrounded bycerebrospinal fluid, which suspends it within the skull and safeguards it by acting as a motion dampener. Carlson categorizes the brain components into three groups; the Forebrain, Midbrain and Hindbrain. Anatomically it can be divided into three main structures (Carlson, 2007): brain stem (hindbrain), cerebrum and cerebellum (forebrain) have shown in Figure 1. The functions are summarized as follows (Table 1 and Table 2).

BCI COMPONENTS

The BCI framework consists of several stages, which are shown in Figure 2. The main five stages are:

Table 1. Functions of the different part of the human brain

Name of the Component	Function
Brainstem	Controls the autonomic nerve functions (respiration, heart rate, blood pressure etc.) and reflexes.
Cerebrum	It assimilates information from all of the sense organs, controls emotions; higher thought processes, holds memory and initiates motor functions.
Cerebellum	Assimilates information from the vestibular system that indicates position and movement. By using this information maintains balance and coordinate limb movements.
Hypothalamus	Pituitary gland controls body temperature, visceral functions, and behavioral responses such as drinking, feeding, sexual response, aggression and pleasure.
Thalamus	The thalamic sensory input is crucial to generate and modulate the rhythmic cortical activity.

Table 2. Cortical areas of the brain and their function

Cortical Area	Function
Auditory association area	Complex processing of auditory information
Auditory cortex	Detection of sound quality (loudness, tone)
Broca's area (speech center)	Speech production and articulation
Prefrontal cortex	Problem solving, emotion, complex thought
Premotor cortex	Coordination of complex movement
Primary Motor cortex	Initiation of voluntary movement
Primary somatosensory cortex	Receives tactile information from the body
Sensory association area	Processing of multisensory information
Gustatory area	Processing of taste information
Wernicke's area	Language comprehension
Primary Visual Cortex	Complex processing of visual information

Figure 1. Functional areas of the brain

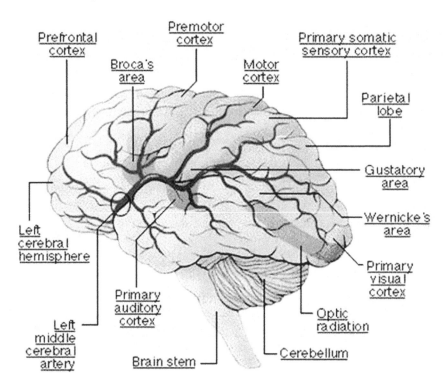

Signal Acquisition

The Electrophysiological brain signals are recorded using signal acquisition systems. The main components of the signal acquisition systems are the sensors or electrodes. The signal acquisition system does some low level filtering. It converts a continuous signal into a discrete signal and passes the data into the next stage [3-4]. Different signal acquisition processes of the EEG signal have been stated in (Hochberg, 2006) Leigh R. et. al. and (Vigário, 2000)R. Vigario et. al.

Preprocessing

This stage includes amplification, artifact removal and initial filtering of the recorded signals through the signal acquisition systems. In this stage the discrete signal is converted to a digital signal (Bashashati et. al., 2007). Various preprocessing methods like regression based EOG, common spatial patterns (CSP), principal component analysis (PCA), singular value decomposition (SVD), short time Fourier transform (STFT), recurrent quantum neural network (RQNN) etc.[depicted in (Schlögl et.al., 2007) A. Schlogl et. al. and (Srinivasuluet.al., 2012) A. Srinivasulu et.al., (Mukul et.al., 2010) M. K. Mukul et.al, (Bhattacharyya et.al., 2014) S. Bhattacharyya et.al., (Gandhi et.al., 2014) Vaibhav Gandhi et.al.]

Feature Extraction

Features are extracted from the preprocessed brain signals. Typically the features are different statistical properties of the signal like mean, variance, correlation, cross correlation, standard deviation, power spectral density, relative spectral power (RSP), temporal relative spectral power (TRSP), hjorth parameter, time frequency representation (TFR), cepstral coefficient, cepstrum, etc. stated in (Machavarapu et. al., 2014) Sarath Chandra Machavarapu et. al., (Hjorth, 1970) Bo Hjorth,(Bhattacharyya et.al., 2016) S. Bhattacharyya et.al, (Bhattacharyya et.al., 2014) S. Bhattacharyya et.al., (Ngoc et. al., 2013) H. T. Ngoc et.al., (Bhattacharyya et.al., 2016) S. Bhattacharyya et.al.. The goal of the feature extraction is to form a distinct set of features for different mental tasks. If the feature sets of the different mental tasks overlap each other, then it is very difficult to classify those mental tasks. If the feature sets are distinct enough, then any classifier can classify those features.

Classification

The extracted features from the previous stage are the input for the classifier. The BCIs can be classified by a different number of classes; typically 2 to 5 classes. The mainly two type linear and nonlinear classifiers e.g. Linear Discriminant Analysis (LDA), Support Vector Machine (SVM), Bayesian Classifier etc. mentioned in (Bhattacharyya et.al., 2014),(Bhattacharyya et.al., 2016) S. Bhattacharyya et.al (Duda et. al., 2001) R. Duda, P. Hart, et al.. Classifiers are trained to recognize different mental tasks.

Device Control

Output of the classifiers is the input for the device control. The device control transforms the classification to a particular action. The action can be, e.g., an up or down, left or right movement of different parts etc. (Long et. al., 2012).

Figure 2. BCI components

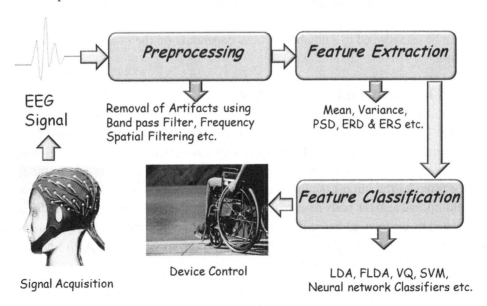

FUNDAMENTAL APPROACHES TO BCI DESIGN

BCI systems interpret human desires directly into the enormous potential for the widespread population. The BCI researchers have utilized knowledge of electrophysiology of brain's to analyze brain activity.

There exist two basic approaches for the BCI design. The first one is the *pattern recognition approach* (PR) based on identification of the brain activity in response to performing a mental task. The second one is the *operant conditioning approach*(OC) based on the self-regulation of the BCI signals.

PR Approach

The activity of the BCI associated with certain mental tasks, localized to specific regions of the brain. BCI researchers guide the user to generate distinguishable brain patterns in response to different mental tasks. The PR approach uses different signal processing algorithms for feature extraction and classification of different brain activity in response to these mental tasks. The mental tasks used in the BCI framework have included motor imagery, visual, arithmetic and baseline tasks. Challenges in the PR approach are to recognize distinguishable patterns from brain activity in a specific brain region related to different mental tasks (Machavarapu et. al., 2014)-(Long et. al., 2012).

OC Approach

The OC approach of the BCI design requires the user to perform lengthy training sessions. Rhythmic brain activity, event-related potentials are the most common method of categorizing brain signal patterns for use in the BCI system. The OC approach is the effective use of biofeedback in the training scenario for a subject to develop the ability to self-regulate rhythmic property of the brain signal (Birbaumer et. al., 1999).

CATEGORIZATION OF THE BCI SYSTEMS DEPENDS ON VARIOUS ASPECTS AND METHODOLOGIES

BCI systems can be categorized in a number of ways depending on their various BCI aspects or methodologies applied.

Invasive, Non-Invasive, and Partially Invasive

Depending on the data acquisition systems, the BCIs is classified in three categories; Invasive, Non-invasive and Partially invasive. Invasive BCI systems are implemented by implanting sensors directly into the grey matter of the human brain through neurosurgery. As the sensors lie in the grey matter, invasive device provides the utmost quality signals to BCI devices. However they are prone to cause scar-tissue build-up, and also the body reacts to a foreign object in the brain. Scalp recorded electromagnetic waves created by the neuron; based BCI systems are most commonly known as non-invasive BCI. Due to the signals measured from the outside of the scalp, non-invasive BCI systems have poor spatial resolution, high temporal resolution and are relatively inexpensive. The partially invasive BCI systems are implanted by implanting sensors inside the skull, but they rest outside the brain rather than within the grey matter. They provide better spatial resolution signals than non-invasive BCIs where the bone tissue of the cranium deflects and deforms signals, and have a minor risk of forming scar-tissue in the brain compared to fully invasive BCIs ((Bashashati et. al., 2007).

Online and Offline

Depending on the data analysis systems, the BCI framework has been classified into two categories; online and offline. The fundamental aspect of the online BCIs is that to facilitate the actual real-time atmosphere. Offline BCI systems are for hypothetical simulations of an existent BCI system to facilitate investigative studies of the BCI components like different electrode positions, preprocessing, feature extraction and classification methods etc. (Gandhi et.al., 2014) -(Bhattacharyya et.al., 2016).

Synchronous and Asynchronous

Depending on the cue used in the time of the data acquisition, BCI has been categorized into two types synchronous (cued) and asynchronous (un-cued). A synchronous BCI system is the mental activity triggered by the external stimuli. When the user decides to control a mental task and the resultant control signal is generated, is called an 'asynchronous BCI system'. The synchronous BCI systems are less demanding in the feature extraction and classification steps compared with the asynchronous systems. The cued BCIs offer a less normal method of control because someone must wait for the suitable cue in order to make a decision. Un-cued BCIs are user driven (i.e. the control is not system-generated, but user-initiated). This offers whole control to the user (Bashashati et. al., 2007).

Universal and Individual

Depending on the gathering of the signal or data from the number of subjects, the BCI is categorized into two types; universal and individual. Universal BCI systems assume to be the gathering of the data from multiple users to find features and a classification function which will be valid in general for every user. Individual BCI systems are personalized to the individual and the fact is that no two persons are the same, both physiologically and psychologically. Adaptive BCI systems such as the Adaptive Brain Interface systems (Bashashati et. al., 2007)-(Bhattacharyya et.al., 2016) provide the adaptability of the system to user for time and psychological variations.

Design of a universal BCI system is moreover simple, but it will have poor performance level.

Dependent and Independent

Depending on the dependency on ocular activity, the BCI is categorized in two types; independent and dependent. Dependent BCI systems depend on the ocular activity or artifacts (Bashashati et. al., 2007). The ocular activity-based communication offers better performance than BCI systems. Independent BCIs do not require any ocular intervention.

Paradigm

Depending on the mental tasks of the users, the BCI system is categorized into different types; motor imagery, arithmetic or spatial relational, visual related, etc. (Bashashati et. al., 2007)

BCI CATEGORIZATION DEPENDS ON DATA ACQUISITION METHODOLOGIES

Broadly, the BCI system is categorized by the data acquisition methods depicted in Figure 3.

Electroencephalography (EEG)

EEG signals measure the brain activity caused by the flow of electrons during synaptic excitations of the dendrites in neurons (Bhattacharyya et.al., 2016). EEG signals are recorded in a non-invasive manner through electrodes placed on the scalp. The EEG signals are measured as the potential differences over time between signals or active electrodes and reference electrodes. An extra electrode present in the system, known as the ground electrode, is used to measure the differential voltage between the active and reference points.

The minimal configuration for EEG measurement consists of one active, one reference, and one ground electrode. The multi-channel configurations comprise up to 128 or 256 active electrodes (Wolpaw et. al., 1994). These electrodes are usually made of silver chloride (AgCl) (Hochberg, 2006). Electrode-scalp contact impedance should be between 1 kΩ and 10 kΩ (less than 5kΩ) to record an accurate signal (Hochberg, 2006).

Magneto Encephalography (MEG)

MEG is a non-invasive brain imaging technique that records the brain's magnetic activity by means of magnetic induction. MEG measures the intracellular currents flowing through the dendrites which

Figure 3. BCI categorization

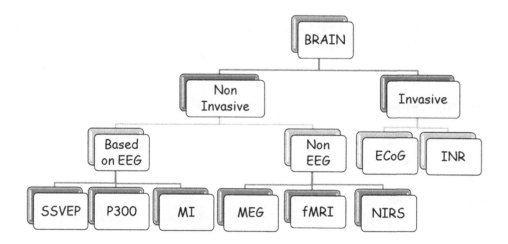

generates magnetic fields that are measurable from the outside of the head. The neuro-physiological processes that produce MEG signals are similar to those that produce EEG signals. The MEG offers signals with higher spatiotemporal resolution than EEG, which reduces the training time needed to control a BCI system. MEG-based BCIs, as compared with EEG-based BCIs, are still at an early stage (Mellinger et. al., 2007).

Electrocorticography (ECoG)

ECoG is a technique that measures electrical activity in the cerebral cortex by means of electrodes placed directly inside the brain. Compared to EEG, ECoG provides higher temporal and spatial resolution, as well as higher amplitudes and a lower vulnerability to artifacts such as blinks and eye movement (Waldert et. al., 2009).

Intracortical Neuron Recording (INR)

Intracortical neuron data recording is a neuroimaging technique. INR measures electrical activity inside the gray matter of the brain. It is an invasive recording modality that needs to implant microelectrode arrays inside the cortex to capture spike signals and local field potentials from neurons. Three signals can be obtained by intracortical neuron recording: single-unit activity (SUA), multi-unit activity (MUA), and local field potentials (LFPs) (Wolpaw et. al., 2009).

Table 3. Neuroimaging methods

Neuroimaging method	Activity Measured	Direct/Indirect Measurement	Temporal resolution	Spatial resolution	Risk	Portability
EEG	Electrical	Direct	~0.05 s	~10 mm	Non-invasive	Portable
MEG	Magnetic	Direct	~0.05 s	~5 mm	Non-invasive	Non-portable
ECoG	Electrical	Direct	~0.003 s	~1 mm	Invasive	Portable
Intracortical neuron recording	Electrical	Direct	~0.003 s	~0.5 mm (LFP) ~0.1mm (MUA) ~0.05mm (SUA)	Invasive	Portable
fMRI	Metabolic	Indirect	~1 s	~1 mm	Non-invasive	Non-portable
NIRS	Metabolic	Indirect	~1 s	~5 mm	Non-invasive	Portable

Table 4. Non-invasive recording of the brain signals

Non Invasive Recording of Brain Signal				
	fMRI	NIRS	MEG	EEG
Spatial Resolution (SR)	HH	H	?	?
Temporal Resolution (TR)	M	M	HH	HH
Portability	L	HH	L	HH
Safety	H	HH	HH	HH
?=ill posed, H=High, L=Low, M=Medium, HH=Very High				

Functional Magnetic Resonance Imaging (fMRI)

fMRI is a non-invasive neuroimaging technique which detects changes in local cerebral blood volume, cerebral blood flow and oxygenation levels during neural activation by means of electromagnetic fields. fMRI is generally performed using MRI scanners which apply electromagnetic fields of strength in the order of 3**T** or 7**T**. The main advantage of the use of fMRI is high space resolution. For that reason, fMRI have been applied for localizing active regions inside the brain (Christopher et. al., 2004).

Near Infrared Spectroscopy (NIRS)

NIRS is an optical spectroscopy method that employs infrared light to characterize noninvasively acquired fluctuations in the cerebral metabolism during neural activity. Infrared light penetrates the skull to a depth of approximately 1–3 cm below its surface, where the intensity of the attenuated light allows alterations in oxy-hemoglobin and deoxy-hemoglobin concentrations to be measured. Due to shallow light penetration in the brain, this optical neuroimaging technique is limited to the outer cortical layer (Bashashati et. al., 2007).

REASON BEHIND THE SELECTION OF EEG AS THE BCI INPUT MODALITY

There exist a number of technologies that can monitor brain activity. These include, for example fMRI, MEG, PET, SPECT and EEG. EEG is the only practical noninvasive brain imaging technology for the following reasons:

1. Inexpensiveness
2. Ease of acquisition
3. High temporal resolution (i.e. almost instantaneous representations of brain activity, within 1ms)
4. Real-time implementation possible
5. Direct correlation of functional brain activity with EEG recordings

Almost all BCIs reported to date have been based on EEG for these reasons. Research reported in this book chapter focuses for these reasons on EEG-based BCI system design and implementation.

BCI EVALUATION PARAMETERS

The performance of BCI systems has been evaluated by a large variety of parameters. The evaluation criteria's are very necessary to compare different BCI systems and approaches. The most common BCI evaluation parameters shown in Figure 4.

Table 5. Normal EEG rhythms characteristics

Brain Rhythm	Typical Frequency range (Hz)	Normal Amp. (μV)	Where It Can Be Found	Reactivity	Comments
Delta	0.1 - 4	<100	Dominant in infants, during deep stages of adult sleep and serious organic brain disease. Central cerebrum and parietal lobes	Focal in pathologies. Occur after transactions of the upper brain stem separating the reticular activating system from the cerebral cortex	Polymorphic delta: severe, acute, ongoing injury to cortical neurons. Rhythmic discharge: psychophysiology dysfunction
Theta	4 – 8	<100	In drowsy normal adults, in frontal, parietal and temporal regions. In children when awake	Rare in EEG of awake adults During emotional stress in some adults sudden removal of something causing pleasure will cause about 20s of theta waves	Nieder meyer lists some studies in which theta activity of 6-7 Hz over frontal midline region had been correlated with mental activity Focal or lateralized theta indicates focal pathology, Diffuse theta more generalized neurologic syndrome.
Alpha	8 - 13	20-60	The most prominent rhythm in the normal alert adult brain. Most prominent at occipital and parietal regions. About 25% stronger over the right hemisphere.	Fully present when a subject is mentally inactive, alert, with eyes closed. Blocked or attenuated by deep sleep, attention, especially visual, and mental effort When a person is alert and their attention is directed to a specific activity, the alpha waves are replaced by asynchronous waves of higher frequency and lower amplitude. Eye opening/closure offers the most effective manipulation	Location of central alpha peak declines with age and in dementia. Alpha waves are usually attributed to summated dendrite potentials. Slowing is considered a non-specific abnormality in metabolic, toxic, and infectious conditions. Asymmetries unilateral lesions. Loss of reactivity a lesion in the temporal lobe. Loss of alpha - brainstem lesion.
Mu	10 - 12	<50	Central electrodes, over motor and somatosensory cortex	Does not react to opening of eyes like alpha rhythm Blocking before movement of the contra lateral hand. Blocking for light tactile stimuli. Blocking for readiness or imagination to move limbs	Physiologically and topographically different to alpha rhythm Not clinically useful. Useful as a BCI input in relation to actual and imagined limb movement Typically appears as part of a background rhythm.
Beta	14 – 30	<20	Three basic types frontal beta widespread posterior	Frontal beta blocked by movement Widespread beta often nonreactive Posterior beta shows reactivity to eye opening	Beta I waves, lower frequencies, which disappear during mental activity Beta II waves, higher frequencies, appearing tension and intense mental activity Under intense mental activity beta can extend as far as 50Hz
Gamma	> 30	<2	Widespread	Found when the subject is paying attention or is having some other sensory stimulation	Due to its really low amplitude it is very difficult to isolate without band-pass filtering

Classification Accuracy

The Classification Accuracy is the most widely used BCI evaluation criteria in BCI research. The Classification Accuracy has denoted as ACC. This parameter has been easily calculated and interpreted.

$$ACC = p_0 = \frac{\sum_{i=1}^{M} n_{ii} \rightarrow \text{Correctly classified sample}}{N \rightarrow \text{Total number of sample}}$$

The maximum classification accuracy can never exceed 100%.

Cohen's Kappa Coefficient

Cohen's Kappa Coefficient addresses several of the analyses on the accuracy measurement. The calculation of the Cohen's Kappa Coefficient uses the overall agreement $p_0 = ACC$ and the chance agreement:

$$p_e = \frac{\sum_{i=1}^{M} n_{:i} n_{i:} \rightarrow \text{Sum of i-th column}}{N^2 \rightarrow \text{Sum of i-th row}}$$

$$K = \frac{p_o - p_e}{1 - p_e} \tag{1}$$

K= 0 Predicted classes show no correlation with actual classes

K= 1 Perfect classification

K< 0 Different assignment between output and the true classes

$$\sigma_e(\kappa) = \frac{\sqrt{(p_o + p_e^2 - \sum_{i=1}^{M} [n_{:i} n_{i:} (n_{:i} + n_{i:})] / N^3)}}{(1 - p_e)\sqrt{N}} \tag{2}$$

Mutual Information

Mutual Information measures the mutual dependency of different random variable. One of the goals of a BCI system is to provide an additional way of communication from the subjects' brains to their environment.

Information transfer for M classes can be calculated as:

$$I = \log_2(M) \tag{3}$$

Figure 4. BCI evaluation parameter

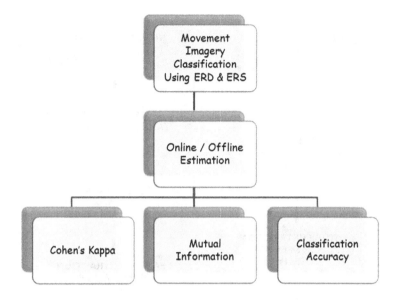

BACKGROUND: CHALLENGES IN BCI

The BCI researchers have explored different methodologies with variable success rates to achieve the goal of developing new alternatives for communication and control technologies of the BCI. A few challenges of the BCI research are;

- Clustering of Neurons
- Signal Acquisition
- Noise Filtering
- Feature Identification
- Feature Classification
- User Interface Design

PROPOSED BCI METHODOLOGY

The author's main goal is to emphasize different BCI parameters. Two different algorithms are applied in EEG-based non-invasive BCI research work. Comparative performance of two algorithms has been analyzed in result in a discussion section.

The proposed methods of EEG signal preprocessing are shown in Figure 5 A and B. The recorded EEG signals (displayed in block 1 in Figure 5 A and B).The FIR filter and FIR filter with BSS has been applied for EOG correction to remove artifacts (displays in block II in Figure 5 A and block II, III in Figure 5 B). The EOG corrected EEG signal was processed to the feature extraction method (displays in block III in Figure 5A and block IV in Figure 5B) using PSD. The extracted feature was further subjected to classification techniques through the LDA classifier (displays in block IV in Figure 5 A and block V in Figure 5 B).

Figure 5. Proposed method for the motor imagery classification

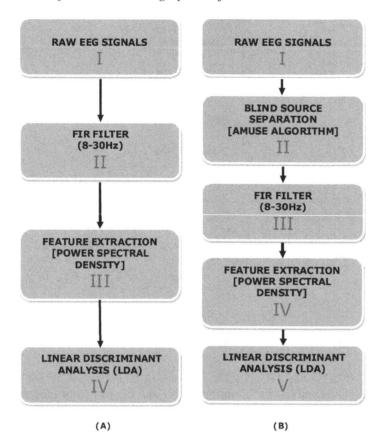

(A)   (B)

RESULTS AND DISCUSSIONS

Data Set Description and EOG Correction

In order to understand the EOG correction by the ICA (Choi et. al., 2005) method, the author has been using their own recorded EEG signals in their institute laboratory. The authors are interested in finding the preprocessing method for the movement imagery EEG time series data for eliminating the eye artifacts, the muscles noise, and cardiac signal, and extract the hidden information related to the movement imagery in the frequency band alpha and beta. Each subject was asked to do a mental task related to the movement imagination for eighteen seconds. Initial five seconds of data have been discarded, because the recording environment was MATLAB SIMULINK which set the amplifier characteristics at the beginning of the recording for each trail so its characteristics are transient. Each subject was trying to keep his concentration during the whole recording duration. The subject was verbally asked to concentrate on the mental task of the imagination of the left, the right hand and the straight movement. For each subject a total of 12 trials were recorded (three trials of each type of movement imagery). The recording was made using a G. Tec amplifier (http://www.gtec.at) and Ag/AgCl electrodes. All signals were sampled at 128 Hz and filtered between 0.5 and 30 Hz. The sixteen unipolar EEG channels were measured using the sixteen electrodes placed according to the 10/20 electrode placement system (Gutberlet et. al., 2009) positioning nomenclature which have been shown in Figure 8. All the channels have been referenced to the vertex Cz. The ground electrode was placed at Fz that is located at the forehead. The sensor layout used in the recordings is shown in Figure 6.

A sixteen channel raw EEG signals shown in Figure 7.

Now the standard AMUSE (Choi et. al., 2005) algorithm is implemented on the recorded EEG signals and the AMUSE filtered signals have been shown in Figure 8 and Figure 9 represents the eye blink artifacts.

For the mental task the relaxed eye was closed, so the eye blink artifacts are not present in the AMUSE filtered signal. For the mental task left, right and straight hand movement imagination, the authors have the eye blink artifacts. The Eye blink artifact has high amplitude compared to other EEG and artifact signals present in the raw EEG signals. The AMUSE filtered signals are sorted by the decreasing Eigenvalue decomposition of the covariance matrix of a single time lagged covariance matrix. The first Eigenvalue corresponds to the eye blink artifact. This artifact should be eliminated before the feature extraction or from the deflated signals.

Feature Extraction and Classification

In this problem, the authors have used the Graze dataset III of the BCI Competition II (BCI Competition II, 2003). There was a single subject in this dataset and the data were recorded for the left and right hand movement imageries. The total number of trials recorded for the EEG signals are 280. Out of 280 trials, 140 trials belong to the training data and the remaining 140 trials belong to the testing data. The train-

Figure 6. The sensor layout for recording the EEG signals

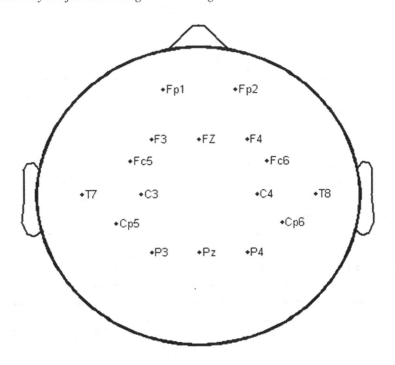

Figure 7. A sixteen channel raw EEG signals

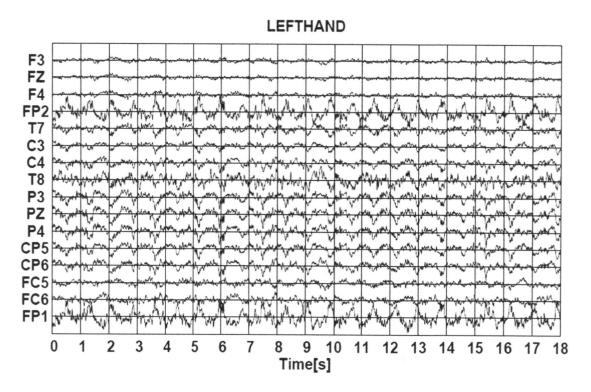

Figure 8. The AMUSE filtered EEG signals

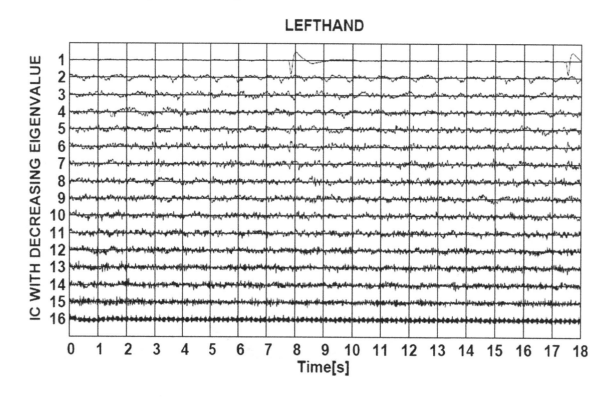

Figure 9. The eye blink (EOG) components extracted from the raw EEG signals

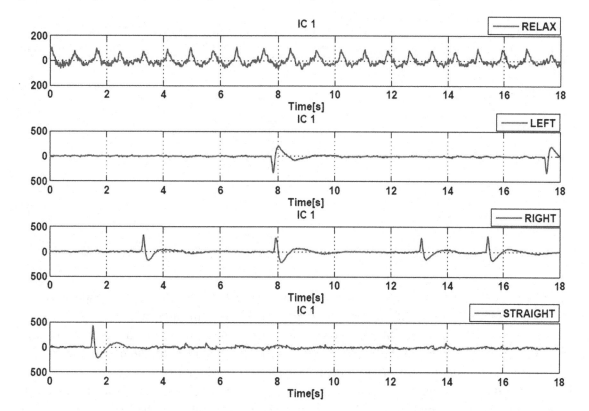

ing data contains 70 trials for the left hand movement imagery and 70trials for the right hand movement imagery. The authors have applied two approaches of signal preprocessing to the recorded EEG signals, and the preprocessed signals were subjected to the feature extraction using PSD. In the first approach, the standard AMUSE algorithm has been applied to the recorded EEG signals. The AMUSE filtered signals were partitioned into signal subspace and noise subspace components based on the Eigenvalues. The parts of the AMUSE filtered signals which correspond to the lowest Eigenvalues were discarded and other parts of the AMUSE filtered signals which correspond to the dominant Eigenvalues were used to deflate the channel signals. To select the rhythmic band information's from the deflated channel signals, the FIR digital filter was applied. The PSD was considered as a feature. In the second approach, the FIR filtered signals from Channels C3 andC4 were subjected to the PSD estimation. The batch processing of the signals was considered. The extracted features are further subjected to the linear classifier to estimate the classifier weight parameter over the training data. The same preprocessing techniques were applied over the testing data. Only the classifier weight parameter estimated over the training data was applied to the testing data classification. The extracted features over the testing data are further classified by the estimated classifier weight parameter over the training data. The FIR filter order was set to 16. The effectiveness of the applied methods was evaluated in terms of the classification accuracy, the specific accuracy, the Cohen's kappa coefficient and the mutual information or information transfer rate.

The estimated PSD of the channels C3 and C4 by the Welch's method is shown in Figure 10 for the left and the right hand movement imagination (FIR filtered only). Looking at the plot of the PSD curve, the authors got the spectral modulation at 10Hz, 15Hz and 20Hz frequency components for both the AMUSE

Figure 10. The PSD of the FIR filtered EEG signals estimated by the Welch's method

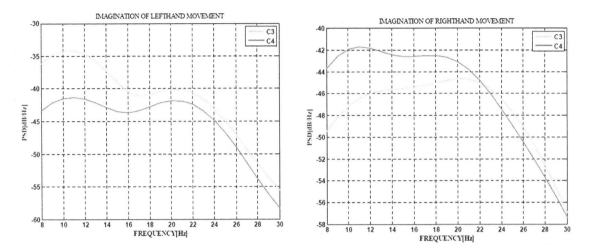

and the FIR filtered signals. The spectral modulation is observed at 10Hz frequency components when the parametric approach of the PSD estimation was applied, while in the nonparametric approach there was no spectral modulation at the 10Hz frequency. The reason why there was not a spectral modulation at 10Hz frequency band is due to short data length. For the short data length, the parametric approach is the best method in order to find out the hidden characteristics present in the signals.

Figure 11 and Figure 12 show the classification output over the training and testing data, when the EEG signals are processed by the FIR filter and the PSD was estimated by the Welch's periodogram

Figure 11. The classification output of the FIR filtered training data when the PSD was estimated by the Welch's method

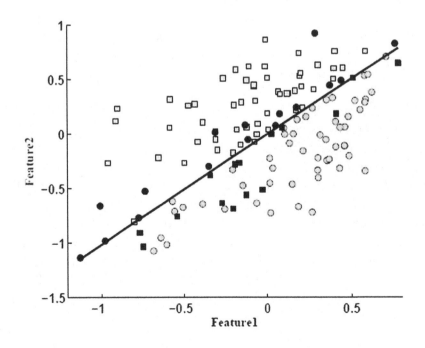

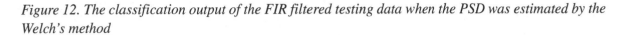

Figure 12. The classification output of the FIR filtered testing data when the PSD was estimated by the Welch's method

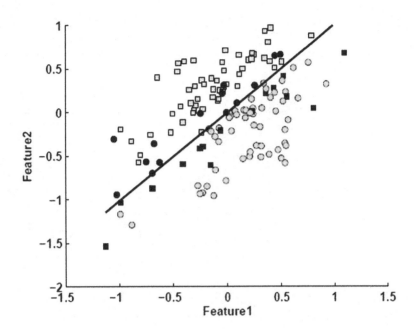

methods. The Feature1 corresponds to the mean of the channel C3 PSD magnitude and Feature2 corresponds to the mean of the channel C4 PSD magnitude. The green color circles indicate the correctly classified left class data while the gray color squares show the correctly classified right class data. The black circles indicate the incorrectly classified left class trials as right class trials, while black squares indicate the incorrectly classified right class trials as left class trials. The straight line is called the boundary line, which separates two classes. Evaluation parameters were described in BCI evaluation parameter.

The Eigenvalue decomposition of the covariance matrix of a three channel EEG signals gives us three Eigenvalues. In among a three Eigenvalues, two are the dominant and others are the non-dominant Eigenvalue. The channels signals were reconstructed in terms of components which belong to the dominant Eigenvalues. The whole procedure is known as deflation. From these deflated signals, the rhythmic information's were extracted by applying the FIR digital filter. The extracted information was further subjected to the feature extraction step. The extracted features were further subjected to estimate the classifier weight parameter over the training data.

The extracted classifier weight parameter was further subjected to classify the testing data. The PSD curve estimated is shown in Figure13, which was estimated for the FIR filtered information' of deflated signals by the Welch's method.

Figure 14 and 15 show the classification output for the training and testing data, when the EEG signals were processed by the AMUSE algorithm and the PSD was estimated by the Welch's method. These PSD curves do not show amplitude modulation at 10Hz, 15 Hz and 20Hz frequency clearly. It has been observed that in the whole frequency band of 8-30Hz, there was a lateralized spectral difference for each frequency. For both spectrum estimation methods, there were differences in the spectral contents on the contra-lateral channels for each frequency too. The classification output of the AMUSE filtered testing data when the PSD was estimated by the Welch's method displayed in Figure 15.

Figure 13. The PSD of the AMUSE filtered EEG signals when the PSD was estimated by the Welch's method

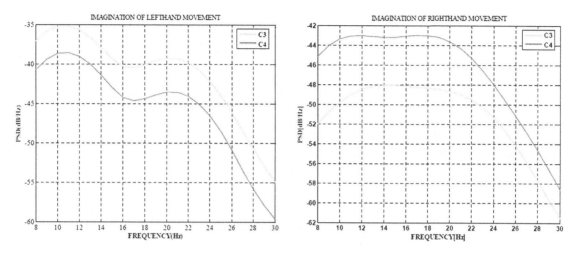

Figure 14. The classification output of the AMUSE filtered training data when the PSD was estimated by the Welch's method

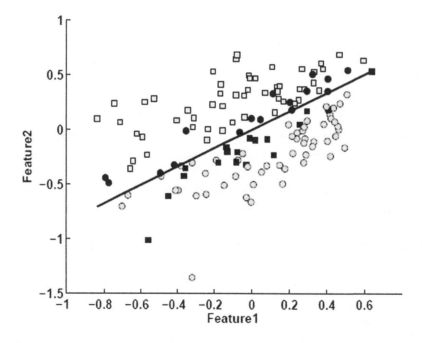

Figure 16 shows the receiver operator characteristics (ROC) curve for the training and the testing data respectively, when the EEG signals were processed by the AMUSE algorithm and the PSD was estimated by the Welch's method.

The classification performance was evaluated using the 10×10 cross validation procedures. This validation procedure mixes the feature set randomly and divides it into ten equally-sized distinct sets.

Figure 15. The classification output of the AMUSE filtered testing data when the PSD was estimated by the Welch's method

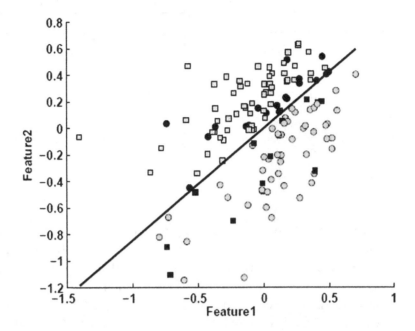

Figure 16. The ROC curve of the AMUSE filtered signals when the PSD was estimated by the Welch's method, left figure for the training data and right figure for the testing data

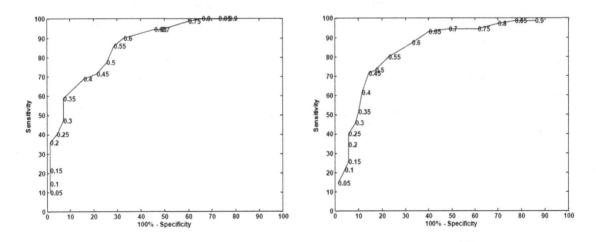

Each set was then used for the testing purpose while other sets were used for the training purpose. This results in ten different error rates, or accuracy, which were averaged. To further improve the estimate, this procedure was repeated 10 times and all error rates over these ten runs were again averaged. When the PSD was estimated for the AMUSE filtered signals, there was a maximum value of the MI and the Cohen's kappa coefficient for both the training and the testing data. Maximum value of the MI and the Cohen's kappa coefficient are listed in Table 6-7. There was poor performance for the FIR filtered sig-

Table 6. The BCI evaluation parameters over the training data.(PSD as a feature.)

Methods	К	ACC(%)	ACC_L(%)	ACC_R (%)	MI
AMUSE	0.55	77	76	78	0.24
FIR	0.58	79	79	79	0.26

Table 7. The BCI evaluation parameters over the testing data.(PSD as a feature.)

Methods	К	ACC(%)	ACC_L(%)	ACC_R (%)	MI
AMUSE	0.50	75	78	75	0.18
FIR	0.54	77	76	77	0.22

nals. When the PSD was estimated by the Welch periodogram method, there was a slight improvement in the evaluation parameters for the testing data compared to the AMUSE filtered signals. Figure15 shows the ROC curve for the training data. Still the conventional AMUSE algorithm along with the FIR filter for rhythmic band selection does not achieve 100% classification accuracy.

In order to do this analysis, the authors have utilized the MATLAB platform for simulation purposes. There are various open source MATLAB based toolboxes available for BCI simulation. The work highlighted in this chapter is completely inter-disciplinary in nature, and consists of signal acquisition, preprocessing, feature extraction and classification. There are different well-known MATLAB functions and toolboxes available for the purpose of signal processing, pattern classification and statistical signal analysis. For example, the MATLAB inbuilt function "load" has been utilized to access the pre-recorded signal for further analysis. The g-Tech amplifier has been utilized for the purpose of EEG signal recording. The authors used the "load" command along with the path of the stored EEG data to load the data into the MATLAB workspace. The "load" function represents the time domain information of the recorded EEG data through specific channel or electrode. The recorded data has been stored in the form of a matrix. The dimension of the recorded data indicates the number of channels as rows and number of sample points as columns. The MATLAB inbuilt function "size" may be applied to know the number of column and number of rows. The time information of the recorded signal can be estimated through the sampling frequency and number of sample points. For example, a very simple MATLAB code to represent the recorded EEG signals which are kept in some computer directory with a file name EEGDATA.

```
Clear all;
Close all;
RData=load ('D/EEGDATA');
[M N]= size (RData);
fs=x; % x is the sampling frequency of the recorded EEG data
t=0:1/fs: (N-1)/fs;
plot (t, RData);
```

This above example is used to plot the recoded EEG signal. The information regarding particular tasks is observed in the particular frequency band of the recorded EEG data. A filter based on a particular frequency band can be designed by a MATLAB code of desired filter of desired response with the help of signal processing in built function 'fdatool'. The fdatool is a Graphical User Interface (GUI) that allows to design, import, and analyze digital FIR and IIR filters. The MATLAB function "fir" and "iir" are used to design finite impulse response filter or infinite impulse response filter. The spectrum of the filtered EEG data has been estimated through parametric as well as nonparametric approaches. Spectrums of the signal by using parametric as well as after filtering of the desired signal. The Welch periodogram and fast Fourier transform based non-parametric approach has been applied for spectrum analysis. The MATLAB built in functions like "pwelch" and "fft" are used for that spectrum analysis. The autoregressive based parametric method is applied for spectrum estimation. The MATLAB built-in functions like "pburg" or "pyulear" functions are used to calculate power spectrum of the signal. The BIOSIG toolbox (Biosig) has been applied to extract feature from the spectrum from the EEG signal. The MATLAB platform also contains a pattern classification toolbox for classifying different tasks. The ICALAB toolbox (ICA Lab) from RIKEN JAPAN has been applied for the spatial filtering operation of recorded data. This toolbox is very important from the spatial filtering point of view. The EEG signals of the nearby channels are highly correlated because the channel distances are very small. The EEG signals are de-correlated before any operations. The ICALAB toolbox has been used to de-correlate EEG signals. All Multiple Unknown Signal Extraction (AMUSE) algorithm has been used to extract original information sources which are mixed instantaneously at sensor points. This is the first basic algorithm in blind source separation (BSS) which exploits second order statistics of original source signals to extract it from multichannel signals. The Objective of the BSS algorithm is to estimate the separating matrix, which is the inverse of mixing matrix.

FUTURE RESEARCH DIRECTIONS

The objective of this research work is to examine the areas of the BCI/BMI with respect to classification accuracy, and the information transfer rate, for real time control of an electric wheelchair for a disabled person. In order to develop the real time control of electric wheelchair a good quality EEG amplifier along with readymade electric wheelchair are needed. In this research work, the authors proposed to investigate the approach which will maximize the classification accuracy, the information transfer rate and minimize the processing for the real time control of the external machine. These are the fundamental problems and require some advanced signal analysis and feature extraction methods, which will efficiently solve these fundamental problems. Many researchers have estimated the periodic wave forms from the recorded sensor signals. Instead of sensor signals, one can use the uncorrelated sensor signals for the detection of a sinusoidal periodic waveform, which will give a good estimation of certain frequency signals. For the same, researchers can apply the blind source separation algorithm for the decorrelation of sensor signals. The authors are also interested to investigate the best power spectral density approach in order to get the peak value of signal at desired frequency. Also the authors are interested to apply an adaptive filtering algorithm to estimate the desired frequency component signals. During sanctioned period of project, the authors are planning to develop and investigate the novel idea of signal processing, which will maximize the information transfer rate for real time control of electric wheelchair for disabled person. Recent trends of the BCI research is based on neuro fuzzy, ssvep, p300 stated in Ankit

Kumar Das et al. (2016), Hao-Teng Hsu et al. (2016), Haiqiang Wang et al. (2016), Ko Watanabe et al. (2016), Erwei Yin et al. (2015), Sameer Kishore et al. (2014), Yeou-Jiunn Chen et al. (2014), Christoph Groenegress et al. (2010).

CONCLUSION

The concept of thought generation in the human brain is a very complex phenomenon and has not been accessible yet directly, as the biological processing and the format of the signal in the brain is not clearly understood. However, the levels of thoughts and types of thoughts have been broadly investigated as change in the rhythm and the patterns of the EEG signals are captured at the surface of the skull. Although, the EEG signals are not the direct access to the levels of thoughts and thought related actions, but it represents the shadow of it and hence to some extent, thought related patterns can be inferred and used for a controlling action. However, 100% thought recognition will remain untouched for either of the statistical classifiers using a single feature vector. For the real-time control, the information transfer rate is not sufficient to control an external machine such as a robot, an electric wheelchair or a computer cursor. The challenges are usability of the EEG signals for the cognitive task selection. If it can be used, what will be the best approach of signal processing, feature extraction; will maximize the information transfer rate.

REFERENCES

Bashashati, A., Fatourechi, M., Ward, R. K., & Birch, G. E. (2007). A survey of signal processing algorithms in brain–computer interfaces based on electrical brain signals. *Journal of Neural Engineering*, 4(2), R32–R57. doi:10.1088/1741-2560/4/2/R03 PMID:17409474

Birbaumer, N., Ghanayim, N., & Flor, H. (1999). A spelling device for the paralysed. *Nature*, 398(6725), 297–298. doi:10.1038/18581 PMID:10192330

Bhattacharyya, S., & Mukul, M. K. (2017). Temporal Relative Spectral Power Based Real Time Motor Imagery Classification. *International Journal of Engineering Sciences & Research Technology*, 33-38.

Bhattacharyya, S., & Mukul, M. K. (2016). Cepstral Coefficients Based Feature for Real Time Movement Imagery Classification. *International Journal of Engineering and Technology*, 8(1), 117-123.

Bhattacharyya Sumanta Mukul, M. K. (2016). Short Time Fourier Transform based Dominant Frequency Extraction Algorithm for Brain Computer Interface. *International Journal of Scientific Research & Technology*, 2(1), 67-74.

Bhattacharyya, S., & Mukul, M. K. (2016, September). Cepstrum Based Algorithm for Motor Imagery Classification. *International Conference on Micro-Electronics and Telecommunication Engineering (ICMETE 2016)* (pp. 397-402). IEEE. doi:10.1109/ICMETE.2016.140

Carlson, N. R. (2007). *Foundations of physiological psychology*. Allyn and Bacon. Available from: http://www.bbci.de/competition/ii/

Biosig for Matlab and Octave – An open source software library for biomedical signal processing. (2005). Available from: http://biosig.sf.net

Christopher de Charms, R., Christoff, K., Glover, G. H., Pauly, J. M., Whitfield, S., & Gabrieli, J. D. (2004). Learned regulation of spatially localized brain activation using real-time fMRI. *NeuroImage*, *21*(1).

Choi, S., Cichocki, A., Park, H. M., & Lee, S. Y. (2005). Blind source separation and independent component analysis: A review. *Neural Information Processing-Letters and Reviews*, *6*(1), 1–57.

Das, A. K., Sundaram, S., & Sundararajan, N. (2016). A Self-Regulated Interval Type-2 Neuro-Fuzzy Inference System for Handling Nonstationarities in EEG Signals for BCI. *IEEE Transactions on Fuzzy Systems*, *24*(6), 1565–1577. doi:10.1109/TFUZZ.2016.2540072

Duda, R. O., Hart, P. E., & Stork, D. G. (2001). *2nd Pattern Classification*. Academic Press.

Gandhi, V., Prasad, G., Coyle, D., Behera, L., &McGinnity, T. M. (2014). Quantum neural network-based EEG filtering for a brain–computer interface. *IEEE Transactions on Neural Networks and Learning Systems*, *25*(2), 278-288.

Groenegress, C., Holzner, C., Guger, C., & Slater, M. (2010). Effects of P300-based BCI use on reported presence in a virtual environment. *Presence (Cambridge, Mass.)*, *19*(1), 1–11. doi:10.1162/pres.19.1.1

Gutberlet, I., Debener, S., Jung, T. P., &Makeig, S. (2009). Techniques of EEG recording and preprocessing. *Quantative EEG Analysis Methods and Clinical Applications*, 23-49.

Hochberg, L. R., & Donoghue, J. P. (2006). Sensors for brain-computer interfaces. *IEEE Engineering in Medicine and Biology Magazine*, *25*(5), 32–38. doi:10.1109/MEMB.2006.1705745 PMID:17020197

Hjorth, B. (1970). EEG analysis based on time domain properties. *Electroencephalography and Clinical Neurophysiology*, *29*(3), 306–310. doi:10.1016/0013-4694(70)90143-4 PMID:4195653

Hsu, H. T., Lee, I. H., Tsai, H. T., Chang, H. C., Shyu, K. K., Hsu, C. C., & Lee, P. L. (2016). Evaluate the feasibility of using frontal SSVEP to implement an SSVEP-based BCI in young, Elderly and ALS Groups. *IEEE Transactions on Neural Systems and Rehabilitation Engineering*, *24*(5), 603–615. doi:10.1109/TNSRE.2015.2496184 PMID:26625417

ICA Lab – an open source software library for biomedical signal processing. (n.d.). Available from: http://www.bsp.brain.riken.jp/ICALAB/

Kishore, S., González-Franco, M., Hintemüller, C., Kapeller, C., Guger, C., Slater, M., & Blom, K. J. (2014). Comparison of SSVEP BCI and eye tracking for controlling a humanoid robot in a social environment. *Presence (Cambridge, Mass.)*, *23*(3), 242–252. doi:10.1162/PRES_a_00192

Long, J., Li, Y., Wang, H., Yu, T., Pan, J., & Li, F. (2012). A hybrid brain computer interface to control the direction and speed of a simulated or real wheelchair. *IEEE Transactions on Neural Systems and Rehabilitation Engineering*, *20*(5), 720–729. doi:10.1109/TNSRE.2012.2197221 PMID:22692936

Machavarapu, S. C., Mukul, M. K., & Kumar, D. (2014, March). EEG classification based on variance. In *Green Computing Communication and Electrical Engineering (ICGCCEE), 2014 International Conference on* (pp. 1-4). IEEE. doi:10.1109/ICGCCEE.2014.6922216

Mellinger, J., Schalk, G., Braun, C., Preissl, H., Rosenstiel, W., Birbaumer, N., & Kübler, A. (2007). An MEG-based brain-computer interface (BCI). *NeuroImage, 36*(3), 581–593. doi:10.1016/j.neuroimage.2007.03.019 PMID:17475511

Mukul, M. K., & Matsuno, F. (2010, December). Comparative study between subband and standard ICA/BSS method in context with EEG signal for movement imagery classification. In *System Integration (SII), 2010 IEEE/SICE International Symposium on* (pp. 341-346). IEEE.

Ngoc, H. T., Nguyen, T. H., & Ngo, C. (2013). Average partial power spectrum density approach to feature extraction for EEG-based motor imagery classification. *American Journal of Biomedical Engineering, 3*(6), 208–219.

Schlögl, A., Keinrath, C., Zimmermann, D., Scherer, R., Leeb, R., & Pfurtscheller, G. (2007). A fully automated correction method of EOG artifacts in EEG recordings. *Clinical Neurophysiology, 118*(1), 98–104. doi:10.1016/j.clinph.2006.09.003 PMID:17088100

Srinivasulu, A., & Reddy, M. S. (2012). Artifacts Removing From EEG Signals by ICA Algorithms. *IOS Journal of Electrical and Electronics Engineering, 2*(4), 11–16. doi:10.9790/1676-0241116

Vigário, R., Sarela, J., Jousmiki, V., Hamalainen, M., & Oja, E. (2000). Independent component approach to the analysis of EEG and MEG recordings. *IEEE Transactions on Bio-Medical Engineering, 47*(5), 589–593. doi:10.1109/10.841330 PMID:10851802

Wang, H., Zhang, Y., Waytowich, N. R., Krusienski, D. J., Zhou, G., Jin, J., & Cichocki, A. (2016). Discriminative feature extraction via multivariate linear regression for SSVEP-based BCI. *IEEE Transactions on Neural Systems and Rehabilitation Engineering, 24*(5), 532–541. doi:10.1109/TNSRE.2016.2519350 PMID:26812728

Watanabe, K., Tanaka, H., Takahashi, K., Niimura, Y., Watanabe, K., & Kurihara, Y. (2016). NIRS-Based Language Learning BCI System. *IEEE Sensors Journal, 16*(8), 2726–2734. doi:10.1109/JSEN.2016.2519886

Waldert, S., Pistohl, T., Braun, C., Ball, T., Aertsen, A., & Mehring, C. (2009). A review on directional information in neural signals for brain-machine interfaces. *Journal of Physiology, Paris, 103*(3), 244–254. doi:10.1016/j.jphysparis.2009.08.007 PMID:19665554

Wolpaw, J. R., Birbaumer, N., McFarland, D. J., Pfurtscheller, G., & Vaughan, T. M. (2002). Brain–computer interfaces for communication and control. *Clinical Neurophysiology, 113*(6), 767–791. doi:10.1016/S1388-2457(02)00057-3 PMID:12048038

Wolpaw, J. R., Birbaumer, N., Heetderks, W. J., McFarland, D. J., Peckham, P. H., Schalk, G., & Vaughan, T. M. (2000). Brain-computer interface technology: A review of the first international meeting. *IEEE Transactions on Rehabilitation Engineering, 8*(2), 164–173. doi:10.1109/TRE.2000.847807 PMID:10896178

Wolpaw, J. R., & McFarland, D. J. (1994). Multichannel EEG-based brain-computer communication. *Electroencephalography and Clinical Neurophysiology, 90*(6), 444–449. doi:10.1016/0013-4694(94)90135-X PMID:7515787

Chen, Y.-J., & Aaron, R. A. S. (2014). SSVEP-based BCI classification using power cepstrum analysis. *MIT Press Journals*, *50*(10), 735–737.

Yin, E., Zhou, Z., Jiang, J., Yu, Y., & Hu, D. (2015). A dynamically optimized SSVEP brain–computer interface (BCI) speller. *IEEE Transactions on Bio-Medical Engineering*, *62*(6), 1447–1456. doi:10.1109/TBME.2014.2320948 PMID:24801483

KEY TERMS AND DEFINITIONS

Asymmetry: Asymmetry exists when the two halves of something don't match or are unequal. lack or absence of symmetry in spatial arrangements or in mathematical or logical relations.

Blind Source Separation: Blind signal separation (BSS), also known as blind source separation, is the separation of a set of source signals from a set of mixed signals, without the aid of information (or with very little information) about the source signals or the mixing process.

Brain-Computer Interface: A Brain Computer Interface is a communication system that does not depend on the Brain's normal output pathways of peripheral nerves and muscles. Brain computer interface (BCI) is a collaboration between a brain and a device that enables signals from the brain to direct some external activity, such as control of a cursor or a prosthetic limb. The interface enables a direct communications pathway between the brain and the object to be controlled.

Classification Accuracy: It is the number of correct predictions made divided by the total number of predictions made, multiplied by 100 to turn it into a percentage.

Cohen's Kappa Coefficient: Cohen's kappa coefficient is a statistic which measures inter-rater agreement for qualitative (categorical) items. It is generally thought to be a more robust measure than simple percent agreement calculation, since κ takes into account the possibility of the agreement occurring by chance.

Electroencephalogram: An electroencephalogram (EEG) is a test that detects electrical activity in your brain using small, flat metal discs (electrodes) attached to your scalp.

Independent Component Analysis: Independent component analysis (ICA) is a statistical and computational technique for revealing hidden factors that underlie sets of random variables, measurements, or signals.

Mutual Information: In probability theory and information theory, the mutual information (MI) of two random variables is a measure of the mutual dependence between the two variables. More specifically, it quantifies the "amount of information" (in units such as bits) obtained about one random variable, through the other random variable.

Chapter 19
A Case–Based–Reasoning System for Feature Selection and Diagnosing Asthma

Somayeh Akhavan Darabi
Azad University of Tehran Shomal, Iran

Babak Teimourpour
Tarbiat Modares University, Iran

ABSTRACT

Asthma is a chronic disease of the airways in the lungs. The differentiation between asthma, COPD and bronchiectasis in the early stage of disease is very important for the adoption of appropriate therapeutic measures. In this research, a case-based-reasoning (CBR) model is proposed to assist a physician to therapy. First of all, features and symptoms are determined and patients' data is gathered with a questionnaire, then CBR algorithm is run on the data which leads to the asthma diagnosis. The system was tested on 325 asthmatic and non-asthmatic adult cases and the accuracy was eighty percent. The consequences were promising. This study was performed in order to determine risk factors for asthma in a specific society and the results of research showed that the most important variables of asthma disease are symptoms hyper-responsive, frequency of cough and cough.

INTRODUCTION

Asthma is the most prevalent chronic disease in children and adolescents which causes much morbidity increase, mortality and health care expenditure. In addition to the mortality augmentation caused by this disease, asthma has a lot of effects on the life quality and children's educational activities. It is clear that false diagnosis and inappropriate therapy are two factors which help morbidity and mortality increase in asthmatic illness which both occur for the reason of lack of knowledge in the patients and the families. Studies show that there is a considerable difference between accepted asthma prevalence by physicians and the asthma related to symptoms in medical researches which it shows the lack of asthma recognition by physicians in Iran (Tootoonchi, 2004). By better identification of pathogenic mechanisms

DOI: 10.4018/978-1-5225-2515-8.ch019

in asthma ailment and the efficient communication in effective variables in asthma and determining the most important of them, one can promote people and patients' knowledge and this trend causes the disease symptoms and the asthmatic patient's life quality to be connected intensity as scoring searches. Feedbacks with their significance accept the transferable relationships (Akhavan Darabi et al., 2014). Asthma has also more morbidity in the developed countries, but it has more asthmatic mortalities which can be ascribed to the third world countries. The other reasons can be attributed to the nonexistence of sufficient specialists, the lack of necessary facilities for diagnosis and the ignorance of people in this field which is more significant than other reasons.

The prevalence of asthma varies widely in different regions of the world due to distinct genetic, environmental and occupational risk factors. However, this disparity appears to be closing as the prevalence in high-income countries is reaching a plateau, whereas the prevalence in low and middle-income countries continues to rise. Worldwide, it is estimated that approximately 334 million people currently suffer from asthma, and 250,000 deaths are attributed to the disease each year. The prevalence of the disease is continuing to grow, and the overall prevalence is estimated to increase by 100 million by 2025 (Yolanda Smith & BPharm, 2016).

Within the medical community, there has been significant research into preventing clinical deterioration among hospital patients. Data mining on electronic medical records has attracted a lot of attention, but it is still at an early stage in practice. Clinical study has found that 4–17% of patients undergo cardiopulmonary or respiratory arrest while in the hospital (Commission, 2008). Early detection and intervention are essential to preventing these serious, often life-threatening events. Indeed, early detection and treatment of patients with sepsis has already shown promising results, resulting in significantly lower mortality rates (Joans and Brown, 2008).

Case based reasoning (CBR) technique is one of the data mining tools which are applied for the medical diagnosis, anticipating the chronological order and so forth.

LITERATURE REVIEW

There are different kinds of studies for Data Mining techniques in medical databases. We identify the following categories:

Data Mining Techniques and Healthcare

Lee et al. (2015), used new data mining mechanism for the purpose of asthma attack disease prediction. These two methods are called the tree decision depended upon the law-based pattern. The accuracy of this system is 84.12 percent.

Nordquist et al. (1996), studied about the rendering of the learning operation. As a matter of fact, the aim was to determine the success level of performing the learning process on the basis of the sample. In another article, Chae and Hoo (1996), compared the two nervous lattices algorithms and case based reasoning (CBR).

Misra and Dehuri (2007), in their study, Functional Link Artificial Neural Network for Classification Task in Data Mining created a Functional Link Artificial Neural network and compared its classification performance with other machine learning algorithms. Their FLANN has given 21.87% misclassification performance and MLP has given 24.8% classification performance.

Delen (2009), used three popular data mining techniques (decision trees, artificial neural networks and support vector machines) along with the most commonly used statistical analysis technique logistic regression to develop prediction models for prostate cancer survivability. The data set contained around 120,000 records and 77 variables. A k-fold cross-validation methodology was used in building, evaluating and comparing the model. The results showed that support vector machines are the most accurate predictor (with a testing set accuracy of 92.85%) for this domain, followed by artificial neural networks and decision trees.

Karaolis et al. (2010), developed a data-mining system for the assessment of heart event-related risk factors targeting in the reduction of CHD events. The risk factors investigated were: 1) before the event: a) non modifiable-age, sex, and family history for premature CHD, b) modifiable-smoking before the event, history of hypertension, and history of diabetes; and 2) after the event: modifiable-smoking after the event, systolic blood pressure, diastolic blood pressure, total cholesterol, high-density lipoprotein, low-density lipoprotein, triglycerides and glucose. The events investigated were: myocardial infarction (MI), percutaneous coronary intervention (PCI) and coronary artery bypass graft surgery (CABG). A total of 528 cases were collected from the Paphos district in Cyprus, most of them with more than one event. Data mining analysis was carried out using the C4.5 decision tree algorithm for the aforementioned three events using five different splitting criteria. The most important risk factors, as extracted from the classification rules analysis were: 1) for MI, age, smoking and history of hypertension; 2) for PCI, family history, history of hypertension and history of diabetes; and 3) for CABG, age, history of hypertension and smoking. Most of these risk factors were also extracted by other investigators. The highest percentages of correct classifications achieved were 66%, 75%, and 75% for the MI, PCI, and CABG models, respectively. It is anticipated that data mining could help in the identification of high and low risk subgroups of subjects, a decisive factor for the selection of therapy, i.e., medical or surgical. However, further investigation with larger datasets is still needed.

Kumari and Godara (2011), in their research used data mining classification techniques RIPPER classifier, Decision Tree, Artificial neural networks (ANNs) and Support Vector Machine (SVM) that have been applied on cardiovascular disease dataset. The performance of these techniques was compared through sensitivity, specificity, accuracy, error rate, True Positive Rate and False Positive Rate. In their study, 10-fold cross validation method was used to measure the unbiased estimate of these prediction models. Their analysis showed that out of these four classification models SVM predicts cardiovascular disease with least error rate and highest accuracy.

They demonstrated an overview of the current research being carried out using the data mining techniques to enhance heart disease diagnosis and prediction including decision trees, Naive Bayes classifiers, K-nearest neighbour classification (KNN), support vector machine (SVM) and artificial neural networks techniques. Results showed that SVM and neural networks perform positively high to predict the presence of coronary heart diseases (CHD). Decision trees after features reduction is the best recommended classifier to diagnose cardiovascular disease (CVD). Still the performance of data mining techniques to detect coronary arteries diseases (CAD) is not encouraging (between 60%-75%) and further improvements should be pursued (Salha M. Alzahani et al, 2014).

AiswaryaIyer et al. (2015), found the solutions to diagnose the disease by analyzing the patterns found in the data through classification analysis by employing Decision Tree and Naïve Bayes algorithms. The research hopes to propose a quicker and more efficient technique of diagnosing the disease, leading to timely treatment of the patients.

Jaya et al. (2015), studied the data mining techniques, methods, tools and applications in various industries. In their study, the following chapters are presented- various data mining techniques, merits and demerits of data mining, open source data mining tools available, and also domains or industries applied DM.

Sheenal Pate and Hardik Patel (2016), conducted a survey on the data mining techniques that are used in Healthcare domain. They used various data mining techniques such as classification, clustering, association and also highlighted related work to analyze and predict human disease.

Haripriya and Porkodi (2016), investigated mainly the data mining techniques used in DICOM (Medical Imaging) which are stored in distributed storage. Data mining on DICOM enables quick retrieval.

Krishnaiah et al. (2016), studied different papers in which one or more algorithms of data mining used for the prediction of heart disease. Based on the study, it is observed that the fuzzy intelligent techniques increase the accuracy of the heart disease prediction system. The generally used techniques for heart disease prediction and their complexities are summarized in this article.

CBR and Healthcare

Schmidt et al. (1999), discussed the importance of creating prototypes automatically within Case-Based Reasoning systems. They presented some general ideas about prototypes deduced from analyses of their experiences with prototype designs in domain specific medical CBR systems. Four medical Case-Based Reasoning systems are described. As they used prototypes for different purposes, the gained improvement is different as well. Furthermore, they claimed that the generation of prototypes is an adequate technique to learn the intrinsic case knowledge, especially if the domain theory is weak.

Sefion et al. (2003), chose case-based reasoning paradigm to develop medical decision support system. Intelligent data analysis methods have been used to determine the case model for their system. Their similarity metric is based on the MVDM method. They developed two methods to reuse retrieved cases. They presented their data analysis results and similarity metric from which they designed case based system for asthmatic patient's health care: ADEMA.

Jaulent et al. (2005), presented the functional architecture of a Case-Based-Reasoning system in this domain. The main procedure is the selection of similar previous cases that has been implemented. The selection of the procedure was based on an original similarity measure that takes into account both semantic and structural resemblances and differences between the cases. The first evaluation of the system was performed on a base of 35 pathological cases of specimen of breast palpable tumors.

Ying Shen et al. (2015), depicted the methodological steps and tools about the combined operation of case-based reasoning (CBR) and multi-agent system (MAS) to expose the ontological application in the field of clinical decision support. The multi-agent architecture works for the consideration of the whole cycle of clinical decision-making adaptable to many medical aspects such as the diagnosis, prognosis, treatment and therapeutic monitoring of gastric cancer. In the multi-agent architecture, the ontological agent type employs the domain knowledge to ease the extraction of similar clinical cases and provide treatment suggestions to patients and physicians. Ontological agent is used for the extension of domain hierarchy and the interpretation of input requests. Case-based reasoning memorizes and restores experience data for solving similar problems, with the help of matching approach and defined interfaces of ontologies. A typical case is developed to illustrate the implementation of the knowledge acquisition and restitution of medical experts.

Asthma

Chooi et al. (2001), demonstrated that there are not necessary feasibilities for evaluating the respiration by using the computer program which causes more ascension for the asthma diagnosis accuracy. Nevertheless, the present study focuses on developing a computer program model to help diagnose asthma. Bibi et al. (2001), created a nervous lattice for the target of foretelling the asthma respiratory symptoms and COPD disease and bronchiectasis.

Zolnoori et al. (2010), created a computer-aided intelligent system for diagnosing pediatric asthma ((age range 6-18) as a phase-proficient system for asthma diagnosis in 6-18 year olds which showed a system sensitivity of 88% and specificity of 100%.

Behrouz Alizadeh et al. (2015), developed an intelligent system for the diagnosis of asthma based on artificial neural network. The study population is the patients who had visited one of the Lung Clinics in Tehran. According to the analysis performed by means of SPSS to select the top factors, 13 effective factors were selected, in different performances, data was mixed in various forms, so the different modes was made for the training data and testing networks. In all different modes, the network was able to predict correctly 100% of all cases.

Abhinav et al. (2016), tried to integrate the data preprocessing technique with data classification technique to mine the big data of the asthma based patients. They used cloud based data mining model. Cloud computing provides the software on pay-per-use option which make it easier for the people who are not able to meet the economic requirements. Since the whole scenario is beneficial to big industries such as facebook, google, orkut and etc., various order fields are also getting dependent on cloud computing. Since tons of data are uploaded every second to the cloud server, they need to be mined properly for efficient data storage.

The input variable of this system is the air pollution. This system is able to predict 12 percent of error. The designed system of asthma diagnosis helps save time and money, so this system causes saving in time and expense.

The CBR system methodology is discussed in the following section followed by a discussion on the system performance test and evaluation in the "system performance evaluation section. The "Discussion and Conclusion" section will summarize and conclude the article.

METHODOLOGY

In the present research, a case-based-reasoning system for the purpose of diagnosing the disease more truly and accurately followed by appropriation therapy has been designed. For the sake of creating and developing this system, at first the data collected from the lungs specialized hospital with questionnaire and the efficient variables in the asthma disease have been identified. Features are divided into 5 categories such as Symptoms, Genetic Factors, Medical History, Allergy Factors and Social Factors, as shown in Table 1. The creation of this system includes determining the system inputs, weighting the variables, ascertaining CBR algorithm structure, evaluating and performance testing which are discussed in this study. The overall framework of the model is illustrated in Figure 1.

After identifying the variables, a questionnaire was arranged in conformity with it and after that filling out the questionnaire through the patient's enquiry under the physician surveillance. The data gathering has been conducted. The data includes asthmatic and non asthmatic patients that have been brought

Table 1. Features

Diagnosis of Asthma				
Symptoms	**Genetic Factors**	**Medical History**	**Allergy Factors**	**Social Factors**
1. Cough	8. Allergy rhinitis in Father or Mother	17. Sinusitis	23. Allergies	27. Location: village or city
2. Just nocturnal	9. Allergy rhinitis in Father & Mother	18. GER	24. Irritant	28. Exposure to chemical materials
3. Just daily cough	10. Allergy rhinitis in immediate	19. Allergy rhinitis	25. Food allergies	29. Air pollution
4. Phlegm	11. Eczema in Father or mother	20. Cold	26. Emotional	30. High density of dust
5. Seasonal cough	12. Eczema in father and mother	21. Eczema	23. Allergies	31. Exposure to smoking
6. Wheeze	13. Eczema in immediate	22. BMI	24. Irritant	32. Exposure to water cooler
7. Symptoms exercise	14. Asthma in Father or Mother		25. Food allergies	33. Precedent of pets
36. Time of cough	15. Asthma in Father and Mother		26. Emotional	34. Humidity in house
37. Frequency of cough	16. Asthma in immediate			35. Climate with humidity
38. Time of wheeze				
39. Frequency of wheeze				
40. Type of wheeze				
41. Chest tightness				
42. Dyspnea				

as a database in the excel table. Data processing: the data is preprocessed in order to be applied in the (CBR) system. This section is very important and time consuming, and it involves the following steps:

1. Deleting the data columns, file code, computer code, age, gender and the number of the patient's column.
2. We made the multi substandard variables ordinal in order to decrease the number of variables (ordinal in order to decrease cough, wheeze, ... column)
3. Improving and repairing of noise and error data
4. Filling the missing data by Knn Imputation
5. Outliers data identification and deletion
6. Editing the duplications
7. Mixing up the genetic factors which blend with each other for the reason of identical significance
8. Data normalization: the variables are classified into the classes of medical history (Ernst et al., 2002), environmental factors (Bousquet et al., 2003), allergic rhinitis (Shapiro et al., 2006) and genetic factors.

Figure 1. Fundamental method

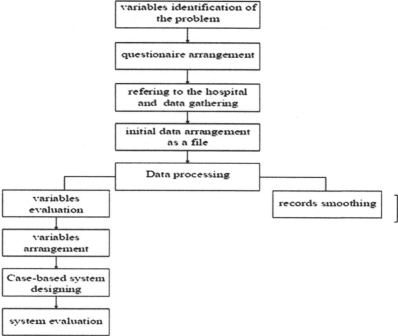

FEATURE EVALUATION

Variables evaluation is an important problem in statistical research and machine learning methods. Feature selection algorithms provide a more effective set of data.

Feature evaluation algorithms attribute one rank to each variable that shows the effect of that variable in the classification of the classes.

The more the rank of a variable is, the more share that rank has in the calculations. In fact, some sort of weighting variables is performed.

For weighting variables, two methods of weighting named RandomForest and P-value have been applied. The system was evaluated by both methods. The RandomForest method yielded better results. In the test with assumption of $x^2=0$, there exists two independent variables and if P-valuebe comes less than the pre-determined amount of a = 0.05 or 0.1.

Terminated to the zero test refusal, this means that the less the amount of P-values, the more dependent those both variables are. On the other hand, the more a variable is closer to the target variable, the more influence it has on it. Thus, the inverted values of P-value as a feature weight are used. With obeying the rest of the weight vector provision like when total weights becomes one. Random forests can be used to rank the importance of variables in a regression or classification problem in a natural way.

The first step in measuring the variable importance in a data set $D= (X_i, Y_i)[i=1$ to n] is to fit a random forest to the data. During the fitting process the out-of-bag error for each data point is recorded and averaged over the forest (errors on an independent test set can be substituted if bagging is not used during training).

To measure the importance of the j-th feature after training, the values of the j-th feature are permuted among the training data and the out-of-bag error is again computed on this perturbed data set. The importance score for the j-th feature is computed by averaging the difference in out-of-bag error before and after the permutation over all trees. The score is normalized by the standard deviation of these differences.

Smoothing the Records

By applying the smoothing method (minimizing large classes and creating artificial data for smaller classes), some changes were made in the data number. Data arrangement: for multilevel variables changed into the ordinal ones.

CBR Algorithm Structure

Case-based-reasoning method has been formed on the basis of using the previous problem response for the solution of the new identical problems.

CBR is known as a method which has modeled the human behavior quality in conformity with the new problems; hence it uses the acquired experiences in solving the previous problems as a guide for the new problem solution.

A CBR system is used to find a solution for the new difficulty passes through a four step process. The steps of this process form a ring which has been illustrated in Figure 2.

- Retrieving the identical previous cases.
- Reusing the cases for new problem solution.
- Revising the suggested solution in cases of necessity.
- Retaining the given solutions as a new case.

Case: It determines a description in series of questions which must be asked and the possible responses for them, also the operations that must be done for each of them. In this study, the sort of database is smooth, in other words, it means that all the cases have a series of identical features.

Retrieving step: In the retrieve phase of the CBR cycle, one or several cases from the case base are selected, based on the modeled similarity. In a nutshell, the retrieval task is defined as finding a small number of cases from the case base with the highest similarity to the query. Hence, this is a k-nearest-neighbor retrieval task considering a specific similarity function. However, when the case base grows, the efficiency of retrieval decreases, because an increasing number of cases must be taken into account to find the most similar case. Thus one sub-branch of CBR research deals with methods that improve retrieval efficiency, e.g. by using specific index structures such as kd-trees, case-retrieval nets, or discrimination networks (Bergmann, 2002). This step includes retrieving the existed identical cases in the cases library in which a similar difficulty was confronted; thus, the closest neighborhood method was considered to be the most fundamental method of distance based learning method. After summing up the similarity among the various variables by using the algorithm (1), the similarity between the two records is calculated (Bagherjeiran et al., 2006).

Figure 2. Case based reasoning processing

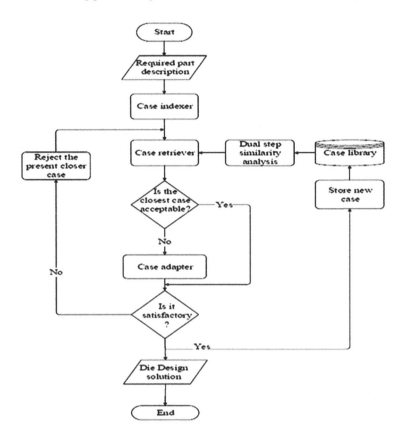

Algorithm (1) shows the similarity among the records with heterogeneous variables:

1.   For K_{th} variable, calculate and normalize the similarity between the two records of $S(X, Y)$.

2.   For K_{th} variable defines the k pointer as follows: $\delta_k = \begin{cases} 0 \\ 1 \end{cases}$

3.   Calculate the overall similarity between the two records by applying the following:

$$\text{Phrase: Similarity}(x, y) = \frac{\sum_{k=1}^{n} wk \times \partial k \times sk}{\sum_{k=1}^{n} \partial k} \tag{1}$$

$$\sum_{k=1}^{n} wk = 1$$

Phase 2 and 3 exhibit that at first every feature weight must be included in the distance calculation. Secondly, when the K_{th} variable of one or both records is lost or for asymmetric variables when both records have the sum of zero, that K_{th} variable does not enter the calculations. Thirdly, the gained distances must eventually be normalized as well.

Evaluating the System Performance and Result

As a result, 325 samples of asthmatic and none asthmatic patients were gathered in 2014 -2015.

These patients were adults (men and women are both included). For the purpose of increasing system accuracy, the non asthmatic patients sample had difficulty in their lungs. For performing the CBR system the R software was used.

R Software is one of the best tools for data mining. For this study, some of the functions is implemented in R software. In order to select the features, RandomForest and p-value techniques are used. For weighting the criteria, RANDOM and P-VALUE function are used in R and most importantly, the CBR is implemented in R software completely.

The previous methods tried to find a compact representation of the data that can be used for future prediction. In case-based reasoning, the training examples (the cases) are stored and accessed to solve a new problem. To get a prediction for a new example, those cases that are similar or close to the new example are used to predict the value of the target features of the new example. This is at one extreme of the learning problem where unlike decision trees and neural networks, relatively little work must be done offline, and virtually all of the work is performed at query time.

Case-based reasoning can be used for classification and regression. It is also applicable when the cases are complicated, such as in legal cases, where the cases are complex legal rulings, and in planning, where the cases are previous solutions to complex problems.

If the cases are simple, one algorithm that works well is to use the k-nearest neighbors for some given number k. Given a new example, the k training examples that have the input features closest to that example are used to predict the target value for the new example. The prediction can be the mode, average, or some interpolation between the predictions of these k training examples, perhaps weighting closer examples more than distant examples.

For this method to work, a distance metric is required to measure the closeness of two examples. First define a metric for the domain of each feature, in which the values of the features are converted to a numerical scale that can be used to compare values. Suppose $val(e,X_i)$ is a numerical representation of the value of feature X_i for the example e. Then $(val(e_1,X_i) - val(e_2,X_i))$ is the difference between example e_1 and e_2 on the dimension defined by feature X_i. The Euclidean distance, the square root of the sum of the squares of the dimension differences, can be used as the distance between two examples. One important issue is the relative scales of different dimensions; increasing the scale of one dimension increases the importance of that feature. Let w_i be a non-negative real-valued parameter that specifies the weight of feature X_i. The distance between examples e_1 and e_2 is then:

$$d(e_1, e_2) = sqrt(\sum i.w_i.(val(e_1, X_i) - val(e_2, X_i))^2).$$

The feature weights can be provided as an input. It is also possible to learn these weights. The learning agent can try to find a parameter setting that minimizes the error in predicting the value of each element of the training set, based on every other instance in the training set. This is called the leave-one-out cross-validation error measure.

The system performance was tested and evaluated by the specialist physicians. The system evaluation standards are specificity, sensitivity and accuracy.

After deleting the data, 30 percent of the database data was selected randomly to test the system and the remaining 70 percent were used for making the system cases.

The consequences given in this section is the result of the system experiment on the testing data (as shown in Table 2).

Sensitivity: Represents the ratio of the positive cases which mark their model as a plus or positive mark.

Specificity: Represents the ratio of the negative cases that the experiment marks them truly as a negative mark or minus.

As these results display, the RandomForest gives more favorite conclusions (as shown in Table 3). In the feature selection step, the computerized and the statistical methods of p-value and the Random-Forest have been used, and a weight has been given to each feature. By applying the rFCV order and R software, the weights were gained from the RandomForest and where it gave the least error, the features numbers were selected. The model selected 32 variables with least error.

With regards to the point that the system accuracy is better by using RandomForest method, according to the gathered data, the selection of the risk factors of the asthma disease has been identified in accordance with this table. Filling the lost amounts by using the closest neighborhood method, With K=10 for 209 series patient sample (as shown in Table 4):

All data values must be completed before they are weighted by running the Random Forest Method. The missing values were filled out in the tables using KnnImpt method.

DISCUSSION AND CONCLUSION

This system is in the first step diagnoses of the adult asthmatic patients and identifies the risk factors in a specific society. The main goal of using the case-based reasoning system is to assist the physician for the purpose of diagnosing the disease and select the therapy more effectively. The next step is creating a system for the sake of helping the general practitioners and medical students in the adult's asthma diagnosis. The asthma diagnosis system development is to assist in warning the potential asthmatic patients for personal hygiene and health as well as the disease prevention. The application of this system is in the health ministry medical learning and therapy and it is used by the physicians and the medical students. Through this system analysis in diagnosing the adult's asthma disease, the amount of 80% accuracy, 65% sensitivity and 84% specificity were obvious. For elevating the system accuracy through the data gathering step, Physicians talked with patients to fill out the questionnaire in order to collect

Table 2. System evaluation results based on test data

Weighting with Random Forest	Weighting with P-value
K=5 Accuracy = 80 percent Sensitivity = 65 percent Specificity = 84 percent	K=5 for each Accuracy = 68 percent Sensitivity = 17 percent Specificity = 76 percent

Table 3. Ranking features with RandomForest and p-value

Ranking Features with RandomForest	Ranking Features with P-value
symptoms.heperresponsivity.3 Frequency of cough	symptoms.heperresponsivity.3
Cough	BMI
symptoms.heperresponsivity.2 frequency of wheeze	Just nocturnal cough without any pattern
Wheeze	Phlegm.1
Dyspnoea	Genetic factors.1
Chest tightness	Frequency of cough
Type of wheeze	Just daily cough without any pattern
symptoms.heperresponsivity.4 symptoms.heperresponsivity.1 allergic rhinitis severity	cold.3
GER	symptoms.heperresponsivity4
phlegm.2	cold.2
exercise.2	Allergic rhinitis severity
Genetic factors.6	cold.1
cold.3	Eczema
Genetic factors.4	cough
Sinusitis	social.factores.1
Social factores.5	Symptoms heperresponsivity.1
exercise.1	Symptoms heperresponsivity.2
Social factores.3	exercise.2
cold.1	Phlegm.2
BMI	exercise.1
Allergic rhinitis time	Social factores.4
cold.2	Sinusitis
eczema	Chest tightness
phlegm.5	Allergic rhinitis time
Just daily cough	Type of wheeze
Social factores.1	Frequency of cough
phlegm.3	Seasonal cough
Phlegm.1	GER
social.factores.4	Genetic factors.2
Just nocturnal cough	Dyspnoea
genetic factor.3	Genetic factors.3
genetic factor.2	Wheeze
genetic factor.5	Genetic factors.6
seasonal cough	Social factores.2
genetic factor.1	Genetic factors.4
Phlegm.4	Social factores.3

Table 4. Filling the missing data

1	0	NA	NA	NA	NA	NA	NA	NA	NA	NA	NA	3	2	1
1	0	0	1	1	0	1	0	0	1	0	0	3	2	1

Table 5. The data balancing results

	Before Balancing	After Balancing
Number of Class One (Asthma)	209	287
Number of Class One (Non Asthma)	115	230

data on the relevant variables. The patient's files have been referenced. The data is without the laboratory information. The results of research showed that the most important variables of asthma disease are symptoms hyper responsive, frequency of cough, cough. The selected variables by the system have conformity with the physician's point of view. This system is also applicable to diagnose other diseases and depends upon the kind of the endemic variables in every country, one can add new variables and delete the old ones. Finally, assessment was performed by pulmonary specialists.

FUTURE STUDIES

Proposed future studies includes:

- Investigating non adult's asthmatic patients.
- Using fuzzy variables.
- Comparison of the different classification algorithms.

REFERENCES

Abhinav, H., Sukhdeep, K., & Navdeep, S. (2016). Cloud Based Data Mining Model for Asthma Diagnosis. *International Journal of Grid and Distributed Computing, 9*(9), 317–326. doi:10.14257/ijgdc.2016.9.9.27

Aiswarya, I., Jeyalatha,S., & Ronak, S. (2015). Diagnosis of diabetes using classification mining techniques. *International Journal of Data Mining & Knowledge Management Process, 5*(1).

Akhavan Darabi, S., Teymourpour, B., Heydarnejad, H., & Safi Samghabadi, A. (2014). A New Method For Feature Selection in Diagnosis Using DEMATEL and ANP: Case Study: Asthma. *Journal of Information Engineering and Applications, 4*(4).

Alizadeh, B., Safdari, R., Zolnoori, M., & Bashiri, A. (2015). Developing an Intelligent System for Diagnosis of Asthma Based on Artificial Neural Network. *Acta inform Med, 23*(4), 220–223.

Bagherjeiran, A., Christoph, F., Rouhana, A., & Vilalta, R. (2006). *Distance Function Learning for Supervised Similarity Assessment*. Department of Computer Science University of Houston.

Bergmann, R. (2002). Experience Management - Foundations, Development Methodology, and Internet-Based Applications. *LNAI, 2432*.

Bibi, M., Nutman, A., Nutman, A., Shoseyov, D., Shalom, M., Peled, R., & Nutman, J. et al. (2001). Prediction of Emergency Department Visits for Respiratory Symptoms Using an Artificial Neural Network. *Chest Journal, 5*(122), 1627–132. PMID:12426263

Bousquet, J., Vignola, A. M., & Demoly, P. (2003). Links Between Rhinitis and Asthma. *Allergy, 58*(8), 691–706. doi:10.1034/j.1398-9995.2003.00105.x PMID:12859545

Chae, Y. M., Ho, S. H., Hong, C. S., & Kim, C. W. (1996). Comparison of Alternative Knowledge Model for Diagnosis of asthma. *Expert Systems with Applications, 4*(11), 423–429. doi:10.1016/S0957-4174(96)00057-7

Ernst, P., Ghezzo, H., & Becklake, M. R. (2002). Risk Factors for Bronchial. Hyper responsiveness in Late Childhood and Early adolescence. *The European Respiratory Journal, 20*(3), 635–639. doi:10.11 83/09031936.02.00962002 PMID:12358340

Haripriya, R., & Porkodi. (2016). A Survey Paper on Data mining Techniques and Challenges in Distributed DICOM. *International Journal of Advanced Research in Computer and Communication Engineering, 5*(3).

Lee, C. H., Chen, J. C., & Tseng, V. S. (2010). *A Novel Data Mining Mechanism Considering Bio-Signal and Environmental Data with Applications on Asthma Monitoring*. Comput Methods Programs Biom.

Misra, B. B., & Dehuri, S. (2007). Functional Link Artificial Neural Network for Classification Task in Data Mining. *Journal of Computer Science, 3*(12), 948–955. doi:10.3844/jcssp.2007.948.955

Riedler, J., Braun-Fahrländer, C., Eder, W., Schreuer, M., Waser, M., Maisch, S., & Al, E. X. et al. (2001). Study Team, Exposure to farming in early life and development of asthma and allergy: A cross-sectional survey. *Journal Lattice, 358*, 1129–1133. PMID:11597666

Sefion, I., & Ennaji, A. (2003). Gailhardou M, Canu S. ADEMA: A decision support system for asthma health care. *Studies in Health Technology and Informatics, 95*, 623–628. PMID:14664057

Shapiro, G. G. (2006). Among Young Children Who Wheeze, Which Children will have Persistent Asthma. *The Journal of Allergy and Clinical Immunology, 118*(3), 562–564. doi:10.1016/j.jaci.2006.07.011 PMID:16950270

Tan, P., Steinbach, M., & Kumar, V. (2006). *Introduction to Data Mining*. Pearson Addison Wesley.

Zolnoori, M., Fazelzarandi, M., Moin, M., & Heydarnejad, H. (2010). Computer-Aided Intelligent System for Diagnosing Pediatric Asthma. *Journal of Medical Systems*. PMID:20703652

Zolnoori, M., Fazel Zarandi, M. H., Moin, M., & Kazemnejad, A. (2010). Computer Aided Intelligence System for Diagnosing Pediatric Asthma. *Journal of Medical Systems*.

Salha, M., Alzahani Afnan, A., Ashwag, A., Boushra, A., & Suheer, A. (2014). An Overview of Data Mining Techniques Applied for Heart Disease Diagnosis and Prediction. *Notes on Information Theory, 2*(4).

Kumari, M., & Godara, S. (2011). Comparative Study of Data Mining Classification Methods in Cardiovascular Disease Prediction. *International Journal of Clothing Science and Technology, 2*(2), 304–308.

Delen, D. (2009). Analysis of cancer data: a data mining approach. *Expert System, 26*(1), 100–112.

Karaolis, M. A., Moutiris, J. A., Hadjipanayi, D., & Pattichis, C. S. (2010). Assessment of the risk factors of coronary heart events based on data mining with decision trees. *IEEE Transactions on Information Technology in Biomedicine, 14*(3), 559–566. doi:10.1109/TITB.2009.2038906 PMID:20071264

Jaulent, M., Le Bozec, C., Zapletal, E., & Degoulet, P. (2005). A Case-Based Reasoning method for computer-assisted diagnosis in histopathology, Diagnostic Problem Solving. *Artificial Intelligence in Medicine, 1211*, 239–242.

Schmidt, R., Pollwein, B., & Gierl, L. (1999). Experiences with Case-Based Reasoning Methods and Prototypes for Medical Knowledge-Based Systems. *Artificial Intelligence in Medicine, 1620*, 124–132.

Shena, Y., Colloc, J., Jacquet-Andrieub, A., & Leia, K. (2015). Emerging medical informatics with case-based reasoning for aiding clinical decision in multi-agent system. *Journal of Biomedical Informatics, 56*, 307–317. doi:10.1016/j.jbi.2015.06.012 PMID:26133480

KEY TERMS AND DEFINITIONS

Asthma: Asthma is a chronic (long-term) lung disease that inflames and narrows the airways. Asthma causes recurring periods of wheezing (a whistling sound when you breathe), chest tightness, shortness of breath, and coughing. The coughing often occurs at night or early in the morning.

Case-Based Reasoning: Process of arriving at the solution of a new problem on the basis of the solutions of previously-solved similar problems, such as when a doctor, lawyer, or mechanic relies on experience to remedy a current situation. In comparison to rule based systems (see expert system) which are useful where only one or a few solutions to a problem are possible, case based systems are useful in solving complex problems with many alternative solutions.

Classification: Classification is a general process related to categorization, the process in which ideas and objects are recognized, differentiated, and understood.

Data Mining: Data mining, also called knowledge discovery in databases, in computer science, the process of discovering interesting and useful patterns and relationships in large volumes of data. The field combines tools from statistics and artificial intelligence (such as neural networks and machine learning) with database management to analyze large digital collections, known as data sets.

Differential Diagnosis: The process of weighing the probability of one disease versus that of other diseases possibly accounting for a patient's illness.

Feature Selection: In machine learning and statistics, feature selection, also known as variable selection, attribute selection or variable subset selection, is the process of selecting a subset of relevant features (variables, predictors) for use in model construction. Feature selection techniques are used for four reasons: Simplification of models to make them easier to interpret by researchers/users, Shorter training times, To avoid the curse of dimensionality, Enhanced generalization by reducing over fitting.

Random Forest: Random Forest consists of a collection or ensemble of simple tree predictors, each capable of producing a response when presented with a set of predictor values. For classification problems, this response takes the form of a class membership, which associates, or classifies, a set of independent predictor values with one of the categories present in the dependent variable. Alternatively, for regression problems, the tree response is an estimate of the dependent variable given the predictors. A Random Forest consists of an arbitrary number of simple trees, which are used to determine the final outcome. For classification problems, the ensemble of simple trees vote for the most popular class. In the regression problem, their responses are averaged to obtain an estimate of the dependent variable. Using tree ensembles can lead to significant improvement in prediction accuracy.

Compilation of References

Abbas, A. L. B. K. (2014). Simulation Models Of Emergency Department In Hospital. *Journal of Engineering and Development, 18*(2).

Abdar, M., Zomorodi-Moghadam, M., Das, R., & Ting, I. H. (2016). (in press). Performance analysis of classification algorithms on early detection of Liver disease. *Expert Systems with Applications*.

Abdi, M. J., & Giveki, D. (2013b). Automatic detection of erythemato-squamous diseases using PSO–SVM based on association rules. *Engineering Applications of Artificial Intelligence, 26*(1), 603–608. doi:10.1016/j.engappai.2012.01.017

Abdi, M. J., Hosseini, S. M., & Rezghi, M. (2012a). A novel weighted support vector machine based on particle swarm optimization for gene selection and tumor classification. *Computational and Mathematical Methods in Medicine*.

Abhinav, H., Sukhdeep, K., & Navdeep, S. (2016). Cloud Based Data Mining Model for Asthma Diagnosis. *International Journal of Grid and Distributed Computing, 9*(9), 317–326. doi:10.14257/ijgdc.2016.9.9.27

Abo-Hamad, W., & Arisha, A. (2013). Simulation-based framework to improve patient experience in an emergency department. *European Journal of Operational Research, 224*(1), 154–166. doi:10.1016/j.ejor.2012.07.028

Abu-Laban, R. B. (2006). The junkyard dogs find their teeth: Addressing the crisis of admitted patients in Canadian emergency departments. *Canadian Journal of Emergency Medical Care, 8*(06), 388–391. doi:10.1017/S1481803500014160 PMID:17209487

Adams, J., & Klein, J. (2011). Business Intelligence and Analytics in Health Care - A Primer. Washington, DC: The Advisory Board Company. Retrieved from http://www.advisory.com/Research/IT-Strategy-Council/Research-Notes/2011/Business-Intelligence-and-Analytics-in-Health-Care

Agustinos, A., & Voros, S. (2016). 2D/3D Real-Time Tracking of Surgical Instruments Based on Endoscopic Image Processing. In X. Luo, T. Reichl, A. Reiter, & G. M. Mariottini (Eds.), *Computer-Assisted and Robotic Endoscopy* (pp. 90–100). Springer. doi:10.1007/978-3-319-29965-5_9

Ahmadi, A., Gupta, S., Karim, R., & Kumar, U. (2010). Selection of maintenance strategy for aircraft systems using multi-criteria decision making methodologies. *International Journal of Reliability Quality and Safety Engineering, 17*(3), 223–243. doi:10.1142/S0218539310003779

Ahmed, M. A., & Alkhamis, T. M. (2009). Simulation optimization for an emergency department healthcare unit in Kuwait. *European Journal of Operational Research, 198*(3), 936–942. doi:10.1016/j.ejor.2008.10.025

Ahonen, T., & Pietikainen, M. (2009). Image description using joint distribution of filter bank responses. *Pattern Recognition Letters, 30*(4), 368–376. doi:10.1016/j.patrec.2008.10.012

Aiswarya, I., Jeyalatha,S., & Ronak, S. (2015). Diagnosis of diabetes using classification mining techniques. *International Journal of Data Mining & Knowledge Management Process, 5*(1).

Akbari, H., & Kosugi, Y. (2007). Neural Network Blood Vessel Detection in Laparoscopy. *International Journal of Bioelectromagnetism, 9*(1), 37–38.

Akhavan Darabi, S., Teymourpour, B., Heydarnejad, H., & Safi Samghabadi, A. (2014). A New Method For Feature Selection in Diagnosis Using DEMATEL and ANP: Case Study: Asthma. *Journal of Information Engineering and Applications, 4*(4).

Alam, S. K., Feleppa, E. J., Rondeau, M., Kalisz, A., & Garra, B. S. (2011). Ultrasonic multi-feature analysis procedure for computer-aided diagnosis of solid breast lesions. *Ultrasonic Imaging, 33*(1), 17–38. doi:10.1177/016173461103300102 PMID:21608446

Alberta Health. (2013). *Public Health Notifiable Disease Management Guidelines; Measles.* Retrieved 21 January 2017 from http://www.health.alberta.ca/documents/Guidelines-Measles-2013.pdf

Alberta Health. (2014). *Public health notifiable disease management guidelines; salmonellosis.* Retrieved from http://www.health.alberta.ca/documents/Guidelines-Salmonellosis-2014.pdf

Alemany, M. M. E., Boj, J. J., Mula, J., & Lario, F. (2009). Mathematical programming model for centralized master planning in ceramic tile supply chains. *International Journal of Production Research, 48*(17), 5053–5074. doi:10.1080/00207540903055701

Alessandro, P., Adriano, T., Annunziata, M., & Oscar, T. (2015). A Simulation Model For Analyzing The Nurse Workload In A University Hospital Ward. *Proceedings of the 2015 Winter Simulation Conference.*

Alexandru, A. et al.. (2016). Healthcare, Big Data and Cloud Computing. *WSEAS Transactions on Computer Research, 4*, 123–131.

Alger, P. W., Niederberger, C. S., & Turk, T. M. (2009). Neural Network to Predict Stone Free Rate Status After SWL, PCNL or Ureteroscopy. *The Journal of Urology, 181*(4), 492. doi:10.1016/S0022-5347(09)61391-4 PMID:19110280

Alizadeh, B., Safdari, R., Zolnoori, M., & Bashiri, A. (2015). Developing an Intelligent System for Diagnosis of Asthma Based on Artificial Neural Network. *Acta inform Med, 23*(4), 220–223.

Aljumah, A. A., Ahamad, M. G., & Siddiqui, M. K. (2011a). Predictive Analysis on Hypertension Treatment Using Data Mining Approach in Saudi Arabia. *Intelligent Information Management, 3*(6), 252–261. doi:10.4236/iim.2011.36031

Aljumah, A. A., Ahamad, M. G., & Siddiqui, M. K. (2013b). Application of data mining: Diabetes health care in young and old patients. *Journal of King Saud University-Computer and Information Sciences, 25*(2), 127–136. doi:10.1016/j.jksuci.2012.10.003

Al-Kattan, I. (2009). Disaster recovery plan development for the emergency department-Case study. *Public Administration and Management, 14*(1), 75.

Almeida, A. T., & Bohoris, A. T. (1995). Decision theory in maintenance decision making. *Journal of Quality in Maintenance Engineering, 1*(1), 39–45. doi:10.1108/13552519510083138

Al-Najjar, B., & Alsyouf, I. (2003). Selecting the most efficient maintenance approach using fuzzy multiple criteria decision making. *International Journal of Production Economics, 84*(1), 85–100. doi:10.1016/S0925-5273(02)00380-8

Alpaydin, E. (2014). *Introduction to machine learning.* MIT Press.

Alsyouf, I. (2009). Maintenance practices in Swedish industries: Survey results. *International Journal of Production Economics, 121*(1), 212–223. doi:10.1016/j.ijpe.2009.05.005

Altiok, T., & Melamed, B. (2007). Simulation Modeling and Analysis with Arena. Academic Press.

Amaro, A.C.S., & Barbosa-Po'voa, A.P.F.D. (2008). Planning and scheduling of industrial supply chains with reverse flows: A real pharmaceutical case study. *Computers and Chemical Engineering 32*, 2606-2625.

Ameri, H., & Alizadeh, S. (2015). Predicting complications of type 2 diabetes using decision tree algorithms. *Journal of Mitteilungen Saechsischer Entomologen, 114*, 1011–1028.

Amin, S. U., Agarwal, K., & Beg, R. (2013, April). Genetic neural network based data mining in prediction of heart disease using risk factors. In *Information & Communication Technologies (ICT), IEEE Conference on* (pp. 1227-1231). IEEE.

Amini Khoyi, K., Mirbagheri, A., & Farahmand, F. (2016). Automatic tracking of laparoscopic instruments for autonomous control of a cameraman robot. *Minimally Invasive Therapy & Allied Technologies, 25*(3), 121–128. doi:10.3109/13645706.2016.1141101 PMID:26872883

Amodeo, A., L., Q. A., J.V., J., E., B., & H.R., P. (2009). 2009, Robotic laparoscopic surgery: Cost and training. *The Italian journal of urology and Nephrology, 61*(2), 121-128.

Anbananthen, S. K., Sainarayanan, G., Chekima, A., & Teo, J. (2005, November). Data mining using Artificial Neural network tree. In *Computers, Communications, & Signal Processing with Special Track on Biomedical Engineering, 2005. CCSP 2005. 1st International Conference on* (pp. 160-164). IEEE.

Anbarasi, M., Anupriya, E., & Iyengar, N. C. S. N. (2010). Enhanced prediction of heart disease with feature subset selection using genetic algorithm. *International Journal of Engineering Science and Technology, 2*(10), 5370–5376.

Anderson, D. R., Burnham, K. P., Gould, W. R., & Cherry, S. (2011). Concerns about finding effects that are actually spurious. *Wildlife Society Bulletin, 29*, 311–316.

Andrés, A., Polanco, N., Cebrian, M. P., Sol Vereda, M., Vazquez, S., Nuño, E., . . . Leiva, O. Aguirre, & F., Diaz, R. (2009). Kidneys From Elderly Deceased Donors Discarded for Transplantation. Proceedings of Transplantation, 41(6), 2379-2381.

Antonelli, D., Baralis, E., Bruno, G., Cerquitelli, T., Chiusano, S., & Mahoto, N. (2013). Analysis of diabetic patients through their examination history. *Expert Systems with Applications, 40*(11), 4672–4678. doi:10.1016/j.eswa.2013.02.006

Anvari, F., & Edwards, R. (2011). Maintenance engineering in capital-intensive manufacturing systems. *Journal of Quality in Maintenance Engineering, 17*(4), 351–370. doi:10.1108/13552511111180177

Aphinyanaphongs, Y., Fu, L. D., & Aliferis, C. F. (2012). Identifying unproven cancer treatments on the health web: Addressing accuracy, generalizability and scalability. *Studies in Health Technology and Informatics, 192*, 667–671. PMID:23920640

APQC (American Productivity & Quality Center). (2013). *Benchmarking.* Retrieved May 22, 2013, from http://www.apqc.org/benchmarking

Arafa, A. A. M., Rida, S. Z., & Khalil, M. (2011). Fractional order model of human T-cell lymphotropic virus I (HTLV-I) infection of CD4+ T-cells lymphotropic virus type 1 (HTLV-I). *Advanced Studies in Biology, 3*(7), 347–353.

Archenaa, J., & Mary Anita, E. A. (2015). A Survey of Big Data Analytics in Healthcare and Government. *Procedia Computer Science, 50*, 408–413. doi:10.1016/j.procs.2015.04.021

Armony, M., Shlomo, I., Mandelbaum, A., Marmor, Y., Tseytlin, Y., & Yom-Tov, G. (2010). *On Patient Flow in Hospitals: A Data-Based Queuing-Science Perspective.* Working paper. New York University.

Arodz, T., Yuen, D. A., & Dudek, A. Z. (2006). Ensemble of linear models for predicting drug properties. *Journal of Chemical Information and Modeling, 46*(1), 416–423. doi:10.1021/ci050375+

Aruna, S., Nandakishore, L. V., & Rajagopalan, S. P. (2012). A hybrid feature selection method based on IGSBFS and naïve bayes for the diagnosis of erythemato-squamous diseases. *International Journal of Computers and Applications, 41*(7).

Arunraj, N. S., & Maiti, J. (2010). Risk-based maintenance policy selection using AHP and goal programming. *Safety Science, 48*(2), 238–247. doi:10.1016/j.ssci.2009.09.005

Asadayyoobi, N., & Niaki, S. T. A. (2016). Monitoring patient survival times in surgical systems using a risk-adjusted AFT regression chart. *Quality Technology & Quantitative Management,* 1–12.

Asadzadeh, S., Aghaie, A., & Niaki, S. T. A. (2013). AFT regression-adjusted monitoring of reliability data in cascade processes. *Quality & Quantity, 47*(6), 3349–3362. doi:10.1007/s11135-012-9723-2

Ashour, O. M., & Kremer, G. E. O. (2013). A simulation analysis of the impact of FAHP–MAUT triage algorithm on the Emergency Department performance measures. *Expert Systems with Applications, 40*(1), 177–187. doi:10.1016/j.eswa.2012.07.024

Asquith, B., & Bangham, C. R. M. (2008). How does HTLV-I persist despite a strong cell-mediated immune response? *Trends in Immunology, 29*(1), 4–11. doi:10.1016/j.it.2007.09.006 PMID:18042431

Asquith, B., Mosley, A. J., Heaps, A., Tanaka, Y., Taylor, G. P., McLean, A. R., & Bangham, C. R. M. (2005). Quantification of the virus-host interaction in human T lymphotropic virus I infection. *Retrovirology, 2*(75), 1–9. PMID:16336683

Atay, M. T., Başbük, M., & Eryılmaz, A. (2016). A geometric integration based on magnus series expansion for human T cell lymphotropic virus I (HTLV-I) infection of CD4$^+$T cells model. *Journal of Advances in Applied Mathematics, 1*(2), 98–106. doi:10.22606/jaam.2016.12002

Audit Commission. (1996). By accident or design Improving A& E services in England and Wales. London: HMSO.

Avci, E. (2009). A new intelligent diagnosis system for the heart valve diseases by using genetic-SVM classifier. *Expert Systems with Applications, 36*(7), 10618–10626. doi:10.1016/j.eswa.2009.02.053

Azadeh, A., Rouhollah, F., Davoudpour, F., & Mohammadfam, I. (2013). Fuzzy modelling and simulation of an emergency department for improvement of nursing schedules with noisy and uncertain inputs. *International Journal of Services and Operations Management, 15*(1), 58–77. doi:10.1504/IJSOM.2013.053255

Azaiez, M. N. (2002). A multi-attribute preventive replacement model. *Journal of Quality in Maintenance Engineering, 8*(3), 213–225. doi:10.1108/13552510210439793

Azam, M., Qureshi, M. N., & Talib, F. (2015). AHP Model for Identifying Best Health Care Establishment. *International Journal of Productivity Management and Assessment Technologies, 3*(2), 34–66. doi:10.4018/IJPMAT.2015070104

Azari, A., Janeja, V. P., & Mohseni, A. (2012, December). Predicting hospital length of stay (PHLOS): A multi-tiered data mining approach. In *2012 IEEE 12th International Conference on Data Mining Workshops* (pp. 17-24). IEEE.

Babaoğlu, I., Fındık, O., & Bayrak, M. (2010a). Effects of principle component analysis on assessment of coronary artery diseases using support vector machine. *Expert Systems with Applications, 37*(3), 2182–2185. doi:10.1016/j.eswa.2009.07.055

Babaoglu, İ., Findik, O., & Ülker, E. (2010b). A comparison of feature selection models utilizing binary particle swarm optimization and genetic algorithm in determining coronary artery disease using support vector machine. *Expert Systems with Applications, 37*(4), 3177–3183. doi:10.1016/j.eswa.2009.09.064

Bach, C., & Buchholz, N. (2011). Shock Wave Lithotripsy for Renal and Ureteric Stones. *European Urology Supplements, 10*(5), 423–432. doi:10.1016/j.eursup.2011.07.004

Badrinath, N., Gopinath, G., Ravichandran, K. S., & Soundhar, R. G. (2016). Estimation of automatic detection of erythemato-squamous diseases through adaboost and its hybrid classifiers. *Artificial Intelligence Review, 45*(4), 471–488. doi:10.1007/s10462-015-9436-8

Baesler, F. F., Jahnsen, H. E., & DaCosta, M. (2003, December). Emergency departments I: the use of simulation and design of experiments for estimating maximum capacity in an emergency room. *Proceedings of the 35th conference on Winter simulation: driving innovation*, 1903-1906.

Bagherjeiran, A., Christoph, F., Rouhana, A., & Vilalta, R. (2006). *Distance Function Learning for Supervised Similarity Assessment*. Department of Computer Science University of Houston.

Bagust, A., Place, M., & Posnett, J. W. (1999). Dynamics of bed use in accommodating emergency admissions: Stochastic simulation model. *BMJ (Clinical Research Ed.), 319*(7203), 155–158. doi:10.1136/bmj.319.7203.155 PMID:10406748

Bakar, A. A., Kefli, Z., Abdullah, S., & Sahani, M. (2011, July). Predictive models for dengue outbreak using multiple rulebase classifiers. In *Electrical Engineering and Informatics (ICEEI), 2011 International Conference on* (pp. 1-6). IEEE. doi:10.1109/ICEEI.2011.6021830

Balakrishnan, S., Narayanaswamy, R., Savarimuthu, N., & Samikannu, R. (2008, October). SVM ranking with backward search for feature selection in type II diabetes databases. In *Systems, Man and Cybernetics, 2008. SMC 2008. IEEE International Conference on* (pp. 2628-2633). IEEE. doi:10.1109/ICSMC.2008.4811692

Balakrishnan, V., Shakouri, M. R., & Hoodeh, H. (2013). Developing a hybrid predictive system for retinopathy. *Journal of Intelligent & Fuzzy Systems, 25*(1), 191–199.

Ballantyne, G. H. (2002). Robotic surgery, telerobotic surgery, telepresence, and telementoring. *Surgical Endoscopy and Other Interventional Techniques, 16*(10), 1389-1402.

Bana e Costa, C. A., & Carvalho, R. (2002). Assigning priorities for maintenance, repair and refurbishment in managing a municipal housing stock. *European Journal of Operational Research, 138*(2), 380–391. doi:10.1016/S0377-2217(01)00253-3

Bana e Costa, C. A., Correa, E., De Corte, J. M., & Vansnick, J. C. (2002). Facilitating bid evaluation in public call for tenders: A socio-technical approach. *Omega, 30*(3), 227–242. doi:10.1016/S0305-0483(02)00029-4

Bana e Costa, C. A., De Corte, J. M., & Vansnick, J. C. (2011). MACBETH (Measuring Attractiveness by a Categorical Based Evaluation Technique). In J. J. Cochran, L. A. Cox Jr, P. Keskinocak, J. P. Kharoufeh, & J. C. Smith (Eds.), *Encyclopedia of Operations Research and Management Science*. New York, NY: John Wiley & Sons. doi:10.1002/9780470400531.eorms0970

Bana e Costa, C. A., De Corte, J. M., & Vansnick, J. C. (2012). MACBETH. *International Journal of Information Technology & Decision Making, 11*(2), 359–387. doi:10.1142/S0219622012400068

Bana e Costa, C. A., & Vansnick, J. C. (1997). Applications of the MACBETH approach in the framework of an additive aggregation model. *Journal of Multi-Criteria Decision Analysis, 6*(2), 107–114. doi:10.1002/(SICI)1099-1360(199703)6:2<107::AID-MCDA147>3.0.CO;2-1

Bandyopadhyay, S., Wolfson, J., Vock, D. M., Vazquez-Benitez, G., Adomavicius, G., Elidrisi, M., ... O'Connor, P. J. (2015). Data mining for censored time-to-event data: a Bayesian network model for predicting cardiovascular risk from electronic health record data. *Data Mining and Knowledge Discovery, 29*(4), 1033–1069. https://doi.org/10.1007/s10618-014-0386-6

Banerjee, A., Mbamalu, D., &Hinchley, G. (2008). The impact of process re-engineering on patient throughput in emergency departments in the UK. *International Journal of Emergency Medicine, 1*(3), 189-192.

Bangham, C. R. M. (2000). The immune response to HTLV-I. *Current Opinion in Immunology, 12*(4), 397–402. doi:10.1016/S0952-7915(00)00107-2 PMID:10899027

Bangham, C. R., Meekings, K., Toulza, F., Nejmeddine, M., Majorovits, E., Asquith, B., & Taylor, G. P. (2009). The immune control of HTLV-I infection: Selection forces and dynamics. *Frontiers in Bioscience (Landmark Edition), 14,* 28892903. PMID:19273242

Bangham, C. R., & Osame, M. (2005). Cellular immune response to HTLV-I. *Oncogene, 24*(39), 6035–6046. doi:10.1038/sj.onc.1208970 PMID:16155610

Banihashemi, B., Vlad, R., Debeljevic, B., Giles, A., Kolios, M. C., & Czarnota, G. J. (2008). Ultrasound imaging of apoptosis in tumor response: Novel preclinical monitoring of photodynamic therapy effects. *Cancer Research, 68*(20), 8590–8596. doi:10.1158/0008-5472.CAN-08-0006 PMID:18922935

Banks, J., Carson, J. S., Nelson, B. L., & Nicol, D. M. (2004). *Discrete-Event System Simulation* (4th ed.). Upper Saddle River, NJ: Prentice-Hall, Inc.

Banu, M. N., & Gomathy, B. (2013). Disease Predicting System Using Data Mining Techniques. *International Journal of Technical Research and Applications, 1*(5), 41–45.

Barakat, N., Bradley, A. P., & Barakat, M. N. H. (2010). Intelligible support vector machines for diagnosis of diabetes mellitus. *IEEE Transactions on Information Technology in Biomedicine, 14*(4), 1114–1120. doi:10.1109/TITB.2009.2039485

Baraldi, A., & Parmiggiani, F. (1995). An investigation of texture characteristics associated with gray level co-occurrence matrix structural parameters. *IEEE Transactions on Geoscience and Remote Sensing, 33*(2), 293–304. doi:10.1109/36.377929

Barati, E., Saraee, M., Mohammadi, A., Adibi, N., & Ahmadzadeh, M. R. (2011). A survey on utilization of data mining approaches for dermatological (skin) diseases prediction. *Journal of Selected Areas in Health Informatics, 2*(3), 1–11.

Barnes, E., Harcourt, G., Brown, D., Lucas, M., Phillips, R., Dusheiko, G., & Klenerman, P. (2002). The dynamics of T-lymphocyte responses during combination therapy for chronic hepatitis C virus infection. *Hepatology (Baltimore, Md.), 36*(3), 743–754. doi:10.1053/jhep.2002.35344 PMID:12198669

Bashar, M. K., Kitasaka, T., Suenaga, Y., Mekada, Y., & Mori, K. (2010). Automatic detection of informative frames from wireless capsule endoscopy images. *Medical Image Analysis, 14*(3), 449–470. doi:10.1016/j.media.2009.12.001 PMID:20137998

Bashashati, A., Fatourechi, M., Ward, R. K., & Birch, G. E. (2007). A survey of signal processing algorithms in brain–computer interfaces based on electrical brain signals. *Journal of Neural Engineering, 4*(2), R32–R57. doi:10.1088/1741-2560/4/2/R03 PMID:17409474

Bate, A. (2007). Bayesian confidence propagation neural network. *Drug Safety, 30*(7), 623–625. doi:10.2165/00002018-200730070-00011

Bates, D. W., Saria, S., Ohno-Machado, L., Shah, A., & Escobar, G. (2014). Big Data In Health Care: Using Analytics To Identify And Manage High-Risk And High-Cost Patients. *Health Affairs*, *33*(7), 1123–1131. doi:10.1377/hlthaff.2014.0041 PMID:25006137

Baumhauer, M., Simpfendörfer, T., Müller-Stich, B. P., Teber, D., Gutt, C. N., Rassweiler, J., & Wolf, I. et al. (2008). Soft tissue navigation for laparoscopic partial nephrectomy. *International Journal of Computer Assisted Radiology and Surgery*, *3*(3-4), 307–314. doi:10.1007/s11548-008-0216-7

BC Enteric Policy Working Group. (2007). *Enteric diseases requiring follow-up in BC and standard follow - forms.* Retrieved from http://www.bccdc.ca/resource-gallery/Documents/Guidelines and Forms/Guidelines and Manuals/Epid/CD Manual/Chapter 6 - SCD/BC enteric disease prioritisation_2007.pdf

Beaulieu, H., Ferland, J. A., Gendron, B., & Michelon, P. (2000). A mathematical programming approach for scheduling physicians in the emergency room. *Health Care Management Science*, *3*(3), 193–200. doi:10.1023/A:1019009928005 PMID:10907322

Begg, R., Kamruzzaman, J., & Sarkar, R. (2006). Neural Networks in Healthcare: Potential and Challenges. Idea Group Publishing.

Bekkering, F. C., Stalgis, C., McHutchison, J. G., Brouwer, J. T., & Perelson, A. S. (2001). Estimation of early hepatitis C viral clearance in patients receiving daily interferon and ribavirin therapy using a mathematical model. *Hepatology (Baltimore, Md.)*, *33*(2), 419–423. doi:10.1053/jhep.2001.21552 PMID:11172344

Belciug, S., Salem, A. B., Gorunescu, F., & Gorunescu, M. (2010b, November). Clustering-based approach for detecting breast cancer recurrence. In *2010 10th International Conference on Intelligent Systems Design and Applications* (pp. 533-538). IEEE.

Belciug, S. (2009a). Patient's length of stay grouping using the hierarchical clustering algorithm. *Annals of the University of Craiova-Mathematics and Computer Science Series*, *36*(2), 79–84.

Belle, A., Thiagarajan, R., Soroushmehr, S. M., Navidi, F., Beard, D. A., &Najarian, K. (2015). *Big Data Analytics in Healthcare.* BioMed Research International.

Ben-Ari, A., & Hammond, K. (2015). Text mining the EMR for modeling and predicting suicidal behavior among US veterans of the 1991 Persian Gulf War. *2015 48th Hawaii International Conference on System Sciences*, 3168–75.

Benazon, N. R., Mamdani, M. M., & Coyne, J. C. (2005). Trends in the prescribing of antidepressants following acute myocardial infarction, 1993–2002. *Psychosomatic Medicine*, *67*(6), 916–920. doi:10.1097/01.psy.0000188399.80167.aa PMID:16314596

Benchimol, E. I., Smeeth, L., Guttmann, A., Harron, K., Moher, D., & Petersen, I. (2015). The REporting of studies Conducted using Observational Routinely-collected health Data (RECORD) Statement. *PLoS Med, 12*(10), e1001885. https://doi.org/10.1371/journal.pmed.1001885

Bennett, C., & Doub, T. (2011). *Data mining and electronic health records: selecting optimal clinical treatments in practice.* arXiv preprint arXiv:1112.1668

Benson, D. A., Karsch-Mizrachi, I., Clark, K., Lipman, D. J., Ostell, J., & Sayers, E. W. (2012, January 01). GenBank. *Nucleic Acids Research*, *40*(D1), D48–D53. doi:10.1093/nar/gkr1202 PMID:22144687

Bergmann, R. (2002). Experience Management - Foundations, Development Methodology, and Internet-Based Applications. *LNAI, 2432*.

Berka, P., Rauch, J., & Zighed, D. A. (2009). *Data Mining and Medical Knowledge Management: Cases and Applications*. IGI Global. doi:10.4018/978-1-60566-218-3

Berrada, I. (1993). *Planificationd'horaires du personnel infirmierdansunétablissementhospitalier* (Doctoral dissertation). Departement d" Inforrnatique et de RechercheOpe'rationnelle, Université de Montreal.

Bertolini, M., & Bevilacqua, M. (2006). A combined goal programming-AHP approach to maintenance selection problem. *Reliability Engineering & System Safety, 91*(7), 839–848. doi:10.1016/j.ress.2005.08.006

Bertsimas, D., Bjarnadóttir, M. V., Kane, M. A., Kryder, J. C., Pandey, R., Vempala, S., & Wang, G. (2008). Algorithmic prediction of health-care costs. *Operations Research, 56*(6), 1382–1392. doi:10.1287/opre.1080.0619

Bevilacqua, M., & Braglia, M. (2000). The analytic hierarchy process applied to maintenance strategy selection. *Reliability Engineering & System Safety, 70*(1), 71–83. doi:10.1016/S0951-8320(00)00047-8

Bhattacharyya Sumanta Mukul, M. K. (2016). Short Time Fourier Transform based Dominant Frequency Extraction Algorithm for Brain Computer Interface. *International Journal of Scientific Research & Technology, 2*(1), 67-74.

Bhattacharyya, S., & Mukul, M. K. (2016). Cepstral Coefficients Based Feature for Real Time Movement Imagery Classification. *International Journal of Engineering and Technology, 8*(1), 117-123.

Bhattacharyya, S., & Mukul, M. K. (2017). Temporal Relative Spectral Power Based Real Time Motor Imagery Classification. *International Journal of Engineering Sciences & Research Technology*, 33-38.

Bhattacharyya, S. P., Chapellat, H., & Keel, L. H. (1995). *Robust Control: The Parametric Approach*. Prentice Hall.

Bhattacharyya, S., & Mukul, M. K. (2016, September). Cepstrum Based Algorithm for Motor Imagery Classification. *International Conference on Micro-Electronics and Telecommunication Engineering (ICMETE 2016)* (pp. 397-402). IEEE. doi:10.1109/ICMETE.2016.140

Bhowmik, D. M., Dinda, A. K., Mahanta, P., & Agarwal, S. K. (2010). The evolution of the Banff classification schema for diagnosing renal allograft rejection and its implications for clinicians. *Indian Journal of Nephrology, 20*(1), 2–8. doi:10.4103/0971-4065.62086 PMID:20535263

Bibault, J. E., Fumagalli, I., Ferté, C., Chargari, C., Soria, J. C., & Deutsch, E. (2013). Personalized radiation therapy and biomarker-driven treatment strategies: A systematic review. *Cancer and Metastasis Reviews, 32*(3-4), 479–492. doi:10.1007/s10555-013-9419-7 PMID:23595306

Bibault, J.-E., Giraud, Ph., & Burgun, A. (2016). Big Data and machine learning in radiation oncology: State of the art and future prospects. *Cancer Letters*, 1–8. PMID:27241666

Bibi, M., Nutman, A., Nutman, A., Shoseyov, D., Shalom, M., Peled, R., & Nutman, J. et al. (2001). Prediction of Emergency Department Visits for Respiratory Symptoms Using an Artificial Neural Network. *Chest Journal, 5*(122), 1627–132. PMID:12426263

Bickel, P., & Levina, E. (2008). Covariance regularization by thresholding. *Annals of Statistics, 36*(6), 2577–2604. doi:10.1214/08-AOS600

Biosig for Matlab and Octave – An open source software library for biomedical signal processing. (2005). Available from: http://biosig.sf.net

Birbaumer, N., Ghanayim, N., & Flor, H. (1999). A spelling device for the paralysed. *Nature, 398*(6725), 297–298. doi:10.1038/18581 PMID:10192330

Bisgaard, S., & Kulahci, M. (2011). *Time series analysis and forecasting by example*. John Wiley & Sons. doi:10.1002/9781118056943

Biswas, P., & Kalbfleisch, J. D. (2008). A risk-adjusted CUSUM in continuous time based on the Cox model. *Statistics in Medicine*, *27*(17), 3382–3406. doi:10.1002/sim.3216 PMID:18288785

Blagojević, M. D., Radović, M. D., Radović, M. M., & Filipović, N. D. (2015, November). Neural network based approach for predicting maximal wall shear stress in the artery. In *Bioinformatics and Bioengineering (BIBE), 2015 IEEE 15th International Conference on* (pp. 1-5). IEEE.

Blasak, R. E., Starks, D. W., Armel, W. S., & Hayduk, M. C. (2003, December). Healthcare process analysis: The use of simulation to evaluate hospital operations between the emergency department and a medical telemetry unit. *Proceedings of the 35th conference on Winter simulation: driving innovation*, 1887-1893.

Blattner, W. A., Blayney, D. W., Robert-Guroff, M., Sarngadharan, M. G., Kalyanaraman, V. S., Sarin, P. S., & Gallo, R. C. et al. (1983). Epidemiology of human T cell leukemia/lymphoma virus. *The Journal of Infectious Diseases*, *147*(3), 406–416. doi:10.1093/infdis/147.3.406 PMID:6300254

Blattner, W. A., Kalyanaraman, V. S., Robert-Guroff, M., Lister, T. A., Galton, D. A. G., Sarin, P. S., & Gallo, R. C. et al. (1982). The human type-C retrovirus, HTLV, in Blacks from the Caribbean region, and relationship to adult T cell leukemia/lymphoma. *International Journal of Cancer*, *30*(3), 257–264. doi:10.1002/ijc.2910300302 PMID:6290401

Blecker, S., Bhatia, R. S., You, J. J., Lee, D. S., Alter, D. A., Wang, J. T., & Tu, J. V. et al. (2013). Temporal trends in the utilization of echocardiography in Ontario, 2001 to 2009. *JACC: Cardiovascular Imaging*, *6*(4), 515–522. doi:10.1016/j.jcmg.2012.10.026 PMID:23579013

Blomer, F., & Gunther, H.-O. (2000). LP-based heuristics for scheduling chemical batch processes. *International Journal of Production Research*, *38*(5), 1029–1051. doi:10.1080/002075400189004

Blum, T., Feuner, H., & Navab, N. (2010). *Modeling and segmentation of surgical workflow from laparoscopic video*. Paper presented at the 13th international conference on Medical image computing and computer assisted intervention, Beijing, China. doi:10.1007/978-3-642-15711-0_50

Bock, N., Scholz, M., Piller, G., & Böhm, K. (2016). Capture and Analysis of Sensor Data for Asthma Patients (Research-in-Progress). In *ECIS 2016 Proceedings*. Istanbul, Turkey: Association for Information Systems.

Boender, C. G. E., de Grann, J. G., & Lootsma, F. A. (1989). Multicriteria decision analysis with fuzzy pairwise comparison. *Fuzzy Sets and Systems*, *29*(2), 133–143. doi:10.1016/0165-0114(89)90187-5

Bofill, M., Janossy, G., Lee, C. A., MacDonald-Burns, D., Phillips, A. N., Sabin, C., & Kernoff, P. B. A. et al. (1992). Laboratory control values for CD4 and CD8 T lymphocytes. Implications for HIV-1 diagnosis. *Clinical and Experimental Immunology*, *88*(2), 243–252. doi:10.1111/j.1365-2249.1992.tb03068.x PMID:1349272

Bollier, D., & Firestone, C. M. (2010). *The promise and peril of big data, Communications and Society Program*. Washington, DC: Aspen Institute.

Booth, G. L., Kapral, M. K., Fung, K., & Tu, J. V. (2006). Recent trends in cardiovascular complications among men and women with and without diabetes. *Diabetes Care*, *29*(1), 32–37. doi:10.2337/diacare.29.01.06.dc05-0776 PMID:16373892

Borghans, J. A., De Boer, R. J., Sercarz, E., & Kumar, V. (1998). T cell vaccination in experimental autoimmune encephalomyelitis: A mathematical model. *Journal of Immunology (Baltimore, MD.: 1950)*, *161*, 1087–1093. PMID:9686566

Borghans, J. A., Noest, A. J., & De Boer, R. J. (1999). How specific should immunological memory be? *Journal of Immunology (Baltimore, MD.: 1950)*, *163*, 569–575. PMID:10395642

Borghans, J. A., Taams, L. S., Wauben, M. H., & De Boer, R. J. (1999). Competition for antigenic sites during T cell proliferation: A mathematical interpretation of in vitro data. *Proceedings of the National Academy of Sciences of the United States of America*, *96*(19), 10782–10787. doi:10.1073/pnas.96.19.10782 PMID:10485903

Borsotti, M., Campadelli, P., & Schettini, R. (1998). Quantitative evaluation of color image segmentation results. *Pattern Recognition Letters*, *19*(8), 741–747. doi:10.1016/S0167-8655(98)00052-X

Bouarfa, L., & Dankelman, J. (2012). Workflow mining and outlier detection from clinical activity logs. *Journal of Biomedical Informatics*, *45*(6), 1185–1190. doi:10.1016/j.jbi.2012.08.003 PMID:22925724

Bousquet, J., Vignola, A. M., & Demoly, P. (2003). Links Between Rhinitis and Asthma. *Allergy*, *58*(8), 691–706. doi:10.1034/j.1398-9995.2003.00105.x PMID:12859545

Bozbura, F. T., Beskese, A., & Kahraman, C. (2007). Prioritization of human capital measurement indicators using fuzzy AHP. *Expert Systems with Applications*, *32*(4), 1100–1112. doi:10.1016/j.eswa.2006.02.006

Braga, M., Frasson, M., Zuliani, W., Vignali, A., Pecorelli, N., & Di Carlo, V. (2010). Randomized clinical trial of laparoscopic versus open left colonic resection. *Br J Surg, 97*(8), 1180-1186.

Brammer, T., Murray, E., Fukuda, K., Hall, H., Klimov, A., & Cox, N. (2002). Surveillance for influenza; United States 1997/98, 1998/99, and 1999 to 2000 seasons. *Morbidity & Mortality Weekly Report*, *51*(SS07), 1–10. Retrieved from https://www.cdc.gov/mmwr/preview/mmwrhtml/ss5107a1.htm PMID:12418623

Brenner, S., Zeng, Z., Liu, Y., Wang, J., Li, J., & Howard, P. K. (2010). Modeling and analysis of the emergency department at University of Kentucky Chandler Hospital using simulations. *Journal of Emergency Nursing: JEN*, *36*(4), 303–310. doi:10.1016/j.jen.2009.07.018 PMID:20624562

Brewer, D. D., Potterat, J. J., Muth, S. Q., Malone, P. Z., Montoya, P., Green, D. L., … Cox, P. A. (2005). Randomized trial of supplementary interviewing techniques to enhance recall of sexual partners in contact interviews. *Sexually Transmitted Diseases, 32*(3), 189–193.

Brewer, D. D. (2002). Supplementary Interviewing Techniques to Maximize Output in Free Listing Tasks. *Field Methods*, *14*(1), 108–118. doi:10.1177/1525822X02014001007

Brewer, D. D. (2005). Case-finding effectiveness of partner notification and cluster investigation for sexually transmitted diseases/HIV. *Sexually Transmitted Diseases*, *32*(2), 78–83. doi:10.1097/01.olq.0000153574.38764.0e PMID:15668612

Brewer, D. D., Garrett, S. B., & Kulasingam, S. (1999). Forgetting as a cause of incomplete reporting of sexual and drug injection partners. *Sexually Transmitted Diseases, 26*(3), 166–176. doi:10.1097/00007435-199903000-00008 PMID:10100775

Brewer, D. D., & Webster, C. M. (1999). Forgetting of friends and its effect on measuring friendship networks. *Social Networks*, *21*(4), 361–373. doi:10.1016/S0378-8733(99)00018-0

Brindle, K. (2008). New approaches for imaging tumour responses to treatment. *Nature Reviews. Cancer*, *8*(2), 94–107. doi:10.1038/nrc2289 PMID:18202697

British Columbia. (2016). *Public Health Act*. Vancouver, Canada: British Columbia.

Brownstein, J. S., Freifeld, C. C., & Madoff, L. C. (2009). Digital disease detection - harnessing the Web for public health surveillance. *The New England Journal of Medicine*, *360*(21), 2153–2157. doi:10.1056/NEJMp0900702 PMID:19423867

Brownstein, J. S., Freifeld, C. C., Reis, B. Y., & Mandl, K. D. (2008). Surveillance sans frontieres: Internet-based emerging infectious disease intelligence and the HealthMap project. *PLoS Medicine*, *5*(7), e151. doi:10.1371/journal. pmed.0050151 PMID:18613747

Bruballa, E., Taboada, M., Cabrera, E., Rexachs, D., & Luque, E. (2014, August). Simulation and Big Data: A Way to Discover Unusual Knowledge in Emergency Departments: Work-in-Progress Paper. In *Future Internet of Things and Cloud (FiCloud), 2014 International Conference on* (pp. 367-372). IEEE. doi:10.1109/FiCloud.2014.65

Bryant, R. E. (2007). *Data-intensive supercomputing: The case for DISC*. Pittsburgh, PA: School of Computer Science, Carnegie Mellon University.

Buckley, J. J. (1985). Fuzzy hierarchical analysis. *Fuzzy Sets and Systems*, *17*(3), 233–247. doi:10.1016/0165-0114(85)90090-9

Budía, A., Lopez-Acon, J. D., Trassierra, M., & Boronat, F. (2015). Is an Increase in the Number of Shock Waves per Session Effective and Safe in Extracorporeal Lithotripsy? A Randomized, Prospective and Comparative Study. *European Urology Supplements*, *193*(4), 454–455.

Bullard, M. J., Villa-Roel, C., Bond, K., Vester, M., Holroyd, B. R., & Rowe, B. H. (2009). Tracking emergency department overcrowding in a tertiary care academic institution. *Healthcare Quarterly*, *12*(3), 99–106. doi:10.12927/hcq.2013.20884 PMID:19553772

Burroni, M., Corona, R., Dell'Eva, G., Sera, F., Bono, R., Puddu, P., ... Rubegni, P. (2004). Melanoma Computer-Aided Diagnosis: Reliability and Feasibility Study. *American Association for Cancer Research, 10*(6), 1881–1886. https://doi.org/10.1158/1078-0432.CCR-03-0039

Butler, S. M., &Owcharenko, N. (2007). *Making Health Care Affordable: Bush's Bold Health Tax Reform Plan*. Heritage Foundation.

Butler, G. J., & Waltman, P. (1986). Persistence in dynamical systems. *Proceedings of the American Mathematical Society*, *96*, 425–428. doi:10.1090/S0002-9939-1986-0822433-4

Büyüközkan, G., Kahraman, C., & Ruan, D. (2004). A fuzzy multicriteria decision approach for software development strategy selection. *International Journal of General Systems*, *33*(2-3), 259–280. doi:10.1080/03081070310001633581

Cai, L., Li, X., & Ghosh, M. (2011). Global dynamics of a mathematical model for HTLV-I infection of CD4+T cells. *Applied Mathematical Modelling*, *35*(7), 3587–3595. doi:10.1016/j.apm.2011.01.033

Cai, T., Liu, W., & Luo, X. (2011). A constrained l_1 . *Journal of the American Statistical Association*, *106*(494), 594–607. doi:10.1198/jasa.2011.tm10155 PMID:22844169

Cai, W., Chen, S., & Zhang, D. (2007). Fast and robust fuzzy c-means clustering algorithms incorporating local information for image segmentation. *Pattern Recognition*, *40*(3), 825–838. doi:10.1016/j.patcog.2006.07.011

Callender, C. O., Cherikh, W. S., Traverso, P., Hernandez, A., Oyetunji, T., & Chang, D. (2009). Effect of Donor Ethnicity on Kidney Survival in Different Recipient Pairs: An Analysis of the OPTN/UNOS Database. Proceedings of Transplantation, 41(10), 4125-4130.

Calzavara, L. M., Burchell, A. N., Myers, T., Bullock, S. L., Escobar, M., & Cockerill, R. (1998). Condom use among Aboriginal people in Ontario, Canada. *International Journal of STD & AIDS, 9*(5), 272–279. doi:10.1258/0956462981922205 PMID:9639205

Cameron, P. (2006). Hospital overcrowding: A threat to patient safety?. *The Medical Journal of Australia, 184*(5), 203–204. PMID:16515426

Camila, E., Francisco, R., Jimena, P., & Daniel, B. (2014). Real-Time Simulation As A Way To Improve Daily Operations In An Emergency Room. *Proceedings of the 2014 Winter Simulation Conference.*

Campbell, A. (2004). The SARS Commission Interim Report: SARS and Public Health in Ontario' What went right. *Biosecurity and Bioterrorism: Biodefence Strategy, Practice and Science, 2*(2), 118–126.

Campbell, A. (2006). *The SARS Commission; the spring of fear.* Retrieved from http://www.archives.gov.on.ca/en/e_records/sars/report/v1-pdf/Volume1.pdf

Campos, G. S., Bandeira, A. C., & Sardi, S. I. (2015). Zika Virus Outbreak, Bahia, Brazil. *Emerging Infectious Diseases, 21*(10), 1885–1886. doi:10.3201/eid2110.150847 PMID:26401719

Canabarro, A. A., Gléeria, I. M., & Lyra, M. L. (2004). Periodic solutions and chaos in a nonlinear model for the delayed cellular immune response. *Physica A, 342*(1-2), 234–241. doi:10.1016/j.physa.2004.04.083

Canadian Hospital Epidemiology Committee. (2012). *The Canadian Nosocomial Infection Surveillance Program.* Retrieved from http://www.phac-aspc.gc.ca/nois-sinp/survprog-eng.php

Cann, A. J., & Chen, I. S. Y. (1996). Human T cell leukemia virus types I and II. Philadelphia: Lippincott-Raven Publishers.

Cano González, A., Vara Beceiro, I., Sánchez González, P., Pozo Guerrero, F. D., & Gómez Aguilera, E. J. (2008). Laparoscopic image analysis for automatic tracking of surgical tools. *Computer Assisted Radiology and Surgery 22nd International Congress and Exhibition (CARS 2008).*

Carlson, N. R. (2007). *Foundations of physiological psychology.* Allyn and Bacon. Available from: http://www.bbci.de/competition/ii/

Carnero, M. C., & Gómez, A. (2017). Multicriteria model for the selection of maintenance policies in subsystems of an operating theatre. In Optimum decision making in asset management. IGI Global.

Carnero, M. C. (2005). Selection of diagnostic techniques and instrumentation in a predictive maintenance program. A case study. *Decision Support Systems, 38*(4), 539–555. doi:10.1016/j.dss.2003.09.003

Carnero, M. C. (2007). Model for the selection of predictive maintenance techniques. *INFOR, 45*(2), 83–94.

Carnero, M. C. (2012). Condition Based Maintenance in small industries. In *Proceeding of the 2nd International Workshop on Advanced Maintenance Engineering*, 21-23.

Carnero, M. C. (2014). MCDA Techniques in Maintenance Policy Selection. In J. Wang (Ed.), *Encyclopedia of Business Analytics and Optimization* (Vol. III, pp. 406–415). Hershey, PA: IGI Global.

Carnero, M. C. (2014a). A Decision Support system for Maintenance Benchmarking in big buildings. *European Journal of Industrial Engineering, 8*(3), 388–420. doi:10.1504/EJIE.2014.061064

Carnero, M. C. (2014b). Multicriteria model for Maintenance Benchmarking. *Journal of Manufacturing Systems, 33*(2), 303–321. doi:10.1016/j.jmsy.2013.12.006

Carnero, M. C., & Gómez, A. (2016). A multicriteria decision making approach applied to improving maintenance policies in healthcare organizations. *BMC Medical Informatics and Decision Making, 16*(1), 47. doi:10.1186/s12911-016-0282-7 PMID:27108234

Carter, A. J., & Chochinov, A. H. (2007). A systematic review of the impact of nurse practitioners on cost, quality of care, satisfaction and wait times in the emergency department. *Canadian Journal of Emergency Medical Care, 9*(04), 286–295. doi:10.1017/S1481803500015189 PMID:17626694

Carter, M. W., & Lapierre, S. D. (2001). Scheduling emergency room physicians. *Health Care Management Science*, *4*(4), 347–360. doi:10.1023/A:1011802630656 PMID:11718465

Case, C., Kandola, K., Chui, L., Li, V., Nix, N., & Johnson, R. (2013). Examining DNA fingerprinting as an epidemiology tool in the tuberculosis program in the Northwest Territories, Canada. *International Journal of Circumpolar Health*, *72*(1), 1–8. doi:10.3402/ijch.v72i0.20067 PMID:23671837

Castellucci, S. A., Curcillo, P. G., Ginsberg, P. C., Saba, S. C., Jaffe, J. S., & Harmon, J. D. (2008). Single port access adrenalectomy. *J Endourol, 22*(8), 1573-1576.

Cataloluk, H., & Kesler, M. (2012, July). A diagnostic software tool for skin diseases with basic and weighted K-NN. In *Innovations in Intelligent Systems and Applications (INISTA), 2012 International Symposium on* (pp. 1-4). IEEE. doi:10.1109/INISTA.2012.6246999

Cavalcante, C. A. V., & Lopes, R. S. (2015). Multi-criteria model to support the definition of opportunistic maintenance policy: A study in a cogeneration system. *Energy*, *80*, 32–40. doi:10.1016/j.energy.2014.11.039

Cebeci, U. (2009). Fuzzy AHP-based decision support system for selecting ERP systems in textile industry by using balanced scorecard. *Expert Systems with Applications*, *36*(5), 8900–8909. doi:10.1016/j.eswa.2008.11.046

Ceglowski, A. (2006). *An investigation of emergency department overcrowding using data mining and simulation* (Doctoral dissertation). Monash University.

CEI IEC 61165:2006. (n.d.). *Application of Markov techniques, International Electrotechnical Commission*. IEC.

Celada, F., & Seiden, P. E. (1992). A computer model of cellular interactions in the immune system. *Immunology Today*, *13*(2), 56–62. doi:10.1016/0167-5699(92)90135-T PMID:1575893

Celada, F., & Seiden, P. E. (1996). Affinity maturation and hypermutation in a simulation of the humoral immune response. *European Journal of Immunology*, *26*(6), 1350–1358. doi:10.1002/eji.1830260626 PMID:8647216

Celebi, M. E., Aslandogan, Y. A., & Bergstresser, P. R. (2005, April). Mining biomedical images with density-based clustering. In *International Conference on Information Technology: Coding and Computing (ITCC'05): Vol. 2.* (Vol. 1, pp. 163-168). IEEE.

Centeno, M. A., Giachetti, R., Linn, R., & Ismail, A. M. (2003, December). Emergency departments II: a simulation-ilp based tool for scheduling ER staff. *Proceedings of the 35th conference on Winter simulation: driving innovation*, 1930-1938.

Centeno, A. P., Martin, R., & Sweeney, R. (2013, December). REDSim: A spatial agent-based simulation for studying emergency departments. In *Simulation Conference (WSC)* (pp. 1431-1442). IEEE. doi:10.1109/WSC.2013.6721528

Centers for Disease Control and Prevention. (2001). Updated U.S. Public Health Service Guidelines for the Management of Occupational Exposures to HBV, HCV, and HIV and Recommendations for Postexposure Prophylaxis. *Morbidity and Mortality Weekly Report*, *50*(RR11), 1–42. PMID:11442229

Centers for Disease Control and Prevention. (2006). Guide to confirming an etiology in a foodborne disease outbreak. *Morbidity & Mortality Weekly Report*, *49*(SS-1).

Chae, Y. M., Ho, S. H., Hong, C. S., & Kim, C. W. (1996). Comparison of Alternative Knowledge Model for Diagnosis of asthma. *Expert Systems with Applications*, *4*(11), 423–429. doi:10.1016/S0957-4174(96)00057-7

Chae, Y. M., Kim, H. S., Tark, K. C., Park, H. J., & Ho, S. H. (2003). Analysis of Healthcare Quality Indicators Using Data Mining and Decision Support System. *Expert Systems with Applications*, *24*(2), 167–172. doi:10.1016/S0957-4174(02)00139-2

Chan, C. L., Liu, Y. C., & Luo, S. H. (2008, June). Investigation of diabetic microvascular complications using data mining techniques. In *2008 IEEE International Joint Conference on Neural Networks (IEEE World Congress on Computational Intelligence)* (pp. 830-834). IEEE. doi:10.1109/IJCNN.2008.4633893

Chandra, S., Bhat, R., Singh, H., & Chauhan, D. S. (2009). Detection of brain tumors from MRI using gaussian RBF kernel based support vector machine. *IJACT: International Journal of Advancements in Computing Technology, 1*(1), 46–51. doi:10.4156/ijact.vol1.issue1.7

Chang, Y. J., Chen, C. C., Ho, J. M., & Chen, C. L. (2012). De Novo Assembly of High-Throughput Sequencing Data with Cloud Computing and New Operations on String Graphs. Cloud Computing, 155–161. doi:10.1109/CLOUD.2012.123

Chang, C. D., Wang, C. C., & Jiang, B. C. (2011). Using data mining techniques for multi-diseases prediction modeling of hypertension and hyperlipidemia by common risk factors. *Expert Systems with Applications, 38*(5), 5507–5513. doi:10.1016/j.eswa.2010.10.086

Chang, C. L., & Chen, C. H. (2009). Applying decision tree and neural network to increase quality of dermatologic diagnosis. *Expert Systems with Applications, 36*(2), 4035–4041. doi:10.1016/j.eswa.2008.03.007

Chang, D. Y. (1996). Applications of the extent analysis method on fuzzy AHP. *European Journal of Operational Research, 95*(3), 649–655. doi:10.1016/0377-2217(95)00300-2

Chang, P. L., & Teng, W. G. (2007, June). Exploiting the self-organizing map for medical image segmentation. In *Twentieth IEEE International Symposium on Computer-Based Medical Systems (CBMS'07)* (pp. 281-288). IEEE. doi:10.1109/CBMS.2007.48

Chang, R.-F., Wu, W.-J., Moon, W.-K., Chou, Y.-H., & Chen, D.-R. (2003). Improvement in breast tumour discrimination by support vector machines and speckle-emphasis texture analysis. *Ultrasound in Medicine & Biology, 29*(5), 679–686. doi:10.1016/S0301-5629(02)00788-3 PMID:12754067

Chan, S. S., Cheung, N. K., Graham, C. A., & Rainer, T. H. (2015). Strategies and solutions to alleviate access block and overcrowding in emergency departments. *Hong Kong Medical Journal, 21*(4), 345–352. PMID:26087756

Chanthaweethip, W., & Guha, S. (2012). Temporal data mining and visualization for treatment outcome prediction in HIV patients. *Procedia Computer Science, 13*, 68–79. doi:10.1016/j.procs.2012.09.115

Chaurasia, V., & Pal, S. (2013). Early prediction of heart diseases using data mining techniques. *Carib. j. Sciences et Techniques (Paris), 1*, 208–217.

Chaussy, C. H., Brendel, W., & Schmiedt, E. (1980). Extracorporeally induced destruction of kidney stones by shock waves. *Lancet, 2*(8207), 1265–1268. doi:10.1016/S0140-6736(80)92335-1 PMID:6108446

Chazard, E., Ficheur, G., Bernonville, S., Luyckx, M., & Beuscart, R. (2011). Data mining to generate adverse drug events detection rules. *IEEE Transactions on Information Technology in Biomedicine, 15*(6), 823–830. doi:10.1109/TITB.2011.2165727

Chee, B. W., Berlin, R., & Schatz, B. (2011, December). Predicting adverse drug events from personal health messages. *AMIA ... Annual Symposium Proceedings / AMIA Symposium. AMIA Symposium, 2011*, 217–226.

Chen, C. C., Hsu, C. C., Cheng, Y. C., & Li, S. T. (2009, June). Knowledge Discovery on In Vitro Fertilization Clinical Data Using Particle Swarm Optimization. In *Bioinformatics and BioEngineering, 2009. BIBE'09. Ninth IEEE International Conference on* (pp. 278-283). IEEE.

Chen, C. J., Huang, W., & Song, K. T. (2013). *Image tracking of laparoscopic instrument using spiking neural networks.* Paper presented at the Control, Automation and Systems (ICCAS), Gwangju, China. doi:10.1109/ICCAS.2013.6704052

Chen, J., Xing, Y., Xi, G., Chen, J., Yi, J., Zhao, D., & Wang, J. (2007, June). A comparison of four data mining models: Bayes, neural network, SVM and decision trees in identifying syndromes in coronary heart disease. In *International Symposium on Neural Networks* (pp. 1274-1279). Springer Berlin Heidelberg. doi:10.1007/978-3-540-72383-7_148

Chen, B. H., Kopylov, A., Huang, S. C., Seredin, O., Karpov, R., Kuo, S. Y., & Hung, P. C. et al. (2016). Improved global motion estimation via motion vector clustering for video stabilization. *Engineering Applications of Artificial Intelligence, 54*, 39–48. doi:10.1016/j.engappai.2016.05.004

Chen, D. S., Batson, R. G., & Dang, Y. (2010). *Applied integer programming: modeling and solution.* John Wiley & Sons.

Chen, D.-R., Chang, R.-F., Chen, C.-J., Ho, M.-F., Kuo, S.-J., Chen, S.-T., & Moon, W.-K. et al. (2005). Classification of breast ultrasound images using fractal feature. *Clinical Imaging, 29*(4), 235–245. doi:10.1016/j.clinimag.2004.11.024 PMID:15967313

Cheng, C. H. (1996). Evaluating naval tactical missile systems by fuzzy AHP based on the grade value of membership function. *European Journal of Operational Research, 96*(2), 343–350. doi:10.1016/S0377-2217(96)00026-4

Cheng, H. D., Shan, J., Ju, W., Guo, Y., & Zhang, L. (2010). Automated breast cancer detection and classification using ultrasound images: A survey. *Pattern Recognition, 43*(1), 299–317. doi:10.1016/j.patcog.2009.05.012

Chen, H.-J., Chen, R., Yang, M., Teng, G.-J., & Herskovits, E. H. (2015). Identification of Minimal Hepatic Encephalopathy in Patients with Cirrhosis Based on White Matter Imaging and Bayesian Data Mining. *AJNR. American Journal of Neuroradiology, 36*(3), 481–487. doi:10.3174/ajnr.A4146 PMID:25500314

Chen, H., Zhang, J., Xu, Y., Chen, B., & Zhang, K. (2012). Performance comparison of artificial neural network and logistic regression model for differentiating lung nodules on CT scans. *Expert Systems with Applications, 39*(13), 11503–11509. doi:10.1016/j.eswa.2012.04.001

Chen, L., Liu, R., Liu, Z. P., Li, M., & Aihara, K. (2012). Detecting early-warning signals for sudden deterioration of complex diseases by dynamical network biomarkers. *Scientific Reports, 2*, 1–8. doi:10.1038/srep00342 PMID:22461973

Chen, L., Wang, R., & Zhang, X. (Eds.). (2009). *Biomolecular networks: methods and applications in systems biology.* Hoboken, NJ: John Wiley & Sons. doi:10.1002/9780470488065

Chen, P. C., Liu, Y. T., Hsieh, J. H., & Wang, C. C. (2016). *A practical formula to predict the stone-free rate of patients undergoing extracorporeal shock wave lithotripsy.* Urological Science. doi:10.1016/j.urols.2016.05.004

Chen, R., Mias, G., Li-Pook-Than, J., Jiang, L., Lam, H. Y. K., Chen, R., & Snyder, M. et al. (2012). Personal omics profiling reveals dynamic molecular and medical phenotypes. *Cell, 148*(6), 1293–1307. doi:10.1016/j.cell.2012.02.009 PMID:22424236

Chen, T., Chen, J., & Zhou, B. (2012). A System for Parallel data mining service on cloud. *Second International Conference on Cloud and Green Computing.* doi:10.1109/CGC.2012.49

Chen, W.-P., Hung, C.-L., Tsai, S.-J. J., & Lin, Y.-L. (2014). Novel and efficient tag SNPs selection algorithms. *Bio-Medical Materials and Engineering, 24*(1), 1383–1389. PMID:24212035

Chen, Y.-J., & Aaron, R. A. S. (2014). SSVEP-based BCI classification using power cepstrum analysis. *MIT Press Journals, 50*(10), 735–737.

Chen, Z., Li, J., & Wei, L. (2007). A multiple kernel support vector machine scheme for feature selection and rule extraction from gene expression data of cancer tissue. *Artificial Intelligence in Medicine, 41*(2), 161–175. doi:10.1016/j.artmed.2007.07.008

Chiavetta, J. A., Escobar, M., Newman, A., He, Y., Driezen, P., Deeks, S., & Sher, G. et al. (2003). Incidence and estimated rates of residual risk for HIV, hepatitis C, hepatitis B and human T-cell lymphotropic viruses in blood donors in Canada 1990-2000. *Canadian Medical Association Journal, 169*(8), 767–773. PMID:14557314

Chien, C., & Pottie, G. J. (2012, August). A universal hybrid decision tree classifier design for human activity classification. In *2012 Annual International Conference of the IEEE Engineering in Medicine and Biology Society* (pp. 1065-1068). IEEE.

Chiu, R. K., Chen, R. Y., Wang, S. A., Chang, Y. C., & Chen, L. C. (2013). Intelligent systems developed for the early detection of chronic kidney disease. *Advances in Artificial Neural Systems, 2013,* 1–7. doi:10.1155/2013/539570

Cho, B. H., Yu, H., Kim, K. W., Kim, T. H., Kim, I. Y., & Kim, S. I. (2008). Application of irregular and unbalanced data to predict diabetic nephropathy using visualization and feature selection methods. *Artificial Intelligence in Medicine, 42*(1), 37–53. doi:10.1016/j.artmed.2007.09.005

Choi, S. I., Lee, K. Y., Park, S. J., & Lee, S. H. (2010). Single port laparoscopic right hemicolectomy with D3 dissection for advanced colon cancer. *World J Gastroenterol, 16*(2), 275-278.

Choi, J. W., Song, P. H., & Kim, H. T. (2012). Predictive factors of the outcome of extracorporeal shockwave lithotripsy for ureteral stones. *Korean J Urol, 53*(6), 424–430. doi:10.4111/kju.2012.53.6.424 PMID:22741053

Choi, S., Cichocki, A., Park, H. M., & Lee, S. Y. (2005). Blind source separation and independent component analysis: A review. *Neural Information Processing-Letters and Reviews, 6*(1), 1–57.

Chopra, S., & Meindl, P. (2004). *Supply chain management: Strategy, planning, and operation.* Pearson, Prentice-Hall.

Chorba, T. L., Berkelman, R. L., Safford, S. K., Gibbs, N. P., & Hull, H. F. (1989). Mandatory reporting of infectious diseases by clinicians. *Journal of the American Medical Association, 262*(21), 3018–3026. doi:10.1001/jama.1989.03430210060031 PMID:2810646

Christopher de Charms, R., Christoff, K., Glover, G. H., Pauly, J. M., Whitfield, S., & Gabrieli, J. D. (2004). Learned regulation of spatially localized brain activation using real-time fMRI. *NeuroImage, 21*(1).

Chun, T. W., Stuyver, L., Mizell, S. B., Ehler, L. A., Mican, J. A., Baseler, … Fauci, A.S. (1997). Presence of an inducible HIV-1 latent reservoir during highly active antiretroviral therapy. *Proceedings of the National Academy of Sciences USA, 94,* 13193–13197. doi:10.1073/pnas.94.24.13193

Chung, C. A. (2004). *Simulation Modeling Handbook A Practical Approach.* CRC Press.

Climent, J., & Hexsel, R. A. (2012). Particle filtering in the Hough space for instrument tracking. *Computers in Biology and Medicine, 42*(5), 614–623. doi:10.1016/j.compbiomed.2012.02.007 PMID:22425691

Climent, J., & Mars, P. (2010). Automatic instrument localization in laparoscopic surgery. In H. Bunke, J. J. Villanueva, G. Sanchez, & X. Otazu (Eds.), *Progress in computer vision and image analysis* (Vol. 73). Singapore: World Scientific Publishing Co.

Cohen, J., Kiss, R., & Pertsemlidis, A. (2004). Multiple rare alleles contribute to low plasma levels of HDL cholesterol. *Science, 305*(5685), 869–872. doi:10.1126/science.1099870 PMID:15297675

Coleman, D. J., Lizzi, F. L., Silverman, R. H., Helson, L., Torpey, J. H., & Rondeau, M. J. (1985). A model for acoustic characterization of intraocular tumors. *Investigative Ophthalmology & Visual Science, 26*(4), 545–550. PMID:3884539

Collins, T., Compte, B., & Bartoli, A. (2011). *Deformable Shape-From-Motion in Laparoscopy using a Rigid Sliding Window.* Paper presented at the MIUA.

Colosimo, M. E., Peterson, M. W., Mardis, S. A., & Hirschman, L. (2011). Nephele: Genotyping via complete composition vectors and MapReduce. *Source Code for Biology and Medicine*, 6–13. PMID:21851626

Colvin, M., & Maravelias, C. T. (2008). A stochastic programming approach for clinical trial planning in new drug development. *Computers & Chemical Engineering*, *32*(11), 2626–2642. doi:10.1016/j.compchemeng.2007.11.010

Colvin, M., & Maravelias, C. T. (2010). Modeling methods and a branch and cut algorithm for pharmaceutical clinical trial planning using stochastic programming. *European Journal of Operational Research*, *203*(1), 205–215. doi:10.1016/j.ejor.2009.07.022

Commonwealth of Australia. National Health Security Act 2007, Pub. L. No. 174. (2010). Retrieved from https://www.legislation.gov.au/Details/C2013C00147

Communicable Disease Network Australia. (2015a). *Protocol for making a change to the national notifiable disease list in Australia.* Retrieved January 4, 2017, from http://www.health.gov.au/internet/main/publishing.nsf/Content/ohp-protocol-NNDL-list.htm

Communicable Disease Network Australia. (2015b). *Protocol for making a change to the national notifiable diseases list (NNDL) in Australia.* Retrieved 21 Jnauary 2017 from http://www.health.gov.au/internet/main/publishing.nsf/Content/8DF6148BCAC589D6CA257EE5001D0DF7/$File/Protocol-change-NNDL.pdf

Conde, R. (2007). El benchmarking en la industria química. In *Proceedings of the Jornada sobre Benchmarking en Mantenimiento Industrial.* Madrid: Spanish Maintenance Association.

Cooke, M., Fisher, J., Dale, J., McLeod, E., Szczepura, A., Walley, P., & Wilson, S. (2004). *Reducing attendances and waits in emergency departments: A systematic review of present innovations.* Academic Press.

Cook, V. J., Shah, L., & Gardy, J. (2012). Modern contact investigation methods for enhancing tuberculosis control in aboriginal communities. *International Journal of Circumpolar Health*, *71*(1), 18643. doi:10.3402/ijch.v71i0.18643

Cooper, J. N., Wei, L., Fernandez, S. A., Minneci, P. C., & Deans, K. J. (2015). Pre-operative prediction of surgical morbidity in children: Comparison of five statistical models. *Computers in Biology and Medicine*, *57*, 54–65. doi:10.1016/j.compbiomed.2014.11.009

Coppel, W. A. (1965). *Stability and asymptotical behavior of differential equations, Heath Mathematical Monographs.* Boston: D.C. Heath and Company.

Coulouris, G. F., Dollimore, J., & Kindberg, T. (2005). *Distributed Systems: Concepts and Design.* Pearson Education.

Cowdell, F., Lees, B., & Wade, M. (2002). Discharge planning. *Armchair fan. The Health Service Journal*, *112*(5807), 28–29. PMID:12073514

Criminisi, A., & Shotton, J. (2013). *Decision forests for computer vision and medical image analysis.* London: Springer. doi:10.1007/978-1-4471-4929-3

Cromley, E., & McLafferty, S. (2012). *GIS and Public Health* (2nd ed.). New York: The Guidford Press.

Cronin, J. G., & Wright, J. (2006). Breach avoidance facilitator–managing the A&E 4-hour target. *Accident and Emergency Nursing*, *14*(1), 43–48. doi:10.1016/j.aaen.2005.11.005 PMID:16377191

Cula, O. G., & Dana, K. J. (2004). 3D texture recognition using bidirectional feature histograms. *International Journal of Computer Vision*, *59*(1), 33–60. doi:10.1023/B:VISI.0000020670.05764.55

Cullen, P. (2001). *Feature Selection Methods for Intelligent Systems Classifiers in Healthcare (PhD Dissertation).* Chicago: Loyola University of Chicago.

Curiac, D. I., Vasile, G., Banias, O., Volosencu, C., & Albu, A. (2009, June). Bayesian network model for diagnosis of psychiatric diseases. In *Information Technology Interfaces, 2009. ITI'09. Proceedings of the ITI 2009 31st International Conference on* (pp. 61-66). IEEE. doi:10.1109/ITI.2009.5196055

Czarnota, G. J., & Kolios, M. C. (2010). Ultrasound detection of cell death. *Imaging in Medicine, 2*(1), 17–28. doi:10.2217/iim.09.34

Czarnota, G. J., Kolios, M. C., Abraham, J., Portnoy, M., Ottensmeyer, F. P., Hunt, J. W., & Sherar, M. D. (1999). Ultrasound imaging of apoptosis: High-resolution non-invasive monitoring of programmed cell death in vitro, in situ and in vivo. *British Journal of Cancer, 81*(3), 520–527. doi:10.1038/sj.bjc.6690724 PMID:10507779

Czernin, J., & Phelps, M. E. (2002). Positron emission tomography scanning: Current and future applications. *Annual Review of Medicine, 53*(1), 89–112. doi:10.1146/annurev.med.53.082901.104028 PMID:11818465

D'Alessio, A., Piro, E., Tadini, B., & Beretta, F. (2002). One-trocar transumbilical laparoscopic-assisted appendectomy in children: our experience. *Eur J Pediatr Surg, 12*(1), 24-27.

Dadi, Z., & Alizade, S. (2016). Codimension-one bifurcation and stability analysis in an immunosuppressive infection model. SpringerPlus, 5, 106-121.

Dadi, Z., & Alizade, S. (2016). Codimension-one bifurcation and stability analysis in an immunosup-pressive infection model. SpringerPlus, 5, 106-121.

Dai, L., Gao, X., Guo, Y., Xiao, J., & Zhang, Z. (2012). Bioinformatics clouds for big data manipulation. *Biology Direct, 7*(1), 43. doi:10.1186/1745-6150-7-43 PMID:23190475

Dana, K. J., van Ginneken, B., Nayar, S. K., & Koenderink, J. J. (1999). Reflectance and texture of real-world surfaces. *ACM Transactions on Graphics, 18*(1), 1–34. doi:10.1145/300776.300778

Dangare, C. S., & Apte, S. S. (2012). Improved study of heart disease prediction system using data mining classification techniques. *International Journal of Computers and Applications, 47*(10), 44–48. doi:10.5120/7228-0076

DAngelo-Scott, H., Cutler, J., Friedman, D., Hendriks, A., & Jolly, A. M. (2015). Social network investigation of a syphilis outbreak in ottawa, Ontario. *The Canadian Journal of Infectious Diseases & Medical Microbiology, 26*(5), 268–272. doi:10.1155/2015/705720 PMID:26600816

Das, A. K., Sundaram, S., & Sundararajan, N. (2016). A Self-Regulated Interval Type-2 Neuro-Fuzzy Inference System for Handling Nonstationarities in EEG Signals for BCI. *IEEE Transactions on Fuzzy Systems, 24*(6), 1565–1577. doi:10.1109/TFUZZ.2016.2540072

Das, R., Turkoglu, I., & Sengur, A. (2009). Effective diagnosis of heart disease through neural networks ensembles. *Expert Systems with Applications, 36*(4), 7675–7680. doi:10.1016/j.eswa.2008.09.013

De Boer, R. J., & Perelson, A. S. (1993). How diverse should the immune system be? *Proceedings. Biological Sciences, 252*(1335), 171–175. doi:10.1098/rspb.1993.0062 PMID:8394577

De Cos Juez, F. J., Suárez-Suárez, M. A., Lasheras, F. S., & Murcia-Mazón, A. (2011). Application of neural networks to the study of the influence of diet and lifestyle on the value of bone mineral density in post-menopausal women. *Mathematical and Computer Modelling, 54*(7), 1665–1670. doi:10.1016/j.mcm.2010.11.069

De Domenico, M., Lima, A., & Musolesi, M. (2013). Interdependence and predictability of human mobility and social interactions. *Pervasive and Mobile Computing, 9*(6), 798–807. doi:10.1016/j.pmcj.2013.07.008

De Oliveira Branco, M. (2009). *Distributed Data Management for Large Scale Applications*. Southampton, UK: University of Southampton.

Dean, J., & Ghemawat, S. (2008). MapReduce: Simplified data processing on large clusters. *Communications of the ACM, 51*(1), 107–113. doi:10.1145/1327452.1327492

DeBoer, R. J., & Perelson, A. S. (1998). Target cell limited and immune control models of HIV infection: A comparison. *Journal of Theoretical Biology, 190*(3), 201–214. doi:10.1006/jtbi.1997.0548 PMID:9514649

Deeny, S. R., & Steventon, A. (2015). Making sense of the shadows: Priorities for creating a learning healthcare system based on routinely collected data. *BMJ Quality & Safety, 24*(8), 505–515. doi:10.1136/bmjqs-2015-004278 PMID:26065466

Delen, D. (2009). Analysis of cancer data: a data mining approach. *Expert System, 26*(1), 100–112.

Delen, D., Walker, G., & Kadam, A. (2005). Predicting breast cancer survivability: A comparison of three data mining methods. *Artificial Intelligence in Medicine, 34*(2), 113–127. doi:10.1016/j.artmed.2004.07.002

De, P., Singh, A. E., Wong, T., Yacoub, W., & Jolly, A. M. (2004). Sexual network analysis of a gonorrhoea outbreak. *Sexually Transmitted Infections, 80*(4), 280–285. doi:10.1136/sti.2003.007187 PMID:15295126

Department of Health Government of Australia. (2014). *National framework for communicable disease control*. Retrieved 21 January 2017 from http://www.health.gov.au/internet/main/publishing.nsf/Content/E5134F29919E9D74CA257CFB0082C7C5/$File/National-framework.pdf

Derlet, R. W., & Richards, J. R. (2000). Overcrowding in the nations emergency departments: Complex causes and disturbing effects. *Annals of Emergency Medicine, 35*(1), 63–68. doi:10.1016/S0196-0644(00)70105-3 PMID:10613941

Derlet, R. W., Richards, J. R., & Kravitz, R. L. (2001). Frequent overcrowding in US emergency departments. *Academic Emergency Medicine, 8*(2), 151–155. doi:10.1111/j.1553-2712.2001.tb01280.x PMID:11157291

Detours, V., & Perelson, A. S. (1999). Explaining high alloreactivity as a quantitative consequence of affinity-driven thymocyte selection. *Proceedings of the National Academy of Sciences of the United States of America, 96*(9), 5153–5158. doi:10.1073/pnas.96.9.5153 PMID:10220434

Detours, V., & Perelson, A. S. (2000). The paradox of alloreactivity and self MHC restriction: Quantitative analysis and statistics. *Proceedings of the National Academy of Sciences of the United States of America, 97*(15), 8479–8483. doi:10.1073/pnas.97.15.8479 PMID:10900009

Díaz-Uriarte, R., & De Andres, S. A. (2006). Gene selection and classification of microarray data using random forest. *BMC Bioinformatics, 7*(1), 3. doi:10.1186/1471-2105-7-3 PMID:16398926

Diebold, F. X., Cheng, X., Diebold, S., Foster, D., Halperin, M., Lohr, S., & Schorfheide, F. (2012). *A Personal Perspective on the Origin (s) and Development of "Big Data"*. The Phenomenon, the Term, and the Discipline.

Diepolder, H. M., Jung, M. C., Keller, E., Schraut, W., Gerlach, J. T., Gruner, N., & Pape, G. R. et al. (1998). A vigorous virus specific CD4+ T cell response may contribute to the association of HLA-DR13 with viral clearance in hepatitis B. *Clinical and Experimental Immunology, 113*(2), 244–251. doi:10.1046/j.1365-2249.1998.00665.x PMID:9717974

Ding, R., Chen, X., Wu, D., Wei, R., Hong, Q., Shi, S., & Xie, Y. et al. (2013). Effects of Aging on Kidney Graft Function, Oxidative Stress and Gene Expression after Kidney Transplantation. *Journal of Public Library of Science, 8*(6), e65613. PMID:23824036

Dinov, I. D. (2016). Methodological challenges and analytic opportunities for modeling and interpreting Big Healthcare Data. *GigaSci, 5*-12.

Dinov, I. D. (2016). Volume and Value of Big Healthcare Data. *J Med Stat Inform, 4*(1), 1–15. doi:10.7243/2053-7662-4-3 PMID:26998309

Diu, M., Gangeh, M. J., & Kamel, M. S. (2013). Unsupervised visual changepoint detection using maximum mean discrepancy. In *Proceedings of the 10th International Conference on Image Analysis and Recognition* (pp. 336–345). Berlin: Springer-Verlag. doi:10.1007/978-3-642-39094-4_38

Doherty, J. A. (2000). Establishing priorities for national communicable disease surveillance. *The Canadian Journal of Infectious Diseases, 11*(1), 21–4. Retrieved January 4 2017 from http://www.pubmedcentral.nih.gov/articlerender.fcgi?artid=2094737&tool=pmcentrez&rendertype=abstract

Doherty, J.-A. (2006). Final report snd recommendations from the national notifiable diseases working group. *Canada Communicable Disease Report, 32*(19), 211–225. PMID:17076030

Doignon, C., Graebling, P., & Mathelin, M. D. (2005). Real-time segmentation of surgical instruments inside the abdominal cavity using a joint hue saturation color feature. *Real Time Imaging, 11*(5-6), 429–442. doi:10.1016/j.rti.2005.06.008

Donohue, K. D., Huang, L., Burks, T., Forsberg, F., & Piccoli, C. W. (2001). Tissue classification with generalized spectrum parameters. *Ultrasound in Medicine & Biology, 27*(11), 1505–1514. doi:10.1016/S0301-5629(01)00468-9 PMID:11750750

Dosis, A., Bello, F., Gillies, D., Undre, S., Aggarwal, R., & Darzi, A. (2005). Laparoscopic task recognition using Hidden Markov Models. *Studies in Health Technology and Informatics, 111*, 115–122. PMID:15718711

Dou, J., & Li, J. (2014). Robust human action recognition based on spatio-temporal descriptors and motion temporal templates. *Optik - International Journal for Light and Electron Optics, 125*(7), 1891-1896.

Dowling, P. (2011). Health care supply chains in developing countries: Situational Analysis. Arlington, VA: Academic Press.

Duan, X., Wang, J., Qu, M., Leng, S., Liu, Y., Krambeck, A., & McCollough, C. (2012). Kidney Stone Volume Estimation from Computerized Tomography Images Using a Model Based Method of Correcting for the Point Spread Function. *The Journal of Urology, 188*(3), 989–995. doi:10.1016/j.juro.2012.04.098 PMID:22819107

Dua, S., & Du, X., Sree, S. V., & Vi, T. A. (2012). Novel classification of coronary artery disease using heart rate variability analysis. *Journal of Mechanics in Medicine and Biology, 12*(04), 1240017. doi:10.1142/S0219519412400179

Duda, R. O., Hart, P. E., & Stork, D. G. (2001). *2nd Pattern Classification*. Academic Press.

Duda, R. O., Hart, P. E., & Stork, D. G. (2001). *Pattern Classification (2nd ed.)*. New York: John Wiley & Sons.

Duggan, E. (2011, January). Dairy farmer to challenge raw milk rules. *Globe and Mail*. Retrieved 21 January 2017 from http://www.theglobeandmail.com/news/british-columbia/dairy-farmer-to-challenge-raw-milk-rules/article562804/

Dunmirea, B., Harperb, J. D., Cunitza, B. W., Leeb, F. C., Hsib, R., Liud, Z., & Sorensen, M. D. et al. (2016). Use of the Acoustic Shadow Width to Determine Kidney Stone Size with Ultrasound. *The Journal of Urology, 195*(1), 171–177. doi:10.1016/j.juro.2015.05.111 PMID:26301788

Dunn, R. L. (1999). *Basic guide to maintenance benchmarking*. Retrieved June 3, 2016, from http://www.plantengineering.com

Dunn, R. L. (2001). Benchmarking maintenance. *Plant Engineering, 55*, 68–70.

Dunn, S., Anderson, G. M., & Bierman, A. S. (2009). Temporal and regional trends in IUD insertion: A population-based study in Ontario, Canada. *Contraception, 80*(5), 469–473. doi:10.1016/j.contraception.2009.04.004 PMID:19835722

Durairaj, M., & NandhaKumar, R. (2013). Data Mining Application on IVF Data for the Selection of Influential Parameters on Fertility. *Int J Eng Adv Technol*, *2*(6), 278–283.

Durán, O. (2011). Computer-aided maintenance management systems selection based on a fuzzy AHP approach. *Advances in Engineering Software*, *42*(10), 821–829. doi:10.1016/j.advengsoft.2011.05.023

Eagle, N., Pentland, A. S., & Lazer, D. (2009). Inferring friendship network structure by using mobile phone data. *Proceedings of the National Academy of Sciences of the United States of America*, *106*(36), 15274–15278. doi:10.1073/pnas.0900282106 PMID:19706491

Easton, J. F., Stephens, C. R., & Angelova, M. (2014). Risk factors and prediction of very short term versus short/intermediate term post-stroke mortality: A data mining approach. *Computers in Biology and Medicine*, *54*, 199–210. doi:10.1016/j.compbiomed.2014.09.003 PMID:25303114

Eisenhauer, E. A., Therasse, P., Bogaerts, J., Schwartz, L. H., Sargent, D., Ford, R., & Verweij, J. et al. (2009). New response evaluation criteria in solid tumours: Revised {RECIST} guideline (version 1.1). *European Journal of Cancer*, *45*(2), 228–247. doi:10.1016/j.ejca.2008.10.026 PMID:19097774

El Emam, K., Hu, J., Mercer, J., Peyton, L., Kantarcioglu, M., Malin, B., & Earle, C. et al. (2011). A secure protocol for protecting the identity of providers when disclosing data for disease surveillance. *Journal of the American Medical Informatics Association*. PMID:21486880

Elaiw, A. M. (2010). Global properties of a class of HIV models. *Nonlinear Analysis Real World Applications*, *11*(4), 2253–2263. doi:10.1016/j.nonrwa.2009.07.001

El-Dahshan, E. S. A., Hosny, T., & Salem, A. B. M. (2010). Hybrid intelligent techniques for MRI brain images classification. *Digital Signal Processing*, *20*(2), 433–441. doi:10.1016/j.dsp.2009.07.002

El-Nahas, A. R., El-Assmy, A. M., Mansour, O., & Sheir, K. Z. (2007). A Prospective Multivariate Analysis of Factors Predicting Stone Disintegration by Extracorporeal Shock Wave Lithotripsy: The Value of High-Resolution Noncontrast Computed Tomography. *European Urology*, *51*(6), 1688–1694. doi:10.1016/j.eururo.2006.11.048 PMID:17161522

Emblemsvag, J., & Tonning, L. (2003). Decision support in selecting maintenance organization. *Journal of Quality in Maintenance Engineering*, *9*(1), 11–24. doi:10.1108/13552510310466765

EN15341. (2007). *Maintenance. Maintenance key performance indicators*. CEN.

Ernst, P., Ghezzo, H., & Becklake, M. R. (2002). Risk Factors for Bronchial. Hyper responsiveness in Late Childhood and Early adolescence. *The European Respiratory Journal*, *20*(3), 635–639. doi:10.1183/09031936.02.00962002 PMID:12358340

Escudero, J., Zajicek, J. P., & Ifeachor, E. (2011, August). Early detection and characterization of Alzheimer's disease in clinical scenarios using Bioprofile concepts and K-means. In *2011 Annual International Conference of the IEEE Engineering in Medicine and Biology Society* (pp. 6470-6473). IEEE. doi:10.1109/IEMBS.2011.6091597

Eshima, N., Iwata, O., Iwata, S., Tabata, M., Higuchi, Y., Matsuishi, T., & Karukaya, S. (2009). Age and gender specific prevalence of HTLV-I. *Journal of Clinical Virology*, *45*(2), 135–138. doi:10.1016/j.jcv.2009.03.012 PMID:19386541

Eshima, N., Tabata, M., Okada, T., & Karukaya, S. (2003). Population dynamics of HTLV-I infection: A discrete-time mathematical epidemic model approach. *Mathematical Medicine and Biology*, *20*(1), 29–45. doi:10.1093/imammb/20.1.29 PMID:12974497

Eskandari, H., Riyahifard, M., Khosravi, S., & Geiger, C. D. (2011, December). Improving the emergency department performance using simulation and MCDM methods. *Simulation Conference (WSC) Proceedings*, 1211–1222.

Estabrooks, A., Jo, T., & Japkowicz, N. (2004). A multiple resampling method for learning from imbalanced data sets. *Computational Intelligence*, *20*(1), 18–36. doi:10.1111/j.0824-7935.2004.t01-1-00228.x

Evirgen, H., & Çerkezi, M. (2014). Prediction and Diagnosis of Diabetic Retinopathy using Data Mining Technique. *Turkish Online Journal of Science & Technology*, *4*(3).

Falou, O., Soliman, H., Sadeghi-Naini, A., Iradji, S., Lemon-wong, S., Zubovits, J., & Czarnota, G. J. et al. (2012). Diffuse optical spectroscopy evaluation of treatment response in women with locally advanced breast cancer receiving. *Translational Oncology*, *5*(4), 238–246. doi:10.1593/tlo.11346 PMID:22937175

Faltin, F., Kenett, R. S., & Ruggeri, F. (Eds.). (2012). *Statistical methods in healthcare*. John Wiley & Sons. doi:10.1002/9781119940012

Fan, J., & Fan, Y. (2008). High dimensional classification using features annealed independence rules. *Annals of Statistics*, *36*(6), 2605–2637. doi:10.1214/07-AOS504 PMID:19169416

Fan, J., Guo, S., & Hao, N. (2012). Variance estimation using refitted cross-validation in ultrahigh dimensional regression. *Journal of the Royal Statistical Society. Series B. Methodological*, *74*(1), 37–65. doi:10.1111/j.1467-9868.2011.01005.x PMID:22312234

Fan, J., Han, F., & Liu, H. (2014). Challenges of Big Data analysis. *National Science Review*, *1*(2), 293–314. doi:10.1093/nsr/nwt032 PMID:25419469

Fan, J., Liao, Y., & Mincheva, M. (2011). High dimensional covariance matrix estimation in approximate factor models. *Annals of Statistics*, *39*(6), 3320–3356. doi:10.1214/11-AOS944 PMID:22661790

Fan, J., Liao, Y., & Mincheva, M. (2013). Large covariance estimation by thresholding principal orthogonal complements (with discussion). *Journal of the Royal Statistical Society. Series B, Statistical Methodology*, *75*(4), 603–680. doi:10.1111/rssb.12016 PMID:24348088

Fan, J., & Liu, H. (2013). *Statistical Analysis of Big Data on Pharmacogenomics. Advanced Drug Delivery Reviews*.

Fei, S. W. (2010). Diagnostic study on arrhythmia cordis based on particle swarm optimization-based support vector machine. *Expert Systems with Applications*, *37*(10), 6748–6752. doi:10.1016/j.eswa.2010.02.126

Feleppa, E. J., Kalisz, A., Sokil-Melgar, J. B., Lizzi, F. L., Liu, T., Rosado, A. L., & Heston, W. D. W. et al. (1996). Typing of prostate tissue by ultrasonic spectrum analysis. *IEEE Transactions on Ultrasonics, Ferroelectrics, and Frequency Control*, *43*(4), 609–619. doi:10.1109/58.503779

Fengqi, Y., Grossmann, I., & Wassick, J. (2003). Multi-Site Capacity, Production and Distribution Planning with Reactor Modifications: MILP Model, Bi-level Decomposition Algorithm vs. Lagrangean Decomposition Scheme. *Industrial & Engineering Chemistry Research*, *50*(9), 4831–4849.

Fenton, A., Lello, J., & Bonsall, M. B. (2006). Pathogen responses to host immunity: The impact of time delays and memory on the evolution of virulence. *Proceedings. Biological Sciences*, *273*(1597), 2083–2090. doi:10.1098/rspb.2006.3552 PMID:16846917

Fetter, R. B., & Thompson, J. D. (1965). The Simulation Of Hospital Systems. *Opns Res*, *13*(5), 689–711. doi:10.1287/opre.13.5.689

First Things First—Highmark makes healthcare-fraud prevention top priority with SAS. (2006). SAS. Retrieved from http://www.sas.com/ success/pdf/highmarkfraud.pdf

Flahault, A., Blanchon, T., Dorleans, Y., Toubiana, L., Vibert, J. F., & Valleron, A. J. (2006). Virtual surveillance of communicable diseases: A 20-year experience in France. *Statistical Methods in Medical Research*, *15*(5), 413–421. doi:10.1177/0962280206071639 PMID:17089946

Foege, W. H., Hogan, R. C., & Newton, L. H. (1976). Surveillance projects for selected diseases. *International Journal of Epidemiology*, *5*(1), 29–37. doi:10.1093/ije/5.1.29 PMID:944166

Fong, S., Wang, D., Fiaidhi, J., Mohammed, S., Chen, L., & Ling, L. (2016). Clinical Pathways Inference from Decision Rules by Hybrid Stream Mining and Fuzzy Unordered Rule Induction Strategy. *Computerized Medical Imaging and Graphics*. doi:10.1016/j.compmedimag.2016.06.008

Forero, R., Hillman, K. M., McCarthy, S., Fatovich, D. M., Joseph, A. P., & Richardson, D. B. (2010). Access block and ED overcrowding. *Emergency Medicine Australasia*, *22*(2), 119–135. doi:10.1111/j.1742-6723.2010.01270.x PMID:20534047

Foster, I., & Kesselman, C. (2003). *The Grid 2: Blueprint for a new Computing Infrastructure*. Houston, TX: Elsevier.

Fouladgar, M. M., Yazdani-Chamzini, A., Lashgari, A., Zavadskas, E. K., & Turskis, Z. (2012). maintenance strategy selection using AHP and COPRAS under fuzzy environment. *International Journal of Strategic Property Management*, *16*(1), 85–104. doi:10.3846/1648715X.2012.666657

Fritsch, V., Varoquaux, G., Thyreau, B., Poline, J.-B., & Thirion, B. (2012). Detecting outliers in high dimensional neuroimaging datasets with robust covariance estimators. *Medical Image Analysis*, *16*(7), 1359–1370. doi:10.1016/j.media.2012.05.002 PMID:22728304

Fu, L. D., & Zhang, Y. F. (2010, November). Medical image retrieval and classification based on morphological shape feature. In *Intelligent Networks and Intelligent Systems (ICINIS), 2010 3rd International Conference on* (pp. 116-119). IEEE.

Fumagalli, L., & Macchi, M. (2009). A state of the art of CBM in the Italian industry. *Proceedings of the 22nd International Congress on Condition Monitoring and Diagnostic Engineering Management - COMADEM*, 173-180.

Galar, M., Fernández, A., Barrenechea, E., Bustince, H., & Herrera, F. (2012). A review on ensembles for the class Imbalance problem: Bagging-, boosting-, and hybrid-based approaches. *IEEE Trans. on Systems, Man, and Cybernetics, Part C: Applications and Reviews*, *42*(4), 463–484. doi:10.1109/TSMCC.2011.2161285

Gandhi, V., Prasad, G., Coyle, D., Behera, L., &McGinnity, T. M. (2014). Quantum neural network-based EEG filtering for a brain–computer interface. *IEEE Transactions on Neural Networks and Learning Systems*, *25*(2), 278-288.

Gangeh, M. J., Raheem, A., Tadayyon, H., Liu, S., Hadizad, F., & Czarnota, G. J. (2016). Breast tumour visualization using 3-D quantitative ultrasound methods. SPIE Medical Imaging, 979006.

Gangeh, M. J., Sørensen, L., Shaker, S. B., Kamel, M. S., & de Bruijne, M. (2010). Multiple classifier systems in texton-based approach for the classification of CT images of lung. In *Proceedings of the Medical Computer Vision: Recognition Techniques and Applications in Medical Imaging (MCV)* (pp. 153–163). Berlin: Springer-Verlag.

Gangeh, M. J., El Kaffas, A., Hashim, A., Giles, A., & Czarnota, G. J. (2015). Advanced machine learning and textural methods in monitoring cell death using quantitative ultrasound spectroscopy. *Proceedings of the International Symposium on Biomedical Imaging: From Nano to Macro (ISBI)*, 646–650. doi:10.1109/ISBI.2015.7163956

Gangeh, M. J., Fung, B., Tadayyon, H., Tran, W. T., & Czarnota, G. J. (2016). Response monitoring using quantitative ultrasound methods and supervised dictionary learning in locally advanced breast cancer. *Proceedings of SPIE Medical Imaging*, 978406.

Gangeh, M. J., Hashim, A., Giles, A., & Czarnota, G. J. (2014). Cancer therapy prognosis using quantitative ultrasound spectroscopy and a kernel-based metric. *Proceedings of SPIE Medical Imaging*, 903406.

Gangeh, M. J., Hashim, A., Giles, A., Sannachi, L., & Czarnota, G. J. (2016). Computer aided prognosis for cell death categorization and prediction in vivo using quantitative ultrasound and machine learning techniques. *Medical Physics, 43*(12), 6439–6454. doi:10.1118/1.4967265 PMID:27908167

Gangeh, M. J., Sadeghi-Naini, A., Diu, M., Tadayyon, H., Kamel, M. S., & Czarnota, G. J. (2014). Categorizing extent of tumour cell death response to cancer therapy using quantitative ultrasound spectroscopy and maximum mean discrepancy. *IEEE Transactions on Medical Imaging, 33*(6), 1390–1400. doi:10.1109/TMI.2014.2312254 PMID:24893261

Gangeh, M. J., Sadeghi-Naini, A., Kamel, M. S., & Czarnota, G. J. (2013). Assessment of cancer therapy effects using texton-based characterization of quantitative ultrasound parametric images. *Proc. of the International Symposium on Biomedical Imaging: From Nano to Macro (ISBI)*, 1372–1375. doi:10.1109/ISBI.2013.6556788

Gangeh, M. J., Sørensen, L., Shaker, S. B., Kamel, M. S., de Bruijne, M., & Loog, M. (2010). A texton-based approach for the classification of lung parenchyma in CT images. In *Proceedings of the International Conference on Medical Image Computing and Computer Assisted Intervention (MICCAI)* (pp. 595–602). Berlin: Springer-Verlag. doi:10.1007/978-3-642-15711-0_74

Gangeh, M. J., Tadayyon, H., Sannachi, L., Sadeghi-Naini, A., & Czarnota, G. J. (2015). Quantitative ultrasound spectroscopy and a kernel-based metric in clinical cancer response monitoring. *Proceedings of the International Symposium on Biomedical Imaging: From Nano to Macro (ISBI)*, 255–259. doi:10.1109/ISBI.2015.7163862

Gangeh, M. J., Tadayyon, H., Sannachi, L., Sadeghi-Naini, A., Tran, W. T., & Czarnota, G. J. (2016). Computer aided theragnosis using quantitative ultrasound spectroscopy and maximum mean discrepancy in locally advanced breast cancer. *IEEE Transactions on Medical Imaging, 35*(3), 778–790. doi:10.1109/TMI.2015.2495246 PMID:26529750

Gao, Z., Hong, W., Xu, Y., Zhang, T., Song, Z., & Liu, J. (2010, September). Osteoporosis Diagnosis Based on the Multifractal Spectrum Features of Micro-CT Images and C4. 5 Decision Tree. In *Pervasive Computing Signal Processing and Applications (PCSPA), 2010 First International Conference on* (pp. 1043-1047). IEEE.

Garay, J., Cartagena, R., Esensoy, A. V., Handa, K., Kane, E., Kaw, N., & Sadat, S. (2014). Strategic analytics: towards fully embedding evidence in healthcare decision-making. *Healthcare Quarterly (Toronto, Ont.), 17*, 23-27.

García, M. L., Centeno, M. A., Rivera, C., & DeCario, N. (1995, December). Reducing time in an emergency room via a fast-track. *In Simulation Conference Proceedings, 1995. Winter* (pp. 1048-1053). IEEE. doi:10.1109/WSC.1995.478898

Gardner, R. C., Burke, J. F., Nettiksimmons, J., Kaup, A., Barnes, D. E., & Yaffe, K. (2014). Dementia risk after traumatic brain injury vs nonbrain trauma: The role of age and severity. *JAMA Neurology, 71*(12), 1490–1497. doi:10.1001/jamaneurol.2014.2668 PMID:25347255

Gardy, J. L., Johnston, J. C., Ho Sui, S. J., Cook, V. J., Shah, L., Brodkin, E., & Tang, P. et al. (2011). Whole-genome sequencing and social-network analysis of a tuberculosis outbreak. *The New England Journal of Medicine, 364*(8), 730–739. doi:10.1056/NEJMoa1003176 PMID:21345102

Garifullin. (2015). *Simulating Wait Time In Healthcare: Accounting For Transition Process Variability Using Survival Analyses*. Academic Press.

Gatica, G., Papageorigio, L. G., & Shah, N. (2011). Capacity Planning Under Uncertainty for the Pharmaceutical Industry. *Chemical Engineering Research & Design, 81*(6), 665–678.

Geelhoed, G. C., & de Klerk, N. H. (2012). Emergency department overcrowding, mortality and the 4-hour rule in Western Australia. *The Medical Journal of Australia, 196*(2), 122–126. doi:10.5694/mja11.11159 PMID:22304606

Geng, J. H., Tu, H. P., Shih, P. M. C., Shen, J. T., Jang, M. Y., Wu, W. J., & Juan, Y. S. et al. (2015). Noncontrast computed tomography can predict the outcome of shockwave lithotripsy via accurate stone measurement and abdominal fat distribution determination. *The Kaohsiung Journal of Medical Sciences*, *31*(1), 34–41. doi:10.1016/j.kjms.2014.10.001 PMID:25600918

Gennings, C., Ellis, R., & Ritter, J. K. (2012). Linking empirical estimates of body burden of environmental chemicals and wellness using NHANES data. *Environment International*, *39*(1), 56–65. doi:10.1016/j.envint.2011.09.002

Geraci, J. M., Johnson, M. L., Gordon, H. S., Peterson, N. J., Daley, J., Hur, K., & Wray, N. P. et al. (2000). Mortality after non-cardiac surgery: Prediction from administrative versus clinical data. *Journal of Investigative Medicine*, *48*(2).

Gershon, A. S., Guan, J., Wang, C., & To, T. (2010a). Trends in asthma prevalence and incidence in Ontario, Canada, 1996–2005: A population study. *American Journal of Epidemiology*. PMID:20716702

Gershon, A. S., Wang, C., Wilton, A. S., Raut, R., & To, T. (2010b). Trends in chronic obstructive pulmonary disease prevalence, incidence, and mortality in Ontario, Canada, 1996 to 2007: A population-based study. *Archives of Internal Medicine*, *170*(6), 560–565. doi:10.1001/archinternmed.2010.17 PMID:20308643

Ghosh, D., & Roy, S. (2010). A decision-making framework for process plant maintenance. *European Journal of Industrial Engineering*, *4*(1), 78–98. doi:10.1504/EJIE.2010.029571

Giannarou, S., Visentini-Scarzanella, M., & Yang, G. Z. (2012). *Probabilistic tracking of affine-invariant anisotropic regions*. Paper presented at the IEEE Trans Pattern Anal Mach Intell.

Giri, D., Acharya, U. R., Martis, R. J., Sree, S. V., Lim, T. C., Ahamed, T., & Suri, J. S. (2013). Automated diagnosis of coronary artery disease affected patients using LDA, PCA, ICA and discrete wavelet transform. *Knowledge-Based Systems*, *37*, 274–282. doi:10.1016/j.knosys.2012.08.011

Gokdogan, A., & Merdan, M. (2011). A multistage homotopy perturbation method for solving human T cell lymphotropic virus I (HTLV-I) infection of CD4+T cells model. *Middle-East Journal of Scientific Research*, *9*(4), 503–509.

Goktas, C., Akca, O., Horuz, R., Gokhan, O., Albayrak, S., & Sarica, K. (2011). SWL in Lower Calyceal Calculi: Evaluation of the Treatment Results in Children and Adults. *Urology*, *78*(6), 1402–1406. doi:10.1016/j.urology.2011.08.005 PMID:21962877

Goldman, D., Fastenau, J., Dirani, R., Helland, E., Joyce, G., & Conrad, R. et al.. (2014). Medicaid prior authorization policies and imprisonment among patients with schizophrenia. *The American Journal of Managed Care*, *20*, 577–586. PMID:25295404

Gómez de León, F. C., & Ruiz, J. J. (2006). Maintenance strategy based on a multicriterion classification of equipments. *Reliability Engineering & System Safety*, *91*(4), 444–451. doi:10.1016/j.ress.2005.03.001

Gómez-Acevedo, H., & Li, Y. M. (2005). Backward bifurcation in a model for HTLV-I infection of CD4+ T Cells. *Bulletin of Mathematical Biology*, *67*(1), 101–114. doi:10.1016/j.bulm.2004.06.004 PMID:15691541

Gómez-Vaquero, C., Soler, A. S., Pastor, A. J., Mas, J. P., Rodriguez, J. J., & Virós, X. C. (2009). Efficacy of a holding unit to reduce access block and attendance pressure in the emergency department. *Emergency Medicine Journal*, *26*(8), 571–572. doi:10.1136/emj.2008.066076 PMID:19625552

Gomez, W., Pereira, W. C. A., & Infantosi, A. F. C. (2012). Analysis of co-occurrence texture statistics as a function of gray-level quantization for classifying breast ultrasound. *IEEE Transactions on Medical Imaging*, *31*(10), 1889–1899. doi:10.1109/TMI.2012.2206398 PMID:22759441

Goossens, A. J. M., & Basten, R. J. I. (2015). Exploring maintenance policy selection using the Analytic Hierarchy Process; An application for naval ships. *Reliability Engineering & System Safety, 142*, 31–41. doi:10.1016/j.ress.2015.04.014

Goplani, K. R., Kute, V. B., Vanikar, A. V., Shah, P. R., Gumber, M. R., Patel, H. V., . . . Trivedi, H. L. (2010). Expanded Criteria Donor Kidneys for Younger Recipients: Acceptable Outcomes. In Proceedings of Transplantation, 42(10), 3931–3934.

Gorunow, M., Gunther, H.-O., & Yang, G. (2003). Plant co-ordination in pharmaceutics supply networks. *Operational Research Spectrum, 25*(1), 109–141. doi:10.1007/s00291-002-0117-z

Gostin, L. O. (2004). Health of the people: The highest law?. *Journal of Law Medicine & Ethics, 32*(3), 509. http://doi.org/DOI 10.1111/j.1748-720X.2004.tb00164.x

Gostin, L. O. (2000). Public health law in a new century: part I: law as a tool to advance the communitys health. *Journal of the American Medical Association, 283*(21), 2837–2841. doi:10.1001/jama.283.21.2837 PMID:10838654

Government of Saskatchewan. (2014a). *Communicable Disease Control Manual; Blood and body fluid pathogens; hepatitis C.* Retrieved 21 January 2017 from https://www.ehealthsask.ca/services/manuals/Documents/cdc-section-6.pdf#page=18

Government of Saskatchewan. (2014b). *Communicable Disease Control Manual; Respiratory and direct contact; measles.* Retrieved 21 January 2017 from http://www.ehealthsask.ca/services/manuals/Documents/cdc-section-2.pdf#page=87

Goyal, S. K., & Giri, B. C. (2001). Recent trends in modeling of deteriorating inventory. *European Journal of Operational Research, 134*(1), 1–16. doi:10.1016/S0377-2217(00)00248-4

Granville, V. (2014). *Developing Analytic Talent: Becoming a Data Scientist*. John Wiley & Sons.

Grasso, M. A., Finin, T., Zhu, X., Joshi, A., & Yesha, Y. (2009). *Video Summarization of Laparoscopic Cholecystectomies*. Paper presented at the the AMIA 2009 Annual Symposium.

Grayling, T. (1999). *Guidelines for safe disposal of unwanted pharmaceutical in and after emergencies*. Geneva: WHO.

Grether, J. K., Anderson, M. C., Croen, L. A., Smith, D., & Windham, G. C. (2009). Risk of autism and increasing maternal and paternal age in a large North American population. *American Journal of Epidemiology, 170*(9), 1118–1126. doi:10.1093/aje/kwp247 PMID:19783586

Gretton, A., Borgwardt, K. M., Rasch, M. J., Schölkopf, B., & Smola, A. (2012). A kernel two-sample test. *Journal of Machine Learning Research, 13*, 723–773.

Gretton, A., Borgwardt, K., Rasch, M., Schölkopf, B., & Smola, A. (2006). A kernel method for the two-sample-problem. *Advances in Neural Information Processing Systems, 19*, 513–520.

Grigg, O. A., & Farewell, V. T. (2004). A risk-adjusted Sets method for monitoring adverse medical outcomes. *Statistics in Medicine, 23*(10), 1593–1602. doi:10.1002/sim.1763 PMID:15122739

Grigg, O. A., Farewell, V. T., & Spiegelhalter, D. J. (2003). Use of risk-adjusted CUSUM and RSPRT charts for monitoring in medical contexts. *Statistical Methods in Medical Research, 12*(2), 147–170. doi:10.1177/096228020301200205 PMID:12665208

Grigg, O. A., & Spiegelhalter, D. J. (2007). A simple risk-adjusted exponentially weighted moving average. *Journal of the American Statistical Association, 102*(477), 140–152. doi:10.1198/016214506000001121

Grigg, O., & Farewell, V. (2004). An overview of risk-adjusted charts. *Journal of the Royal Statistical Society. Series A, (Statistics in Society), 167*(3), 523–539. doi:10.1111/j.1467-985X.2004.0apm2.x

Groenegress, C., Holzner, C., Guger, C., & Slater, M. (2010). Effects of P300-based BCI use on reported presence in a virtual environment. *Presence (Cambridge, Mass.), 19*(1), 1–11. doi:10.1162/pres.19.1.1

Grossman, R., Bailey, S., Ramu, A., Malhi, B., Hallstrom, P., Pulleyn, I., & Qin, X. (1999). The management and mining of multiple predictive models using the predictive modeling markup language. *Information and Software Technology, 41*(9), 589–595. doi:10.1016/S0950-5849(99)00022-1

Groves, P., Kayyali, B., Knott, D., & Van Kuiken, S. (2013). *The 'big data' revolution in healthcare: Accelerating value and innovation. McKinsey & Company.*

Guh, R. S., Wu, T. C. J., & Weng, S. P. (2011). Integrating genetic algorithm and decision tree learning for assistance in predicting in vitro fertilization outcomes. *Expert Systems with Applications, 38*(4), 4437–4449. doi:10.1016/j. eswa.2010.09.112

Gul, M., & Guneri, A. F. (2015). A comprehensive review of emergency department simulation applications for normal and disaster conditions. *Computers & Industrial Engineering, 83*, 327–344. doi:10.1016/j.cie.2015.02.018

Gunal, M. M., & Pidd, M. (2006, December). Understanding accident and emergency department performance using simulation. *In Simulation Conference, 2006. WSC 06. Proceedings of the Winter* (pp. 446-452). IEEE. doi:10.1109/WSC.2006.323114

Günal, M., & Pidd, M. (2010). Discrete event simulation for Performance Modelling in Health care: A review of the Literature. *Journal of Simulation, 4*(1), 42–51. doi:10.1057/jos.2009.25

Guo, H., Goldsman, D., Tsui, K. L., Zhou, Y., & Wong, S. Y. (2016). Using simulation and optimisation to characterise durations of emergency department service times with incomplete data. *International Journal of Production Research, 54*(21), 6494–6511. doi:10.1080/00207543.2016.1205760

Gupta, A., & Maranas, C. (2000). A Two-Stage Modeling and Solution Framework for Multisite Midterm Planning under Demand Uncertainty. *Industrial & Engineering Chemistry Research, 39*(10), 3799–3813. doi:10.1021/ie9909284

Gürbüz, E., & Kılıç, E. (2014). A new adaptive support vector machine for diagnosis of diseases. *Expert Systems: International Journal of Knowledge Engineering and Neural Networks, 31*(5), 389–397. doi:10.1111/exsy.12051

Gurmankin, A. D., Baron, J., & Armstrong, K. (2004). The effect of numerical statements of risk on trust and comfort with hypothetical physician risk communication. *Medical Decision Making, 24*(3), 265–271. doi:10.1177/0272989X04265482 PMID:15155015

Gutberlet, I., Debener, S., Jung, T. P., &Makeig, S. (2009). Techniques of EEG recording and preprocessing. *Quantative EEG Analysis Methods and Clinical Applications*, 23-49.

Hachesu, P. R., Ahmadi, M., Alizadeh, S., & Sadoughi, F. (2013). Use of data mining techniques to determine and predict length of stay of cardiac patients. *Healthcare Informatics Research, 19*(2), 121-129.

Hadjidemetriou, E., Grossberg, M. D., & Nayar, S. K. (2004). Multiresolution histograms and their use for recognition. *IEEE Transactions on Pattern Analysis and Machine Intelligence, 26*(7), 831–847. doi:10.1109/TPAMI.2004.32 PMID:18579943

Haferlach, T., Kohlmann, A., Wieczorek, L., Basso, G., Kronnie, G. T., Bene, M.-C., & Fo, R. et al. (2010). Clinical utility of microarray-based gene expression profiling in the diagnosis and subclassification of leukemia: Report from the international microarray innovations in leukemia study group. *Journal of Clinical Oncology, 28*(15), 2529–2537. doi:10.1200/JCO.2009.23.4732 PMID:20406941

Hale, J. K. (1969). *Ordinary differential equations.* New York: Wiley Interscience.

Halevy, A., Norvig, P., & Pereira, F. (2009). The unreasonable effectiveness of data. *IEEE Intelligent Systems, 24*(2), 8–12. doi:10.1109/MIS.2009.36

Hamrock, E., Paige, K., Parks, J., Scheulen, J., & Levin, S. (2012). Discrete Event Simulation for Healthcare Organizations: A Tool for Decision Making. *Journal of Healthcare Management, 58*(2), 110–124. PMID:23650696

Han, F., & Pan, W. (2010). A data-adaptive sum test for disease association with multiple common or rare variants. *Human Heredity, 70*(1), 42–54. doi:10.1159/000288704 PMID:20413981

Han, J., & Kamber, M. (2001). *Data Mining: Concepts and Techniques Morgan Kaufmann.* San Francisco: International Thomson.

Han, J., & Kamber, M. (2006). *Data Mining: Concepts and Techniques* (2nd ed.). San Francisco: Morgan Kaufman Publisher.

Han, J., Rodriguez, J. C., & Beheshti, M. (2008, December). Diabetes data analysis and prediction model discovery using rapidminer. In *2008 Second International Conference on Future Generation Communication and Networking* (Vol. 3, pp. 96-99). IEEE. doi:10.1109/FGCN.2008.226

Hannan, E. L., Giglio, R. J., & Sadowski, R. S. (1974, January). A simulation analysis of a hospital emergency department. In *Proceedings of the 7th conference on winter simulation* (vol. 1, pp. 379-388). ACM. doi:10.1145/800287.811199

Hansen, M. M., Miron-Shatz, T., Lau, A. Y. S., & Paton, C. (2014). Big Data in Science and Healthcare: A Review of Recent Literature and Perspectives Contribution of the IMIA Social Media Working Group. *IMIA Yearbook of Medical Informatics, 9*(1), 21–26. doi:10.15265/IY-2014-0004 PMID:25123717

Hardin, J. M., & Chhieng, D. C. (2007). Data Mining and Clinical Decision Support Systems. In E. S. B. E. Fhimss Facmi (Ed.), *Clinical Decision Support Systems* (pp. 44–63). Springer New York. doi:10.1007/978-0-387-38319-4_3

Haripriya, R., & Porkodi. (2016). A Survey Paper on Data mining Techniques and Challenges in Distributed DICOM. *International Journal of Advanced Research in Computer and Communication Engineering, 5*(3).

Harpaz, R., DuMouchel, W., Shah, N. H., Madigan, D., Ryan, P., & Friedman, C. (2012). Novel data mining methodologies for adverse drug event discovery and analysis. *Clinical Pharmacology and Therapeutics, 91*(6), 1010–1021. doi:10.1038/clpt.2012.50 PMID:22549283

Harper, P. R. (2005). A review and comparison of classification algorithms for medical decision making. *Health Policy (Amsterdam), 71*(3), 315–331. doi:10.1016/j.healthpol.2004.05.002

Harrison, R. F., & Kennedy, R. L. (2005). Artificial neural network models for prediction of acute coronary syndromes using clinical data from the time of presentation. *Annals of Emergency Medicine, 46*(5), 431–439. doi:10.1016/j.annemergmed.2004.09.012

Hart, G. K., Mullany, D., Cook, D. A., Pilcher, D., & Duke, G. (2008). Review of the application of risk-adjusted charts to analyse mortality outcomes in critical care. *Critical Care and Resuscitation, 10*, 239–251. PMID:18798724

Hay, A. M., Valentin, E. C., & Bijlsma, R. A. (2006, December). Modeling emergency care in hospitals: a paradox-the patient should not drive the process. In *Simulation Conference, 2006. WSC 06. Proceedings* (pp. 439-445). IEEE.

Hayashi, Y., Misawa, K., Hawkes, D. J., & Mori, K. (2016). Progressive internal landmark registration for surgical navigation in laparoscopic gastrectomy for gastric cancer. *International Journal of Computer Assisted Radiology and Surgery, 1*(5), 837–845. doi:10.1007/s11548-015-1346-3 PMID:26811079

Hay, S. I., George, D. B., Moyes, C. L., & Brownstein, J. S. (2013). Big Data Opportunities for Global Infectious Disease Surveillance. *PLoS Medicine, 10*(4), e1001413. doi:10.1371/journal.pmed.1001413 PMID:23565065

Healthways Heads Off Increased Costs with SAS. (2009). SAS. Retrieved from http://www.sas.com/success/pdf/healthways.pdf

He, H., & Garcia, E. A. (2009). Learning from imbalanced data. *IEEE Transactions on Knowledge and Data Engineering, 21*(9), 1263–1284. doi:10.1109/TKDE.2008.239

Heikes, K. E., Eddy, D. M., Arondekar, B., & Schlessinger, L. (2008). Diabetes Risk Calculator A simple tool for detecting undiagnosed diabetes and pre-diabetes. *Diabetes Care, 31*(5), 1040–1045. doi:10.2337/dc07-1150

Hemant, P., & Pushpavathi, T. (2012, July). A novel approach to predict diabetes by Cascading Clustering and Classification. In *Computing Communication & Networking Technologies (ICCCNT), 2012 Third International Conference on* (pp. 1-7). IEEE. doi:10.1109/ICCCNT.2012.6396069

Hermon, R., & Williams, P. A. H. (2014). Big data in healthcare: what is it used for?. *Proceedings of the 3rd Australian eHealth Informatics and Security Conference*, 40-49.

Hillier, F., & Lieberman, G. (2002). *Introduction to operations research*. New York, NY: McGraw-Hill Science.

Hill, N. R., Fatoba, S. T., Oke, J. L., Hirst, J. A., OCallaghan, C. A., Lasserson, D. S., & Hobbs, F. R. (2016). Global Prevalence of Chronic Kidney Disease–A Systematic Review and Meta-Analysis. *PLoS ONE, 11*(7), e0158765. doi:10.1371/journal.pone.0158765 PMID:27383068

Hillner, B. E., Smith, T. J., & Desch, C. E. (2000). Hospital and physician volume or specialization and outcomes in cancer treatment: Importance in quality of cancer care. *Journal of Clinical Oncology, 18*(11), 2327–2340. doi:10.1200/JCO.2000.18.11.2327 PMID:10829054

Hiroyasu, T., Tanaka, N., Hagiwara, A., & Ozamoto, Y. (2015). *Emphasizing mesenteric blood vessels in laparoscopic colon cancer surgery video images*. Paper presented at the 37th Annual International Conference of the IEEE Engineering in Medicine and Biology Society (EMBC), Milan, Italy. doi:10.1109/EMBC.2015.7318780

Hjorth, B. (1970). EEG analysis based on time domain properties. *Electroencephalography and Clinical Neurophysiology, 29*(3), 306–310. doi:10.1016/0013-4694(70)90143-4 PMID:4195653

Hlavacek, W. S., Redondo, A., Metzger, H., Wofsy, C., & Goldstein, B. (2001). Kinetic proofreading models for cell signaling predict ways to escape kinetic proofreading. *Proceedings of the National Academy of Sciences of the United States of America, 98*(13), 7295–7300. doi:10.1073/pnas.121172298 PMID:11390967

Hochberg, L. R., & Donoghue, J. P. (2006). Sensors for brain-computer interfaces. *IEEE Engineering in Medicine and Biology Magazine, 25*(5), 32–38. doi:10.1109/MEMB.2006.1705745 PMID:17020197

Hoffenberg, S., Hill, M. B., & Houry, D. (2001). Does Sharing Process Differences Reduce Patient Length of Stay in the Emergency Department? *Annals of Emergency Medicine, 38*(5), 533–540. doi:10.1067/mem.2001.119426 PMID:11679865

Hoge, C. W., McGurk, D., Thomas, J. L., Cox, A. L., Engel, C. C., & Castro, C. A. (2008). Mild traumatic brain injury in U.S. soldiers, returning from Iraq. *The New England Journal of Medicine, 358*(5), 15–27. doi:10.1056/NEJMoa072972 PMID:18234750

Holmes, A. (2012). *Hadoop in practice*. Manning Publications Co.

Holte, R. C., Acker, L. E., & Porter, B. W. (1989). Concept learning and the problem of small disjuncts. In *Proceedings of the 11th International Joint Conference on Artificial Intelligence* (pp. 813–818). Morgan Kaufmann.

Houshmand, E., Ebrahimipour, H., Doosti, H., Vafaei, N. A., Mahmoudian, P., & Hosseini, S. E. (2016). *Validity and reliability of the Persian version of quality assessment questionnaire (SERVUSE model).* Academic Press.

Houthooft, R., Ruyssinck, J., van der Herten, J., Stijven, S., Couckuyt, I., Gadeyne, B., & De Turck, F. et al. (2015). Predictive modelling of survival and length of stay in critically ill patients using sequential organ failure scores. *Artificial Intelligence in Medicine, 63*(3), 191–207. doi:10.1016/j.artmed.2014.12.009

Hoyt, R.E., & Yoshihashi, A. (2014). *Healthcare Data Analytics. Health Informatics: Practical Guide for Healthcare and Information Technology Professionals.* Academic Press.

Hsu, H. T., Lee, I. H., Tsai, H. T., Chang, H. C., Shyu, K. K., Hsu, C. C., & Lee, P. L. (2016). Evaluate the feasibility of using frontal SSVEP to implement an SSVEP-based BCI in young, Elderly and ALS Groups. *IEEE Transactions on Neural Systems and Rehabilitation Engineering, 24*(5), 603–615. doi:10.1109/TNSRE.2015.2496184 PMID:26625417

Huang, C. L., Liao, H. C., & Chen, M. C. (2008). Prediction model building and feature selection with support vector machines in breast cancer diagnosis. *Expert Systems with Applications, 34*(1), 578–587. doi:10.1016/j.eswa.2006.09.041

Huang, I. B., Keisler, J., & Linkov, I. (2011). Multi-criteria decision analysis in environmental sciences: Ten years of applications and trends. *The Science of the Total Environment, 409*(19), 3578–3594. doi:10.1016/j.scitotenv.2011.06.022 PMID:21764422

Huang, M. J., Chen, M. Y., & Lee, S. C. (2007). Integrating data mining with case-based reasoning for chronic diseases prognosis and diagnosis. *Expert Systems with Applications, 32*(3), 856–867. doi:10.1016/j.eswa.2006.01.038

Huang, Y.-L., & Chen, D.-R. (2005). Support vector machines in sonography: Application to decision making in the diagnosis of breast cancer. *Clinical Imaging, 29*(3), 179–184. doi:10.1016/j.clinimag.2004.08.002 PMID:15855062

Huang, Y., McCullagh, P., Black, N., & Harper, R. (2007). Feature selection and classification model construction on type 2 diabetic patients data. *Artificial Intelligence in Medicine, 41*(3), 251–262. doi:10.1016/j.artmed.2007.07.002

Huang, Z., Juarez, J. M., Duan, H., & Li, H. (2013a). Length of stay prediction for clinical treatment process using temporal similarity. *Expert Systems with Applications, 40*(16), 6330–6339. doi:10.1016/j.eswa.2013.05.066

Huang, Z., Juarez, J. M., Duan, H., & Li, H. (2014b). Reprint of Length of stay prediction for clinical treatment process using temporal similarity. *Expert Systems with Applications, 41*(2), 274–283. doi:10.1016/j.eswa.2013.08.036

Hughes, G. (2015). *How big is 'big data' in healthcare?.* Retrieved 27 Sep, 2015, from http://blogs.sas.com/content/hls/2011/10/21/how-big-is-big-data-in-healthcare/

Hung, R. (1995). Hospital nurse scheduling. *The Journal of Nursing Administration, 25*(7-8), 21–23. doi:10.1097/00005110-199507000-00010 PMID:7636569

Husain, M., (2014). Big Data: could it ever cure Alzheimer's disease?. *Brain, a Journal of Neurology, 137*, 2623–2624.

Iakovidis, D. K., Tsevas, S., & Polydorou, A. (2010). Reduction of capsule endoscopy reading times by unsupervised image mining. *Computerized Medical Imaging and Graphics, 34*(6), 471–478. doi:10.1016/j.compmedimag.2009.11.005 PMID:19969440

IBM. (2017). *IBM SPSS Software.* Retrieved January 15, 2017, from http://www.ibm.com/analytics/us/en/technology/spss/

Ibrahim, H., Saad, A., Abdo, A., & Eldin, A. S. (2016). Mining association patterns of drug-interactions using post marketing FDAs spontaneous reporting data. *Journal of Biomedical Informatics, 60*, 294–308. doi:10.1016/j.jbi.2016.02.009

ICA Lab – an open source software library for biomedical signal processing. (n.d.). Available from: http://www.bsp.brain.riken.jp/ICALAB/

Igarashi, T., Suzuki, H., & Naya, Y. (2009). Computer-based endoscopic image-processing technology for endourology and laparoscopic surgery. *International Journal of Urology*, *16*(6), 533–543. doi:10.1111/j.1442-2042.2009.02258.x PMID:19226356

Ilangkumaran, M., & Kumanan, S. (2009). Selection of maintenance policy for textile industry using hybrid multi-criteria decision making approach. *Journal of Manufacturing Technology Management*, *20*(7), 1009–1022. doi:10.1108/17410380910984258

Ilango, B. S., & Ramaraj, N. (2010, September). A hybrid prediction model with F-score feature selection for type II Diabetes databases. In *Proceedings of the 1st Amrita ACM-W Celebration on Women in Computing in India* (p. 13). ACM. doi:10.1145/1858378.1858391

Ilayaraja, M., & Meyyappan, T. (2015). Efficient Data Mining Method to Predict the Risk of Heart Diseases Through Frequent Itemsets. *Procedia Computer Science*, *70*, 586–592. doi:10.1016/j.procs.2015.10.040

Il-Chul, M., Won, B. J., Junseok, L., Doyun, K., Hyunrok, L., Taesik, L., & Woon, K. G. et al. (2015). EMSSIM: Emergency Medical Service Simulator With Geographic And Medical Details. *Proceedings of the 2015 Winter Simulation Conference*.

Inan, O., Uzer, M. S., & Yılmaz, N. (2013). A new hybrid feature selection method based on association rules and PCA for detection of breast cancer. *International Journal of Innovative Computing, Information, & Control*, *9*(2), 727–729.

Insana, M. F., & Oelze, M. (2006). *Advanced ultrasonic imaging techniques for breast cancer research* (J. Suri, R. Rangayyan, & S. Laxminarayan, Eds.). Valencia, CA: American Scientific Publishers.

Institute of Medicine Committee on the Future of Emergency Care in the United States Health System. (2007). *Hospital-based emergency care: At the Breaking Point*. Washington, DC: National Academies Press. Available from: http://www.nap.edu/catalog/11621.html

Institute of Medicine. (2006). *Emergency Medical Services: At the Crossroads*. Washington, DC: National Academies Press.

International Association of Food Protection. (2011). Procedures to investigate foodborne illness (6th ed.). New York: Springer.

Isaai, M. T., Kanani, A., Tootoonchi, M., & Afzali, H. R. (2011). Intelligent timetable evaluation using fuzzy AHP. *Expert Systems with Applications*, *38*(4), 3718–3723. doi:10.1016/j.eswa.2010.09.030

Isa, N. A. M., Salamah, S. A., & Ngah, U. K. (2009). Adaptive fuzzy moving K-means clustering algorithm for image segmentation. *IEEE Transactions on Consumer Electronics*, *55*(4), 2145–2153. doi:10.1109/TCE.2009.5373781

Iskrant, A., & Khan, H. (1948). Statistical indices used in the evaluation of syphilis contact investigation. *Journal of Venereal Disease Information*, *29*(1), 1–6. PMID:18917634

Izady, N., & Worthington, D. (2012). Setting staffing requirements for time dependent queueing networks: The case of accident and emergency departments. *European Journal of Operational Research*, *219*(3), 531–540. doi:10.1016/j.ejor.2011.10.040

Jacobsen, S., Hall, S., & Swisher, J. (2006). Discrete-Event Simulation of Health Care Systems. In R. Hall (Ed.), *Patient Flow: Reducing Delay in Healthcare Delivery* (pp. 211–252). Springer. doi:10.1007/978-0-387-33636-7_8

Jacquez, J., & Simon, C. (2002). Qualitative theory of compartmental systems with lags. *Mathematical Biosciences*, *180*(1-2), 329–362. doi:10.1016/S0025-5564(02)00131-1 PMID:12387931

Jaffa, M. A., Woolson, R. F., Lipsitz, S. R., Baliga, P. K., Lopes-Virella, M., & Lackland, D. T. (2010). Analyses of renal outcome following transplantation Adjusting for informative right censoring and demographic factors: A longitudinal study. *Journal of Renal Failure*, *32*(6), 691–698. doi:10.3109/0886022X.2010.486495 PMID:20540637

Jain, A. K., & Farrokhnia, F. (1991). Unsupervised texture segmentation using gabor filters. *Pattern Recognition*, *24*(12), 1167–1186. doi:10.1016/0031-3203(91)90143-S

Jajosky, R. A., & Groseclose, S. L. (2004). Evaluation of reporting timeliness of public health surveillance systems for infectious diseases. *BMC Public Health*, *4*(1), 29. doi:10.1186/1471-2458-4-29 PMID:15274746

Jaulent, M., Le Bozec, C., Zapletal, E., & Degoulet, P. (2005). A Case-Based Reasoning method for computer-assisted diagnosis in histopathology, Diagnostic Problem Solving. *Artificial Intelligence in Medicine*, *1211*, 239–242.

Jaumard, B., Semet, F., & Vovor, T. (1998). A generalized linear programming model for nurse scheduling. *European Journal of Operational Research*, *107*(1), 1–18. doi:10.1016/S0377-2217(97)00330-5

Jayalakshmi, T., & Santhakumaran, A. (2010, February). A novel classification method for diagnosis of diabetes mellitus using artificial neural networks. In *Data Storage and Data Engineering (DSDE), 2010 International Conference on* (pp. 159-163). IEEE. doi:10.1109/DSDE.2010.58

Jayaprakash, N., O'Sullivan, R., Bey, T., Ahmed, S. S., &Lotfipour, S. (2009). Crowding and delivery of healthcare in emergency departments: the European perspective. *Western Journal of Emergency Medicine*, *10*(4).

Jen, C. H., Wang, C. C., Jiang, B. C., Chu, Y. H., & Chen, M. S. (2012). Application of classification techniques on development an early-warning system for chronic illnesses. *Expert Systems with Applications*, *39*(10), 8852–8858. doi:10.1016/j.eswa.2012.02.004

Jerbi, B., & Kamoun, H. (2009). Using simulation and goal programming to reschedule emergency department doctors shifts: Case of a Tunisian hospital. *Journal of Simulation*, *3*(4), 211–219. doi:10.1057/jos.2009.6

Jha, V., Garcia-Garcia, G., Iseki, K., Li, Z., Naicker, S., Plattner, B., & Yang, C. W. et al. (2013). Chronic kidney disease: Global dimension and perspectives. *Lancet*, *382*(9888), 260–272. doi:10.1016/S0140-6736(13)60687-X PMID:23727169

Ji, Y., Ying, H., Dews, P., Farber, M. S., Mansour, A., Tran, J., . . . Massanari, R. M. (2010a, July). A fuzzy recognition-primed decision model-based causal association mining algorithm for detecting adverse drug reactions in postmarketing surveillance. In *Fuzzy Systems (FUZZ), 2010 IEEE International Conference on* (pp. 1-8). IEEE.

Ji, Y., Ying, H., Tran, J., Dews, P., Mansour, A., & Massanari, R. M. (2011c, December). Mining Infrequent Causal Associations in Electronic Health Databases. In *2011 IEEE 11th International Conference on Data Mining Workshops* (pp. 421-428). IEEE.

Jilani, T. A., Yasin, H., Yasin, M., & Ardil, C. (2009). Acute coronary syndrome prediction using data mining techniques-an application. *World Academy of Science. Engineering and Technology*, *59*(4), 295–299.

Ji, Y., Ying, H., Dews, P., Mansour, A., Tran, J., Miller, R. E., & Massanari, R. M. (2011b). A potential causal association mining algorithm for screening adverse drug reactions in postmarketing surveillance. *IEEE Transactions on Information Technology in Biomedicine*, *15*(3), 428–437. doi:10.1109/TITB.2011.2131669

Ji, Y., Ying, H., Tran, J., Dews, P., Mansour, A., & Massanari, R. M. (2013d). A method for mining infrequent causal associations and its application in finding adverse drug reaction signal pairs. *IEEE Transactions on Knowledge and Data Engineering*, *25*(4), 721–733. doi:10.1109/TKDE.2012.28

Jolly, A. M., Moffatt, M. E. K., Fast, M. V., & Brunham, R. C. (2005). Sexually transmitted disease thresholds in Manitoba, Canada. *Annals of Epidemiology*, *15*(10), 781–788. doi:10.1016/j.annepidem.2005.05.001 PMID:16168671

Jolly, A. M., & Wylie, J. L. (2001). Sampling individuals with large sexual networks - An evaluation of four approaches. *Sexually Transmitted Diseases*, 28(4), 200–207. doi:10.1097/00007435-200104000-00003 PMID:11318250

Jolly, A., & Wylie, J. L. (2013). Sexual networks and sexually transmitted infections; the strength of weak (long distance) ties. In S. O. Aral, K. A. Fenton, & J. Lipshutz (Eds.), *The New Public Health and STD/HIV Prevention: Personal, Public and Health Systems Approaches* (pp. 77–109). Springer-Verlag. doi:10.1007/978-1-4614-4526-5_5

Jonas, M., Solangasenathirajan, S., & Hett, D. (2014). Patient Identification, A Review of the Use of Biometrics in the ICU. In Annual Update in Intensive Care and Emergency Medicine (pp. 679-688). New York: Springer.

Jones, S. L. P. (1987). *The Implementation of Functional Programming Languages*. Prentice-Hall International Series in Computer Science.

Joo, S., Yang, Y. S., Moon, W. K., & Kim, H. C. (2004). Computer-aided diagnosis of solid breast nodules: Use of an artificial neural network based on multiple sonographic features. *IEEE Transactions on Medical Imaging*, 23(10), 1292–1300. doi:10.1109/TMI.2004.834617 PMID:15493696

Jose, J. S., Sivakami, R., Maheswari, N. U., & Venkatesh, R. (2012). An efficient diagnosis of kidney images using association rules. Int. J. Comput. Technol. Electron. *Eng*, 12(2), 14–20.

Joshi, A. J., & Rys, M. J. (2011). Study on the effect of different arrival patterns on an emergency department capacity using discrete event simulation. *International journal of industrial engineering. Theory Applications and Practice*, 18(1), 40–50.

Joshi, R., Banwet, D. K., & Shankar, R. A. (2011). Delphi-AHP-TOPSIS based benchmarking framework for performance improvement of a cold chain. *Expert Systems with Applications*, 38(8), 10170–10182. doi:10.1016/j.eswa.2011.02.072

Juan, G., Sen-lin, L., Hong-bo, J., Tie-mei, Z., & Yi-wen, H. (2007, May). Type 2 diabetes data processing with EM and C4. 5 algorithm. In *Complex Medical Engineering, 2007. CME 2007. IEEE/ICME International Conference on* (pp. 371-377). IEEE.

Juang, C. F. (2004). A hybrid of genetic algorithm and particle swarm optimization for recurrent network design. *IEEE Transactions on Systems, Man, and Cybernetics. Part B, Cybernetics*, 34(2), 997–1006. doi:10.1109/TSMCB.2003.818557 PMID:15376846

Julesz, B. (1981). Textons, the elements of texture perception, and their interactions. *Nature*, 290(5802), 91–97. doi:10.1038/290091a0 PMID:7207603

Jünger, M., Liebling, T. M., Naddef, D., Nemhauser, G. L., Pulleyblank, W. R., Reinelt, G., & Wolsey, L. A. (Eds.). (2009). *50 Years of integer programming 1958-2008: From the early years to the state-of-the-art*. Springer Science & Business Media.

Jun, J. B., Jacobson, S. H., & Swisher, J. R. (1999). Application of Discrete-Event Simulation in Health Care Clinics: A Survey. *The Journal of the Operational Research Society*, 50(2), 109–123. doi:10.1057/palgrave.jors.2600669

Kadri, F., Harrou, F., Chaabane, S., & Tahon, C. (2014). Time series modelling and forecasting of emergency department overcrowding. *Journal of Medical Systems*, 38(9), 1–20. doi:10.1007/s10916-014-0107-0 PMID:25053208

Kahn, J., Svantesson, T., Olver, D., & Poling, A. (2009). Global Maintenance and Reliability Indicators: Fitting the Pieces Together (2nd ed.). European Federation of National Maintenance Societies and the Society of Maintenance & Reliability Professionals.

Kahraman, C., Cebeci, U., & Ruan, D. (2004). Multi-attribute comparison of catering service companies using fuzzy AHP: The case of Turkey. *International Journal of Production Economics*, 87(2), 171–184. doi:10.1016/S0925-5273(03)00099-9

Kajabadi, A., Saraee, M. H., & Asgari, S. (2009, October). Data mining cardiovascular risk factors. In *Application of Information and Communication Technologies, 2009. AICT 2009. International Conference on* (pp. 1-5). IEEE.

Kalams, S. A., & Walker, B. D. (1998). The critical need for CD4 help in maintaining effective cytotoxic T lymphocyte responses. *The Journal of Experimental Medicine, 188*(12), 2199–2204. doi:10.1084/jem.188.12.2199 PMID:9858506

Kang, D. H., Chung, D. Y., Cho, K. S., Lee, D. H., Han, J. H., Kang, H. W., & Lee, J. Y. et al. (2015). Impact of colic pain as a significant factor for predicting the stone free rate of one-session shock wave lithotripsy for treating ureter stones: A Bayesian logistic regression model analysis. *European Urology Supplements, 14*.

Kang, H., Nembhard, H., Rafferty, C., & DeFlitch, C. (2014). Patient Flow In The Emergency Department: A Classification And Analysis Of Admission Process Policies. *Annals of Emergency Medicine, 64*(4), 335–342. doi:10.1016/j.annemergmed.2014.04.011 PMID:24875896

Karabatak, M., & Ince, M. C. (2009). An expert system for detection of breast cancer based on association rules and neural network. *Expert Systems with Applications, 36*(2), 3465–3469. doi:10.1016/j.eswa.2008.02.064

Karaolis, M. A., Moutiris, J. A., Hadjipanayi, D., & Pattichis, C. S. (2010). Assessment of the risk factors of coronary heart events based on data mining with decision trees. *IEEE Transactions on Information Technology in Biomedicine, 14*(3), 559–566. doi:10.1109/TITB.2009.2038906

Karegowda, A. G., Jayaram, M. A., & Manjunath, A. S. (2012). Cascading k-means clustering and k-nearest neighbor classifier for categorization of diabetic patients. *International Journal of Engineering and Advanced Technology, 1*(3), 147–151.

Karim, G., Oualid, J., Zied, J., Mathias, W., Romain, H., Valérie, T., & Ger, K. (2014). A Comprehensive Simulation Modeling Of An Emergency Department: A Case Study For Simulation Optimization Of Staffing Levels. *Proceedings of the 2014 Winter Simulation Conference*.

Karimi, M., Amirfattahi, R., Sadri, S., & Marvasti, S. A. (2005, November). Noninvasive detection and classification of coronary artery occlusions using wavelet analysis of heart sounds with neural networks. In *Medical Applications of Signal Processing, 2005. The 3rd IEE International Seminar on (Ref. No. 2005-1119)* (pp. 117-120). IET.

Karlik, B., & Harman, G. (2013, April). Computer-aided software for early diagnosis of eerythemato-squamous diseases. In *Electronics and Nanotechnology (ELNANO), 2013 IEEE XXXIII International Scientific Conference* (pp. 276-279). IEEE. doi:10.1109/ELNANO.2013.6552035

Kasemthaweesab, P., & Kurutach, W. (2012, July). Association analysis of diabetes mellitus (DM) with complication states based on association rules. In *2012 7th IEEE Conference on Industrial Electronics and Applications (ICIEA)* (pp. 1453-1457). IEEE.

Kassebaum, N. J., Arora, M., Barber, R. M., Bhutta, Z. A., Brown, J., Carter, A., & Cornaby, L. et al. (2016). Global, regional, and national disability-adjusted life-years (DALYs) for 315 diseases and injuries and healthy life expectancy (HALE), 1990–2015: A systematic analysis for the Global Burden of Disease Study 2015. *Lancet, 388*(10053), 1603–1658. doi:10.1016/S0140-6736(16)31460-X PMID:27733283

Katri, P., & Ruan, S. (2004). Dynamics of human T cell lymphotropic virus I (HTLV-I) infection of CD4$^+$ T cells. *Comptes Rendus Biologies, 327*(11), 1009–1016. doi:10.1016/j.crvi.2004.05.011 PMID:15628223

Kavitha, K., & Sarojamma, R. M. (2012). Monitoring of diabetes with data mining via CART Method. *International Journal of Emerging Technology and Advanced Engineering, 2*(11), 157–162.

Kavitha, M. S., Ganesh Kumar, P., Park, S. Y., Huh, K. H., Heo, M. S., Kurita, T., & Chien, S. I. et al. (2016). Automatic detection of osteoporosis based on hybrid genetic swarm fuzzy classifier approaches. *Dento Maxillo Facial Radiology*, *45*(7), 20160076. doi:10.1259/dmfr.20160076

Kaw, N., Esensoy, A. V., Sadat, S., Liu, A., Bastedo, S., & Nesrallah, G. (2016). *Planning for dialysis capacity and bundled patient-based funding in Ontario, Canada.* Unpublished Manuscript.

Keeney, R. L. (1996). *Value-focused Thinking: A Path to Creative Decision making.* Cambridge, MA: Harvard.

Kelen, G. D., Kraus, C. K., McCarthy, M. L., Bass, E., Hsu, E. B., Li, G., & Green, G. B. et al. (2006). Inpatient disposition classification for the creation of hospital surge capacity: A multiphase study. *Lancet*, *368*(9551), 1984–1990. doi:10.1016/S0140-6736(06)69808-5 PMID:17141705

Kelessidis, V. (2000). *Benchmarking.* Report produced for the EC funded project INNOREGIO: dissemination of innovation management and knowledge techniques.

Kelle, P., Woosley, J., & Schneider, H. (2012). Pharmaceutical supply chain specifics and inventory solutions for a hospital case. *Operations Research for Health Care*, *1*(2-3), 54–63. doi:10.1016/j.orhc.2012.07.001

Kelton, W. D., Sadowski, R. P., & Sadowski, D. A. (2002). *Simulation with ARENA.* McGraw-Hill, School Education Group.

Kelton, W. D., Sadowski, R. P., & Sadowski, D. A. (2004). *Simulation with Arena.* McGraw Hill.

Kepler, T. B., & Perelson, A. S. (1993). Cyclic re-entry of germinal center B cells and the efficiency of affinity maturation. *Immunology Today*, *14*(8), 412–415. doi:10.1016/0167-5699(93)90145-B PMID:8397781

Kesmir, C., & De Boer, R. J. (1999). A mathematical model on germinal center kinetics and termination. *Journal of Immunology (Baltimore, MD.: 1950)*, *163*, 2463–2469. PMID:10452981

Kessler, R. C., Warner, C. H., Ivany, C., Petukhova, M. V., Rose, S., Bromet, E. J., & Ursano, R. J. et al. (2015). Predicting suicides after psychiatric hospitalization in US Army soldiers: The army study to assess risk and resilience in service members (Army STARRS). *JAMA Psychiatry*, *72*(1), 49–57. doi:10.1001/jamapsychiatry.2014.1754 PMID:25390793

Khairudin, Z., Mohd, N., & Hamid, H. (2012, September). Predictive models of prolonged stay after Coronary Artery Bypass surgery. *In Statistics in Science, Business, and Engineering (ICSSBE), 2012 International Conference on* (pp. 1-5). IEEE.

Khan, M. U., Choi, J. P., Shin, H., & Kim, M. (2008, August). Predicting breast cancer survivability using fuzzy decision trees for personalized healthcare. In *2008 30th Annual International Conference of the IEEE Engineering in Medicine and Biology Society* (pp. 5148-5151). IEEE.

Khanna, S., & Agarwal, S. (2013, December). An Integrated Approach towards the prediction of Likelihood of Diabetes. In *Machine Intelligence and Research Advancement (ICMIRA), 2013 International Conference on* (pp. 294-298). IEEE. doi:10.1109/ICMIRA.2013.62

Kharitonov, V. L. (1978). Asymptotic stability of an equilibrium position of a family of systems of linear differential equations. *Differensial'nye Uravnenya*, *14*, 2086–2088.

Khatibi, T., Sepehri, M. M., & Shadpour, P. (2013). SIDF: A Novel Framework for Accurate Surgical Instrument Detection in Laparoscopic Video Frames. *International Journal of Hospital Research*, *2*(4), 163–170.

Khatibi, T., Sepehri, M. M., & Shadpour, P. (2014). A novel unsupervised approach for minimally-invasive video segmentation. *Medical Signals and Sensors*, *4*(1), 53–71. PMID:24695410

Kim, T. B., Lee, S. C., Kim, K. H., Jung, H., Yoon, S. J., & Oh, J. K. (2013). The feasibility of shockwave lithotripsy for treating solitary, lower calyceal stones over 1 cm in size. *Canadian Urological Association, 7*(3), 156–160. doi:10.5489/cuaj.473 PMID:23589749

Kirby Institute for infection and immunity in society 2015. (2015). *HIV, viral hepatitis and sexually transmitted infections in Australia; annual surveillance report 2015.* Retrieved 21 January 2015 from http://kirby.unsw.edu.au/sites/default/files/hiv/resources/NBBVSTI%20Surveillance%20and%20Monitoring%20Report%202015_0.pdf

Kirubakaran, B., & Ilangkumaran, M. (2016). Selection of optimum maintenance strategy based on FAHP integrated with GRA-TOPSIS. *Annals of Operations Research, 245*(1), 285–313. doi:10.1007/s10479-014-1775-3

Kishore, S., González-Franco, M., Hintemüller, C., Kapeller, C., Guger, C., Slater, M., & Blom, K. J. (2014). Comparison of SSVEP BCI and eye tracking for controlling a humanoid robot in a social environment. *Presence (Cambridge, Mass.), 23*(3), 242–252. doi:10.1162/PRES_a_00192

Kliegr, T., Vojíř, S., & Rauch, J. (2011). Background knowledge and PMML: first considerations. *Proceedings of the 2011 workshop on Predictive markup language modeling.* doi:10.1145/2023598.2023606

Klovdahl, A. S. (1985). Social networks and the spread of infectious diseases: The AIDS example. *Social Science & Medicine, 21*(11), 1203–1216. doi:10.1016/0277-9536(85)90269-2 PMID:3006260

Klovdahl, A. S., Graviss, E. A., Yaganehdoost, A., Ross, M. W., Wanger, A., Adams, G. J., & Musser, J. M. (2001). Networks and tuberculosis: An undetected community outbreak involving public places. *Social Science & Medicine, 52*(5), 681–694. doi:10.1016/S0277-9536(00)00170-2 PMID:11218173

Koh, H. C., & Tan, G. (2011). Data mining applications in healthcare. *Journal of Healthcare Information Management, 19*(2), 64–72.

Kohlwey, E., Sussman, A., Trost, J., & Maurer, A. (2011). Leveraging the cloud for big data biometrics: Meeting the performance requirements of the next generation biometric systems. *IEEE World Congress on Services (SERVICES),* 597–601. doi:10.1109/SERVICES.2011.95

Kolachalama, V. B., Bressloff, N. W., & Nair, P. B. (2007). Mining data from hemodynamic simulations via Bayesian emulation. *Biomedical Engineering Online, 6*(1), 1. doi:10.1186/1475-925X-6-47

Kolb, E. M., Schoening, S., Peck, J., & Lee, T. (2008, December). Reducing emergency department overcrowding: five patient buffer concepts in comparison. *Proceedings of the 40th conference on winter simulation,* 1516-1525. doi:10.1109/WSC.2008.4736232

Koley, S., & Majumder, A. (2011, May). Brain MRI segmentation for tumor detection using cohesion based self-merging algorithm. In *Communication Software and Networks (ICCSN), 2011 IEEE 3rd International Conference on* (pp. 781-785). IEEE.

Kolios, M. C., & Czarnota, G. J. (2009). Potential use of ultrasound for the detection of cell changes in cancer treatment. *Future Oncology (London, England), 5*(10), 1527–1532. doi:10.2217/fon.09.157 PMID:20001791

Komarova, N. L., Barnes, E., Klenerman, P., & Wodarz, D. (2003). Boosting immunity by antiviral d rug therapy: A simple relationship among timing, efficacy, and success. *Proceedings of the National Academy of Sciences of the United States of America, 100*(4), 1855–1860. doi:10.1073/pnas.0337483100 PMID:12574516

Komashie, A., & Mousavi, A. (2005, December). Modeling emergency departments using discrete event simulation techniques. *Proceedings of the 37th conference on Winter simulation,* 2681-2685. doi:10.1109/WSC.2005.1574570

Komonen, K. (2002). A cost model of industrial maintenance for profitability analysis and benchmarking. *International Journal of Production Economics*, *79*(1), 15–31. doi:10.1016/S0925-5273(00)00187-0

Kosinski, M., Stillwell, D., & Graepel, T. (2013). Private traits and attributes are predictable from digital records of human behaviour. *Proceedings of the National Academy of Sciences of the United States of America*, *110*(15), 5802–5805. doi:10.1073/pnas.1218772110 PMID:23479631

Kourou, K., Rigas, G., Exarchos, K. P., Goletsis, Y., Exarchos, T. P., Jacobs, S., & Fotiadis, D. I. et al. (2016). Prediction of time dependent survival in HF patients after VAD implantation using pre-and post-operative data. *Computers in Biology and Medicine*, *70*, 99–105. doi:10.1016/j.compbiomed.2016.01.005

Kowalczuk, J., Meyer, A., Carlson, J., Psota, E. T., Buettner, S., Pérez, L. C., & Oleynikov, D. et al. (2012). Real-time three-dimensional soft tissue reconstruction for laparoscopic surgery. *Surgical Endoscopy*, *26*(12), 3413–3417. doi:10.1007/s00464-012-2355-8 PMID:22648119

Kraemer, M. U. G., Sinka, M. E., Duda, K. A., Mylne, A. Q. N., Shearer, F. M., Barker, C. M., & Hay, S. I. et al. (2015). The global distribution of the arbovirus vectors Aedes aegypti and Ae. Albopictus. *eLife*, *4*, 1–18. doi:10.7554/eLife.08347 PMID:26126267

Krishnamachari, S., & Chellappa, R. (1997). Multiresolution Gauss-Markov random field models for texture segmentation. *IEEE Transactions on Image Processing*, *6*(2), 251–267. doi:10.1109/83.551696 PMID:18282921

Krupa, A., Doignon, C., Gangloff, J., & Mathelin, M. D. (2002). *Combined image-based and depth visual servoing applied to robotized laparoscopic surgery*. Paper presented at the IEEE/RSJ International Conference on Intelligent Robots and Systems, Lausanne, Switzerland. doi:10.1109/IRDS.2002.1041409

Kulldorff, B. M. (2015). *SaTScan User Guide V9.4*. Retrieved 21 January 2017 from http://www.unc.edu/~emch/gisph/SaTScan.pdf

Kumar, A., & Niu, F., & Hazy, R. C. (2013). Making it easier to build and maintain big-data analytics. *Communications of the ACM*, *56*(3), 40–49. doi:10.1145/2428556.2428570

Kumari, M., & Godara, S. (2011). Comparative Study of Data Mining Classification Methods in Cardiovascular Disease Prediction. *International Journal of Clothing Science and Technology*, *2*(2), 304–308.

Kuo, Y. H., Leung, J. M., & Graham, C. A. (2012, December). Simulation with data scarcity: Developing a simulation model of a hospital emergency department. *Simulation Conference (WSC) Proceedings*, 1–12.

Kuo, Y. H., Rado, O., Lupia, B., Leung, J. M., & Graham, C. A. (2016). Improving the efficiency of a hospital emergency department: A simulation study with indirectly imputed service-time distributions. *Flexible Services and Manufacturing Journal*, *28*(1-2), 120–147. doi:10.1007/s10696-014-9198-7

Kurosaki, M., Matsunaga, K., Hirayama, I., Tanaka, T., Sato, M., Yasui, Y., & Nakanishi, H. et al. (2010). A predictive model of response to peginterferon ribavirin in chronic hepatitis C using classification and regression tree analysis. *Hepatology Research*, *40*(3), 251–260. doi:10.1111/j.1872-034X.2009.00607.x

Kurt, I., Ture, M., & Kurum, A. T. (2008). Comparing performances of logistic regression, classification and regression tree, and neural networks for predicting coronary artery disease. *Expert Systems with Applications*, *34*(1), 366–374. doi:10.1016/j.eswa.2006.09.004

Kusiak, A., Dixon, B., & Shah, S. (2005). Predicting survival time for kidney dialysis patients: A data mining approach. *Computers in Biology and Medicine*, *35*(4), 311–327. doi:10.1016/j.compbiomed.2004.02.004

Kviatkovsky, I., Rivlin, E., & Shimshoni, I. (2014). Online action recognition using covariance of shape and motion. *Computer Vision and Image Understanding, 129*, 15–26. doi:10.1016/j.cviu.2014.08.001

Lahane, A., Yesha, Y., Grasso, M. A., Joshi, A., Park, A., & Lo, A. (2012). *Detection of unsafe action from laparoscopic cholecystectomy video.* Paper presented at the ACM SIGHIT International Health Informatics Symposium (ACM IHI). doi:10.1145/2110363.2110400

Lahsasna, A., Ainon, R. N., Zainuddin, R., & Bulgiba, A. (2012). Design of a fuzzy-based decision support system for coronary heart disease diagnosis. *Journal of Medical Systems, 36*(5), 3293–3306. doi:10.1007/s10916-012-9821-7

Lai, J. H. K., & Yik, F. W. H. (2008). Benchmarking operation and maintenance costs of luxury hotels. *Journal of Facilities Management, 6*(4), 279–289. doi:10.1108/14725960810908145

Laínez, J. M., Schaefer, E., & Reklaitis, G. V. (2012). Challenges and opportunities in enterprise-wide optimization in the pharmaceutical industry. *Computers & Chemical Engineering, 47*, 19–28. doi:10.1016/j.compchemeng.2012.07.002

Lakshmi, K. S., & Kumar, G. S. (2014, February). Association rule extraction from medical transcripts of diabetic patients. In *Applications of Digital Information and Web Technologies (ICADIWT), 2014 Fifth International Conference on the* (pp. 201-206). IEEE.

Lal Mohan, T., & Roh, T. (2013). Simulation in Healthcare. In J. A. Larson (Ed.), *A Book Management Engineering: A Guide to Best Practices for Industrial Engineering in Health Care* (1st ed.). Taylor and Francis Group.

Lambin, P., van Stiphout, R. G. P. M., Starmans, M. H. W., Rios-Velazquez, E., Nalbantov, G., Aerts, H. J. W. L., & Dekker, A. et al. (2013). Predicting outcomes in radiation oncology–multifactorial decision support systems. *Nat. Rev. Clin. Oncol, 10*(1), 27–40. doi:10.1038/nrclinonc.2012.196 PMID:23165123

Lämmel, R. (2008). Googles MapReduce programming model—Revisited. *Science of Computer Programming, 70*(1), 1–30. doi:10.1016/j.scico.2007.07.001

Lane, D. C., Monefeldt, C., & Rosenhead, J. V. (2000). Looking in the wrong place for healthcare improvements: A system dynamics study of an accident and emergency department. *The Journal of the Operational Research Society, 51*(5), 518–531. doi:10.1057/palgrave.jors.2600892

Lang, J. (2009). *Periodic Solutions and Bistability in a Model for Cytotoxic T-Lymphocyte (CTL) Response to Human T-Cell* (M.Sc. dissertation). University of Alberta, Canada.

Lang, J., & Li, M. Y. (2012). Stable and transient periodic oscillations in a mathematical model for CTL response to HTLV-I infection. *Journal of Mathematical Biology, 65*(1), 181–199. doi:10.1007/s00285-011-0455-z PMID:21792554

Langmuir, A. (1963). The surveillance of communicable diseases of public health importance. *The New England Journal of Medicine, 268*(4), 182–194. doi:10.1056/NEJM196301242680405 PMID:13928666

Laroque, C., Himmelspach, J., Pasupathy, R., Rose, O., & Uhrmacher, A. M. (2012). Simulation with data scarcity: developing a simulation model of a hospital emergency department. *WSC '12 Proceedings of the Winter Simulation Conference.*

Law, A. M. (2007). *Simulation Modeling and Analysis* (4th ed.). McGraw Hill.

Leachman, R., Johnston, L., Li, S., & Shen, L. (2014). An automated planning engine for biopharmaceutical production. *European Journal of Operational Research, 238*(1), 327–338. doi:10.1016/j.ejor.2014.03.002

Lechner, F., Sullivan, J., Spiegel, H., Nixon, D. F., & Ferrari, B., Davis,... Klenerman, P. (. (2000). Why do cytotoxic T lymphocytes fail to eliminate HCV? Lessons from studies using MHC class I tetramers. *Philosophical Transactions of the Royal Society of London. Series B, Biological Sciences, 355*, 1085–1092. doi:10.1098/rstb.2000.0646 PMID:11186310

Lechner, F., Wong, D. K., Dunbar, P. R., Chapman, R., Chung, R. T., Dohrenwend, P., & Walker, B. D. et al. (2000). Analysis of Successful Immune Responses in Persons Infected with Hepatitis C Virus. *The Journal of Experimental Medicine*, *191*(9), 1499–1512. doi:10.1084/jem.191.9.1499 PMID:10790425

Lee, E. C., Asher, J. M., Goldlust, S., Kraemer, J. D., Lawson, A. B., & Bansal, S. (2016). *Mind the scales: Harnessing spatial big data for infectious disease surveillance and inference*. Retrieved 2016, from https://arxiv.org/abs/1605.08740

Lee, H. G., Noh, K. Y., & Ryu, K. H. (2007, May). Mining biosignal data: coronary artery disease diagnosis using linear and nonlinear features of HRV. In *Pacific-Asia Conference on Knowledge Discovery and Data Mining* (pp. 218-228). Springer Berlin Heidelberg. doi:10.1007/978-3-540-77018-3_23

Lee, P. Y., Yan, S. L., Hu, M. H., & Marescaux, J. (2015). *A computed stereoscopic method for laparoscopic surgery by using feature tracking*. Paper presented at the IEEE international conference on Consumer Electronics, Taipai, Taiwan. doi:10.1109/ICCE-TW.2015.7217046

Lee, A., Lau, F. L., Hazlett, C. B., Kam, C. W., Wong, P., Wong, T. W., & Chow, S. (1999). Measuring the inappropriate utilization of accident and emergency services? *International Journal of Health Care Quality Assurance*, *12*(7), 287–292. doi:10.1108/09526869910287558 PMID:10724572

Lee, C. H., Chen, J. C., & Tseng, V. S. (2010). *A Novel Data Mining Mechanism Considering Bio-Signal and Environmental Data with Applications on Asthma Monitoring*. Comput Methods Programs Biom.

Lee, E. C., Viboud, C., Simonsen, L., Khan, F., & Bansal, Sh. (2015). Detecting Signals of Seasonal Influenza Severity through Age Dynamics. *BMC Infectious Diseases*, *15*(587), 1–19. PMID:26715193

Lee, H. G., Choi, M. K., Shin, B. S., & Lee, S. C. (2013). Reducing redundancy in wireless capsule endoscopy videos. *Computers in Biology and Medicine*, *43*(6), 670–682. doi:10.1016/j.compbiomed.2013.02.009 PMID:23668342

Lee, H. Y., Yang, Y. H., Lee, Y. L., Shen, J. T., Jang, M. Y., Shih, P. M. C., & Juan, Y. S. et al. (2015). Noncontrast computed tomography factors that predict the renal stone outcome after shock wave lithotripsy. *Clinical Imaging*, *39*(5), 845–850. doi:10.1016/j.clinimag.2015.04.010 PMID:25975631

Lee, J., Karshafian, R., Papanicolau, N., Giles, A., Kolios, M. C., & Czarnota, G. J. (2012). Quantitative ultrasound for the monitoring of novel microbubble and ultrasound radiosensitization. *Ultrasound in Medicine & Biology*, *38*(7), 1212–1221. doi:10.1016/j.ultrasmedbio.2012.01.028 PMID:22579547

Lee, S. K., Mogi, G., Lee, S. K., & Kim, J. W. (2011). Prioritizing the weights of hydrogen energy Technologies in the sector of the hydrogen economy by using a fuzzy AHP approach. *International Journal of Hydrogen Energy*, *36*(2), 1897–1902. doi:10.1016/j.ijhydene.2010.01.035

Lee, S. L., Lerotic, M., Vitiello, V., Giannarou, S., Kwok, K. W., Visentini-Scarzanella, M., & Yang, G. Z. (2010). From medical images to minimally invasive intervention: Computer assistance for robotic surgery. *Computerized Medical Imaging and Graphics*, *34*(1), 33–45. doi:10.1016/j.compmedimag.2009.07.007 PMID:19699056

Lee, W. J., Chong, K., Chen, J. C., Ser, K. H., Lee, Y. C., Tsou, J. J., & Chen, S. C. (2012). Predictors of diabetes remission after bariatric surgery in Asia. *Asian Journal of Surgery*, *35*(2), 67–73. doi:10.1016/j.asjsur.2012.04.010

Lee, W. P., Hsiao, Y. T., & Hwang, W. C. (2014). Designing a parallel evolutionary algorithm for inferring gene networks on the cloud computing environment. *BMC Systems Biology*, *8*(1), 5. doi:10.1186/1752-0509-8-5 PMID:24428926

Lefebvre, F., Meunier, M., Thibault, F., Laugier, P., & Berger, G. (2000). Computerized ultrasound B-scan characterization of breast nodules. *Ultrasound in Medicine & Biology*, *26*(9), 1421–1428. doi:10.1016/S0301-5629(00)00302-1 PMID:11179616

Lejeune, M. A. (2006). A variable neighborhood decomposition search method for supply chain management planning problems. *European Journal of Operational Research*, *175*(2), 959–976. doi:10.1016/j.ejor.2005.05.021

Lekkas, S., & Mikhailov, L. (2010). Evolving fuzzy medical diagnosis of Pima Indians diabetes and of dermatological diseases. *Artificial Intelligence in Medicine*, *50*(2), 117–126. doi:10.1016/j.artmed.2010.05.007

Le, Q. T., & Courter, D. (2008). Clinical biomarkers for hypoxia targeting. *Cancer and Metastasis Reviews*, *27*(3), 351–362. doi:10.1007/s10555-008-9144-9 PMID:18483785

Leroi, I., Burns, A., Aarsland, D., Brønnick, K., Ehrt, U., De Deyn, P. P., & Cummings, J. et al. (2007). Neuropsychiatric symptoms in patients with Parkinsons disease and dementia: Frequency, profile and associated care giver stress. *Journal of Neurology, Neurosurgery, and Psychiatry*, *78*(1). doi:10.1136/jnnp.2006.101162

Letham, K., & Gray, A. (2012). The four-hour target in the NHS emergency departments: A critical comment. *Emergencias*, *24*(1), 69–72.

Leung, T., & Malik, J. (2001). Representing and recognizing the visual appearance of materials using three-dimensional textons. *International Journal of Computer Vision*, *43*(1), 29–44. doi:10.1023/A:1011126920638

Lewin Group. (2005). *TrendWatchChartbook 2005: Trends Affecting Hospitals and Health Systems*. American Hospital Association.

Lewin, S. R., Ribeiro, R. M., Walters, T., Lau, G. K., Bowden, S., Locarnini, S., & Perelson, A. S. (2001). Analysis of hepatitis B viral load decline under potent therapy: Complex decay profiles observed. *Hepatology (Baltimore, Md.)*, *34*(5), 1012–1020. doi:10.1053/jhep.2001.28509 PMID:11679973

Lewis, S., Csordas, A., Killcoyne, S., Hermjakob, H., Hoopmann, M. R., Moritz, R. L., & Boyle, J. et al. (2012). Hydra: A scalable proteomic search engine which utilizes the Hadoop distributed computing framework. *BMC Bioinformatics*, *13*(1), 3–24. doi:10.1186/1471-2105-13-324 PMID:23216909

Li, B., & Meng, M. Q. H. (2009). Computer-based detection of bleeding and ulcer in wireless capsule endoscopy images by chromaticity moments. *Computers in Biology and Medicine*, *39*(2), 141–147. doi:10.1016/j.compbiomed.2008.11.007 PMID:19147126

Lifson, J. D., Rossio, J. L., Arnaout, R., Li, L., Parks, T. L., Schneider, D. K., & Wodarz, D. et al. (2000). Containment of simian immunodeficiency virus: Cellular immune responses and protection from rechallenge following transient postinoculation antiretroviral treatment. *Journal of Virology*, *74*(6), 2584–2593. doi:10.1128/JVI.74.6.2584-2593.2000 PMID:10684272

Lifson, J. D., Rossio, J. L., Piatak, M., Parks, T., Li, L., Kiser, R., & Wodarz, D. et al. (2001). Role of CD8(+) lymphocytes in control of simian immunodeficiency virus infection and resistance to rechallenge after transient early antiretroviral treatment. *Journal of Virology*, *75*(21), 10187–10199. doi:10.1128/JVI.75.21.10187-10199.2001 PMID:11581387

Li, M. Y., & Muldowney, J. S. (1996). A geometric approach to the global-stability problems. *SIAM Journal on Mathematical Analysis*, *27*(4), 1070–1083. doi:10.1137/S0036141094266449

Li, M. Y., & Shu, H. (2010a). Impact of intracellular delays and target-cell dynamics on in vivo viral infections. *SIAM Journal on Applied Mathematics*, *70*(7), 2434–2448. doi:10.1137/090779322

Li, M. Y., & Shu, H. (2010b). Global dynamics of an in-host viral model with intracellular delay. *Bulletin of Mathematical Biology*, *72*(6), 1492–1505. doi:10.1007/s11538-010-9503-x PMID:20087671

Li, M. Y., & Shu, H. (2011). Multiple stable periodic oscillations in a mathematical model of CTL response to HTLV-I infection. *Bulletin of Mathematical Biology*, *73*(8), 1774–1793. doi:10.1007/s11538-010-9591-7 PMID:20976566

Li, M. Y., & Shu, H. (2012). Joint effects of mitosis and intracellular delay on viral dynamics: Two parameter bifurcation analysis. *Journal of Mathematical Biology, 64*(6), 1005–1020. doi:10.1007/s00285-011-0436-2 PMID:21671033

Lim, A. G., & Maini, P. K. (2014). HTLV-I infection: A dynamic struggle between viral persistence and host immunity. *Journal of Theoretical Biology, 352*, 92–108. doi:10.1016/j.jtbi.2014.02.022 PMID:24583256

Lima, F. R., Osiro, L., & Carpinetti, L. C. R. (2014). A comparison between Fuzzy AHP and Fuzzy TOPSIS method to suplier selection. *Applied Soft Computing, 21*, 194–209. doi:10.1016/j.asoc.2014.03.014

Lim, M. E., Nye, T., Bowen, J. M., Hurley, J., Goeree, R., & Tarride, J. E. (2012). Mathematical modeling: The case of emergency department waiting times. *International Journal of Technology Assessment in Health Care, 28*(02), 93–109. doi:10.1017/S0266462312000013 PMID:22559751

Lim, M. E., Worster, A., Goeree, R., & Tarride, J. E. (2012). PRM28 physicians as pseudo-agents in a hospital emergency department discrete event simulation. *Value in Health, 15*(4), A163. doi:10.1016/j.jval.2012.03.884

Lin, C. C., Hsu, Y. S., & Chen, K. K. (2008). Predictive Factors of Lower Calyceal Stone Clearance After Extracorporeal Shockwave Lithotripsy (ESWL): The Impact of Radiological Anatomy. *Chinese Medical Associations, 71*(10), 496-501.

Lin, H. C., Shafran, I., Yuh, D., & Hager, G. D. (2006). Towards automatic skill evaluation: Detection and segmentation of robot-assisted surgical motions. *Computer Aided Surgery, 11*(5), 220-230.

Lin, Y. L. (2013). Implementation of a parallel protein structure alignment service on cloud. *Int J Genomics*, 1–8.

Linares, C., Martinez-Martin, P., Rodríguez-Blázquez, C., Forjaz, M. J., Carmona, R., & Díaz, J. (2016). Effect of heat waves on morbidity and mortality due to Parkinsons disease in Madrid: A time-series analysis. *Environment International, 89*, 1–6. doi:10.1016/j.envint.2016.01.017

Lin, C. C., Ou, Y. K., Chen, S. H., Liu, Y. C., & Lin, J. (2010). Comparison of artificial neural network and logistic regression models for predicting mortality in elderly patients with hip fracture. *Injury, 41*(8), 869–873. doi:10.1016/j.injury.2010.04.023

Lin, Z., Uemura, M., Zecca, M., & Sessa, S. (2012). Objective Skill Evaluation for Laparoscopic Training Based on Motion Analysis. *IEEE Transactions on Bio-Medical Engineering, 60*(4), 977–985. PMID:23204271

Liu, J., Yuan, X., & Buckles, B. P. (2008, August). Breast cancer diagnosis using level-set statistics and support vector machines. In *2008 30th Annual International Conference of the IEEE Engineering in Medicine and Biology Society* (pp. 3044-3047). IEEE.

Liu, K. F., & Lu, C. F. (2009, August). BBN-based decision support for health risk analysis. In *INC, IMS and IDC, 2009. NCM'09. Fifth International Joint Conference on* (pp. 696-702). IEEE.

Liu, B. (2004). *Uncertainty theory: An introduction to its axiomatic foundations*. Berlin: Springer-Verlag. doi:10.1007/978-3-540-39987-2

Liu, B., & Liu, Y. K. (2002). Expected value of fuzzy variable and fuzzy expected value models. *IEEE Transactions on Fuzzy Systems, 10*(4), 445–450. doi:10.1109/TFUZZ.2002.800692

Liu, B., Yuan, Z., Aihara, K., & Chen, L. (2014). Reinitiation enhances reliable transcriptional responses in eukaryotes. *Journal of the Royal Society, Interface, 11*(97), 1–11. doi:10.1016/j.jcis.2014.08.014 PMID:24850905

Liu, D. Y., Chen, H. L., Yang, B., Lv, X. E., Li, L. N., & Liu, J. (2012). Design of an enhanced fuzzy k-nearest neighbor classifier based computer aided diagnostic system for thyroid disease. *Journal of Medical Systems, 36*(5), 3243–3254. doi:10.1007/s10916-011-9815-x

Liu, M., Wu, Y., Chen, Y., Sun, J., Zhao, Z., Chen, X. W., & Xu, H. et al. (2012). Large-scale prediction of adverse drug reactions using chemical, biological, and phenotypic properties of drugs. *Journal of the American Medical Informatics Association*, *19*(e1), e28–e35. doi:10.1136/amiajnl-2011-000699

Liu, R., Wang, X., Aihara, K., & Chen, L. (2014). Early diagnosis of complex diseases by molecular biomarkers, network biomarkers, and dynamical network biomarkers. *Medicinal Research Reviews*, *34*(3), 4555–4578. doi:10.1002/med.21293 PMID:23775602

Liu, R., Yu, X., Liu, X., Xu, D., Aihara, K., & Chen, L. (2014). Identifying critical transitions of complex diseases based on a single sample. *Bioinformatics (Oxford, England)*, *30*(11), 1579–1586. doi:10.1093/bioinformatics/btu084 PMID:24519381

Liu, S., & Wang, L. (2010). Global stability of an HIV-1 model with distributed intracellular delays and a combination therapy. *Mathematical Biosciences and Engineering*, *7*(3), 675–685. doi:10.3934/mbe.2010.7.675 PMID:20578792

Liu, T., Hu, L., Ma, C., Wang, Z. Y., & Chen, H. L. (2015). A fast approach for detection of erythemato-squamous diseases based on extreme learning machine with maximum relevance minimum redundancy feature selection. *International Journal of Systems Science*, *46*(5), 919–931. doi:10.1080/00207721.2013.801096

Liu, Z., Sokka, T., Maas, K., Olsen, N. J., & Aune, T. M. (2009). Prediction of disease severity in patients with early rheumatoid arthritis by gene expression profiling. *Human Genomics and Proteomics*, *1*(1).

Li, X., & Liu, B. (2006). A sufficient and necessary condition of credibility measure. *International Journal of Uncertainty & Knowledge-Based System*, *14*(5), 527–535. doi:10.1142/S0218488506004175

Li, Y., & Chen, L. (2014). Big Biological Data: Challenges and Opportunities. *Genomics, Proteomics & Bioinformatics*, *12*(5), 187–189. doi:10.1016/j.gpb.2014.10.001 PMID:25462151

Lizzi, F. L., Ostromogilsky, M., Feleppa, E. J., & Others. (1986). Relationship of ultrasonic spectral parameters to features of tissue microstructure. *IEEE Trans. Ultrason. Ferroelect. Freq. Contr., UFFC-33*, 319–329.

Logan, J. J., Jolly, A. M., & Blanford, J. I. (2016). The sociospatial network: Risk and the role of place in the transmission of infectious diseases. *PLoS ONE*, *11*(2), 1–14. doi:10.1371/journal.pone.0146915 PMID:26840891

Lohr, H. F., Krug, S., Herr, W., Weyer, S., Schlaak, J., Wolfel, T., & Meyer zum Buschenfelde, K. H. et al. (1998). Quantitative and functional analysis of core-specific T helper cell and CTL activities in acute and chronic hepatitis B. *Liver*, *18*(6), 405–413. doi:10.1111/j.1600-0676.1998.tb00825.x PMID:9869395

Loke, C. K., & Gan, F. F. (2012). Joint monitoring scheme for clinical failures and predisposed risks. *Quality Technology & Quantitative Management*, *9*(1), 3–21. doi:10.1080/16843703.2012.11673274

Long, J., Li, Y., Wang, H., Yu, T., Pan, J., & Li, F. (2012). A hybrid brain computer interface to control the direction and speed of a simulated or real wheelchair. *IEEE Transactions on Neural Systems and Rehabilitation Engineering*, *20*(5), 720–729. doi:10.1109/TNSRE.2012.2197221 PMID:22692936

Luo, Z., Wu, X., Guo, S., & Ye, B. (2008, June). Diagnosis of breast cancer tumor based on manifold learning and support vector machine. In *Information and Automation, 2008. ICIA 2008. International Conference on* (pp. 703-707). IEEE.

Luxhej, J., Riis, J. O., & Thorsteinsson, U. (1997). Trends and Perspectives in Industrial Maintenance Management. *Journal of Manufacturing Systems*, *16*(6), 437–453. doi:10.1016/S0278-6125(97)81701-3

Machavarapu, S. C., Mukul, M. K., & Kumar, D. (2014, March). EEG classification based on variance. In *Green Computing Communication and Electrical Engineering (ICGCCEE), 2014 International Conference on* (pp. 1-4). IEEE. doi:10.1109/ICGCCEE.2014.6922216

MacLean, B., Eng, J. K., Beavis, R. C., & McIntosh, M. (2006). General framework for developing and evaluating database scoring algorithms using the TANDEM search engine. *Bioinformatics (Oxford, England)*, *22*(22), 2830–2832. doi:10.1093/bioinformatics/btl379 PMID:16877754

Ma, H., Zhou, T., Aihara, K., & Chen, L. (2014). Predicting time-series from short-term high dimensional data. *International Journal of Bifurcation and Chaos in Applied Sciences and Engineering*, *24*(12), 1–19. doi:10.1142/S021812741430033X

Maini, M. K., & Bertoletti, A. (2000). How Can the Cellular Immune Response Control Hepatitis B Virus Replication? *Journal of Viral Hepatitis*, *7*(5), 321–326. doi:10.1046/j.1365-2893.2000.00234.x PMID:10971819

Mallon, W., & Kassinove, A. (1999). Mandatory Reporting Laws and the Emergency Department. In *Topics in Emergency Medicine*. Aspen Publishers, Inc. Retrieved from http://ovidsp.ovid.com/ovidweb.cgi?T=JS%7B&%7DPAGE=referenc e%7B&%7DD=ovftd%7B&%7DNEWS=N%7B&%7DAN=00007815-199909000-00009

Mamdani, M. M., Parikh, S. V., Austin, P. C., & Upshur, R. E. (2000). Use of antidepressants among elderly subjects: Trends and contributing factors. *The American Journal of Psychiatry*, *157*(3), 360–367. doi:10.1176/appi.ajp.157.3.360 PMID:10698810

Mamou, J., Coron, A., Hata, M., Machi, J., Yanagihara, E., Laugier, P., & Feleppa, E. J. (2010). Three-dimensional high-frequency characterization of cancerous lymph nodes. *Ultrasound in Medicine & Biology*, *36*(3), 361–375. doi:10.1016/j.ultrasmedbio.2009.10.007 PMID:20133046

Manitoba Health. (2008). *Enteric illness protocol.* Retrieved 21 January 2017 from http://www.gov.mb.ca/health/publichealth/cdc/protocol/enteric.pdf

Manitoba Health. (2011). *Communicable Disease Management Protocol; Invasive meningococcal disease.* Retrieved 21 January 2017 from http://www.gov.mb.ca/health/publichealth/cdc/protocol/mid.pdf

Manitoba Health. (2015a). *Communicable Disease Management Protocol; Legionellosis.* Retrieved 21 January 2017 from http://www.gov.mb.ca/health/publichealth/cdc/protocol/legion.pdf

Manitoba Health. (2015b). *Communicable disease management protocol;shigellosis.* Retrieved 21 January 2017 from http://www.gov.mb.ca/health/publichealth/cdc/protocol/shigellosis.pdf

Manitoba. Public Health Act. (2016). Retrieved 21 January 2017, from http://www.gov.mb.ca/health/publichealth/act.html

Manjunath, B. S., & Ma, W. Y. (1996). Texture feature for browsing and retrieval of image data. *IEEE Transactions on Pattern Analysis and Machine Intelligence*, *18*(8), 837–842. doi:10.1109/34.531803

Marcinczak, J. M., & Grigat, R. R. (2013). Closed Contour Specular Reflection Segmentation in Laparoscopic Images. *International Journal of Biomedical Imaging*, 6. PMID:23983675

Marconi, L., Moreira, P., Parada, B., Bastos, C., Roseiro, A., & Mota, A. (2011). Donor Cause of Brain Death in Renal Transplantation: A Predictive Factor for Graft Function. Proceedings of Transplantation, 43(1), 74-76.

Markonis, D., Schaer, R., Eggel, I., Müller, H., & Depeursinge, A. (2012). Using MapReduce for Large-Scale Medical Image Analysis. HISB.

Mark, T. L., Levit, K. R., & Buck, J. A. (2009). Datapoints: Psychotropic drug prescriptions by medical specialty. *Psychiatric Services (Washington, D.C.)*, *60*(9), 1167. doi:10.1176/ps.2009.60.9.1167 PMID:19723729

Marmor, Y. (2010). *Emergency-departments simulation in support of service-engineering: Staffing, design, and real-time tracking* (Doctoral dissertation).

Martin, M., Champion, R., Kinsman, L., & Masman, K. (2011). Mapping patient flow in a regional Australian emergency department: A model driven approach. *International Emergency Nursing*, *19*(2), 75–85. doi:10.1016/j.ienj.2010.03.003 PMID:21459349

Martin, P., Vincent, A., & Xiaolan, X. (2014). Hospitalization Admission Control Of Emergency Patients Using Markovian Decision Processes And Discrete Event Simulation. *Proceedings of the 2014 Winter Simulation Conference*.

Martorell, S., Villanueva, J. F., Carlos, S., Nebot, Y., Sanchez, A., Pitarch, J. L., & Serradell, V. (2005). RAMS+C informed decision-making with application to multiobjective optimization of technical specifications and maintenance using genetic algorithms. *Reliability Engineering & System Safety*, *87*(1), 65–75. doi:10.1016/j.ress.2004.04.009

Marvik, R., Langø, T., Tangen, G. A., Andersen, J. O., Kaspersen, J. H., Ystgaard, B., . . . Nagelhus Hernes, T. A. (2004). Laparoscopic navigation pointer for three-dimensional image-guided surgery. *Surg Endosc, 18*, 1242-1248.

Marx, P., & Antal, P. (2015). Decomposition of Shared Latent Factors Using Bayesian Multi-morbidity Dependency Maps. In *First European Biomedical Engineering Conference for Young Investigators* (pp. 40-43). Springer Singapore. doi:10.1007/978-981-287-573-0_10

Maryland Healthcare Commission. (2007). *Use of Maryland Hospital Emergency Departments: An Update and Recommended Strategies to Address Crowding*. Author.

Masethe, H. D., & Masethe, M. A. (2014, October). Prediction of heart disease using classification algorithms. *Proceedings of the World Congress on Engineering and Computer Science*, *2*, 22-24.

Materka, A., & Strzelecki, M. (1998). *Texture analysis methods - A review*. Academic Press.

Mathur, A. (2014). A new perspective to data processing: Big Data. *Computing for Sustainable Global Development (INDIACom), International IEEE Conference*.

McAfee, A., & Brynjolfsson, E. (2012). Big data: The management revolution. *Harvard Business Review*, *90*, 61–68. PMID:23074865

McBride, J., Zhang, S., Wortley, M., Paquette, M., Klipple, G., Byrd, E., . . . Zhao, X. (2011, March). Neural network analysis of gait biomechanical data for classification of knee osteoarthritis. In Biomedical Sciences and Engineering Conference (BSEC), 2011 (pp. 1-4). IEEE. doi:10.1109/BSEC.2011.5872315

McCarthy, M. L., Aronsky, D., Jones, I. D., Miner, J. R., Band, R. A., Baren, J. M., & Shesser, R. et al. (2008). The emergency department occupancy rate: A simple measure of emergency department crowding? *Annals of Emergency Medicine*, *51*(1), 15–24. doi:10.1016/j.annemergmed.2007.09.003 PMID:17980458

McCarthy, M. L., Zeger, S. L., Ding, R., Levin, S. R., Desmond, J. S., Lee, J., & Aronsky, D. (2009). Crowding delays treatment and lengthens emergency department length of stay, even among high-acuity patients. *Annals of Emergency Medicine*, *54*(4), 492–503. doi:10.1016/j.annemergmed.2009.03.006 PMID:19423188

McKeithan, T. W. (1995). Kinetic proofreading in T-cell receptor signal transduction. *Proceedings of the National Academy of Sciences of the United States of America*, *92*(11), 5042–5046. doi:10.1073/pnas.92.11.5042 PMID:7761445

McKenna, A., Hanna, M., Banks, E., Sivachenko, A., Cibulskis, K., Kernytsky, A., & Daly, M. et al. (2010). The Genome Analysis Toolkit: A MapReduce framework for analyzing next-generation DNA sequencing data. *Genome Research*, *20*(9), 1297–1303. doi:10.1101/gr.107524.110 PMID:20644199

McLean, A. R., Rosado, M. M., Agenes, F., Vasconcellos, R., & Freitas, A. A. (1997). Resource competition as a mechanism for B cell homeostasis. *Proceedings of the National Academy of Sciences of the United States of America*, *94*(11), 5792–5797. doi:10.1073/pnas.94.11.5792 PMID:9159153

Mease, D., Wyner, A. J., & Buja, A. (2007). Boosted classification trees and class probability/quantile estimation. *Journal of Machine Learning Research, 8*, 409–439.

Medeiros, D. J., Swenson, E., & DeFlitch, C. (2008, December). Improving patient flow in a hospital emergency department. *Proceedings of the 40th Conference on Winter Simulation*, 1526-1531. doi:10.1109/WSC.2008.4736233

Meijboom, B., & Obel, B. (2007). Tactical coordination in a multi-location and multi-stage operations structure: A model and a pharmaceutical company case. *Omega, 35*(3), 258–273. doi:10.1016/j.omega.2005.06.003

Meixner, O. (2009). Fuzzy AHP Group Decision Analysis and its Application for the Evaluation of Energy Sources. In *Proceedings of the 10th International Symposium on the Analytic Hierarchy/Network Process*. Pittsburgh, PA: University of Pittsburgh.

Mellinger, J., Schalk, G., Braun, C., Preissl, H., Rosenstiel, W., Birbaumer, N., & Kübler, A. (2007). An MEG-based brain-computer interface (BCI). *NeuroImage, 36*(3), 581–593. doi:10.1016/j.neuroimage.2007.03.019 PMID:17475511

Meng, X. H., Huang, Y. X., Rao, D. P., Zhang, Q., & Liu, Q. (2013). Comparison of three data mining models for predicting diabetes or prediabetes by risk factors. *The Kaohsiung Journal of Medical Sciences, 29*(2), 93–99. doi:10.1016/j.kjms.2012.08.016

Miele, V., Andreoli, C., & Grassi, R. (2006). The management of emergency radiology: Key facts. *European Journal of Radiology, 59*(3), 311–314. doi:10.1016/j.ejrad.2006.04.020 PMID:16806785

Milewski, R., Malinowski, P., Milewska, A. J., Ziniewicz, P., & Wołczyński, S. (2010). The usage of margin-based feature selection algorithm in IVF ICSI/ET data analysis. Studies in Logic. *Grammar and Rhetoric, 21*(34), 35–46.

Miller, M. J., Ferrin, D. M., & Messer, M. G. (2004, December). Fixing the emergency department: A transformational journey with EDSIM. In *Simulation Conference, 2004. Proceedings of the 2004 (Vol. 2*, pp. 1988-1993). IEEE. doi:10.1109/WSC.2004.1371560

Ministry of Health and Long-term Care. (2016). *Quality-Based Procedures Clinical Handbook for Chronic Kidney Disease. January 2016*. Retried December 6, 2016, from: http://www.health.gov.on.ca/en/pro/programs/ecfa/docs/qbp_kidney.pdf

Mirmehdi, M., Xie, X., & Suri, J. E. (2008). *Handbook of Texture Analysis*. London: Imperial Collage Press. doi:10.1142/p547

Miro, O., Sanchez, M., Espinosa, G., Coll-Vinent, B., Bragulat, E., & Milla, J. (2003). Analysis of patient flow in the emergency department and the effect of an extensive reorganisation. *Emergency Medicine Journal, 20*(2), 143–148. doi:10.1136/emj.20.2.143 PMID:12642527

Mirzapour Al-e-hashem, S. M. J., Malekly, H., & Aryanezhad, M. B. (2011). A multi-objective robust optimization model for multi-product multi-site aggregate production planning in a supply chain under uncertainty. *International Journal of Production Economics, 134*(1), 28–42. doi:10.1016/j.ijpe.2011.01.027

Misra, B. B., & Dehuri, S. (2007). Functional Link Artificial Neural Network for Classification Task in Data Mining. *Journal of Computer Science, 3*(12), 948–955. doi:10.3844/jcssp.2007.948.955

Moayedi, F., Azimifar, R., & Boostani, R. (2015). Structured sparse representation for human action recognition. *Neurocomputing, 161*, 38–46. doi:10.1016/j.neucom.2014.10.089

Mohammadian, F., Niaki, S. T. A., & Amiri, A. (2016, February). Phase-I risk-adjusted geometric control charts to monitor health-care systems. *Quality and Reliability Engineering International, 32*(1), 19–28. doi:10.1002/qre.1722

Mohammed, E. A., Far, B. H., & Naugler, C. (2014). Applications of the MapReduce programming framework to clinical big data analysis: current landscape and future trends. *BioData Mining*, 7-22.

Mohan, L. T., Thomas, R., & Todd, H. (2015). Simulation Based Optimization: Applications In Healthcare. *Proceedings of the 2015 Winter Simulation Conference*.

Monteith, S., Glenn, T., Geddes, J., & Bauer, M., (2015). Big data are coming to psychiatry: a general introduction. *Int J Bipolar Disord*, 3-21.

Montignac, F., Noirot, I., & Chaudourne, S. (2009). Multi-criteria evaluation of on-board hydrogen storage technologies using the MACBETH approach. *International Journal of Hydrogen Energy*, 34(10), 4561–4568. doi:10.1016/j.ijhydene.2008.09.098

Moon, S. S., Kang, S. Y., Jitpitaklert, W., & Kim, S. B. (2012). Decision tree models for characterizing smoking patterns of older adults. *Expert Systems with Applications*, 39(1), 445–451. doi:10.1016/j.eswa.2011.07.035

Morales, D. A., Bengoetxea, E., Larrañaga, P., García, M., Franco, Y., Fresnada, M., & Merino, M. (2008). Bayesian classification for the selection of in vitro human embryos using morphological and clinical data. *Computer Methods and Programs in Biomedicine*, 90(2), 104–116. doi:10.1016/j.cmpb.2007.11.018

Morgareidge, D., Hui, C. A. I., & Jun, J. I. A. (2014). Performance-driven design with the support of digital tools: Applying discrete event simulation and space syntax on the design of the emergency department. *Frontiers of Architectural Research*, 3(3), 250–264. doi:10.1016/j.foar.2014.04.006

Mortreux, F., Gabet, A. S., & Wattel, E. (2003). Molecular and cellular aspects of HTLV-I associated leukemogenesis in vivo. *Leukemia*, 17(1), 26–38. doi:10.1038/sj.leu.2402777 PMID:12529656

Mortreux, F., Kazanji, M., Gabet, A. S., de Thoisy, B., & Wattel, E. (2001). Two-step nature of human T-cell leukemia virus type1 replication in experimentally infected squirrel monkeys (Saimiri sciureus). *Journal of Virology*, 75(2), 1083–1089. doi:10.1128/JVI.75.2.1083-1089.2001 PMID:11134325

Moskop, J. C., Sklar, D. P., Geiderman, J. M., Schears, R. M., & Bookman, K. J. (2009). Emergency department crowding, part 2—barriers to reform and strategies to overcome them. *Annals of Emergency Medicine*, 53(5), 612–617. doi:10.1016/j.annemergmed.2008.09.024 PMID:19027194

Moudani, W., Shahin, A., Chakik, F., & Rajab, D. (2011). Intelligent predictive osteoporosis system. *International Journal of Computers and Applications*, 32(5), 28–37.

Mould, G., Bowers, J., Dewar, C., & McGugan, E. (2013). Assessing the impact of systems modeling in the redesign of an Emergency Department. *Health Systems*, 2(1), 3–10. doi:10.1057/hs.2012.15

Mountney, P., & Yang, G. Z. (2012). Context specific descriptors for tracking deforming tissue. *Medical Image Analysis*, 16(3), 550–561. doi:10.1016/j.media.2011.02.010 PMID:21641270

Mousazadeh, M., & Torabi, S. A. (2014). *Green and reverse logistics management under fuzziness*. In C. Kahraman & B. Öztaysi (Eds.), *Supply Chain Management Under Fuzziness, Studies in Fuzziness and Soft Computing* (Vol. 313, pp. 607–637). Springer-Verlag Berlin Heidelberg.

Mousazadeh, M., Torabi, S. A., & Zahiri, B. (2015). A robust possibilistic programming approach for pharmaceutical supply chain network design. *Journal of Computers and Chemical Engineering*, 82, 115–128. doi:10.1016/j.compchemeng.2015.06.008

Mrvar, A., & Batagelj, V. (n.d.). *Pajek: Program for Analysis and Visualization of Large Networks (Reference Manual)* (A. M. V. Batagelj, Ed.). Retrieved from http://pajek.imfm.si/doku.php?id=pajek

Muchiri, P., & Pintelon, L. (2008). Performance measurement using overall equipment effectiveness (OEE): Literature review and practical application discussion. *International Journal of Production Research*, *46*(13), 3517–3535. doi:10.1080/00207540601142645

Mueller, A., Schnuelle, P., Waldherr, R., & van der Woude, F. J. (2000). Impact of the Banff 97 classification for histological diagnosis of rejection on clinical outcome and renal function parameters after kidney transplantation. *Transplantation*, *69*(6), 1123–1127. doi:10.1097/00007890-200003270-00017 PMID:10762217

Mukandavire, Z., Garira, W., & Chiyaka, C. (2007). Asymptotic properties of an HIV/AIDS model with a time delay. *Journal of Mathematical Analysis and Applications*, *330*(2), 916–933. doi:10.1016/j.jmaa.2006.07.102

Mukul, M. K., & Matsuno, F. (2010, December). Comparative study between subband and standard ICA/BSS method in context with EEG signal for movement imagery classification. In *System Integration (SII), 2010 IEEE/SICE International Symposium on* (pp. 341-346). IEEE.

Muldowney, J. S. (1990). Compound matrices and ordinary differential equations. *The Rocky Mountain Journal of Mathematics*, *20*(4), 857–872. doi:10.1216/rmjm/1181073047

Muneeswaran, K., Ganesan, L., Arumugam, S., & Soundar, K. R. (2005). Texture classification with combined rotation and scale invariant wavelet features. *Pattern Recognition*, *38*(10), 1495–1506. doi:10.1016/j.patcog.2005.03.021

Munro, J., Mason, S., & Nicholl, J. (2006). Effectiveness of measures to reduce emergency department waiting times: A natural experiment. *Emergency Medicine Journal*, *23*(1), 35–39. doi:10.1136/emj.2005.023788 PMID:16373801

Münzer, B., Schoeffmann, K., & Böszörmenyi, L. (2013). *Relevance Segmentation of Laparoscopic Videos*. Paper presented at the 2013 IEEE International Symposium on Multimedia (ISM), Anaheim, CA. doi:10.1109/ISM.2013.22

Murdoch, T. B., & Detsky, A. S. (2013). The inevitable application of big data to health care. *Journal of the American Medical Association*, *309*(13), 1351–1352. doi:10.1001/jama.2013.393 PMID:23549579

Murphy, D. R., Meyer, A. N. D., Bhise, V., Russo, E., Sittig, D. F., Wei, L., & Singh, H. et al. (2016). Computerized Triggers of Big Data to Detect Delays in Follow-up of Chest Imaging Results. *Chest*, *150*(3), 613–620. doi:10.1016/j.chest.2016.05.001 PMID:27178786

Murphy, E. L., Figueroa, J. P., Gibbs, W. N., Holding-Cobham, M., Cranston, B., Malley, K., & Blattner, W. A. et al. (1991). Human T lymphotropic virus type I (HTLV-I) seroprevalence in Jamaica: I.demographic determinants. *American Journal of Epidemiology*, *33*(11), 1114–1124. doi:10.1093/oxfordjournals.aje.a115824 PMID:2035515

Musselman, R. P., Gomes, T., Chan, B. P., Auer, R. C., Moloo, H., Mamdani, M., & Boushey, R. P. et al. (2012). Changing trends in rectal cancer surgery in Ontario: 2002–2009. *Colorectal Disease*, *14*(12), 1467–1472. doi:10.1111/j.1463-1318.2012.03044.x PMID:22487101

Nahar, J., Imam, T., Tickle, K. S., & Chen, Y. P. P. (2013). Association rule mining to detect factors which contribute to heart disease in males and females. *Expert Systems with Applications*, *40*(4), 1086–1093. doi:10.1016/j.eswa.2012.08.028

Nahmias, S. (2011). SEAC determines low bidders. *Technical News Bulletin*, *1954*, 38–179.

Narayana, S. A., Pati, R. K., & Vrat, P. (2012). Research on management issues in the pharmaceutical industry: A literature review. *International Journal of Pharmaceutical and Healthcare Marketing*, *6*(4), 351–375. doi:10.1108/17506121211283235

Navarra, G., Pozza, E., Occhionorelli, S., Carcoforo, P., & Donini, I. (1997). One-wound laparoscopic cholecystectomy. *British Journal of Surgery*, *84*(5), 695. doi:10.1002/bjs.1800840536 PMID:9171771

Nazim, S. M., Ather, M. H., & Khan, N. (2014). Measurement of Ureteric Stone Diameter in Different Planes on Multidetector Computed Tomography e Impact on the Clinical Decision Making. *Urology*, *83*(2), 288–293. doi:10.1016/j.urology.2013.09.037 PMID:24275282

Negassa, A., & Monrad, E. S. (2011). Prediction of length of stay following elective percutaneous coronary intervention. *ISRN Surgery*.

Nelson, R., & Millet, I. (2004). *Data Flow Diagrams Versus Use Cases – Student Reactions*. Paper presented at the Tenth Americas Conference on Information Systems, New York, NY.

Nelson, P. W., Murray, J. D., & Perelson, A. S. (2000). A model of HIV-1 pathogenesis that includes an intracellular delay. *Mathematical Biosciences*, *163*(2), 201–215. doi:10.1016/S0025-5564(99)00055-3 PMID:10701304

Nelson, P., & Perelson, A. (2002). A Mathematical analysis of delay differential equation models of HIV- 1 infection. *Mathematical Biosciences*, *179*(1), 73–94. doi:10.1016/S0025-5564(02)00099-8 PMID:12047922

Neshat, M., Sargolzaei, M., Nadjaran Toosi, A., & Masoumi, A. (2012). Hepatitis disease diagnosis using hybrid case based reasoning and particle swarm optimization. *ISRN Artificial Intelligence*.

Neumann, A. U., Lam, N. P., Dahari, H., Gretch, D. R., Wiley, T. E., Layden, T. J., & Perelson, A. S. (1998). Hepatitis C viral dynamics in vivo and the antiviral efficacy of interferon-α therapy. *Science*, *282*(5386), 103–107. doi:10.1126/science.282.5386.103 PMID:9756471

Ngoc, H. T., Nguyen, T. H., & Ngo, C. (2013). Average partial power spectrum density approach to feature extraction for EEG-based motor imagery classification. *American Journal of Biomedical Engineering*, *3*(6), 208–219.

Nguyen, A. V., Wynden, R., & Sun, Y. (2011). HBase, MapReduce, and Integrated Data Visualization for Processing Clinical Signal Data. *AAAI Spring Symposium: Computational Physiology*.

Nicolau, M., James, A., Benny, P. L., Darzi, A., & Yang, G. Z. (2005). *Invisible Shadow for Navigation and Planning in Minimal Invasive Surgery. In Medical Image Computing and Computer-Assisted Intervention – MICCAI 2005* (Vol. 3750, pp. 25–32). Springer. doi:10.1007/11566489_4

Nicolau, S., Soler, L., Mutter, D., & Marescaux, J. (2011). Augmented reality in laparoscopic surgical oncology. *Surgical Oncology*, *20*(3), 189–201. doi:10.1016/j.suronc.2011.07.002 PMID:21802281

Noma, N. G., & Ghani, M. K. A. (2012, December). Discovering pattern in medical audiology data with FP-growth algorithm. In *Biomedical Engineering and Sciences (IECBES), 2012 IEEE EMBS Conference on* (pp. 17-22). IEEE.

Nordberg, H., Bhatia, K., Wang, K., & Wang, Z. (2013). BioPig: A Hadoop-based analytic toolkit for large-scale sequence data. *Bioinformatics (Oxford, England)*, *29*(23), 3014–3019. doi:10.1093/bioinformatics/btt528 PMID:24021384

Northwest Territories. Public Health Act. (2011). *Yellowknife: Territorial Assembly*. Retrieved 21 January 2017 from https://www.justice.gov.nt.ca/en/files/legislation/public-health/public-health.a.pdf

Nova Scotia Department of Health and Wellness. (2013). *Nova Scotia Communicable Diseases Manual; Lyme disease*. Retrieved from 21 January 2017 http://novascotia.ca/dhw/cdpc/cdc/documents/Lyme.pdf

Nova Scotia Department of Health and Wellness. (n.d.). *Nova Scotia Communicable Diseases Manual; West Nile Virus*. Retrieved 21 January 2017 http://novascotia.ca/dhw/cdpc/cdc/documents/West-Nile-Virus.pdf

Nowak, M. A., & Bangham, C. R. M. (1996). Population dynamics of immune responses to persistence viruses. *Science*, *272*(5258), 74–79. doi:10.1126/science.272.5258.74 PMID:8600540

Ntziachristos, V., & Chance, B. (2001). Breast imaging technology: Probing physiology and molecular function using optical imaging - applications to breast cancer. *Breast Cancer Research, 3*(1), 41–46. doi:10.1186/bcr269 PMID:11250744

Nuwangi, S. M., Oruthotaarachchi, C. R., Tilakaratna, J. M. P. P., & Caldera, H. A. (2010a, December). Utilization of Data Mining Techniques in Knowledge Extraction for Diminution of Diabetes. In *Information Technology for Real World Problems (VCON), 2010 Second Vaagdevi International Conference on* (pp. 3-8). IEEE.

Nuwangi, S. M., Oruthotaarachchi, C. R., Tilakaratna, J. M. P. P., & Caldera, H. A. (2010b, November). Usage of association rules and classification techniques in knowledge extraction of diabetes. In *Advanced Information Management and Service (IMS), 2010 6th International Conference on* (pp. 372-377). IEEE.

Oelze, M. L., OBrien, W. D., Blue, J. P., & Zachary, J. F. (2004). Differentiation and characterization of rat mammary fibroadenomas and 4T1 mouse carcinomas using quantitative ultrasound imaging. *IEEE Transactions on Medical Imaging, 23*(6), 764–771. doi:10.1109/TMI.2004.826953 PMID:15191150

Oguma, S. (1990). Simulation of dynamic changes of human T cell leukemia virus type I carriage rates. *Japanese Journal of Cancer Research, 81*(1), 1521. doi:10.1111/j.1349-7006.1990.tb02501.x PMID:2108943

Oh, C., Novotny, A. M., Carter, P. L., Ready, R. K., Campbell, D. D., & Leckie, M. C. (2016). Use of a simulation-based decision support tool to improve emergency department throughput. *Operations Research for Health Care, 9*, 29–39. doi:10.1016/j.orhc.2016.03.002

Oh, H. C., & Karimi, I. A. (2004). Regulatory factors and capacity-expansion planning in global chemical supply chains. *Industrial & Engineering Chemistry Research, 43*(13), 3364–3380. doi:10.1021/ie034339g

Oh, J. H., Hwang, S., Lee, J. K., Tavanapong, W., Wong, J., & Groen, P. C. D. (2007). Informative frame classification for endoscopy video. *Medical Image Analysis, 11*(2), 110–127. doi:10.1016/j.media.2006.10.003 PMID:17329146

Öhsen, U. V., Marcinczak, J. M., Vélez, A. F. M., & Grigat, R. R. (2012). *Keyframe selection for robust pose estimation in laparoscopic videos.* Paper presented at the Medical Imaging 2012: Image-Guided Procedures, Robotic Interventions, and Modeling, San Diego, CA.

Ojala, T., Pietikäinen, M., & Mäenpää, T. (2002). Multiresolution gray-scale and rotation invariant texture classification with local binary patterns. *IEEE Transactions on Pattern Analysis and Machine Intelligence, 24*(7), 971–987. doi:10.1109/TPAMI.2002.1017623

Ojo, A. (2014). Addressing the global burden of chronic kidney disease through clinical and translational research. *Transactions of the American Clinical and Climatological Association, 125*, 229. PMID:25125737

Okunieff, P., Chen, Y., Maguire, D. J., & Huser, A. K. (2008). Molecular markers of radiation related normal tissue toxicity. *Cancer and Metastasis Reviews, 27*(3), 363–374. doi:10.1007/s10555-008-9138-7 PMID:18506399

Olavarria, E. N., Gomes, A. N., Kruschewsky, R. A., Galvão-Castro, B., & Grassi, M. F. R. (2012). Evolution of HTLV-1 proviral load in patients from Salvador, Brazil. *The Brazilian Journal of Infectious Diseases, 16*(4), 357–360. doi:10.1016/j.bjid.2012.06.022 PMID:22846124

Olson, M. (2010). Hadoop: Scalable, flexible data storage and analysis. *IQT Quart, 1*(3), 14–18.

Olston, C., Reed, B., Srivastava, U., Kumar, R., & Tomkins, A. (2008). Pig latin: a not-so-foreign language for data processing. *Proceedings of the 2008 ACM SIGMOD International Conference on Management of Data*, 1099–1110. doi:10.1145/1376616.1376726

Omri, F., Hamila, R., Foufou, S., & Jarraya, M. (2012). Cloud-Ready Biometric System for Mobile Security Access. In *Networked Digital Technologies* (pp. 192–200). New York: Springer. doi:10.1007/978-3-642-30567-2_16

Ontario Ministry of Finance. (2016). *Ontario Fact Sheet. November 2016.* Retried November 30, 2016, from: http://www.fin.gov.on.ca/en/economy/ecupdates/factsheet.html

Ontario Renal Network. (2012). *Ontario Renal Plan.* Retrieved July 6, 2016, from: https://www.cancercare.on.ca/common/pages/UserFile.aspx?fileId=253261

Ontario Renal Network. (2015). *Ontario Renal Plan II.* Retrieved July 6, 2016, from the Ontario Renal Network Website: http://www.renalnetwork.on.ca/ontario_renal_plan/#.V3wczPl97IU

Ontario Renal Network. (2016). *Ontario Renal Reporting System.* Retrieved December 6, 2016, from the Ontario Renal Network Website: http://www.renalnetwork.on.ca/hcpinfo/ontario_renal_reporting_system/#.WE2tsncZOV4

Ontario. Health Protection and Promotion Act. (2015). Ontario Provincial Parliament. Retrieved 21 January 2017 from https://www.ontario.ca/laws/statute/90h07

Orcun, S., Altinel, I. K., & Hortacsua, Ö. (2001). General continuous time models for production planning and scheduling of batch processing plants: Mixed integer linear program formulations and computational issues'. *Computers & Chemical Engineering, 25*(2-3), 371–389. doi:10.1016/S0098-1354(00)00663-3

Ordóñez, C., Matías, J. M., de Cos Juez, J. F., & García, P. J. (2009). Machine learning techniques applied to the determination of osteoporosis incidence in post-menopausal women. *Mathematical and Computer Modelling, 50*(5), 673–679. doi:10.1016/j.mcm.2008.12.024

Orlovska, S., Pedersen, M. S., Benros, M. E., Mortensen, P. B., Agerbo, E., & Nordentoft, M. (2014). Head injury as risk factor for psychiatric disorders: A nationwide register-based follow-up study of 113,906 persons with head injury. *The American Journal of Psychiatry, 171*(4), 463–469. doi:10.1176/appi.ajp.2013.13020190 PMID:24322397

Oropesa, I., Sanchez-Gonzalez, P. J., Chmarra, M. K., Lamata, P., Fernandez, A. I., Sanchez-Margallo, J. A., & Gomez, E. J. et al. (2013). EVA: Laparoscopic Instrument Tracking Based on Endoscopic Video Analysis for Psychomotor Skills Assessment. *Surgical Endoscopy, 27*(3), 1029–1039. doi:10.1007/s00464-012-2513-z PMID:23052495

Ortiz, G. M., Hu, J., Goldwitz, J. A., Chandwani, R., Larsson, M., Bhardwaj, N., & Nixon, D. F. et al. (2002). Residual viral replication during antiretroviral therapy boosts human immunodeficiency virus type 1-specific CD8+ T- cell responses in subjects treated early after infection. *Journal of Virology, 76*(1), 411–415. doi:10.1128/JVI.76.1.411-415.2002 PMID:11739706

O'Shea, J. S. (2007). *The Crisis in America's Emergency Rooms and What Can Be Done.* Heritage Foundation.

Otsu, N. (1979). A Threshold Selection Method from Gray-Level Histograms. *IEEE Transactions on Systems, Man, and Cybernetics, 9*(1), 62–66. doi:10.1109/TSMC.1979.4310076

Özçift, A., & Gülten, A. (2013). Genetic algorithm wrapped Bayesian network feature selection applied to differential diagnosis of erythemato-squamous diseases. *Digital Signal Processing, 23*(1), 230–237. doi:10.1016/j.dsp.2012.07.008

Padoy, N., Blum, T., Essa, I., Feussner, H., Berger, M., & Navab, N. (2007). *A boosted segmentation method for surgical workflow analysis.* Paper presented at the Medical Image Computing and Computer Assisted Intervention. doi:10.1007/978-3-540-75757-3_13

Pagel, C., Utley, M., Crowe, S., Witter, T., Anderson, D., Samson, R., & Brown, K. (2013). Real time monitoring of risk-adjusted paediatric cardiac surgery outcomes using variable life-adjusted display: Implementation in three UK centres. *Heart (British Cardiac Society), 99*(19), 1445–1450. doi:10.1136/heartjnl-2013-303671 PMID:23564473

Palaniappan, S., & Awang, R. (2008, March). Intelligent heart disease prediction system using data mining techniques. In *2008 IEEE/ACS International Conference on Computer Systems and Applications* (pp. 108-115). IEEE. doi:10.1109/AICCSA.2008.4493524

Palmer, G. (1996). Casemix Funding of Hospitals: Objectives and Objections. *Health Care Analysis*, *4*(3), 185–193. doi:10.1007/BF02252878 PMID:10162141

Papageorgiou, L. G. (2009). Supply chain optimization for the process industries: Advances and opportunities. *Computers & Chemical Engineering*, *33*(12), 1931–1938. doi:10.1016/j.compchemeng.2009.06.014

Parameshwaran, R., Srinivasan, P. S. S., Punniyamoorthy, M., Charunyanath, S. T., & Ashwin, C. (2009). Integrating fuzzy analytical hierarchy process and data envelopment analysis for performance management in automobile repair shops. *European Journal of Industrial Engineering*, *3*(4), 450–467. doi:10.1504/EJIE.2009.027037

Pareek, G., Armenakas, N. A., Panagopoulos, G., Bruno, J. J., & Fracchia, J. A. (2005). Extracorporeal shock wave lithotripsy success based on body mass index and Hounsfield units. *Urology, 65*, 33-36.

Park, E. H., Park, J., Ntuen, C., Kim, D., & Johnson, K.Cone Memorial Hospital. (2008). Forecast driven simulation model for service quality improvement of the emergency department in the Moses H. Cone Memorial Hospital. *Asian Journal on Quality*, *9*(3), 1–14. doi:10.1108/15982688200800024

Parsonnet, V., Dean, D., & Bernstein, A. D. (1989). A method of uniform stratifcation of risk for evaluating the results of surgery in acquired adult heart disease. *Circulation*, *79*(6 Pt 2), I3–I12. PMID:2720942

Parthiban, G., Rajesh, A., & Srivatsa, S. K. (2011). Diagnosis of heart disease for diabetic patients using naive bayes method. *International Journal of Computers and Applications*, *24*(3), 7–11. doi:10.5120/2933-3887

Parthiban, G., & Srivatsa, S. K. (2012). Applying machine learning methods in diagnosing heart disease for diabetic patients. *International Journal of Applied Information Systems*, *3*, 2249–0868.

Pascual, J., Zamora, J., & Pirsch, J. D. (2008). A Systematic Review of Kidney Transplantation From Expanded Criteria Donors. *American Journal of Kidney Diseases*, *52*(3), 553–586. doi:10.1053/j.ajkd.2008.06.005 PMID:18725015

Patel, S., Sherrill, D., Hughes, R., Hester, T., Huggins, N., Lie-Nemeth, T., & Bonato, P. et al. (2006, April). Analysis of the severity of dyskinesia in patients with Parkinson's disease via wearable sensors. In *International Workshop on Wearable and Implantable Body Sensor Networks (BSN'06)*. IEEE.

Patil, B. M., Joshi, R. C., & Toshniwal, D. (2010 a, February). Association rule for classification of type-2 diabetic patients. In *Machine Learning and Computing (ICMLC), 2010 Second International Conference on* (pp. 330-334). IEEE.

Patil, B. M., Joshi, R. C., & Toshniwal, D. (2010 b). Hybrid prediction model for Type-2 diabetic patients. *Expert Systems with Applications*, *37*(12), 8102–8108. doi:10.1016/j.eswa.2010.05.078

Patil, S. B., & Kumaraswamy, Y. S. (2009). Extraction of significant patterns from heart disease warehouses for heart attack prediction. *IJCSNS*, *9*(2), 228–235.

Patiño, J., Guilhaumon, F., Whittaker, R. J., Triantis, K. A., Gradstein, S. R., Hedenäs, L., & Vanderpoorten, A. et al. (2013). Accounting for data heterogeneity in patterns of biodiversity: An application of linear mixed effect models to the oceanic island biogeography of spore-producing plants. *Ecography*, *36*(8), 904–913. doi:10.1111/j.1600-0587.2012.00020.x

Patvivatsiri, L. (2006, December). A simulation model for bioterrorism preparedness in an emergency room. *Proceedings of the 38th conference on Winter simulation*, 501-508. doi:10.1109/WSC.2006.323122

Paul, J. A., & Hariharan, G. (2007, December). Hospital capacity planning for efficient disaster mitigation during a bioterrorist attack. In *Proceedings of the 39th conference on Winter simulation: 40 years! The best is yet to come* (pp. 1139-1147). IEEE Press.

Paul, J. A., & Lin, L. (2012). Models for improving patient throughput and waiting at hospital emergency departments. *The Journal of Emergency Medicine*, *43*(6), 1119–1126. doi:10.1016/j.jemermed.2012.01.063 PMID:22902245

Paul, S. A., Reddy, M. C., & DeFlitch, C. J. (2010). A systematic review of simulation studies investigating emergency department overcrowding. *Simulation*, *86*(8-9), 559–571.

Paul, S. A., Reddy, M. C., & DeFlitch, C. J. (2010). A Systematic Review of Simulation Studies Investigating Emergency Department Overcrowding. *Simulation*, *86*(8-9), 559–571.

Paynabar, K., Jionghua, J., & Yeh, A. B. (2012). Phase I risk-adjusted control charts for monitoring surgical performance by considering categorical covariates. *Journal of Quality Technology*, *44*, 39–53.

Pegden, C. D. (1990). *Introduction to Simulation Using SIMAN*. McGraw-Hill, Inc.

Peidro, D., Mula, J., Poler, R., & Verdegay, J.-L. (2009). Fuzzy Optimization for Supply Chain Planning Under Supply, Demand and Process Uncertainties. *Fuzzy Sets and Systems*, *160*(18), 2640–2657. doi:10.1016/j.fss.2009.02.021

Pentland, A., Reid, T. G., & Heibeck, T. (2013). Revolutionizing medicine and Public Health. Report of the Big Data and Health Working Group, Doha.

Percus, J. K., Percus, O. E., & Perelson, A. S. (1993). Predicting the size of the T-cell receptor and antibody combining region from consideration of efficient self-non-self discrimination. *Proceedings of the National Academy of Sciences of the United States of America*, *90*(5), 1691–1695. doi:10.1073/pnas.90.5.1691 PMID:7680474

Perelson, A. S. (2002). Modelling viral and immune system dynamics. *Nature Reviews. Immunology*, *2*(1), 28–36. doi:10.1038/nri700 PMID:11905835

Perelson, A. S., & Nelson, P. W. (1999). Mathematical analysis of HIV-I dynamics in vivo. *SIAM Review*, *41*(1), 3–44. doi:10.1137/S0036144598335107

Perelson, A. S., & Oster, G. F. (1979). Theoretical studies of clonal selection: Minimal antibody repertoire size and reliability of self–non-self discrimination. *Journal of Theoretical Biology*, *81*(4), 645–670. doi:10.1016/0022-5193(79)90275-3 PMID:94141

Perelson, A. S., & Weisbuch, G. (1997). Immunology for physicists. *Reviews of Modern Physics*, *69*(4), 1219–1267. doi:10.1103/RevModPhys.69.1219

Perks, A. E., Schuler, T. D., Lee, J., Ghiculete, D., Chung, D. G., & Honey, R. J. (2008). Stone attenuation and skin-to-stone distance on computed tomography predicts for stone fragmentation by shock wave lithotripsy. *Urology*, *72*(4), 765–769. doi:10.1016/j.urology.2008.05.046 PMID:18674803

Perlis, R. H., Iosifescu, D. V., Castro, V. M., Murphy, S. N., Gainer, V. S., & Minnier, J. (2012). Using electronic medical records to enable large-scale studies in psychiatry: Treatment resistant depression as a model. *Psychological Medicine*, *42*, 41–50.

Perl, J., Pierratos, A., Kandasamy, G., McCormick, B. B., Quinn, R. R., Jain, A. K., & Oliver, M. J. et al. (2014). Peritoneal dialysis catheter implantation by nephrologists is associated with higher rates of peritoneal dialysis utilization: A population-based study. *Nephrology, Dialysis, Transplantation*, gfu359. PMID:25414373

Perou, C. M., Sørlie, T., Eisen, M. B., van de Rijn, M., Jeffrey, S. S., & Rees, C. A. ... Botstein, D. (2000). Molecular portraits of human breast tumours. *Nature, 406*(6797), 747–752. https://doi.org/10.1038/35021093

Petrou, M., & Sevilla, P. G. (2006). *Image Processing Dealing with Texture*. West Sussex, UK: John Wiley & Sons. doi:10.1002/047003534X

Piateski, G., & Frawley, W. (1991). *Knowledge discovery in databases*. MIT Press.

Pidd, M. (2003). *Tools for Thinking: Modelling in Management Science* (2nd ed.). Chichester, UK: Wiley.

Pinjala, S. K., Pintelon, L., & Vereecke, A. (2006). An empirical investigation on the relationship between business and maintenance strategies. *International Journal of Production Economics, 104*(1), 214–229. doi:10.1016/j.ijpe.2004.12.024

Pishvaee, M. S., Razmi, J., & Torabi, S. A. (2012b). Robust possibilistic programming for socially responsible supply chain network design: A new approach. *Fuzzy Sets and Systems, 206*, 1–20. doi:10.1016/j.fss.2012.04.010

Pishvaee, M. S., Torabi, S. A., & Razmi, J. (2012a). Credibility-based fuzzy mathematical programming model for green logistics design under uncertainty. *Computers & Industrial Engineering, 62*(2), 624–632. doi:10.1016/j.cie.2011.11.028

Pittelkow, P. H., & Ghosh, M. (2008). Theoretical measures of relative performance of classifiers for high dimensional data with small sample sizes. *Journal of the Royal Statistical Society. Series B. Methodological, 70*(1), 159–173. doi:10.1111/j.1467-9868.2007.00631.x

Podolsky, E. R., Mouhlas, A., Wu, A. S., Poor, A. E., & Curcillo, P. G. (2010). Single Port Access (SPA) laparoscopic ventral hernia repair: initial report of 30 cases. *Surg Endosc, 24*(7), 1557-1561.

Poiesz, B. J., Ruscetti, F. W., Gazdar, A. F., Bunn, P. A., Minna, J. D., & Gallo, R. C. (1980). Detection and isolation of type C retrovirus particles from fresh and cultured lymphocytes of a patient with cutaneous T-cell lymphoma. *Proceedings of the National Academy of Sciences of the United States of America, 77*(12), 7415–7419. doi:10.1073/pnas.77.12.7415 PMID:6261256

Polat, K. (2012). Application of attribute weighting method based on clustering centers to discrimination of linearly non-separable medical datasets. *Journal of Medical Systems, 36*(4), 2657–2673. doi:10.1007/s10916-011-9741-y

Polat, K., & Güneş, S. (2007). An expert system approach based on principal component analysis and adaptive neuro-fuzzy inference system to diagnosis of diabetes disease. *Digital Signal Processing, 17*(4), 702–710. doi:10.1016/j.dsp.2006.09.005

Polat, K., Güneş, S., & Arslan, A. (2008). A cascade learning system for classification of diabetes disease: Generalized discriminant analysis and least square support vector machine. *Expert Systems with Applications, 34*(1), 482–487. doi:10.1016/j.eswa.2006.09.012

Potash, J. B. (2015). Electronic medical records: Fast track to big data in bipolar disorder. *The American Journal of Psychiatry, 172*(4), 310–321. doi:10.1176/appi.ajp.2015.15010043 PMID:25827027

Potter, R. (2007). *Comparison of classification algorithms applied to breast cancer diagnosis and prognosis*. Presented at the 7th Industrial Conference on Data Mining, ICDM 2007, Leipzig, Germany.

Potterat, J. J., Rothenberg, R. B., Woodhouse, D. E., Muth, J. B., Pratts, C. I., & Fogle, J. S. (1985). Gonorrhea as a social disease. *Sexually Transmitted Diseases, 12*(1), 25–32. doi:10.1097/00007435-198501000-00006 PMID:4002091

Preater, J. (2002). A Bibliography of Queues in Health and Medicine. *Health Care Management Science, 5*(4), 283. doi:10.1023/A:1020334207282

Prince Edward Island. Public Health Act. (2014). Retrieved 21 January 2017 from https://www.princeedwardisland.ca/en/legislation/public-health-act

Privett, N., & Gonsalvez, D. (2015). The top ten global health supply chain issues. *Journal of Operations Research for Health Care.*

Provincial Infectious Disease Advisory Committee on Communicable Disease. (2014). *Recommendations for the public health response to hepatitis C in Ontario.* Retrieved 21 January 2017 from http://www.publichealthontario.ca/en/eRepository/Recommendations_Public_Health_Response_Hepatitis_C.pdf

Public Health Agency of Canada. (2014). *Canadian tuberculosis standards* (VII). Ottawa, Ontario: Public Health Agency of Canada, Canadian Lung Association. Retrieved 21 January 2017 from http://www.respiratoryguidelines.ca/tb-standards-2013

Public Health Ontario. (2014). *Provincial Case Definitions for Reportable Diseases; Chlamydia trachomatis infections.* Retrieved 21 January 2017 from http://www.health.gov.on.ca/en/pro/programs/publichealth/oph_standards/docs/mumps_cd.pdf

Public Health Ontario. (2015). *How to complete the measles and rubella enhanced surveillance form.* Retrieved 21 January 2017 from http://www.publichealthontario.ca/en/eRepository/How_to_complete_MR_Surveillance_Form_2015.pdf

Pugliese, A., & Gandolfi, A. (2008). A simple model o f pathogen-immune dynamics including specific and non-specific immunity. *Mathematical Biosciences, 214*(1-2), 73–80. doi:10.1016/j.mbs.2008.04.004 PMID:18547594

Purnami, S. W., Zain, J. M., & Embong, A. (2010, March). A new expert system for diabetes disease diagnosis using modified spline smooth support vector machine. In *International Conference on Computational Science and Its Applications* (pp. 83-92). Springer Berlin Heidelberg. doi:10.1007/978-3-642-12189-0_8

Pyle, D. (1999). *Data preparation for data mining* (Vol. 1). Morgan Kaufmann.

Quebec. Public Health Act. (2016). Quebec National Assembly. Retrieved 21 January 2017 from http://www.gov.pe.ca/law/statutes/pdf/p-30_1.pdf

Quellec, G., Charrière, K., Lamard, M., Droueche, Z., Roux, C., Cochener, B., & Cazuguel, G. (2014). Real-time recognition of surgical tasks in eye surgery videos. *Medical Image Analysis, 18*(3), 579–590. doi:10.1016/j.media.2014.02.007 PMID:24637155

Quinn, R. R., Laupacis, A., Hux, J. E., Moineddin, R., Paterson, M., & Oliver, M. J. (2009). Forecasting the need for dialysis services in Ontario, Canada to 2011. *Healthcare Policy, 4*(4).

Racusen, L. C., Solez, K., Colvin, R. B., Bonsib, S. M., Castro, M. C., Cavallo, T., & Yamaguchi, Y. et al. (1999). The Banff 97 working classification of renal allograft pathology. *Kidney International, 55*(2), 713–723. doi:10.1046/j.1523-1755.1999.00299.x PMID:9987096

Radhakrishnan, D. K., Dell, S. D., Guttmann, A., Shariff, S. Z., Liu, K., & To, T. (2014). Trends in the age of diagnosis of childhood asthma. *The Journal of Allergy and Clinical Immunology, 134*(5), 1057–1062. doi:10.1016/j.jaci.2014.05.012 PMID:24985402

Radha, P., & Srinivasan, B. (2014, August). Feature Selection Using Particle Swarm Optimization for Predicting the Risk of Cardiovascular Disease in Type-II Diabetic Patients. *International Journal on Recent and Innovation Trends in Computing and Communication., 2*(8), 2503–2509.

Rado, O., Lupia, B., Leung, J. M., Kuo, Y. H., & Graham, C. A. (2014). Using simulation to analyze patient flows in a hospital emergency department in Hong Kong. In *Proceedings of the International Conference on Health Care Systems Engineering* (pp. 289-301). Springer International Publishing. doi:10.1007/978-3-319-01848-5_23

Raghava, N. (2011). Iris recognition on hadoop: A biometrics system implementation on cloud computing. *IEEE International Conference on Cloud Computing and Intelligence Systems*, 482–485.

Raghupathi, W., & Raghupathi, V. (2014). Big data analytics in healthcare: Promise and potential. *Health Information Science and Systems*, 7(2-3), 1-10.

Rajesh, K., & Sangeetha, V. (2012). Application of data mining methods and techniques for diabetes diagnosis. *International Journal of Engineering and Innovative Technology*, 2(3).

Raj, G., Auge, B. K., Weizer, A. Z., Denstedt, J. D., Watterson, J. D., Beiko, D. T., & Preminger, G. M. et al.G.V. (2003). Percutaneous Management of Calculi Within Horseshoe Kidneys. *The Journal of Urology*, 170(1), 48–51. doi:10.1097/01.ju.0000067620.60404.2d PMID:12796642

Raju, D., Su, X., Patrician, P. A., Loan, L. A., & McCarthy, M. S. (2015). Exploring factors associated with pressure ulcers: A data mining approach. *International Journal of Nursing Studies*, 52(1), 102–111. doi:10.1016/j.ijnurstu.2014.08.002 PMID:25192963

Ram, S., Zhang, W., Williams, M., & Pengetnze, Y. (2015). Predicting Asthma-Related Emergency Department Visits Using Big Data. *IEEE Journal of Biomedical and Health Informatics*, 19(4), 1216–1223. https://doi.org/10.1109/JBHI.2015.2404829

Ramirez, D., Maurice, M. J., & Kaouk, J. H. (2016). Robotic Single-port Surgery: Paving the Way for the Future. *Urology*, 95, 5–10. doi:10.1016/j.urology.2016.05.013 PMID:27211930

Ramirez, E., Cartier, L., Torres, M., & Barria, M. (2007). Temporal dynamics of human T lymphotropic virus type I tax mRNA and proviral DNA load in peripheral blood mononuclear cells of human T lymphotropic virus type I associated myelopathy patients. *Journal of Medical Virology*, 79(6), 782–790. doi:10.1002/jmv.20844 PMID:17457906

Randen, T., & Husøy, J. H. (1999). Filtering for texture classification: A comparative study. *IEEE Transactions on Pattern Analysis and Machine Intelligence*, 21(4), 291–310. doi:10.1109/34.761261

Rastgoo, M., Lemaitre, G., Massich, J., Morel, O., Garcia, R., Meriaudeau, F., & Marzani, F. et al. (2016). Tackling the problem of data imbalancing for melanoma classification. *Bioimaging*.

Redheffer, R. (1985). Volterra multipliers I. *SIAM Journal on Algebraic and Discrete Methods*, 6, 592–611.

Reed, T. R., & du Buf, J. M. H. (1993). A Review of recent texture segmentation and feature extraction techniques. *CVGIP. Image Understanding*, 57(3), 359–372. doi:10.1006/ciun.1993.1024

Ren, X., Wang, Y., Chen, L., Zhang, X. S., & Jin, Q. (2013). EllipsoidFN: A tool for identifying a heterogeneous set of cancer biomarkers based on gene expressions. *Nucleic Acids Research*, 41(4), 1–8. doi:10.1093/nar/gks1288 PMID:23262226

Resorlu, B., Unsal, A., Gulec, H., & Oztuna, D. (2012). A New Scoring System for Predicting Stone-free Rate After Retrograde Intrarenal Surgery: The Resorlu-Unsal Stone Score. *Urology*, 80(3), 512–518. doi:10.1016/j.urology.2012.02.072 PMID:22840867

Rezaei, J. (2015). Best-worst multi-criteria decision-making method. *Omega*, 53, 49–57. doi:10.1016/j.omega.2014.11.009

Ribeiro, M. X., Traina, A. J., Traina, C. Jr, & Azevedo-Marques, P. M. (2008). An association rule-based method to support medical image diagnosis with efficiency. *IEEE Transactions on Multimedia, 10*(2), 277–285. doi:10.1109/TMM.2007.911837

Ribeiro, R. M., Mohri, H., Ho, D. D., & Perelson, A. S. (2002). In vivo dynamics of T cell activation, proliferation, and death in HIV-1 infection: Why are CD4+ but not CD8+ T cells depleted? *Proceedings of the National Academy of Sciences of the United States of America, 99*(24), 15572–15577. doi:10.1073/pnas.242358099 PMID:12434018

Rice, S. D., Heinzman, J. M., Brower, S. L., Ervin, P. R., Song, N., Shen, K., & Wang, D. (2010). Analysis of chemotherapeutic response heterogeneity and drug clustering based on mechanism of action using an in vitro assay. *Anticancer Research, 30*(7), 2805–2811. PMID:20683016

Richardson, D. B. (2006). Increase in patient mortality at 10 days associated with emergency department overcrowding. *The Medical Journal of Australia, 184*(5), 213. PMID:16515430

Richardson, J. H., Edwards, A. J., Cruickshank, J. K., Rudge, P., & Dalgleish, A. G. (1990). In vivo cellular tropism of human T cell leukemia virus type I. *Journal of Virology, 64,* 5682–5687. PMID:1976827

Richardson, J. H., Hollsberg, P., Windhagen, A., Child, L. A., Hafler, D. A., & Lever, A. M. (1997). Variable immortalizing potential and frequent virus latency in blood-derived T-cell clones infected with human T-cell leukemia virus type I. *Blood, 89,* 3303–3314. PMID:9129036

Richmond, B. M., Vescuso, P., & Peterson, S. (1990). *iThink™ Software Manuals.* Academic Press.

Rico, F., Salari, E., & Centeno, G. (2007, December). Emergency departments nurse allocation to face a pandemic influenza outbreak. In *Simulation Conference* (pp. 1292-1298). IEEE. doi:10.1109/WSC.2007.4419734

Riedler, J., Braun-Fahrländer, C., Eder, W., Schreuer, M., Waser, M., Maisch, S., & Al, E. X. et al. (2001). Study Team, Exposure to farming in early life and development of asthma and allergy: A cross-sectional survey. *Journal Lattice, 358,* 1129–1133. PMID:11597666

Rieffe, C., Oosterveld, P., Wijkel, D., & Wiefferink, C. (1999). Reasons why patients bypass their GP to visit a hospital emergency department. *Accident and Emergency Nursing, 7*(4), 217–225. doi:10.1016/S0965-2302(99)80054-X PMID:10808762

Robbins, F. W. A. (2010). Mathematical model of HIV infection: Simulating T4, T8, macrophages, antibody, and virus via specific anti-HIV response in the Presence of adaptation and tropism. *Bulletin of Mathematical Biology, 72*(5), 1208–1253. doi:10.1007/s11538-009-9488-5 PMID:20151219

Robertson-Steel, I. (2006). Evolution of triage systems. *Emergency Medicine Journal, 23*(2), 154–155. doi:10.1136/emj.2005.030270 PMID:16439754

Roberts, S. D. (2011). Tutorial on the Simulation of Healthcare Systems. In *Proceedings of the 2011 Winter Simulation Conference.* Piscataway, NJ: Institute of Electrical and Electronics Engineers, Inc. doi:10.1109/WSC.2011.6147860

Robison, R. J. (2014, January 6). *How big is the human genome? In megabytes, not base pairs.* Retrieved September 14, 2016, from https://medium.com/precision-medicine/how-big-is-the-human-genome-e90caa3409b0

Rogers, D. J., Wilson, A. J., Hay, S. I., & Graham, A. J. (2006). The global distribution of yellow fever and dengue. *Advances in Parasitology, 62,* 181–220. doi:10.1016/S0065-308X(05)62006-4 PMID:16647971

Rolfhamre, R., Janson, A., Arneborn, M., & Ekdahl, K. (2006). SmiNet-2: Description of an internet-based surveillance system for communicable diseases in Sweden. *Eurosurveillance, 11*(5). PMID:16757847

Ronaghi, Z., Duffy, E. B., & Kwartowitz, D. M. (2015). Toward real-time remote processing of laparoscopic video. *medical. Imaging, 2*(4).

Roos, L. L., Nickel, N. C., Romano, P. S., & Fergusson, P. (2014). Administrative Databases. In *Wiley StatsRef: Statistics Reference Online*. John Wiley & Sons, Ltd. doi:10.1002/9781118445112.stat05227

Roques, F., Nashef, S. A. M., Michel, P., Gauducheau, E., De Vincentiis, C., Baudet, E., & Gams, E. (1999). Risk factors and outcome in European cardiac surgery: Analysis of the EuroSCORE multinational database of 19030 patients. *European Journal of Cardio-Thoracic Surgery, 15*(6), 816–823. doi:10.1016/S1010-7940(99)00106-2 PMID:10431864

Rosen, J., Solazzo, M., Hannaford, B., & Sinanan, M. (2002). Task Decomposition of Laparoscopic Surgery for Objective Evaluation of Surgical Residents' Learning Curve Using Hidden Markov Model. *Computer Aided Surgery, 7*(1), 49-61.

Rosenberg, E. S., Altfeld, M., Poon, S. H., Phillips, M. N., & Wilkes, B. M. (2000). Immune control of HIV-1 after early treatment of acute infection. *Nature, 407*(6803), 523–526. doi:10.1038/35035103 PMID:11029005

Rosenberg, T., Kendall, O., Blanchard, J., Martel, S., Wakelin, C., & Fast, M. (1997). Shigellosis on Indian Reserves in Manitoba, Canada : Its Relationship to Crowded Housing, Lack of Running Water, and Inadequate Sewage Disposal. *American Journal of Public Health, 87*(9), 1547–1551. doi:10.2105/AJPH.87.9.1547 PMID:9314814

Rothenberg, R. B., McElroy, P. D., Wilce, M. A., & Muth, S. Q. (2003). Contact tracing: Comparing the approaches for sexually transmitted diseases and tuberculosis. *The International Journal of Tuberculosis and Lung Disease, 7*(12Suppl 3), S342–S348. PMID:14677820

Rowan, M., Ryan, T., Hegarty, F., & OHare, N. (2007). The use of artificial neural networks to stratify the length of stay of cardiac patients based on preoperative and initial postoperative factors. *Artificial Intelligence in Medicine, 40*(3), 211–221. doi:10.1016/j.artmed.2007.04.005

Rowe, B. H., Bond, K., Ospina, M. B., Blitz, S., Friesen, C., & Schull, M. (2006). *Emergency department overcrowding in Canada: what are the issues and what can be done?* [Technology overview no 21]. Ottawa: Canadian Agency for Drugs and Technologies in Health.

Ruktanonchai, N. W., DeLeenheer, P., Tatem, A. J., Alegana, V. A., Trevor Caughlin, T., & Zu Erbach-Schoenberg, E. (2016). Identifying Malaria Transmission Foci for Elimination Using Human Mobility Data. *PLoS Computational Biology, 12*(4), 1–19. doi:10.1371/journal.pcbi.1004846 PMID:27043913

Ruohonen, T., Neittaanmaki, P., & Teittinen, J. (2006, December). Simulation model for improving the operation of the emergency department of special health care. *In Simulation Conference, 2006. WSC 06. Proceedings of the Winter* (pp. 453-458). IEEE. doi:10.1109/WSC.2006.323115

Saaty, T. L. (1980). *The Analytic Hierarchy Process*. New York, NY: McGraw Hill.

Saaty, T. L. (2001). *Decision Making with Dependence and Feedback: The Analytic Network Process*. Pittsburgh, PA: RWS Publications.

Sabariah, M. M. K., Hanifa, S. A., & Sa'adah, M. S. (2014, August). Early detection of type II Diabetes Mellitus with random forest and classification and regression tree (CART). In *Advanced Informatics: Concept, Theory and Application (ICAICTA), 2014 International Conference of* (pp. 238-242). IEEE.

Sadeghi-Naini, A., Falou, O., Tadayyon, H., Al-Mahrouki, A., Tran, W., Papanicolau, N., & Czarnota, G. J. et al. (2013). Conventional frequency ultrasonic biomarkers of cancer treatment response in vivo. *Trasnlational Oncology, 6*(3), 234–243. doi:10.1593/tlo.12385 PMID:23761215

Sadeghi-Naini, A., Falou, O., Zubovits, J., Dent, R., Verma, S., Trudeau, M. E., & Czarnota, G. J. et al. (2013). Quantitative ultrasound evaluation of tumour cell death response in locally advanced breast cancer patients receiving chemotherapy. *Clinical Cancer Research*, *19*(8), 2163–2174. doi:10.1158/1078-0432.CCR-12-2965 PMID:23426278

Sadeghi-Naini, A., Sannachi, L., Pritchard, K., Trudeau, M., Gandhi, S., Wright, F. C., & Czarnota, G. J. et al. (2014). Early prediction of therapy responses and outcomes in breast cancer patients using quantitative ultrasound spectral texture. *Oncotarget*, *5*(11), 3497–3511. doi:10.18632/oncotarget.1950 PMID:24939867

Saedi, D., & Moulavi, M. (2012). Association between some CT characteristics of renal stones and extracorporeal shockwave lithotripsy success rate. *Tehran University Medical Journal*, *70*(3), 169–175.

Saghafian, S., Hopp, W. J., Van Oyen, M. P., Desmond, J. S., & Kronick, S. L. (2012). Patient Streaming as a Mechanism for Improving Responsiveness in Emergency Departments. *Operations Research*, *60*(5), 1080–1097. doi:10.1287/opre.1120.1096

Saidi, R. F., Elias, N., Kawai, T., Hertl, M., Farrell, M., Goes, N., & Ko, D. S. C. et al. (2007). Outcome of Kidney Transplantation using Expanded criteria Donors and Donation After Cardiac Death Kidneys: Realities and Costs. *American Journal of Transplantation*, *7*(12), 2769–2774. doi:10.1111/j.1600-6143.2007.01993.x PMID:17927805

Sa-Ing, V., Thongvigitmanee, S. S., Wilasrusmee, C., & Suthakorn, J. (2012). Adaptive Mean-Shift Kalman Tracking of Laparoscopic Instruments. *International Journal of Computer Theory and Engineering*, *4*(5), 685–689. doi:10.7763/IJCTE.2012.V4.557

Salathe, M., Bengtsson, L., Bodnar, T. J., Brewer, D. D., Brownstein, J. S., Buckee, C., & Vespignani, A. et al. (2012). Digital epidemiology. *PLoS Computational Biology*, *8*(7), e1002616. doi:10.1371/journal.pcbi.1002616 PMID:22844241

Salathé, M., & Khandelwal, Sh. (2011). Assessing vaccination sentiments with online social media: Implications for infectious disease dynamics and control. *PLoS Computational Biology*, *7*(10), 2011. doi:10.1371/journal.pcbi.1002199 PMID:22022249

Salazar, R., Roepman, P., Capella, G., Moreno, V., Simon, I., Dreezen, C., & Tollenaar, R. et al. (2011). Gene expression signature to improve prognosis prediction of stage ii and iii colorectal cancer. *Journal of Clinical Oncology*, *29*(1), 17–24. doi:10.1200/JCO.2010.30.1077 PMID:21098318

Salha, M., Alzahani Afnan, A., Ashwag, A., Boushra, A., & Suheer, A. (2014). An Overview of Data Mining Techniques Applied for Heart Disease Diagnosis and Prediction. *Notes on Information Theory, 2*(4).

Samaha, S., Armel, W. S., & Starks, D. W. (2003, December). Emergency departments I: the use of simulation to reduce the length of stay in an emergency department. *Proceedings of the 35th conference on winter simulation: driving innovation*, 1907-1911.

Sanakal, R., & Jayakumari, T. (2014). Prognosis of diabetes using data mining approach-fuzzy C means clustering and support vector machine. *International Journal of Computer Trends and Technology*, *11*(2), 94–98. doi:10.14445/22312803/IJCTT-V11P120

Sánchez-González, P., Cano, A. M., Oropesa, I., Sánchez-Margallo, F. M., Del Pozo, F., Lamata, P., & Gómez, E. J. (2011). Laparoscopic video analysis for training and image-guided surgery. *Minimally Invasive Therapy & Allied Technologies*, *20*(6), 311–320. doi:10.3109/13645706.2010.541921 PMID:21247251

Sa-ngasoongsong, A., & Chongwatpol, J. (2012). An analysis of diabetes risk factors using data mining approach. Oklahoma State University.

Sannachi, L., Tadayyon, H., Sadeghi-Naini, A., Tran, W. T., Gandhi, S., Wright, F., & Czarnota, G. J. et al. (2015). Non-invasive evaluation of breast cancer response to chemotherapy using quantitative ultrasonic backscatter parameters. *Medical Image Analysis*, *20*(1), 224–236. doi:10.1016/j.media.2014.11.009 PMID:25534283

Santhanam, T., & Padmavathi, M. S. (2015). Application of K-means and genetic algorithms for dimension reduction by integrating SVM for diabetes diagnosis. *Procedia Computer Science*, *47*, 76–83. doi:10.1016/j.procs.2015.03.185

Sapna, S., & Tamilarasi, A. (2009, October). Fuzzy relational equation in preventing diabetic heart attack. In *Advances in Recent Technologies in Communication and Computing, 2009. ARTCom'09. International Conference on* (pp. 635-637). IEEE. doi:10.1109/ARTCom.2009.48

Satish, N., Harris, M., & Garland, M. (2009). Designing efficient sorting algorithms for manycore GPUs. *IEEE International Symposium Parallel & Distributed Processing*, 1-10. doi:10.1109/IPDPS.2009.5161005

Satterthwaite, P. S., & Atkinson, C. J. (2012). Using reverse triage to create hospital surge capacity: Royal Darwin Hospitals response to the Ashmore Reef disaster. *Emergency Medicine Journal*, *29*(2), 160–162. doi:10.1136/emj.2010.098087 PMID:21030549

Saunders, C. E., Makens, P. K., & Leblanc, L. J. (1989). Modeling emergency department operations using advanced computer simulation systems. *Annals of Emergency Medicine*, *18*(2), 134–140. doi:10.1016/S0196-0644(89)80101-5 PMID:2916776

Saxena, K., & Sharma, R. (2016). Efficient Heart Disease Prediction System. *Procedia Computer Science*, *85*, 962–969. doi:10.1016/j.procs.2016.05.288

Sazvar, Z., Baboli, A., & Akbari Jokar, M. R. (2013). A replenishment policy for perishable products with non-linear holding cost under stochastic supply lead time. *International Journal of Advanced Manufacturing Technology*, *64*(5-8), 1087–1098. doi:10.1007/s00170-012-4042-2

Schatz, M. C. (2009). CloudBurst: Highly sensitive read mapping with MapReduce. *Bioinformatics (Oxford, England)*, *25*(11), 1363–1369. doi:10.1093/bioinformatics/btp236 PMID:19357099

Schelling, M., Avril, N., Nährig, J., Kuhn, W., Römer, W., Sattler, D., & Schwaiger, M. et al. (2000). Positron emission tomography using [(18)F]Fluorodeoxyglucose for monitoring primary chemotherapy in breast cancer. *Journal of Clinical Oncology*, *18*(8), 1689–1695. doi:10.1200/JCO.2000.18.8.1689 PMID:10764429

Schelter, B., Winterhalder, M., & Timmer, J. (Eds.). (2006). *Handbook of time series analysis: recent theoretical developments and applications*. John Wiley & Sons. doi:10.1002/9783527609970

Schlögl, A., Keinrath, C., Zimmermann, D., Scherer, R., Leeb, R., & Pfurtscheller, G. (2007). A fully automated correction method of EOG artifacts in EEG recordings. *Clinical Neurophysiology*, *118*(1), 98–104. doi:10.1016/j.clinph.2006.09.003 PMID:17088100

Schmid, C. (2004). Weakly supervised learning of visual models and its application to content-based retrieval. *International Journal of Computer Vision*, *56*(1), 7–16. doi:10.1023/B:VISI.0000004829.38247.b0

Schmidt, R., Pollwein, B., & Gierl, L. (1999). Experiences with Case-Based Reasoning Methods and Prototypes for Medical Knowledge-Based Systems. *Artificial Intelligence in Medicine*, *1620*, 124–132.

Schneider, S. M., Gallery, M. E., Schafermeyer, R., & Zwemer, F. L. (2003). Emergency department crowding: A point in time. *Annals of Emergency Medicine*, *42*(2), 167–172. doi:10.1067/mem.2003.258 PMID:12883503

Schols, R. M., Bouvy, N. D., Dam, R. M. V., & Stassen, L. P. S. (2013). Advanced intraoperative imaging methods for laparoscopic anatomy navigation: An overview. *Surgical Endoscopy, 27*(6), 1851–1859. doi:10.1007/s00464-012-2701-x PMID:23242493

Schönherr, S., Forer, L., Weißensteiner, H., Kronenberg, F., Specht, G., & Kloss-Brandstätter, A. (2012). Cloudgene: A graphical execution platform for MapReduce programs on private and public clouds. *BMC Bioinformatics, 13*(1), 200. doi:10.1186/1471-2105-13-200 PMID:22888776

Schull, M. J., Szalai, J. P., Schwartz, B., & Redelmeier, D. A. (2001). Emergency department overcrowding following systematic hospital restructuring trends at twenty hospitals over ten years. *Academic Emergency Medicine, 8*(11), 1037–1043. doi:10.1111/j.1553-2712.2001.tb01112.x PMID:11691665

Schull, M. J., Vermeulen, M. J., Stukel, T. A., Guttmann, A., Leaver, C. A., Rowe, B. H., & Sales, A. (2012). Evaluating the effect of clinical decision units on patient flow in seven Canadian emergency departments. *Academic Emergency Medicine, 19*(7), 828–836. doi:10.1111/j.1553-2712.2012.01396.x PMID:22805630

Schull, M. J., Vermeulen, M., Slaughter, G., Morrison, L., & Daly, P. (2004). Emergency department crowding and thrombolysis delays in acute myocardial infarction. *Annals of Emergency Medicine, 44*(6), 577–585. doi:10.1016/j.annemergmed.2004.05.004 PMID:15573032

Sefion, I., & Ennaji, A. (2003). Gailhardou M, Canu S. ADEMA: A decision support system for asthma health care. *Studies in Health Technology and Informatics, 95*, 623–628. PMID:14664057

Segel, L. A. (1995). Grappling with *complexity. Complexity, 1*(2), 18–25. doi:10.1002/cplx.6130010207

Segel, L.A., & Baror, R. L. (1999). On the role of feedback in promoting conflicting goals of the adaptive immune system. *Journal of Immunology (Baltimore, MD.: 1950), 163*, 1342–1349. PMID:10415033

Sego, L. H., Reynolds, M. R. Jr, & Woodall, W. H. (2009). Risk-adjusted monitoring of survival times. *Statistics in Medicine, 28*(9), 1386–1401. doi:10.1002/sim.3546 PMID:19247982

Seigel, L. J., Nash, W. G., Poiesz, B. J., Moore, J. L., & OBrien, S. J. (1986). Dynamic and nonspecific dispersal of human Tcell leukemia/lymphoma virus type I integration in cultured lymphoma cells. *Virology, 154*(1), 6775. doi:10.1016/0042-6822(86)90430-7 PMID:3019009

Selby, M. G., Vrtiska, T. J., Krambeck, A. E., McCollough, C. H., Elsherbiny, H. E., Bergstralh, E. J., & Rule, A. D. et al. (2015). Quantification of Asymptomatic Kidney Stone Burden by Computed Tomography for Predicting Future Symptomatic Stone Events. *Urology, 85*(1), 45–50. doi:10.1016/j.urology.2014.08.031 PMID:25440821

Selka, F., Nicolau, S., Agnus, V., Bessaid, A., Marescaux, J., & Soler, L. (2015). Context-specific selection of algorithms for recursive feature trackingin endoscopic image using a new methodology. *Computerized Medical Imaging and Graphics, 40*, 49-61.

Semerjian, A., Zettervall, S. L., Amdur, R., Jarrett, T. W., & Vaziri, K. (2015). 30-Day morbidity and mortality outcomes of prolonged minimally invasive kidney procedures compared with shorter open procedures: National surgical quality improvement program analysis. *Journal of Endourology, 29*(7), 830–837. doi:10.1089/end.2014.0795 PMID:25646859

Sepehri, M. M., Rahnama, P., Shadpour, P., & Teimourpour, B. (2009). A data mining based model for selecting type of treatment for kidney stone patients. *Tehran University Medical Journal, 67*(6), 421–427.

Sepulveda, J., Lopez-Cervantes, M., Frenk, J., Gomez de Leon, J., Lezana-Fernandez, M. A., & Santos-Burgoa, C., & (CDC), C. for D. C. (1992). Key issues in public health surveillance for the 1990s. *Morbidity and Mortality Weekly Report, 41*(Suppl), 61–76. PMID:1344267

Seydel, J., & Kramer, A. (1996). Transmission and population dynamics of HTLV-I infection. *International Journal of Cancer, 66*(2), 197–200. doi:10.1002/(SICI)1097-0215(19960410)66:2<197::AID-IJC10>3.0.CO;2-A PMID:8603811

Seydel, J., & Stilianakis, N. I. (2000). HTLV-I Dynamics: A mathematical model. *Sexually Transmitted Diseases, 27*(10), 652–653. doi:10.1097/00007435-200011000-00031

Sezen, H. K., & Günal, M. M. (2009). *Yöneylem Araştırmasında Benzetim*. Bursa: Ekin Yayınevi.

Shafiee, M. (2015). Maintenance strategy selection problem: An MCDM overview. *Journal of Quality in Maintenance Engineering, 21*(4), 378–402. doi:10.1108/JQME-09-2013-0063

Shafii, M., Hosseini, S. M., Arab, M., Asgharizadeh, E., & Farzianpour, F. (2015). Performance Analysis of Hospital Managers Using Fuzzy AHP and Fuzzy TOPSIS: Iranian Experience. *Global Journal of Health Science, 8*(2), 137–155. doi:10.5539/gjhs.v8n2p137 PMID:26383216

Shahin, A., Shirouyehzad, H., & Pourjavad, E. (2012). Optimum maintenance strategy: A case study in the mining industry. *International Journal of Services and Operations Management, 12*(3), 368–386. doi:10.1504/IJSOM.2012.047626

Shah, N. (2004). Pharmaceutical supply chains: Key issues and strategies for optimization. *Computers & Chemical Engineering, 28*(6-7), 929–941. doi:10.1016/j.compchemeng.2003.09.022

Shamsara, E., Mostolizadeh, R., & Afsharnezhad, Z. (2016). Transcritical bifurcation of an immunosuppressive infection model. *Iranian Journal of Numerical Analysis and Optimization, 6*(2), 1–15.

Shannon, R. E. (1975). *Systems Simulation: The Art and Science*. Prentice-Hall.

Shannon, R. E. (1998). Introduction To The Art And Science Of Simulation. *Proceedings of the 1998 Winter Simulation Conference*. doi:10.1109/WSC.1998.744892

Shapiro, G. G. (2006). Among Young Children Who Wheeze, Which Children will have Persistent Asthma. *The Journal of Allergy and Clinical Immunology, 118*(3), 562–564. doi:10.1016/j.jaci.2006.07.011 PMID:16950270

Sharma, N., & Aggrawal, L. (2010). Automated medical image segmentation techniques. *Journal of Medical Physics, 35*(1), 3–14. doi:10.4103/0971-6203.58777 PMID:20177565

Sharma, U., Danishad, K. K. A., Seenu, V., & Jagannathan, N. R. (2009). Longitudinal study of the assessment by MRI and diffusion-weighted imaging of tumor response in patients with locally advanced breast cancer undergoing neoadjuvant chemotherapy. *NMR in Biomedicine, 22*(1), 104–113. doi:10.1002/nbm.1245 PMID:18384182

Shena, Y., Colloc, J., Jacquet-Andrieub, A., & Leia, K. (2015). Emerging medical informatics with case-based reasoning for aiding clinical decision in multi-agent system. *Journal of Biomedical Informatics, 56*, 307–317. doi:10.1016/j.jbi.2015.06.012 PMID:26133480

Shen, S., Sandham, W., Granat, M., & Sterr, A. (2005). MRI fuzzy segmentation of brain tissue using neighborhood attraction with neural-network optimization. *IEEE Transactions on Information Technology in Biomedicine, 9*(3), 459–467. doi:10.1109/TITB.2005.847500

Shi, P., Chou, M., Dai, J., Ding, D., & Sim, J. (2015). Models and Insights for Hospital Inpatient Operations: Time Dependent ED Boarding Time. *Management Science, 24*, 13–14.

Shirdel, A., Hashemzadeh, K., Sahebari, M., Rafatpanah, H., Hatef, M. R., Rezaieyazdi, Z., & Farid-Hosseini, R. et al. (2013). Is there any association between human lymphotropic virus type I (HTLV-I) infection and systemic lupus erythematosus? An Original Research and Literature Review. *Iranian Journal of Basic Medical Sciences., 16*, 252–257. PMID:24470872

Shouman, M., Turner, T., & Stocker, R. (2012, March). Using data mining techniques in heart disease diagnosis and treatment. In *Electronics, Communications and Computers (JEC-ECC), 2012 Japan-Egypt Conference on* (pp. 173-177). IEEE.

Shu, Y., & Cheriet, F. (2005). *Segmentation of Laparoscopic Images: Integrating Graph-Based Segmentation and Multistage Region Merging*. Paper presented at the Computer and Robot Vision.

Shu, H., Wang, L., & Watmough, J. (2014). Sustained and transient oscillation and chaos induced by delayed antiviral immune response in an immunosuppressive infection model. *Journal of Mathematical Biology, 68*(1-2), 477–503. doi:10.1007/s00285-012-0639-1 PMID:23306425

Shvachko, K., Kuang, H., Radia, S., & Chansler, R. (2010). The hadoop distributed file system. In *IEEE 26th Symposium Mass Storage Systems and Technologies*, 1-10. doi:10.1109/MSST.2010.5496972

Shyjith, K., Ilangkumaran, M., & Kumanan, S. (2008). Multi-criteria decision-making approach to evaluate optimum maintenance strategy in textile industry. *Journal of Quality in Maintenance Engineering, 14*(4), 375–386. doi:10.1108/13552510810909975

Siddharthan, K., Jones, W. J., & Johnson, J. A. (1996). A priority queuing model to reduce waiting times in emergency care. *International Journal of Health Care Quality Assurance, 9*(5), 10–16. doi:10.1108/09526869610124993 PMID:10162117

Simon, R., & Canacari, E. (2012). A Practical Guide to Applying Lean Tools and Management Principles to Health Care Improvement Projects. *Association of Perioperative Registered Nurses Journal, 95*(1), 85–100. doi:10.1016/j.aorn.2011.05.021 PMID:22201573

Singh, R. P., Farney, A. C., Rogers, J., Zuckerman, J., Reeves-Daniel, A., Hartmann, E., & Stratta, R. J. et al. (2011). Kidney Transplantation From donation after cardiac death donors: Lack of impact of delayed graft function on post-transplant outcomes. *Journal of Clinical Transplantation, 25*(2), 255–264. doi:10.1111/j.1399-0012.2010.01241.x PMID:20331689

Sinreich, D., & Jabali, O. (2007). Staggered work shifts: A way to downsize and restructure an emergency department workforce yet maintain current operational performance. *Health Care Management Science, 10*(3), 293–308. doi:10.1007/s10729-007-9021-z PMID:17695139

Sinreich, D., & Marmor, Y. (2005). Emergency department operations: The basis for developing a simulation tool. *IIE Transactions, 37*(3), 233–245. doi:10.1080/07408170590899625

Skevofilakas, M., Zarkogianni, K., Karamanos, B. G., & Nikita, K. S. (2010, August). A hybrid Decision Support System for the risk assessment of retinopathy development as a long term complication of Type 1 Diabetes Mellitus. In *2010 Annual International Conference of the IEEE Engineering in Medicine and Biology* (pp. 6713-6716). IEEE.

Skolarikos, A., Alivizatos, G., & Delarosette, J. (2005). Percutaneous Nephrolithotomy and its Legacy. *European Urology, 47*(1), 22–28. doi:10.1016/j.eururo.2004.08.009 PMID:15582245

SMA (Spanish Maintenance Association). (2000). *El Mantenimiento en España*. Barcelona: Spanish Maintenance Association.

Smeulders, A. W. M., Worring, M., Santini, S., Gupta, A., & Jain, R. (2000). Content-based image retrieval at the end of the early years. *IEEE Transactions on Pattern Analysis and Machine Intelligence, 22*(12), 1349–1380. doi:10.1109/34.895972

Smitha, P., Shaji, L., & Mini, M. G. (2011). A review of medical image classification techniques. *International Conference on VLSI, Communication & Instrumentation*, 34-38.

Smith, D. J., Forrest, S., Ackley, D. H., & Perelson, A. S. (1999). Variable efficacy of repeated annual influenza vaccination. *Proceedings of the National Academy of Sciences of the United States of America, 96*(24), 14001–14006. doi:10.1073/pnas.96.24.14001 PMID:10570188

Snow, J. (1855). *On the mode of communication of cholera*. London: UCLA. Retrieved 21 January 2017 from http://www.ph.ucla.edu/epi/snow/snowbook.html

Sockett, P., Garnett, M., & Scott, C. (1996). Communicable disease surveillance; Notification of infectious diseases in Canada. *The Canadian Journal of Infectious Diseases & Medical Microbiology, 7*(5), 293–295. PMID:22514452

Solez, K., Axelsen, R. A., Benediktsson, H., Burdick, J. F., Cohen, A. H., Colvin, R. B., & Yamaguchi, Y. et al. (1993). International standardization of criteria for the histologic diagnosis of renal allograft rejection: The Banff working classification of kidney transplant pathology. *Kidney International, 44*(2), 411–422. doi:10.1038/ki.1993.259 PMID:8377384

Soliman, T. H. A., Sewissy, A. A., & Abdel Latif, H. (2010, November). A gene selection approach for classifying diseases based on microarray datasets. In *Computer Technology and Development (ICCTD), 2010 2nd International Conference on* (pp. 626-631). IEEE. doi:10.1109/ICCTD.2010.5645975

Song, X., & Li, Y. (2006). Global stability and periodic solution of a model for HTLV-I infection and ATL progression. *Applied Mathematics and Computation, 180*(1), 401–410. doi:10.1016/j.amc.2005.12.022

Soni, J., Ansari, U., Sharma, D., & Soni, S. (2011). Predictive data mining for medical diagnosis: An overview of heart disease prediction. *International Journal of Computers and Applications, 17*(8), 43–48. doi:10.5120/2237-2860

Soni, S., & Vyas, O. P. (2010). Using associative classifiers for predictive analysis in health care data mining. *International Journal of Computers and Applications, 4*(5), 33–37. doi:10.5120/821-1163

Sørensen, L., Gangeh, M. J., Shaker, S. B., & de Bruijne, M. (2007). Texture classification in pulmonary CT. In A. El-Baz & J. S. Sure (Eds.), *Lung Imaging and Computer Aided Diagnosis* (pp. 343–367). CRC Press.

Sousa, T., Liu, S., Papageorgiou, L., & Shaha, N. (2011). Global supply chain planning for pharmaceuticals. *Chemical Engineering Research and Design, 8*(9), 2396–2409.

Spaepen, K., Stroobants, S., Dupont, P., Van Steenweghen, S., Thomas, J., Vandenberghe, P., & Verhoef, G. et al. (2001). Prognostic value of positron emission tomography (PET) with fluorine-18 fluorodeoxyglucose ([18F]FDG) after first-line chemotherapy in non-Hodgkins lymphoma: Is [18F]FDG-PET a valid alternative to conventional diagnostic methods? *Journal of Clinical Oncology, 19*(2), 414–419. doi:10.1200/JCO.2001.19.2.414 PMID:11208833

Sparks, R., & Madabhushi, A. (2013). Explicit shape descriptors: Novel morphologic features for histopathology classification. *Medical Image Analysis, 17*(8), 997–1009. doi:10.1016/j.media.2013.06.002 PMID:23850744

Speidel, S., Kroehnert, A., Bodenstedt, S., Kenngott, H., Müller-Stich, B., & Dillmann, R. (2015). *Image-based tracking of the suturing needle during laparoscopic interventions*. Paper presented at the Medical Imaging 2015: Image-based tracking of the suturing needle during laparoscopic interventions, Orlando, FL.

Spicer, N., Aleshkina, J., Biesma, R., Brugha, R., Caceres, C., Chilundo, B., & Ndubani, P. et al. (2010). National and subnational HIV/AIDS coordination: Are global health initiatives closing the gap between intent and practice?. *Globalization and Health, 6*(3). PMID:20196845

Spinello, L., Arras, K. O., Triebel, R., & Siegwart, R. (2010). A Layered Approach to People Detection in 3D Range Data. In *Twenty-Fourth AAAI Conference on Artificial Intelligence*. Atlanta, GA: AAAI Press.

Srihar, D., & Batniji, R. (2008). Misfinancing global health: A case for transparency in disbursements and decision making. *Lancet, 372*(9644), 1185–119. doi:10.1016/S0140-6736(08)61485-3 PMID:18926279

Srinivasan, S., Moser, R. P., Willis, G., Riley, W., Alexander, M., Berrigan, D., & Kobrin, S. (2015). Small is essential: Importance of subpopulation research in cancer control. *American Journal of Public Health, 105*(S3), S371–S373. doi:10.2105/AJPH.2014.302267 PMID:25905825

Srinivas, K., Rani, B. K., & Govrdhan, A. (2010). Applications of data mining techniques in healthcare and prediction of heart attacks. *International Journal on Computer Science and Engineering, 2*(02), 250–255.

Srinivasulu, A., & Reddy, M. S. (2012). Artifacts Removing From EEG Signals by ICA Algorithms. *IOS Journal of Electrical and Electronics Engineering, 2*(4), 11–16. doi:10.9790/1676-0241116

Stadtler, H. (2005). Supply chain management and advanced planning—basics, overview and challenges. *European Journal of Operational Research, 163*(3), 575–588. doi:10.1016/j.ejor.2004.03.001

Stadtler, H., & Kilger, C. (2008). *Supply Chain Management and Advanced Planning* (4th ed.). Springer. doi:10.1007/978-3-540-74512-9

Stanek, S. R., Tavanapong, W., Wonga, J., Oh, J. H., & Groenc, P. C. D. (2012). Automatic real-time detection of endoscopic procedures using temporal features. *Computer Methods and Programs in Biomedicine, 108*, 524-535.

State of New Jersey. (2013). *Communicable disease outbreak manual - vectorborne diseases.* Retrieved from http://njlmn2.rutgers.edu/sites/default/files/Appendix_T3_Vectorborne_outbreak_investigations.pdf

Statistics Canada. (2011). *Postal code conversion file.* Retrieved January 4, 2017, from http://www.statcan.gc.ca/daily-quotidien/110720/dq110720f-eng.htm

Steiner, S. H., Cook, R. J., Farewell, V. T., & Treasure, T. (2000). Monitoring surgical performance using risk-adjusted cumulative sum charts. *Biostatistics (Oxford, England), 1*(4), 441–452. doi:10.1093/biostatistics/1.4.441 PMID:12933566

Steiner, S. H., & Jones, M. (2010). Risk-adjusted survival time monitoring with an updating exponentially weighted moving average (EWMA) control chart. *Statistics in Medicine, 29*(4), 444–454. doi:10.1002/sim.3788 PMID:19908262

Sternberg, K. M., Eisner, B., Larson, T., Hernandez, N., Han, J., & Pais, V. M. (2016). Ultrasonography Significantly Overestimates Stone Size When Compared to Low-dose, Noncontrast Computed Tomography. *Urology, 95*, 67–71. doi:10.1016/j.urology.2016.06.002 PMID:27289025

Stilianakis, N. I., & Seydel, J. (1999). Modeling the T-cell dynamics and pathogenesis of HTLV-I infection. *Bulletin of Mathematical Biology, 61*(5), 935–947. doi:10.1006/bulm.1999.0117 PMID:17886750

Stoyanov, D., & Yang, G. Z. (2011). *Soft tissue deformation tracking for robotic assisted minimally invasive surgery.* Paper presented at the 2009 Annual International Conference of the IEEE Engineering in Medicine and Biology Society, Minneapolis, MN.

Stoyanov, D., Elson, D., & Yang, G. Z. (2009). *Illumination position estimation for 3D soft-tissue reconstruction in robotic minimally invasive surgery.* Paper presented at the 2009 IEEE/RSJ International Conference on Intelligent Robots and Systems, St. Louis, MO. doi:10.1109/IROS.2009.5354447

Stratta, R. J., Rohr, M. S., Sundberg, A. K., Armstrong, G., Hairston, G., Hartmann, E., & Adams, P. L. et al. (2004). Increased Kidney Transplantation Utilizing Expanded Criteria Deceased Organ Donors with Results Comparable to Standard Criteria Donor Transplant. *Annals of Surgery, 239*(5), 688–697. doi:10.1097/01.sla.0000124296.46712.67 PMID:15082973

Strunk, B. C., & Cunningham, P. J. (2002). *Treading water: Americans' access to needed medical care, 1997-2001.* Academic Press.

Subash, F., Dunn, F., McNicholl, B., & Marlow, J. (2004). Team triage improves emergency department efficiency. *Emergency Medicine Journal, 21*(5), 542–544. doi:10.1136/emj.2002.003665 PMID:15333524

Su, C. T., Yang, C. H., Hsu, K. H., & Chiu, W. K. (2006). Data mining for the diagnosis of type II diabetes from three-dimensional body surface anthropometrical scanning data. *Computers & Mathematics with Applications (Oxford, England)*, *51*(6), 1075–1092. doi:10.1016/j.camwa.2005.08.034

Sulaiman, S. N., & Isa, N. A. M. (2010). Adaptive fuzzy-K-means clustering algorithm for image segmentation. *IEEE Transactions on Consumer Electronics*, *56*(4), 2661–2668. doi:10.1109/TCE.2010.5681154

Sun, B. C., Hsia, R. Y., Weiss, R. E., Zingmond, D., Liang, L.-J., Han, W., & Asch, S. M. et al. (2013). Effect of emergency department crowding on outcomes of admitted patients. *Annals of Emergency Medicine*, *61*(6), 605–611. doi:10.1016/j.annemergmed.2012.10.026 PMID:23218508

Sundaramoorthy, A., Xianming, X., Karimi, I. A., & Srinivasan, R. (2006). An integrated model for planning in global chemical supply chains. *16th European Symposium on Computer Aided Process Engineering and 9th International Symposium on Process Systems Engineering*. doi:10.1016/S1570-7946(06)80373-1

Sun, X., & Wei, J. (2013). Global dynamics of a HTLV-I infection model with CTL response. *Electronic Journal of Qualitative Theory of Differential Equations*, *40*(40), 1–15. doi:10.14232/ejqtde.2013.1.40

Suresh, A., Harish, K. V., & Radhika, N. (2015). Particle swarm optimization over back propagation neural network for length of stay prediction. *Procedia Computer Science*, *46*, 268–275. doi:10.1016/j.procs.2015.02.020

Susarla, N., & Karimi, I. A. (2012). Integrated supply chain planning for multinational pharmaceutical enterprises. *Computers & Chemical Engineering*, *42*, 168–177. doi:10.1016/j.compchemeng.2012.03.002

Svantesson, T. (2006). Benchmarking in Europe. Proceedings of EuroMaintenance.

Swisher, J. R., Jacobson, S. H., Jun, J. B., & Balci, O. (2001). Modeling and analyzing a physician clinic environment using discrete-event (visual) simulation. *Computers & Operations Research*, *28*(2), 105–125. doi:10.1016/S0305-0548(99)00093-3

Tabakov, M. (2006, September). A fuzzy clustering technique for medical image segmentation. In *2006 International Symposium on Evolving Fuzzy Systems* (pp. 118-122). IEEE. doi:10.1109/ISEFS.2006.251140

Tadayyon, H., Sadeghi-Naini, A., & Czarnota, G. J. (2014). Noninvasive Characterization of Locally Advanced Breast Cancer Using Textural Analysis of Quantitative Ultrasound Parametric Images. *Translational Oncology*, *7*(6), 759–767. doi:10.1016/j.tranon.2014.10.007 PMID:25500086

Tadayyon, H., Sadeghi-Naini, A., Wirtzfeld, L., Wright, F. C., & Czarnota, G. J. (2014). Quantitative ultrasound characterization of locally advanced breast cancer by estimation of its scatterer properties. *Medical Physics*, *41*(1), 12903. doi:10.1118/1.4852875 PMID:24387530

Tadayyon, H., Sannachi, L., Gangeh, M., Sadeghi-Naini, A., Tran, W. T., Trudeau, M. E., & Czarnota, G. J. et al. (2016). Quantitative ultrasound assessment of breast tumor response to chemotherapy using a multi-parameter approach. *Oncotarget*, *7*(29), 45094–45111. PMID:27105515

Taghipour, S., Banjevic, D., & Jardine, A. K. S. (2011). Prioritization of medical equipment for maintenance decisions. *The Journal of the Operational Research Society*, *62*(9), 1666–1687. doi:10.1057/jors.2010.106

Taha, H. A. (2011). *Operations research. An introduction*. New York, NY: Prentice Hall.

Tai, Y. M., & Chiu, H. W. (2009). Comorbidity study of ADHD: Applying association rule mining (ARM) to National Health Insurance Database of Taiwan. *International Journal of Medical Informatics*, *78*(12), e75–e83. doi:10.1016/j.ijmedinf.2009.09.005

Tajadod, M., Abedini, M., Rategari, A., & Mobin, M. (2016). A Comparison of Multi-Criteria Decision Making Approaches for Maintenance Strategy Selection (A Case Study). *International Journal of Strategic Decision Sciences*, 7(3), 51–69. doi:10.4018/IJSDS.2016070103

Tam, J. (1999). Delay effect in a model for virus replication. *IMA Journal of Mathematics Applied in Medicine and Biology*, 16(1), 29–37. doi:10.1093/imammb/16.1.29 PMID:10335599

Taneja, A. (2013). Heart disease prediction system using data mining techniques. *Orient. J. Comput. Sci. Technol.*

Tan, P., Steinbach, M., & Kumar, V. (2006). *Introduction to Data Mining*. Pearson Addison Wesley.

Tan, S. (2006). *Introduction to Data*. Pearson Addison Wesley.

Taylor, R. C. (2010). An overview of the Hadoop/MapReduce/HBase framework and its current applications in bioinformatics. *BMC Bioinformatics*, 11(Suppl 12), S1. doi:10.1186/1471-2105-11-S12-S1 PMID:21210976

Tekieh, M. H., & Raahemi, B. (2015). Importance of Data Mining in Healthcare: A Survey. In *Proceedings of the 2015 IEEE/ACM International Conference on Advances in Social Networks Analysis and Mining 2015* (pp. 1057–1062). New York: ACM. doi:10.1145/2808797.2809367

Tekieh, M. H., Raahemi, B., & Izad Shenas, S. A. (2015). Analysing healthcare coverage with data mining techniques. *International Journal of Society Systems Science*, 7(3), 198–221. doi:10.1504/IJSSS.2015.071315

Temurtas, H., Yumusak, N., & Temurtas, F. (2009). A comparative study on diabetes disease diagnosis using neural networks. *Expert Systems with Applications*, 36(4), 8610–8615. doi:10.1016/j.eswa.2008.10.032

Terrazas-Moreno, S., & Grossmann, I. (2011). A multiscale decomposition method for the optimal planning and scheduling of multisite continuous multiproduct plants. *Chemical Engineering Science*, 66(19), 4307–4318.

Thacker, S. B., & Berkelman, R. L. (1988). Public health surveillance in the united states. *Epidemiologic Reviews*, 10. PMID:3066626

Thacker, S. B., & Stroup, D. F. (1994). Future Directions for Comprehensive Public Health Surveillance and Health Information Systems in the United States. *American Journal of Epidemiology*, 140(5), 383–397. doi:10.1093/oxfordjournals.aje.a117261 PMID:8067331

The Four V's of Big Data. (2013). Retrieved May 31, 2016, from: http://www.ibmbigdatahub.com/infographic/four-vs-big-data

Thomas, F., Regis, G., Vincent, A., Xiaolan, X., & Emilie, A. (2015). Performance Evaluation Of An Integrated Care For Geriatric Departments Using Discrete-Event Simulation. *Proceedings of the 2015 Winter Simulation Conference*.

Thomopoulos, N. T. (2012). *Essentials of Monte Carlo simulation: Statistical methods for building simulation models.* Springer Science & Business Media.

Thusoo, A., Sarma, J. S., Jain, N., Shao, Z., Chakka, P., Anthony, S., & Murthy, R. et al. (2009). Hive: a warehousing solution over a map-reduce framework. *Proc VLDB Endowment*, 2(2), 1626–1629. doi:10.14778/1687553.1687609

Titiunik, R. (2015). Can big data solve the fundamental problem of causal inference? *PS Polit Sci Polit*, 48(01), 75–79. doi:10.1017/S1049096514001772

Tjandrasa, H., Arieshanti, I., & Anggoro, R. (2014). Classification of non-proliferative diabetic retinopathy based on segmented exudates using K-Means clustering. *International Journal of Image. Graphics and Signal Processing*, 7(1), 1–8. doi:10.5815/ijigsp.2015.01.01

Tollman, P., Morieux, Y., Murphy, J., & Schulze, U. (2011). *Can R&D be fixed? Lessons from Biopharma outliers*. The Boston Consulting Group.

Torricelli, F. C. M., Marchini, G. S., Yamauchi, F. I., Danilovic, A., Vicentini, F. C., Srougi, M., & Mazzucchi, E. et al. (2015). Impact of Renal Anatomy on Shock Wave Lithotripsy Outcomes for Lower Pole Kidney Stones: Results of a Prospective Multifactorial Analysis Controlled by Computerized Tomography. *The Journal of Urology, 193*(6), 2002–2007. doi:10.1016/j.juro.2014.12.026 PMID:25524240

Tortevoye, P., Tuppin, P., Carles, G., Peneau, C., & Gessain, A. (2005). Comparative trends of seropreval-ence and se-roincidence rates of human T cell lymphotropic virus type I and human immunodeficiency virus 1 in pregnant women of various ethnic groups sharing the same environment in French Guiana. *The American Journal of Tropical Medicine and Hygiene, 73*(3), 560565. PMID:16172481

Totten, S., Maclean, R., Payne, E., & Severini, A. (2015). Chlamydia and lymphogranuloma venereum in Canada: 2003- 2013 summary report. *Canada Communicable Disease Report, 41*(2). Retrieved from http://www.phac-aspc.gc.ca/publicat/ccdr-rmtc/15vol41/dr-rm41-02/surv-1-eng.php

Toussi, M., Lamy, J. B., Le Toumelin, P., & Venot, A. (2009). Using data mining techniques to explore physicians therapeutic decisions when clinical guidelines do not provide recommendations: Methods and example for type 2 diabetes. *BMC Medical Informatics and Decision Making, 9*(1), 1. doi:10.1186/1472-6947-9-28

Tranmer, J. E., Colley, L., Edge, D. S., Sears, K., VanDenKerkhof, E., & Levesque, L. (2015). Trends in nurse practitioners prescribing to older adults in Ontario, 20002010: A retrospective cohort study. *CMAJ Open, 3*(3), E299–E304. doi:10.9778/cmajo.20150029 PMID:26457291

Treigny, O. M. D., Nasr, E. B., Almont, T., Tack, I., Rischmann, P., Souli, M., & Huyghe, E. (2015). The Cumulated Stone Diameter: A Limited Tool for Stone Burden Estimation. *Urology, 86*(3), 477–481. doi:10.1016/j.urology.2015.06.018 PMID:26135811

Tromberg, B. J., Shah, N., Lanning, R., Cerussi, A., Espinoza, J., Pham, T., & Butler, J. et al. (2000). Non-Invasive in vivo characterization of breast tumors using photon migration spectroscopy. *Neoplasia (New York, N.Y.), 2*(1–2), 26–40. doi:10.1038/sj.neo.7900082 PMID:10933066

Troyanskaya, O., Cantor, M., Sherlock, G., Brown, P., Hastie, T., Tibshirani, R., & Altman, R. B. et al. (2001). Missing value estimation methods for DNA microarrays. *Bioinformatics (Oxford, England), 17*(6), 520–525. doi:10.1093/bioinformatics/17.6.520 PMID:11395428

Tu, S. C., Wu, C. C., Hung, C. J., & Chen, J. S. (2010, August). A study for anaesthesia methods in total knee arthroplasties based on data mining. In *Electronics and Information Engineering (ICEIE), 2010 International Conference on (Vol. 1*, pp. V1-61). IEEE. doi:10.1109/ICEIE.2010.5559838

Tuceryan, M., & Jain, A. K. (1998). Texture analysis. In C. H. Chen, L. F. Pau, & P. S. P. Wang (Eds.), *Handbook of Pattern Recognition and Computer Vision* (pp. 207–248). World Scientific Publishing Co.

Tuite, A. R., Tien, J., Eisenberg, M., Earn, D. J. D., Ma, J., & Fisman, D. N. (2011). Cholera Epidemic in Haiti, 2010: Using a Transmission Model to Explain Spatial Spread of Disease and Identify Optimal Control Interventions. *Annals of Internal Medicine, 154*(9), 593–601. doi:10.7326/0003-4819-154-9-201105030-00334 PMID:21383314

Übeyli, E. D., & Doğdu, E. (2010). Automatic detection of erythemato-squamous diseases using k-means clustering. *Journal of Medical Systems, 34*(2), 179–184. doi:10.1007/s10916-008-9229-6

Uecker, D. R., Wang, Y. F., Lee, C., & Wang, Y. (1995). Laboratory Investigation:Automated Instrument Tracking in Robotically Assisted Laparoscopic Surgery. *Journal of Image Guided Surgery, 1*(6), 308–325. doi:10.1002/(SICI)1522-712X(1995)1:6<308::AID-IGS3>3.0.CO;2-E PMID:9080352

Uniyal, N., Eskandari, H., Abolmaesumi, P., Sojoudi, S., Gordon, P., Warren, L., & Moradi, M. et al. (2015). Ultrasound RF time series for classification of breast lesions. *IEEE Transactions on Medical Imaging, 34*(2), 652–661. doi:10.1109/TMI.2014.2365030 PMID:25350925

Uthayakumar, R., & Priyan, S. (2013). Pharmaceutical supply chain and inventory management strategies: Optimization for a pharmaceutical company and a hospital. *Operations Research for Health Care, 2*(3), 52–64. doi:10.1016/j.orhc.2013.08.001

Vahdani, B., Hadipour, H., Sadaghiani, J. S., & Amiri, M. (2010). Extension of VIKOR method based on interval-valued fuzzy sets. *International Journal of Advanced Manufacturing Technology, 47*(9-12), 1231–1239. doi:10.1007/s00170-009-2241-2

Valcarce, E. G., Cerrato, A. O., Fuentes, F. L., Mondéjar, J. M., Fernández, G. M., Rubio, E. L., & Roldán, C. G. et al. (2009). Short Cold Ischemia Time Optimises Transplant results for kidneys from expanded criteria donors. *Journal of Nefrologia, 29*(5), 456–463. PMID:19820758

Valuck, R. J., Anderson, H. O., Libby, A. M., Brandt, E., Bryan, C., Allen, R. R., & Pace, W. D. et al. (2012). Enhancing electronic health record measurement of depression severity and suicide ideation: A distributed ambulatory research in therapeutics network (DARTNet) study. *Journal of the American Board of Family Medicine, 25*(5), 582–593. doi:10.3122/jabfm.2012.05.110053 PMID:22956694

van der Heijden, F., Duin, R. P. W., de Ridder, D., & Tax, D. M. J. (2004). *Classification, Parameter Estimation and State Estimation.* John Wiley & Sons, Ltd. doi:10.1002/0470090154

Van Horn, J. D., & Toga, A. W. (2014). Human neuroimaging as a Big Data science. *Brain Imaging and Behavior, 8*(2), 323–331. doi:10.1007/s11682-013-9255-y PMID:24113873

van Laarhoven, P. J. M., & Pedrycz, W. (1983). A fuzzy extension of Saatys priority theory. *Fuzzy Sets and Systems, 11*(1-3), 229–241. doi:10.1016/S0165-0114(83)80082-7

Van Uden, C. J. T., Winkens, R. A. G., Wesseling, G. J., Crebolder, H. F. J. M., & Van Schayck, C. P. (2003). Use of out of hours services: A comparison between two organisations. *Emergency Medicine Journal, 20*(2), 184–187. doi:10.1136/emj.20.2.184 PMID:12642541

van Walraven, C. (2013). Trends in 1-year survival of people admitted to hospital in Ontario, 1994–2009. *Canadian Medical Association Journal.*

Varma, M., & Zisserman, A. (2005). A Statistical approach to texture classification from single images. *International Journal of Computer Vision: Special Issue on Texture Analysis and Synthesis, 62*(1–2), 61–81. doi:10.1007/s11263-005-4635-4

Varma, M., & Zisserman, A. (2009). A statistical approach to material classification using image patch exemplars. *IEEE Transactions on Pattern Analysis and Machine Intelligence, 31*(11), 2032–2047. doi:10.1109/TPAMI.2008.182 PMID:19762929

Varma, V. A., Pekny, J. F., Blau, G. E., & Reklaitis, G. V. (2008). A framework for addressing stochastic and combinatorial aspects of scheduling and resource allocation in pharmaceutical R&D pipelines. *Computers & Chemical Engineering, 32*(4-5), 1000–1015. doi:10.1016/j.compchemeng.2007.05.006

Vieira, I. T., Cheng, R. C. H., Harper, P. R., & Senna, V. (2010). Small world network models of the dynamics of HIV infection. *Annals of Operations Research*, *178*(1), 173–200. doi:10.1007/s10479-009-0571-y

Vigário, R., Sarela, J., Jousmiki, V., Hamalainen, M., & Oja, E. (2000). Independent component approach to the analysis of EEG and MEG recordings. *IEEE Transactions on Bio-Medical Engineering*, *47*(5), 589–593. doi:10.1109/10.841330 PMID:10851802

Vijayarani, S., Dhayanand, M. S., & Phil, M. (2015). Kidney disease prediction using svm and ann algorithms. *International Journal of Computing and Business Research*, 2229-6166.

Villa-Parish, A. R., Lvy, J., King, R. E., & Abel, S. R. (2012). Patient-based pharmaceutical inventory management: A two-stage inventory and production model for perishable products with Markovian demand. *Health Systems*, *1*(1), 69–83. doi:10.1057/hs.2012.2

Vimala, G. A. G., & Mohideen, S. K. (2013, January). Automatic detection of optic disk and exudate from retinal images using clustering algorithm. In *Intelligent Systems and Control (ISCO), 2013 7th International Conference on* (pp. 280-284). IEEE.

Vlad, R. M., Brand, S., Giles, A., Kolios, M. C., & Czarnota, G. J. (2009). Quantitative ultrasound characterization of responses to radiotherapy in cancer mouse models. *Clinical Cancer Research*, *15*(6), 2067–2074. doi:10.1158/1078-0432.CCR-08-1970 PMID:19276277

Vogel, C., & Funk, M. (2008). Measles Quarantine—The Individual and the Public. *Journal of Travel Medicine*, *15*(2), 65–67. doi:10.1111/j.1708-8305.2008.00182.x PMID:18346237

Voros, S., Long, J. A., & Clinquin, P. (2007). Automatic Detection of Instruments in Laparoscopic Images: A First Step Towards High-level Command of Robotic Endoscopic Holders. *The International Journal of Robotics Research*, *26*(11-12), 1173–1190. doi:10.1177/0278364907083395

Waldert, S., Pistohl, T., Braun, C., Ball, T., Aertsen, A., & Mehring, C. (2009). A review on directional information in neural signals for brain-machine interfaces. *Journal of Physiology, Paris*, *103*(3), 244–254. doi:10.1016/j.jphysparis.2009.08.007 PMID:19665554

Wang, L., Chen, D., Ranjan, R., Khan, S. U., KolOdziej, J., & Wang, J. (2012). Parallel Processing of Massive EEG Data with MapReduce. ICPADS, 164–171.

Wang, W., Richards, G., & Rea, S. (2005, September). Hybrid data mining ensemble for predicting osteoporosis risk. *27th Int. Conf. on Engineering in Medicine and Biology*, 886-889. doi:10.1109/IEMBS.2005.1616557

Wang, Y., & Yu, H. (2013). An ultralow-power memory-based big-data computing platform by nonvolatile domain-wall nanowire devices. In *Proceedings of the International Symposium on Low Power Electronics and Design*. IEEE Press.

Wang, F., Lee, R., Liu, Q., Aji, A., Zhang, X., & Saltz, J. (2011). Hadoop-gis: A high performance query system for analytical medical imaging with mapreduce. Emory University.

Wang, H., Naghavi, M., Allen, C., Barber, R. M., Bhutta, Z. A., Carter, A., & Coggeshall, M. et al. (2016). Global, regional, and national life expectancy, all-cause mortality, and cause-specific mortality for 249 causes of death, 1980–2015: A systematic analysis for the Global Burden of Disease Study 2015. *Lancet*, *388*(10053), 1459–1544. doi:10.1016/S0140-6736(16)31012-1 PMID:27733281

Wang, H., Zhang, Y., Waytowich, N. R., Krusienski, D. J., Zhou, G., Jin, J., & Cichocki, A. (2016). Discriminative feature extraction via multivariate linear regression for SSVEP-based BCI. *IEEE Transactions on Neural Systems and Rehabilitation Engineering*, *24*(5), 532–541. doi:10.1109/TNSRE.2016.2519350 PMID:26812728

Wang, J., Fan, K., & Wang, W. (2010). Integration of fuzzy AHP and FPP with TOPSIS methodology for aeroengine health assessment. *Expert Systems with Applications*, *37*(12), 8516–8526. doi:10.1016/j.eswa.2010.05.024

Wang, K., Fan, A., & Torres, A. (2010). Global properties of an improved hepatitis B virus model. *Nonlinear Analysis Real World Applications*, *11*(4), 3131–3138. doi:10.1016/j.nonrwa.2009.11.008

Wang, K., Wang, W., Pang, H., & Liu, X. (2007). Complex dynamic behavior in a viral model with delayed immune response. *Physica D. Nonlinear Phenomena*, *226*(2), 197–208. doi:10.1016/j.physd.2006.12.001

Wang, L., Chu, J., & Wu, J. (2007). Selection of optimum maintenance strategies based on a fuzzy analytic hierarchy process. *International Journal of Production Economics*, *107*(1), 151–163. doi:10.1016/j.ijpe.2006.08.005

Wang, L., Li, M. Y., & Kirschner, D. (2002). Mathematical analysis of the global dynamics of a model for HTLV-I infection and ATL progression. *Mathematical Biosciences*, *179*(2), 207–217. doi:10.1016/S0025-5564(02)00103-7 PMID:12208616

Wang, Q., & Zheng, M. (2010). An improved KNN based outlier detection algorithm for large datasets. *Advanced Data Mining and Applications*, *6440*, 585–592. doi:10.1007/978-3-642-17316-5_56

Wang, S., Cong, Y., Cao, J., Yang, Y., Tang, Y., Zhao, H., & Yu, H. (2016). Scalable gastroscopic video summarization via similar-inhibition dictionary selection. *Artificial Intelligence in Medicine*, *66*, 1–13. doi:10.1016/j.artmed.2015.08.006 PMID:26363682

Wang, T., Guinet, A., Belaidi, A., & Besombes, B. (2009). Modelling and simulation of emergency services with ARIS and Arena. Case study: The emergency department of Saint Joseph and Saint Luc Hospital. *Production Planning and Control*, *20*(6), 484–495. doi:10.1080/09537280902938605

Wang, W., Haerian, K., Salmasian, H., Harpaz, R., Chase, H., & Friedman, C. (2011). A drug-adverse event extraction algorithm to support pharmacovigilance knowledge mining from PubMed citations. In *AMIA Annual Symposium Proceedings* (pp. 14-64). Bethesda, MD: American Medical Informatics Association.

Wang, Y., Goh, W., Wong, L., & Montana, G. (2013). Random forests on Hadoop for genome-wide association studies of multivariate neuroimaging phenotypes. *BMC Bioinformatics*, *14*(16), 1–15. doi:10.1186/1471-2105-14-S4-S1 PMID:24564704

Watanabe, K., Tanaka, H., Takahashi, K., Niimura, Y., Watanabe, K., & Kurihara, Y. (2016). NIRS-Based Language Learning BCI System. *IEEE Sensors Journal*, *16*(8), 2726–2734. doi:10.1109/JSEN.2016.2519886

Wattel, E., Vartanian, J. P., Pannetier, C., & Wain-Hobson, S. (1995). Clonal expansion of human T cell leukemia virus type I-infected cells in asymptomatic and symptomatic carriers without malignancy. *Journal of Virology*, *69*, 2863–2868. PMID:7707509

Way, T. K., Lau, H. C., & Lee, F. C. Y. (2013). Improving Patient Length-Of-Stay In Emergency Department Through Dynamic Queue Management. *Proceedings of the 2013 Winter Simulation Conference*.

Weber, W. A., Petersen, V., Schmidt, B., Tyndale-Hines, L., Link, T., Peschel, C., & Schwaiger, M. (2003). Positron emission tomography in non–small-cell lung cancer: Prediction of response to chemotherapy by quantitative assessment of glucose use. *Journal of Clinical Oncology*, *21*(14), 2651–2657. doi:10.1200/JCO.2003.12.004 PMID:12860940

Wei, G. Q., Arbter, K., & Hirzinger, G. (1997). Real-time visual servoing for laparoscopic surgery. Controlling robot motion with color image segmentation. *IEEE Engineering in Medicine and Biology Magazine*, *16*(1), 40–45. doi:10.1109/51.566151 PMID:9058581

Weil, G., Heus, K., Francois, P., & Poujade, M. (1995). Constraint programming for nurse scheduling. *Engineering in Medicine and Biology Magazine, IEEE, 14*(4), 417–422. doi:10.1109/51.395324

Weiner, M. W., Veitch, D. P., Aisen, P. S., Beckett, L. A., Cairns, N. J., Green, R. C., & Trojanowski, J. Q. et al. (2012). The Alzheimers disease neuroimaging initiative: A review of papers published since its inception. *Alzheimers & Dementia, 8*(1Suppl), S1–S68. doi:10.1016/j.jalz.2011.09.172 PMID:22047634

Weiss, G., & Provost, F. (2001). *The effect of class distribution on classifier learning: An empirical study.* Academic Press.

Weng, S.-J., Cheng, B.-C., Kwong, S. T., Wang, L.-M., & Chang, C.-Y. (2011). Simulation Optimization for Emergency Department Resources Allocation. In *Proceedings of the 2011 Winter Simulation Conference.* Piscataway, NJ: Institute of Electrical and Electronics Engineers. doi:10.1109/WSC.2011.6147845

Weng, S. J., Cheng, B. C., Kwong, S. T., Wang, L. M., & Chang, C. Y. (2011, December). Simulation optimization for emergency department resources allocation. *Simulation Conference (WSC) Proceedings,* 1231–1238.

Wen, Z., Liu, Z. P., Liu, Z., Zhang, Y., & Chen, L. (2013). An integrated approach to identify causal network modules of complex diseases with application to colorectal cancer. *Journal of the American Medical Informatics Association, 20*(4), 659–667. doi:10.1136/amiajnl-2012-001168 PMID:22967703

Whalley, S. A., Murray, J. M., Brown, D., Webster, G. J., Emery, V. C., Dusheiko, G. M., & Perelson, A. S. (2001). Kinetics of acute hepatitis B virus infection in humans. *The Journal of Experimental Medicine, 193*(7), 847–854. doi:10.1084/jem.193.7.847 PMID:11283157

Wheelhouse, P. J. (2009). Benchmarking Maintenance & Asset Management for Performance Improvement. *Proceedings of the 22nd International Congress on Condition Monitoring and Diagnostic Engineering Management - COMADEM 2009,* 81-87.

White, T. (2012). *Hadoop: The Definitive Guide.* Sebastopol, CA: O'Reilly Media, Inc.

WHO. (2017). *Chronic respiratory diseases: Asthma.* Retrieved January 22, 2017, from: http://www.who.int/respiratory/asthma/en/

Wiechers, I. R., Leslie, D. L., & Rosenheck, R. A. (2013). Prescribing of psychotropic medications to patients without a psychiatric diagnosis. *Psychiatric Services (Washington, D.C.), 64*(12), 1243–1248. doi:10.1176/appi.ps.201200557 PMID:23999894

Wiesenthal, J. D., Ghiculete, D., Ray, A., Honey, R. J. D., & Pace, K. T. (2011). A clinical nomogram to predict the successful shockwave lithotripsy of renal and ureteral calculi. *European Urology Supplements, 10*(2), 38. doi:10.1016/S1569-9056(11)60034-1

Wiinamaki, A., & Dronzek, R. (2003, December). Emergency departments I: using simulation in the architectural concept phase of an emergency department design. *Proceedings of the 35th conference on Winter simulation: driving innovation,* 1912-1916.

Williams, A. E., Fang, C. T., Slamon, D. J., Poiesz, B., Sandler, S., Darr, W., & et, et al.. (1988). Seroprevalence and epidemiological correlates of HTLV–I infection in U. S. blood donors. *Science, 240*(4852), 643–646. doi:10.1126/science.2896386 PMID:2896386

Wilson, S. E., Lipscombe, L. L., Rosella, L. C., & Manuel, D. G. (2009). Trends in laboratory testing for diabetes in Ontario, Canada 1995–2005: A population-based study. *BMC Health Services Research, 9*(1), 41. doi:10.1186/1472-6963-9-41 PMID:19250533

Wireman, T. (1990). *World Class Maintenance Management.* New York, NY: Industrial Press Inc.

Wireman, T. (2004). *Benchmarking best practices in maintenance management*. New York, NY: Industrial Press Inc.

Wodarz, D., & Nowak, M. A. (1999). Specific therapy regimes could lead to long-term control of HIV. *Proceedings of the National Academy of Sciences of the United States of America, 96*(25), 14464–14469. doi:10.1073/pnas.96.25.14464 PMID:10588728

Wodarz, D., Page, K. M., Arnaout, R. A., Thomsen, A. R., Lifson, J. D., & Nowak, M. A. (2000). A new theory of cytotoxic T-lymphocyte memory: Implications for HIV treatment. *Philosophical Transactions of the Royal Society of London. Series B, Biological Sciences, 355*(1395), 329–343. doi:10.1098/rstb.2000.0570 PMID:10794051

Wolf, R., Duchateau, J., Cinquin, P., & Voros, S. (2011). *3D Tracking of Laparoscopic Instruments Using Statistical and Geometric Modeling. In Medical Image Computing and Computer-Assisted Intervention-MICCAI 2011* (Vol. 6891, pp. 203–210). Springer. doi:10.1007/978-3-642-23623-5_26

Wolpaw, J. R., Birbaumer, N., Heetderks, W. J., McFarland, D. J., Peckham, P. H., Schalk, G., & Vaughan, T. M. (2000). Brain-computer interface technology: A review of the first international mee ting. *IEEE Transactions on Rehabilitation Engineering, 8*(2), 164–173. doi:10.1109/TRE.2000.847807 PMID:10896178

Wolpaw, J. R., Birbaumer, N., McFarland, D. J., Pfurtscheller, G., & Vaughan, T. M. (2002). Brain–computer interfaces for communication and control. *Clinical Neurophysiology, 113*(6), 767–791. doi:10.1016/S1388-2457(02)00057-3 PMID:12048038

Wolpaw, J. R., & McFarland, D. J. (1994). Multichannel EEG-based brain-computer communication. *Electroencephalography and Clinical Neurophysiology, 90*(6), 444–449. doi:10.1016/0013-4694(94)90135-X PMID:7515787

Woodall, W. H. (2006). The use of control charts in health-care and public-health surveillance. *Journal of Quality Technology, 38*, 89–104.

Woodward, G. L., Iverson, A., Harvey, R., & Blake, P. G. (2014). Implementation of an agency to improve chronic kidney disease care in Ontario: Lessons learned by the Ontario Renal Network. *Healthcare Quarterly (Toronto, Ont.), 17*, 44-47.

World Health Organisation. (1968). *National and global surveillance of communicable disease*. Retrieved 21 January 2017 from http://apps.who.int/iris/bitstream/10665/143764/1/WHA21_TD-2_eng.pdf

World Health Organisation. (2005). *International Health Regulations*. Geneva: Author.

Worthey, E., Mayer, A., Syverson, G., Helbling, D., Bonacci, B. B., Decker, B., & Dimmock, D. P. et al. (2013). Making a definitive diagnosis: Successful clinical application of whole exome sequencing in a child with intractable inflammatory bowel disease. *Genetics in Medicine, 13*(3), 255–262. doi:10.1097/GIM.0b013e3182088158 PMID:21173700

Wren, J. D., & Garner, H. R. (2005). Data-mining analysis suggests an epigenetic pathogenesis for type 2 diabetes. *BioMed Research International, 2005*(2), 104-112.

Wu, C. H., Chen, Y. C., Liu, C. Y., Chang, C. C., & Sun, Y. N. (2004). *Automatic extraction and visualization of human inner structures from endoscopic image sequences*. Paper presented at the SPIE2004. doi:10.1117/12.535880

Wu, C., Hannan, E. L., Walford, G., Ambrose, J. A., Holmes, D. R. Jr, King, S. B. III, & Jones, R. H. et al. (2006). A risk score to predict in-hospital mortality for percutaneous coronary interventions. *Journal of the American College of Cardiology, 47*(3), 654–660. doi:10.1016/j.jacc.2005.09.071

Wu, F. X., Wu, L., Wang, J., Liu, J., & Chen, L. (2014). Transittability of complex networks and its applications to regulatory biomolecular networks. *Scientific Reports, 4*, 1–10. PMID:24769565

Wu, L. T., Gersing, K. R., Swartz, M. S., Burchett, B., Li, T. K., & Blazer, D. G. (2013). Using electronic health records data to assess comorbidities of substance use and psychiatric diagnoses and treatment settings among adults. *Journal of Psychiatric Research*, *47*(4), 555–563. doi:10.1016/j.jpsychires.2012.12.009 PMID:23337131

Wu, Z., & Huang, N. E. (2009). Ensemble empirical mode decomposition: A noise-assisted data analysis method. *Advances in Adaptive Data Analysis*, *1*(1), 1–41. doi:10.1142/S1793536909000047

Wylie, J. L., & Jolly, A. (2001). Patterns of Chlamydia and Gonorrhea Infection in Sexual Networks in Manitoba, Canada. *Sexually Transmitted Diseases*, *28*(1), 14–24. doi:10.1097/00007435-200101000-00005 PMID:11196040

Xiaojing, J. (2010). Google Cloud Computing Platform Technology Architecture and the Impact of Its Cost. *2010 Second WRI World Congress on Software Engineering*, 17–20. doi:10.1109/WCSE.2010.93

Xiao, N., Sharman, R., Rao, H. R., & Dutta, S. (2012). A simulation-based study for managing hospital emergency departments capacity in extreme events. *International Journal of Business Excellence*, *5*(1-2), 140–154. doi:10.1504/IJBEX.2012.044578

Xie, J., Lei, J., Xie, W., Gao, X., Shi, Y., & Liu, X. (2012a, April). Novel hybrid feature selection algorithms for diagnosing erythemato-squamous diseases. In *International Conference on Health Information Science* (pp. 173-185). Springer Berlin Heidelberg. doi:10.1007/978-3-642-29361-0_21

Xie, J., Lei, J., Xie, W., Shi, Y., & Liu, X. (2013b). Two-stage hybrid feature selection algorithms for diagnosing erythemato-squamous diseases. *Health Information Science and Systems*, *1*(1), 1.

Xuan, X., & Liao, Q. (2007, August). Statistical structure analysis in MRI brain tumor segmentation. In *Image and Graphics, 2007. ICIG 2007. Fourth International Conference on* (pp. 421-426). IEEE. doi:10.1109/ICIG.2007.181

Xu, B., Gao, J., & Li, C. (2012). An efficient algorithm for DNA fragment assembly in MapReduce. *Biochemical and Biophysical Research Communications*, *426*(3), 395–398. doi:10.1016/j.bbrc.2012.08.101 PMID:22960169

Xu, R., & Wang, Q. (2015). Large-scale automatic extraction of side effects associated with targeted anticancer drugs from full-text oncological articles. *Journal of Biomedical Informatics*, *55*, 64–72. doi:10.1016/j.jbi.2015.03.009

Xu, Y., Li, D., Chen, Q., & Fan, Y. (2013). Full supervised learning for osteoporosis diagnosis using micro-CT images. *Microscopy Research and Technique*, *76*(4), 333–341. doi:10.1002/jemt.22171

Yalcin, B. (2013). Overview on locally advanced breast cancer: Defining, epidemiology, and overview on neoadjuvant therapy. *Experimental Oncology*, *35*(4), 250–252. PMID:24382433

Yamamoto, N., Okada, M., Koyanagi, Y., Kannagi, M., & Hinuma, Y. (1982). Transformation of human leukocytes by cocultivation with an adult T cell leukemia virus producer cell line. *Science*, *217*(4561), 737–739. doi:10.1126/science.6980467 PMID:6980467

Yang, C. S., Wei, C. P., Yuan, C. C., & Schoung, J. Y. (2010). Predicting the length of hospital stay of burn patients: Comparisons of prediction accuracy among different clinical stages. *Decision Support Systems*, *50*(1), 325–335. doi:10.1016/j.dss.2010.09.001

Yang, M.-C., Moon, W. K., Wang, Y.-C. F., Bae, M. S., Huang, C.-S., Chen, J.-H., & Chang, R.-F. (2013). Robust texture analysis using multi-resolution gray-scale invariant features for breast sonographic tumour diagnosis. *IEEE Transactions on Medical Imaging*, *32*(12), 2262–2273. doi:10.1109/TMI.2013.2279938 PMID:24001985

Yang, M., Krueger, T. M., Miller, J. G., & Holland, M. R. (2007). Characterization of anisotropic myocardial backscatter using spectral slope, intercept and midband fit parameters. *Ultrasonic Imaging*, *29*(2), 122–134. doi:10.1177/016173460702900204 PMID:17679326

Yann, F., Michael, M., & Uday, R. (2010). Comparing Two Operating Room Allocation Policies For Elective And Emergency Surgeries. *Proceedings of the 2010 Winter Simulation Conference.*

Yaramakala, S., & Margaritis, D. (2005). Speculative Markov blanket discovery for optimal feature selection. In *Fifth IEEE International Conference on Data Mining.* IEEE. doi:10.1109/ICDM.2005.134

Yasodha, P., & Kannan, M. (2011). Analysis of a Population of Diabetic Patients Databases in Weka Tool. *International Journal of Scientific & Engineering Research, 2*(5).

Yeh, D. Y., Cheng, C. H., & Chen, Y. W. (2011). A predictive model for cerebrovascular disease using data mining. *Expert Systems with Applications, 38*(7), 8970–8977. doi:10.1016/j.eswa.2011.01.114

Yıldırım, E. G., Karahoca, A., & Uçar, T. (2011). Dosage planning for diabetes patients using data mining methods. *Procedia Computer Science, 3*, 1374–1380. doi:10.1016/j.procs.2011.01.018

Yin, E., Zhou, Z., Jiang, J., Yu, Y., & Hu, D. (2015). A dynamically optimized SSVEP brain–computer interface (BCI) speller. *IEEE Transactions on Bio-Medical Engineering, 62*(6), 1447–1456. doi:10.1109/TBME.2014.2320948 PMID:24801483

Yi, P., George, S. K., Paul, J. A., & Lin, L. (2010). Hospital capacity planning for disaster emergency management. *Socio-Economic Planning Sciences, 44*(3), 151–160. doi:10.1016/j.seps.2009.11.002

Yip, M. C., Lowe, D. G., Salcudean, S. E., Rohling, R. N., & Nguan, C. Y. (2012). Real-Time Methods for Long-Term Tissue Feature Tracking in Endoscopic Scenes. In P. Abolmaesumi, L. Joskowicz, N. Navab, & P. Jannin (Eds.), *Information Processing in Computer-Assisted Interventions* (pp. 33–43). Springer Berlin Heidelberg. doi:10.1007/978-3-642-30618-1_4

Yoon, P., Steiner, I., & Reinhardt, G. (2003). Analysis of factors influencing length of stay in the emergency department. *Canadian Journal of Emergency Medical Care, 5*(03), 155–161. doi:10.1017/S1481803500006539 PMID:17472779

Yousefi Sarmad, M., & Pishvaee, M. S. (n.d.). A robust possibilistic Tactical Planning Model for Pharmaceutical Supply Chain under Disruption considering Lateral Transshipment and Deterioration. *2nd International Conference on Industrial & Systems Engineering (ICIS)*, 394-401.

Youyou, W., Kosinski, M., & Stillwell, D. (2015). Computer-based personality judgments are more accurate than those made by humans. *Proceedings of the National Academy of Sciences of the United States of America, 112*(4), 1036–1040. doi:10.1073/pnas.1418680112 PMID:25583507

Yu, Y., Nieto, J. J., Torres, A., & Wang, K. (2009). A viral infection model with a nonlinear infection rate. Boundary Value Problems, ArticleID 958016.

Yuan, L., Ding, G., Chen, Y. E., Chen, Z., & Li, Y. (2012). A novel strategy for deciphering dynamic conservation of gene expression relationship. *Journal of Molecular Cell Biology, 4*(3), 177–179. doi:10.1093/jmcb/mjs014 PMID:22498922

Yuan, Y., Zheng, X., & Lu, X. (2016). A discriminative representation for human action recognition. *Pattern Recognition, 59*, 88–97. doi:10.1016/j.patcog.2016.02.022

Yun, W. L., & Mookiah, M. R. K. (2013). Detection of diabetic retinopathy using k-means clustering and self-organizing map. *Journal of Medical Imaging and Health Informatics, 3*(4), 575–581. doi:10.1166/jmihi.2013.1207

Yu, X., Li, G., & Chen, L. (2014). Prediction and early diagnosis of complex diseases by edge-network. *Bioinformatics (Oxford, England), 30*(6), 852–859. doi:10.1093/bioinformatics/btt620 PMID:24177717

Yu, Z., Liu, J., Ding, H., Lu, M., Deng, M., Huang, Y., & Li, K. et al. (2015). An Image-Based Method of Uterus Segmentation in Gynecologic Laparoscopy. *Journal of Medical Imaging and Health Informatics, 5*(4), 819–825. doi:10.1166/jmihi.2015.1463

Zadeh, L. A. (1965). L. A. Fuzzy sets. *Information and Control, 8*(3), 338–353. doi:10.1016/S0019-9958(65)90241-X

Zaim, S., Turkyílmaz, A., Acar, M. F., Al-Turki, U., & Demirel, O. F. (2012). Maintenance strategy selection using AHP and ANP algorithms: A case study. *Journal of Quality in Maintenance Engineering, 18*(1), 16–29. doi:10.1108/13552511211226166

Zappella, L., Béjar, B., Hager, G., & Vidal, R. (2013). Surgical gesture classification from video and kinematic data. *Medical Image Analysis, 17*(7), 732–745. doi:10.1016/j.media.2013.04.007 PMID:23706754

Zellner, B. B., Rand, S. D., Prost, R., Krouwer, H., & Chetty, V. K. (2004). A cost-minimizing diagnostic methodology for discrimination between neoplastic and non-neoplastic brain lesions: Utilizing a genetic algorithm scientific reports. *Academic Radiology, 11*(2), 169–177. doi:10.1016/S1076-6332(03)00654-8 PMID:14974592

Zenbutsu, S., Igarashi, T., & Yamaguchi, T. (2013). Development of Blood Vessel Depth Displaying Method for Laparoscopic Surgery Guidance. *Journal of Medical Imaging and Health Informatics, 3*(1), 101–106. doi:10.1166/jmihi.2013.1134

Zeng, T., Zhang, C. C., Zhang, W., Liu, R., Liu, J., & Chen, L. (2014). Deciphering early development of complex diseases by progressive module network. *Methods (San Diego, Calif.), 67*(3), 334–343. doi:10.1016/j.ymeth.2014.01.021 PMID:24561825

Zeng, T., Zhang, W., Yu, X., Liu, X., Li, M., Liu, R., & Chen, L. N. (2014). Edge biomarkers for classification and prediction of phenotypes. *Sci China Life Sci, 57*(11), 1103–1114. doi:10.1007/s11427-014-4757-4 PMID:25326072

Zhang, Y., Wirkert, S. J., Iszatt, J., Kenngott, H., Wagner, M., Mayer, B., . . . Maier-Hein, L. (2016). *Tissue classification for laparoscopic image understanding based on multispectral texture analysis.* Paper presented at the Medical Imaging: Image-Guided Procedures, Robotic Interventions, and Modeling.

Zhang, D., Wang, Y., Zhou, L., Yuan, H., & Shen, D. (2011). Multimodal classification of Alzheimers disease and mild cognitive impairment. *NeuroImage, 55*(3), 856–867. doi:10.1016/j.neuroimage.2011.01.008

Zhang, K., Sun, F., Waterman, M. S., & Chen, T. (2003). Dynamic programming algorithms for haplotype block partitioning: applications to human chromosome 21 haplotype data. *Proceedings of the Seventh Annual International Conference on Research in Computational Molecular Biology*, 332–340. doi:10.1145/640075.640119

Zhang, L., Gan, F. F., & Loke, C. (2012). Phase I study of surgical performances with risk-adjusted Shewhart control charts. *Quality Technology & Quantitative Management, 9*(4), 375–382. doi:10.1080/16843703.2012.11673299

Zhang, W., Zeng, T., & Chen, L. (2014). EdgeMarker: Identifying differentially correlated molecule pairs as edge-biomarkers. *Journal of Theoretical Biology, 362*, 35–43. doi:10.1016/j.jtbi.2014.05.041 PMID:24931676

Zhang, X., & Payandeh, S. (2002). Application of Visual Tracking for Robot-Assisted Laparoscopic Surgery. *Journal of Robotic Systems, 19*(7), 315–328. doi:10.1002/rob.10043

Zhang, Y., Kim, C. W., Tee, K. F., & Lam, J. S. L. (2017). Optimal sustainable life cycle maintenance strategies for port infrastructures. *Journal of Cleaner Production, 142*(4), 1693–1709. doi:10.1016/j.jclepro.2016.11.120

Zhao, Z., & Ma, C. (2008, December). An intelligent system for noninvasive diagnosis of coronary artery disease with EMD-TEO and BP neural network. In *Education Technology and Training, 2008. and 2008 International Workshop on Geoscience and Remote Sensing. ETT and GRS 2008. International Workshop on* (Vol. 2, pp. 631-635). IEEE. doi:10.1109/ETTandGRS.2008.361

Zhao, Z. (2014). Real-time 3D visual tracking of laparoscopic instruments for robotized endoscope holder. *Bio-Medical Materials and Engineering*, *24*, 2665–2672. PMID:25226970

Zheng, B., Yoon, S. W., & Lam, S. S. (2014). Breast cancer diagnosis based on feature extraction using a hybrid of K-means and support vector machine algorithms. *Expert Systems with Applications*, *41*(4), 1476–1482. doi:10.1016/j.eswa.2013.08.044

Zhou, J., Chan, K. L., Chong, V. F. H., & Krishnan, S. M. (2006, January). Extraction of brain tumor from MR images using one-class support vector machine. In 2005 IEEE Engineering in Medicine and Biology 27th Annual Conference (pp. 6411-6414). IEEE.

Zhuang, B., Chen, T., Leung, C., Chan, K., Dixon, J., Dickie, K., & Pelissier, L. (2012). Microcalcification enhancement in ultrasound images from a concave automatic breast ultrasound scanner. *Proceedings of IEEE International Ultrasonics Symposium*, 1662–1665. doi:10.1109/ULTSYM.2012.0417

Zhu, H., Rao, R. S., Zeng, T., & Chen, L. (2012). Reconstructing dynamic gene regulatory networks from sample-based transcriptional data. *Nucleic Acids Research*, *40*(21), 10657–10667. doi:10.1093/nar/gks860 PMID:23002138

Zhu, H., & Zou, X. (2008). Impact of delays in cell infection and virus production o n HIV-1 dynamics. *Mathematical Medicine and Biology*, *25*(2), 99–112. doi:10.1093/imammb/dqm010 PMID:18504248

Zhu, K. (2012). *The Invalidity of Triangular Fuzzy AHP: A Mathematical Justification. Electronic Journal.* doi:10.2139/ssrn.2011922

Zhu, Z., Wang, S., Xi, Q., Bai, J., Yu, X., & Liu, J. (2011). Logistic Regression Model for Predicting Stone-Free Rate After Minimally Invasive Percutaneous Nephrolithotomy. *Endourology and Stones*, *78*(1), 32–36. PMID:21296398

Zolnoori, M., Fazel Zarandi, M. H., Moin, M., & Kazemnejad, A. (2010). Computer Aided Intelligence System for Diagnosing Pediatric Asthma. *Journal of Medical Systems*.

Zolnoori, M., Fazelzarandi, M., Moin, M., & Heydarnejad, H. (2010). Computer-Aided Intelligent System for Diagnosing Pediatric Asthma. *Journal of Medical Systems*. PMID:20703652

Zou, Z. H., Yun, Y., & Sun, J. N. (2006). Entropy method for determination of weight of evaluating indicators in fuzzy synthetic evaluation for water quality assessment. *Journal of Environmental Sciences (China)*, *18*(5), 1020–1023. doi:10.1016/S1001-0742(06)60032-6 PMID:17278765

Zuckerman, J. M., Singh, R. P., Farney, A. C., Rogers, J., & Stratta, R. J. (2009). Single center experience Transplanting kidneys from deceased donors with terminal acute renal failure. *The Journal of Surgery*, *146*(4), 686–695. PMID:19789028

Zuo, W. L., Wang, Z. Y., Liu, T., & Chen, H. L. (2013). Effective detection of Parkinsons disease using an adaptive fuzzy k-nearest neighbor approach. *Biomedical Signal Processing and Control*, *8*(4), 364–373. doi:10.1016/j.bspc.2013.02.006

About the Contributors

Elham Akhond Zadeh Noughabi is a post-doctoral fellow in the Department of Electrical and Computer Engineering at University of Calgary, Canada. Her main research interests include Data Mining, Big Data and Data Science with applications in healthcare and business. Dr. Noughabi's work has appeared in more than 50 peer-reviewed journals and conferences.

* * *

Somayeh Alizadeh is Assistant Professor of K.N.Toosi University. Her primary research and teaching interest is data mining and its application. She was working in healthcare and data mining in the field of predicting success of infertility cycle, predicting complications of type 2 diabetes, predicting length of stay of cardiac patients and some other applications in healthcare.

Hakimeh Ameri is a Master graduate in information technology at K.N.Toosi University of Technology in Tehran, Iran. Her main interests are in bioinformatic systems, Big data, expert systems, and especially the knowledge engineering based on medical databases.

Negin Asadayyoobi received her B.Sc and M.Sc degrees both in Industrial Engineering from Sharif University of Technology in 2012 and 2014, respectively. Since then, she has been working as a consultant in Bazar Academy and as a research expert in Research Institute for Information and Communication Technology, Tehran, Iran, where she currently continues her collaboration. Her research interest includes Applied Statistics, Quality Control and Mathematical Programming.

Sarah Bastedo has worked for over eight years in Ontario's healthcare sector developing expertise in health policy development, health system planning, and performance measurement and management. She holds a Master of Science degree in Health Services Research from the University of Toronto.

Eric Benchimol is a pediatric gastroenterologist and epidemiologist with a focus on the epidemiology, outcomes, and health services research in patients with chronic diseases using health administrative data. Dr. Benchimol also has an interest in the methods used to conduct research using routinely collected health data. He co-chairs the steering committee for the RECORD statement for the REporting of studies Conducted using Observational Routinely collected Data (an extension to the STROBE reporting guidelines) (record-statement.org).

Sumanta Bhattacharyya received his Bachelor of Science from University of Calcutta on 2004, Bachelor of Technology (ECE) (2008) and M.Tech (ECE) from West Bengal University of Technology, India in 2012; currently he is pursuing PhD in the Department of Electronics and Communication, Birla Institute of Technology, Mesra, Ranchi, India. His areas of interest is Signal Processing, Digital Signal Processing, Biomedical Signal Processing, Bio inspired Optimization, Communication.

María Carmen Carnero has a Doctorate in Industrial Engineering from the University of Castilla-La Mancha (2001) and is a lecturer at the Technical School of Industrial Engineering at the University of Castilla-La Mancha. She has published two books, seven chapters in science books, and research articles in Omega, Decision Support System, European Journal of Operational Research, Reliability Engineering and System Safety, Mechanical Systems and Signal Processing, Journal of Manufacturing Systems, BMC Medical Informatics and Decision Making, Production Planning and Control, etc. She was the lead researcher in three projects, and has been a part of 16 other European, national, regional and local projects.

Arzu Eren Şenaras graduated from Uludağ University in 2007. She took her Master and PhD degree in the Department of Econometrics at Uludag University.

Ali Vahit Esensoy is the Manager of the Strategic Analytics team at CCO, which is an inter-disciplinary group that specializes in applying advanced analytics methods to support complex re/design, management and evaluation decisions in the health system. Over the last 10 years, he has been involved in the management and delivery of innovative analytic products to address health system transformation challenges both in industry and academic settings. He holds BASc, MASc and PhD degrees in Industrial Engineering from the University of Toronto, and is an alumni of the Centre for Healthcare Engineering.

Reyhaneh Gamasaee is a Ph.D. candidate at the Department of Industrial Engineering of Amirkabir University of Technology, Tehran, Iran. Her main research interests are pattern recognition, machine learning, supply chain management, soft computing, fuzzy sets and systems, time series, and forecasting methods.

Mehrdad J. Gangeh received his Ph.D. in Electrical and Computer Engineering from the Centre for Pattern Analysis and Machine Intelligence (C-PAMI), University of Waterloo, Canada, in 2013. He is at present Research Associate jointly at the Dept. of Medical Biophysics, University of Toronto and the Depts. of Radiation Oncology, and Imaging Research–Physical Sciences, Sunnybrook Health Sciences Center, Canada. His current research is mainly focused on the design and development of computer-aided-theragnosis (CAT) systems using novel machine learning algorithms in conjunction with quantitative ultrasound methods in order to predict and/or monitor therapeutic cancer responses. Dr. Gangeh has received several prestigious and highly competitive awards and scholarships including Natural Sciences and Engineering Council (NSERC) postdoctoral fellowship (PDF) and NSERC Alexander Graham Bell-Canada Graduate Scholarship (CGS). His research interests are on multiview learning, dictionary learning and sparse representation, kernel methods, and deep belief networks with the applications to medical imaging, pattern recognition, computer vision, data mining, and bioinformatics. He is Senior

Member of IEEE, and currently Associate Editor of IEEE Trans. on Medical Imaging (TMI), Adjunct Professor at the Dept. of System Design Engineering, University of Waterloo, Canada, and the Vice Chair of the IEEE Engineering in Medicine and Biology (EMB) Chapter of Kitchener/Waterloo Section.

Andrés Gómez received his technical industrial engineering degree from the Polytechnic University of Madrid (Spain) and his industrial engineering degree from the University of Castilla-La Mancha. He has a Doctorate in Industrial Engineering from the University of Castilla-La Mancha (2012). He has worked in the Nuclear Power Stations of Ascó and Trillo and Repsol-YPF as maintenance engineer. He was Manager of the Maintenance Service of the Hospital Complex of Ciudad Real until 2004. Currently, he is Vice-director of the Technical Services of the General Hospital of Ciudad Real (Spain). He has published a research articles in Production Planning and Control and BMC Medical Informatics and Decision Making and, has participated in several conferences and research projects supported by Regional Administration.

Ann Jolly was a research scientist at the Public Health Agency of Canada before becoming an Associate Professor at the University of Ottawa. She studies the transmission of infections through social networks of people, incorporating the genetics of the pathogen, the host, and the social context and geography of the social network. She assists in surveillance and outbreak investigations, and teaches introductory and advanced infectious disease epidemiology.

Seifedine Kadry, PhD, has been an Associate Professor with Beirut Arab University in Lebanon since 2017. He is a faculty member in the department of Mathematics and Computer Science. He serves as Editor-in-Chief of the Research Journal of Mathematics and Statistics, the ARPN Journal of Systems and Software, and the International Journal of Mathematical Sciences and Computing (IJMSC). He worked as Head of Software Support and Analysis Unit of First National Bank where he designed and implemented the data warehouse and business intelligence. In addition, he has published several authored and edited books in Elsevier, Springer, IGI, and Taylor and Francis publishers. He is the author of more than 170 papers on applied math, computer science, and stochastic systems in peer-reviewed journals. Since 2008, he is the symposium chair in ICNAAM international conference. He supervised 5 PhD students. He has more than 500 citations and RG score of 27. His Erdős number is 2. At present his research focuses on system prognostics, stochastic systems, and probability and reliability analysis. He received a PhD in computational and applied mathematics in 2007 from the Blaise Pascal University (Clermont-II) - Clermont-Ferrand in France, MS in applied mathematics from École Polytechnique Fédérale de Lausanne (EPFL) and BS in applied mathematics from the Lebanese University.

Neal Kaw is an M.A.Sc. student in the Department of Mechanical and Industrial Engineering at the University of Toronto. His research interests are in the application of operations research methods to problems in healthcare and medicine.

Toktam Khatibi, Assistant Professor and Faculty member in Department of Industrial and Systems Engineering of Tarbiat Modares University, Tehran, Iran. Ms. Khatibi has received her BSc. degree in Software Engineering from Sharif University of Technology, Tehran, Iran, in 2003, her MSc. degree in Socio-Economic Systems Engineering from Tarbiat Modares University, Tehran, Iran, in 2008 and her PhD. degress in industrial engineering from Tarbiat Modares University, Tehran, Iran, in 2014. Her research interests include Healthcare systems engineering, Image Processing, Pattern Recognition, Data Mining and Artificial Intelligence.

Zhihui (Amy) Liu is a biostatistician at Cancer Care Ontario.

James Logan has been interested in the application of geographic information systems (GIS) to the study of infections since learning of Dr. John Snow's 1854 investigation of cholera and the Broad Street Pump. He has an undergraduate degree in GIS and a Masters (MGIS) from Penn State. His most recent research, published in PLoS One, is on spatial patterns among social networks of street people in Winnipeg and the places they frequent.

Soheila Nasiri received her medical degree in general medicine in 2000, her speciality in internal medicine in 2004 and sub-speciality in nephrology in 2006. She has been an assistant professor of Department of Nephrology in Tehran University of Medical Sciences from 2007 to 2012. Dr. Nasiri is currently a research assistant at the Institute of Clinical Evaluative Sciences (ICES), and a graduate student of population health risk assessment at the University of Ottawa. Dr. Nasiri's current research interests include population-based study of immune-based disease, and outcome of kidney transplantation.

Gihad Nesrallah completed his medical training and nephrology fellowship at Western University and Masters' in Clinical Epidemiology and Research Methodology at McMaster University. He was appointed as active staff at Humber River Hospital in 2004, and became Chief and Physician Director of the Nephrology Program in 2014. He holds academic appointments at Western University and the University of Toronto. He serves as the Provincial Medical Lead of the Data, Analytics, and Reporting Program at the Ontario Renal Network. In this role, he oversees the Ontario Renal Reporting System, and supports a wide range of strategic analytics, performance management, and policy and planning initiatives. His major academic contributions include national guideline development and implementation in chronic kidney disease and dialysis care, as well as comparative effectives studies of dialysis therapies.

Mir Saman Pishvaee received his Ph.D. in Industrial Engineering from University of Tehran and now he is assistant professor at Iran University of Science and Technology (IUST). He has published many papers in the area of supply chain management in various journals such as Transportation Research: Part E (TR-E), Computers & Operations Research (COR) and Computers & Industrial Engineering (CAIE) and several book chapters under Springer-Verlag. His research areas are supply chain management, robust optimization and system dynamics.

Somayeh Sadat (Ph.D., University of Toronto) is a health policy and management specialist with more than fifteen years of academic and professional experience in the health care system. Her experience spans various sectors within the health industry, including hospitals, medical device companies, blood banks, medical education, as well as governmental institutions responsible for policy making, funding, and monitoring chronic care systems. She is especially experienced in advising programs on best defining key business questions that can be supported by analytics, leading analytic projects that involve developing data-driven decision making tools, and building analytic capacity organization wide.

Mohammad Mehdi Sepehri, Professor, Faculty of Industrial and Systems Engineering, Tarbiat Modares University (TMU), Tehran, Iran; Founder and Head of The Laboratory for Healthcare Systems Optimization, Engineering, and Informatics (HCSE); Head of Group of Industrial Engineering; Editor-in-Chief, International Journal of Hospital Research, the official peer-reviewed publication of Hospital Management Research Center (HMRC), Iran University of Medical Sciences, Tehran, Iran. Dr. Sepehri obtained his MSc and PhD in Management Science from the University of Tennessee, Knoxville, Tennessee, USA, in 1987 and 1991. His current research focuses on Internet of Things in Healthcare, Operations Research in Medicine and Healthcare, Healthcare Systems Engineering, Mobile Health, Lean Healthcare and Lean Hospital, and Network Optimization.

Hayrettin Sezen is Professor at the Department of Econometrics, Operations Research MSB at Uludag University in Bursa.

Pejman Shadpour, MD, is currently Professor of Urology IUMS. Program director for pediatric urology and laparoscopic surgery at Iran University of Medical Sciences (IUMS) received his MD in 1992 at the age of 23 with highest honors. Board certified as urologic surgeon in 1998 (Highest honors). Followed by fellowships in pediatric urology and laparoscopic surgery. Special interests include pediatric urology, laparoscopic surgery; and applications of data processing & operations research in surgery and laparoscopy. Publications include 17 books and over 60 full text papers in laparoscopy, clinical urology, public health, medical education, hospital management and the surgical applications of operations research.

Hadi Tadayyon received his PhD in Medical Biophysics from The University of Toronto in 2015. His research interests include ultrasound tissue characterization, medical data analytics, and imaging biomarkers of cancer response. From 2012 to 2014, he held an NSERC Canada Graduate Scholarship CGSD-D2, a competitive national award for doctoral candidates. He also has two patents resulting from his PhD and post-doctoral works. Since July 2016, he has been working as a Data Scientist in the IT industry.

Mohammad Hossein Tekieh is a PhD student in E-Business at University of Ottawa, doing research on pediatrics immune-mediated diseases using data mining. He is also an experienced quality assurance analyst at Privacy Analytics Inc. - now with IMS Health. His main duty is testing and verifying the quality of developed privacy preserving tools for anonymizing real-world health datasets containing protected health information, which are used for research and analysis purposes. He received his MSc in Electronic Business Technologies from University of Ottawa, Canada in 2012. His Master's research field was mining healthcare data to provide beneficial recommendations in improving health services and quality. He has also conducted and instructed web design principles and technologies courses for more than two years.

William Tran is a Radiation Therapist, and clinician scientist in the Department of Radiation Oncology. His research focuses on using optical and ultrasound imaging to model predictive markers for chemosensitivity in breast cancer.

M. H. Fazel Zarandi is a Professor at the Department of Industrial Engineering of Amirkabir University of Technology, Tehran, Iran, and a member of the Knowledge Information Systems Laboratory at the University of Toronto, Ontario, Canada. His main research interests focus on intelligent information systems, soft computing, computational intelligence, fuzzy sets and systems, and multi-agent systems.

Seyed Hessameddin Zegordi is Professor of Industrial Engineering in the Faculty of Industrial & Systems Engineering at Tarbiat Modares University, Iran. He received his PhD from Department of Industrial Engineering and management at Tokyo Institute of Technology, Japan in 1994. He holds an MSc in Industrial Engineering and Systems from Sharif University of Technology, Iran and a BSc in Industrial Engineering from Isfahan University of Technology, Iran. His main areas of teaching and research interests include production planning and scheduling, multi-objective optimization problems, meta-heuristics, quality management and productivity. He has published several articles in international conferences and academic journals including European Journal of Operational Research, International Journal of Production Research, Journal of Operational Research Society of Japan, Computers & Industrial Engineering, Amirkabir Journal of Science and Engineering and Scientia Iranica International Journal of Science and Technology.

Index

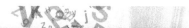
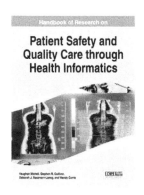
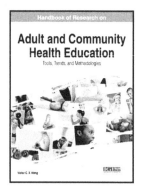
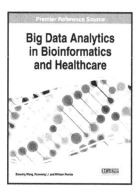
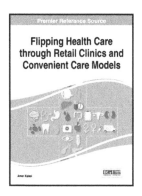
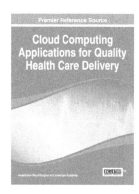
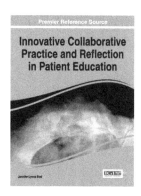
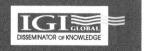

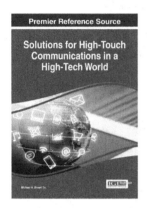 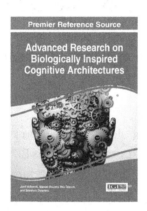 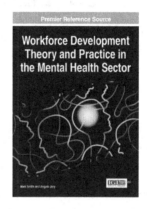 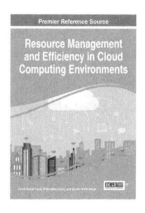

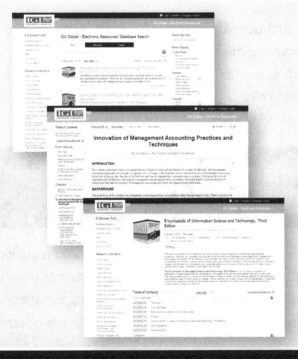
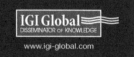

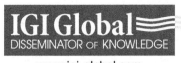
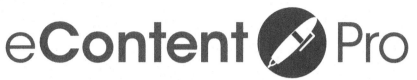
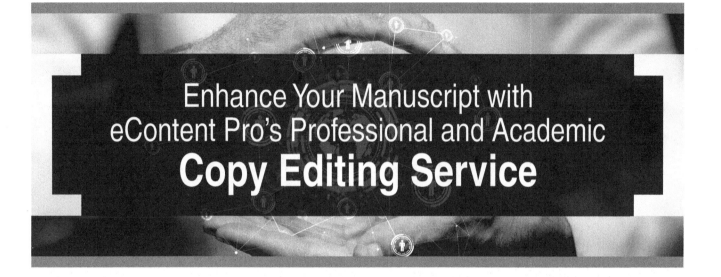

Printed in the United States
By Bookmasters